Clinical Neuroendocrinology: Neuropeptide GPCRs

Clinical Neuroendocrinology: Neuropeptide GPCRs

Edited by Dylan Edwards

STATES
ACADEMIC PRESS
www.statesacademicpress.com

States Academic Press,
109 South 5th Street,
Brooklyn, NY 11249, USA

Visit us on the World Wide Web at:
www.statesacademicpress.com

ISBN: 978-1-63989-112-2

Cataloging-in-Publication Data

Clinical neuroendocrinology : neuropeptide GPCRs / edited by Dylan Edwards.
p. cm.
Includes bibliographical references and index.
ISBN 978-1-63989-112-2
1. Neuroendocrinology. 2. Neuropeptides. 3. G proteins--Receptors. 4. Neurohormones. I. Edwards, Dylan.
QP356.4 .C55 2022
612.8--dc23

Table of Contents

Preface

The branch of biology which focuses on the relationship between the endocrine and the nervous system is termed as neuroendocrinology. The regulation of the activity of the hormones by the brain is studied within this field. The physiological processes in the body are regulated by a process known as neuroendocrine integration, wherein the endocrine and nervous system function together. The major neuroendocrine systems in the body are hypothalamic-pituitary-adrenal axis (HPA axis), hypothalamic-pituitary-thyroid axis (HPT axis), hypothalamic-pituitary-gonadal axis (HPG axis) and hypothalamic-neurohypophyseal system. GPCRs are G protein-coupled receptors, which can bind to numerous neuropeptides. This book is a compilation of chapters that discuss the most vital concepts and emerging trends in the field of neuroendocrinology. It presents the complex subject of neuropeptide GPCRs in the most comprehensible and easy to understand language. The extensive content of this book provides the readers with a thorough understanding of the subject.

The information shared in this book is based on empirical researches made by veterans in this field of study. The elaborative information provided in this book will help the readers further their scope of knowledge leading to advancements in this field.

Finally, I would like to thank my fellow researchers who gave constructive feedback and my family members who supported me at every step of my research.

Editor

1

Mutation of Phe318 within the NPxxY(x)$_{5,6}$F motif in melanin-concentrating hormone receptor 1 results in an efficient signaling activity

Akie Hamamoto*[1], *Manabu Horikawa*[2], *Tomoko Saho*[1] *and Yumiko Saito*[1]

[1] *Graduate School of Integrated Arts and Sciences, Hiroshima University, Hiroshima, Japan*
[2] *Bioorganic Research Institute, Suntory Foundation for Life Sciences, Osaka, Japan*

Edited by:
Hubert Vaudry, University of Rouen, France

Reviewed by:
Jean A. Boutin, Institut de Recherches SERVIER, France
Stewart Clark, University at Buffalo, SUNY, USA

****Correspondence:***
Yumiko Saito, Graduate School of Integrated Arts and Sciences, Hiroshima University, 1-7-1 Kagamiyama, Higashi-hiroshima, Hiroshima 739-8521, Japan.
e-mail: yumist@hiroshima-u.ac.jp

Melanin-concentrating hormone receptor 1 (MCHR1) is a G-protein-coupled receptor (GPCR) that plays an important role in feeding by coupling to Gα_q- and Gα_i-mediated signal transduction pathways. To interrogate the molecular basis for MCHR1 activation, we analyzed the effect of a series of site-directed mutations on rat MCHR1 function. In the highly conserved NPxxY(x)$_{5,6}$F domain of GPCRs, the phenylalanine residue is involved in structural constraints; replacement with alanine generally leads to impaired/lost GPCR function. However, Phe-to-Ala (F318A) mutation in MCHR1 had no significant effect on the level of cell surface expression and receptor signaling. By analyzing a further series of mutants, we found that Phe-to-Lys substitution (F318K) caused the most significant reduction in the EC$_{50}$ value of MCH for calcium mobilization without affecting receptor expression at the cell surface. Interestingly, GTPγS-binding, which monitors Gα_i activation, was not modulated by F318K. Our results, combined with computer modeling, provide new insight into the role of Phe in the NPxxY(x)$_{5,6}$F motif as a structurally critical site for receptor dynamics and a determinant of Gα protein interaction.

Keywords: GPCR, helix 8, melanin-concentrating hormone, NPxxY(x)$_{5,6}$F motif, signal transduction

INTRODUCTION

Mammalian melanin-concentrating hormone (MCH), a cyclic nonadecapeptide produced predominantly by neurons of the lateral hypothalamus, is involved in the regulation of food intake behavior and energy expenditure (Bittencourt et al., 1992; Rossi et al., 1997; Shimada et al., 1998). MCH acts *via* two G-protein-coupled receptors (GPCRs), Melanin-concentrating hormone receptor 1 (MCHR1), and MCHR2 (Chambers et al., 1999; Saito et al., 1999; An et al., 2001), of which MCHR2 is not functionally present in rodents (Tan et al., 2002). MCHR1 is widely expressed at high levels in the brain (Saito et al., 2001). Because mice lacking MCHR1 are lean, hyperactive, hyperphagic, and hypermetabolic (Chen et al., 2002; Marsh et al., 2002), MCHR1 is viewed as the physiologically relevant MCH receptor in rodents. In support of this belief, selective MCHR1 antagonists decrease food intake and body weight in both normal and diet-induced obese rats (Takekawa et al., 2002; Shearman et al., 2003). Moreover, some of these antagonists exhibit anti-depressant and anxiolytic effects (Borowsky et al., 2002; Georgescu et al., 2005). Therefore, the MCH-MCHR1 system could be an important target for the treatment of obesity and certain mood disorders.

Abbreviations: ECL, enhanced chemiluminescence; ER, endoplasmic reticulum; ERK, extracellular signal-regulated kinase; FBS, fetal bovine serum; GPCR, G-protein-coupled receptor; HEK293T, human embryonic kidney 293; helix 8, eighth cytoplasmic helix; i1, intracellular loop 1; i2, intracellular loop 2; i3, intracellular loop 3; MCH, melanin-concentrating hormone; MCHR1, MCHR1 receptor; MCHR2, MCHR2 receptor; PTX, pertussis-toxin; TM, transmembrane.

In mammalian cells transfected with MCHR1, MCH is able to activate multiple signaling pathways including calcium mobilization, activation of extracellular signal-regulated kinase (ERK) and inhibition of cyclic AMP generation through G$\alpha_{i/o}$- and Gα_q-coupled pathways (Chambers et al., 1999; Saito et al., 1999; Hawes et al., 2000). Several studies have reported structural determinants of MCHR1 activation by MCH. Biochemical analysis of MCHR1 using molecular modeling identified Asp123 in the third transmembrane domain (TM3) as being crucial for ligand binding (Macdonald et al., 2000). In addition, Thr255, which is located at the junction of intracellular loop 3 (i3) and transmembrane domain 6 (TM6), is critically important for receptor folding and correct trafficking to the cell surface (Fan et al., 2005). We previously identified that Asn23 in the extracellular N-terminus contributed mainly to N-linked glycosylation of MCHR1 and is necessary for MCHR1 cell surface expression, ligand binding and signal transduction (Saito et al., 2003). We also showed that Arg155 in intracellular loop 2 (i2) and a proximal dibasic motif (Arg319/Lys320) in eighth cytoplasmic helix (helix 8: a common short amphiphilic helical domain in the proximal C-terminal tail) are important for signaling (Tetsuka et al., 2004; Saito et al., 2005), whereas the distal part of the C-terminal tail is necessary for receptor internalization (Saito et al., 2004). However, despite numerous mutagenesis studies, the residues that determine G protein selectivity (Gα_q vs. Gα_i) have yet to be identified.

The NPxxY(x)$_{5,6}$F sequence, located at the junction between TM7 and the connecting cytosolic helix 8, is conserved in most rhodopsin family (class A) GPCRs, including the MCH receptor (Gether, 2000; Huynh et al., 2009). The high degree of conservation of this motif suggests that it must play very important roles in rhodopsin family GPCR functionality. Mutations in the NPxxY(x)$_{5,6}$F motif are reported to affect ligand binding, G protein coupling and receptor phosphorylation. In rhodopsin, the prototypical GPCR, the Tyr and Phe residues within the motif were both found to be critical for proper light-induced conformational changes from the ground state (Acharya and Karnik, 1996). Moreover, the Phe residue is reported to be essential for export of the β1-adrenergic receptor (β1-AR), α2B-adrenergic receptor (α2B-AR) and A1 adenosine receptor from the endoplasmic reticulum (ER) (Delos Santos et al., 2006; Duvernay et al., 2009; Málaga-Diéguez et al., 2010). Indeed, Phe-to-Ala substitution in the α2B-AR dramatically reduced cell-surface expression by 91% compared with their wild-type variants (Duvernay et al., 2009). To determine the role of the conserved Phe residue (F318) in the NPxxY(x)$_{5,6}$F motif present in the MCHR1, we examined the effect of site-directed mutagenesis of this residue on receptor function, and noted a most significant increase in calcium mobilization relative to wild-type after substitution of F318 with a positively-charged lysine residue. Our analyses show that Lys replacement mutation (F318K) produces an efficient signaling property that selectively increases Gα_q-mediated pathway without changing cell surface expression. We further discuss the significance of the position of Phe318 using a homology docking model of MCHR1 with Gα_q and Gα_i proteins, respectively. To date, this is the first study to provide meaningful insights into the relationship between conformational changes in MCHR1 and G protein activation.

MATERIALS AND METHODS

cDNA CONSTRUCTS FOR MCHR1 AND MUTANT RECEPTORS

The generation of a cDNA encoding a Flag epitope tag before the first methionine in rat MCHR1 (NM_031758/GenBank/EMBL) was described previously (Saito et al., 2003). Single-substitution mutations of the NPxxY(x)$_{5,6}$F domain were produced by oligonucleotide-mediated site-directed mutagenesis using a QuikChange site-directed mutagenesis kit (Stratagene, La Jolla, CA, USA). All mutations in the MCHR1 cDNA sequence were confirmed by sequencing analysis. Mutated MCHR1 cDNAs were excised by digestion with EcoRI and XhoI and inserted into the pcDNA3.1 expression vector.

CELL CULTURE AND TRANSIENT TRANSFECTION

HEK293T cells were cultured in DMEM containing 10% fetal bovine serum. The plasmid DNA was mixed with LipofectAMINE PLUS transfection reagent (Life Technologies Corporation, Carlsbad, CA, USA) and the mixture was diluted with OptiMEM and added to the cells (Saito et al., 2003). For western blotting and GTPγS-binding assays, the cells were re-seeded onto 6-well plates. Cells were re-plated onto LAB-TEK 8-well plates (Nunc, Rochester, NY, USA) for immunocytochemistry, and onto 24- and 96-well plates (BIOCOAT, Becton Dickinson, Belford, MA, USA) for FACScan flow cytometric analysis and the calcium influx assay, respectively. The re-plated cells were cultured for a further 18–24 h.

WESTERN BLOTTING FOR MCHR1

To generate whole cell extracts, transiently-transfected HEK293T cells were lysed with ice-cold sodium dodecyl sulfate sample buffer [50 mM Tris-HCl (pH 6.8), 2% sodium dodecyl sulfate, 50 mM β-mercaptoethanol, and 10% glycerol], then homogenized at 4°C by sonication (SONICAOR Ultrasonic processor W-225, Wakenyaku Ltd., Kyoto, Japan) using 5×30 s bursts at 20% power. Aliquots containing 15 μg of total protein were separated by SDS-PAGE and electro-transferred to Hybond-P PVDF membranes (GE Healthcare UK Ltd., Little Chalfont, UK). After blocking with 5% skim milk, membrane-expressed Flag-MCHR1 was detected using 0.5 μg/ml anti-Flag M2 antibody (Wako, Osaka, Japan), followed by a horseradish peroxidase-conjugated goat anti-mouse IgG antibody (Saito et al., 2005). Reactive bands were visualized with enhanced chemiluminescence (ECL) reagent (GE Healthcare UK Ltd.).

FACScan FLOW CYTOMETRIC ANALYSIS OF CELL SURFACE RECEPTORS

Transfected HEK293T cells in 24-well plates were fixed with 1.5% paraformaldehyde-PBS solution for 10 min at room temperature, then incubated with 0.25 μg/ml anti-Flag M2 antibody in PBS containing 20% FBS for 1 h. The cells were washed three times with PBS and then incubated with Alexa Fluor 488-conjugated goat anti-mouse IgG secondary antibody (Molecular Probes, Eugene, OR, USA) for 1 h (Tetsuka et al., 2004; Saito et al., 2005). The cells were washed, harvested with 5 mM EDTA and analyzed using a FACSCalibur flow cytometer (BD, Franklin Lakes, NJ). Cells were gated by light scatter or exclusion of propidium iodide, and 10,000 cells were acquired for each time point. The mean fluorescence of all cells minus the mean cell fluorescence with the Alexa Fluor 488-conjugated secondary antibody only was used for the calculations.

IMMUNOFLUORESCENCE MICROSCOPY

Transfected HEK293T cells were fixed in a 3.7% paraformaldehyde-PBS solution for 10 min. After two washes with PBS, the cells were transferred, either with or without permeabilization using 0.05% Triton X-100 in PBS for 15 min, into a blocking solution (20% goat serum in PBS) for 30 min, then incubated with 0.5 μg/ml anti-Flag M2 antibody for 1 h. The anti-Flag M2 antibody was detected using Alexa Fluor 488-conjugated goat anti-mouse IgG secondary antibody. Fluorescence imaging was performed using a BZ-9000 microscope (Keyence, Tokyo, Japan). For fluorescence imaging of MCH-induced receptor internalization, cells were pre-incubated at 37°C in serum-free DMEM for 3 h. Cells were then incubated with 1 μM rat MCH for 10, 30, and 60 min at 37°C in a 5% CO_2 incubator. Cells were fixed, permeabilized and then incubated with 0.5 μg/ml anti-Flag M2 antibody in PBS containing 20% FBS for 1 h. The cells were washed three times with PBS and then incubated with Alexa Fluor 488-conjugated goat anti-mouse IgG secondary antibody for 1 h. Fluorescence imaging was performed using a FLUOVIEW FV1000 confocal microscope (Olympus, Tokyo, Japan).

MEASUREMENT OF INTRACELLULAR Ca^{2+}

Measurement of intracellular Ca^{2+} was performed as described previously (Saito et al., 2003, 2005; Tetsuka et al., 2004). Transiently transfected cells seeded in 96-well plates were loaded with a non-wash calcium dye (Calcium Assay Kit 5, Molecular Devices Japan, Tokyo, Japan) in Hank's balanced salt solution containing HEPES (pH 7.5) for 1 h at 37°C. For each concentration of MCH, the level of $[Ca^{2+}]_i$ was detected using a FlexStation 3 Microplate Reader (Molecular Devices). The data were expressed as fluorescence (arbitrary units) vs. time. The EC_{50} values for MCH were obtained from sigmoidal fits using a non-linear curve-fitting program (Prism v3.0; GraphPad Software, San Diego, CA, USA). Rat/mouse/human MCH and Compound 15 were purchased from Peptide Institute (Osaka, Japan) and Bachem AG (Bubendorf, Switzerland), respectively.

GTPγS-BINDING ASSAY

GTPγS-binding assay was performed as described previously (Saito et al., 2005). Aliquots (10 μg) of membrane proteins were incubated in GTPγS binding buffer (20 mM HEPES-NaOH pH 7.5, 100 mM NaCl, 5 mM $MgCl_2$, 0.2% BSA and 3 μM GDP) containing 0.2 nM $[^{35}S]$GTPγS (PerkinElmer, Santa Clara, CA, USA) and various concentrations of MCH for 30 min at 30°C. To determine the non-specific binding, unlabeled GTPγS was added to the binding mixtures to a final concentration of 100 μM. Bound $[^{35}S]$GTPγS was separated from free $[^{35}S]$GTPγS by rapid filtration through GF/C filters and washed with ice-cold binding buffer. Filters were then immersed in scintillation cocktail (Emulsion-Scintillator Plus; Packard Bioscience, Groningen, The Netherlands) and trapped radioactivity counted using a liquid scintillation counter.

MOLECULAR MODELING

To generate homology models of rat MCHR1 mutant F318K, we used the X-ray structure of constitutively active rhodopsin bound to the C-terminus peptide of the α-subunit of the G protein, transducin (PDB code 2X72), as a structural template. Alignment analysis in sequences of rat MCHR1 and rhodopsin was performed using CLUSTALW2.0 installed in Genetyx v9.0 (Genetyx Corporation, Tokyo, Japan). Initial models of rat MCHR1 mutant F318K with K341L transducin C-terminus peptide (340–350; ILENLKDCGLF) was constructed using the Modelor module installed in Discovery Studio (DS) v3.0 (Accelrys, Tokyo, Japan). After replacement of L341 and E342 to Lys and Asn, the structure of rat MCHR1(F318K) bound to a C-terminus peptide (343–353; IKNNLKDCGLF) of the $G\alpha_i$ subunit was optimized using the molecular mechanics and molecular dynamics simulation with a CHARMm force field in the DS. Furthermore, replacement of the $G\alpha_i$ peptide with a C-terminus peptide to the $G\alpha_q$ subunit (349–359; LQLNLKEYNLV) and subsequent similar optimization in DS provided the model structure of rat MCHR1(F318K) bound to the $G\alpha_q$ C-terminus peptide. The X-ray structure of rhodopsin (PDB code 2X72) and the two constructed models (rat MCHR1(F318K)-$G\alpha_i$ peptide and rat MCHR1(F318K)-$G\alpha_q$ peptide) were superimposed for comparison.

RESULTS

EFFECTS OF VARIOUS SINGLE-SITE ALA SUBSTITUTION MUTATIONS OF THE CONSERVED $NPxxY(x)_{5,6}F$ motif ON RECEPTOR EXPRESSION AND ACTIVITY

First, to analyze the function of the $NPxxY(x)_{5,6}F$ motif, a series of Ala-substituted mutants were generated, as shown in **Figure 1A**. We transiently transfected Flag-tagged MCHR1 or mutant receptors into HEK293T cells, then examined receptor expression levels by western blotting analysis using an anti-Flag M2 antibody. Several immunoreactive bands were detected in the whole lysate isolated from cells expressing Flag-MCHR1 (**Figure 1B**), some of which corresponded to the predicted molecular masses of MCHR1 variants (approximately 35, 44, 45, and 60 kDa (Saito et al., 2003, 2005; Tetsuka et al., 2004), although additional immunoreactive bands were observed at 45–60 kDa.

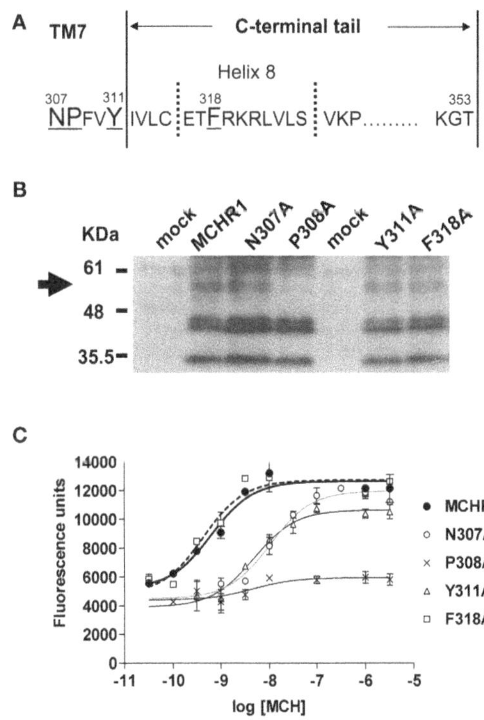

FIGURE 1 | Analysis of the effects of individual substitution mutations in the $NPxxY(x)_{5,6}F$ motif of MCHR1 on receptor function in HEK293T cells. (A) Schematic representation of the conserved $NPxxY(x)_{5,6}F$ motif and the C-terminal tail of the rat MCHR1. The C-terminal tail of rat MCHR1 extends 42 residues from the plasma membrane (residue 312–353) and is predicted to include an eighth cytoplasmic helix (helix 8) (Tetsuka et al., 2004). Amino acid residues targeted for mutational analyses are underlined. TM7; transmembrane 7. **(B)** Protein expression of Flag-MCHR1 and mutant receptors. After lysis of transfected cells with SDS-sample buffer, 15 μg total protein was separated by 15% SDS-PAGE, transferred to a polyvinyl difluoride membrane, and immunoblotted with an anti-Flag M2 antibody. Four major immunoreactive bands of 35, 44, 45, and 60 kDa are present in Flag-MCHR1 and individual mutant receptors. **(C)** Cells transfected with Flag-MCHR1 or substitution mutant receptors were stimulated with the indicated concentrations of MCH, and the subsequent changes in cytoplasmic free Ca^{2+} levels were measured using a FlexStation. Results shown are representative of at least three-independent experiments.

Our previous study revealed that the 35-kDa band is the non-glycosylated form of MCHR1 (Saito et al., 2003), while the three higher molecular mass bands are different *N*-linked glycosylated forms. The migration patterns of N307A, Y311A, and F318A were very similar and no significant reductions in the intensity of the higher molecular mass bands were observed relative to Flag-MCHR1. However, the pattern in P308A was different, with the expression of the higher molecular mass band at 60 kDa apparently drastically reduced (**Figure 1B**, arrow). This phenomenon is likely caused by a lack of appropriate glycosylation of the mutant receptors, as previously shown in an-*N*-linked glycosylation study and other MCHR1 studies (Saito et al., 2003; Aizaki et al., 2009). The cell surface expression levels of Flag-MCHR1 and mutants containing Ala-substitutions in the NPxxY$(x)_{5,6}$F motif were monitored by FACScan flow cytometry using an anti-Flag M2 antibody. Transient transfection of N307A and Y311A gave expression levels of 23% and 30%, respectively, relative to that of Flag-MCHR1, while the F318A mutation was expressed at approximately the same level as the non-mutated control (**Table 1**). Conversely, P308A expression was reduced by more than 90% compared to Flag-MCHR1, suggesting that the mutant was mostly retained intracellularly (**Figure 1B** and **Table 1**).

Next, we assessed the capacity of receptors containing alanine mutations in their NPxxY$(x)_{5,6}$F motif to induce intracellular signals in response to MCH. MCH-induced calcium influx was quantified in transiently transfected cells using a FlexStation 3 Microplate Reader. Mock-transfected HEK293T cells acted as a negative control and did not respond to MCH stimulation (data not shown). Considerable evidence suggests that most single-substitution mutations of highly conserved amino acids (such as the DRY or NPxxY$(x)_{5,6}$F motifs) lead to impairment or inactivation of receptor protein signaling. Indeed, substitution of conserved Pro308 with Ala (P308A) resulted in a dramatic attenuation of cell surface expression (**Table 1**). Therefore, this receptor did not respond to MCH by calcium mobilization (**Figure 1C**, **Table 2**), even when challenged with a high concentration (10 μM) of MCH.

Table 1 | Cell surface expression of Flag-MCHR1 and variants transiently expressed in HEK293T cells.

Receptor	Cell surface expression (FACS, %)
Flag-MCHR1	100
N307A	77.3 ± 0.3^b
P308A	6.3 ± 1.0^b
Y311A	69.3 ± 9.2^a
F318A	91.0 ± 8.7
F318R	90.5 ± 9.5
F318K	96.2 ± 5.8
F318P	90.2 ± 9.1

The data represent the mean ± S.E.M of three or four-independent experiments performed in triplicates.

[a] $P < 0.05$, significantly different from Flag-MCHR1 by Student's t-test.

[b] $P < 0.01$, significantly different from Flag-MCHR1 by Student's t-test.

Substitution of either Asn307 or Tyr311 with Ala also significantly affected MCH-induced calcium mobilization. N307A and Y311A mutant receptors exhibited a maximal response that was 20–30% lower than wild-type receptors and had EC_{50} values that were 21- and 8-fold higher, respectively, than Flag-MCHR1 (**Table 2**). However, the effects of alanine mutation of Phe318 in the highly conserved motif were distinct from other mutants (Delos Santos et al., 2006; Duvernay et al., 2009; Málaga-Diéguez et al., 2010; Kaye et al., 2011). The EC_{50} and maximal response of MCH-induced calcium signaling in cells expressing the F318A mutant were essentially identical to those of Flag-MCHR1. This is consistent with our previous data (Tetsuka et al., 2004). These results indicate that the conserved Phe in MCHR1 has a distinct signaling role as compared with other conserved amino acids in the NPxxY$(x)_{5,6}$F motif.

EFFECTS OF INDIVIDUAL SUBSTITUTION OF HIGHLY CONSERVED PHE ON MCHR1 FUNCTION

To further analyze the effect of the Phe318 substitution in the NPxxY$(x)_{5,6}$F motif, we performed site-directed mutagenesis of Phe318 to proline, a change that is thought to disrupt helix formation and may cause drastic changes in receptor function. We also mutated Phe to Arg and Lys, because these substitutions impart a positive charge to the position. Analysis of receptor expression levels by western blotting analysis with the anti-Flag M2 antibody showed that the migration patterns of F318A, F318P, F318R, and F318K were very similar and no drastic reduction in the intensity of the higher molecular mass bands were observed compared to Flag-MCHR1 (**Figure 2A**). We next determined the expression characteristics of each mutant by quantifying cell surface expression and observing subcellular distribution. The cell surface expression levels of F318A, F318P, F318R, and F318K caused no significant decrease as compared to the Flag-MCHR1 (**Table 1**). Antibody staining in non-permeabilized cells revealed that F318A, F318P, F318R, and F318K were clearly localized in the plasma membrane, and their labeling intensities were approximately equivalent with that of Flag-MCHR1 (**Figure 3**, upper). In permeabilized cells, all four mutants were also predominantly detected in the plasma membrane, as was Flag-MCHR1 (**Figure 3**, bottom). These results confirmed that both the level of cell surface expression and the subcellular localization were unaffected by the Phe318 substitution in the NPxxY$(x)_{5,6}$F motif. This is in marked

Table 2 | Calcium mobilization stimulated by MCH via Flag-MCHR1 and variants [containing various single point mutations in the highly conserved NPxxY$(x)_{5,6}$F motif] expressed in HEK293T cells.

Receptor	EC_{50} of MCH (nM)	Maximum response (%)
Flag-MCHR1	1.5 ± 0.4	100
N307A	32.5 ± 9.0	83.5 ± 5.4
P308A	–	–
Y311A	12.2 ± 2.3	77.3 ± 10.0
F318A	1.2 ± 0.3	101.0 ± 8.2

P308A does not respond to MCH (–). The results represent the mean ± S.E.M. of at least three-independent experiments performed in duplicate.

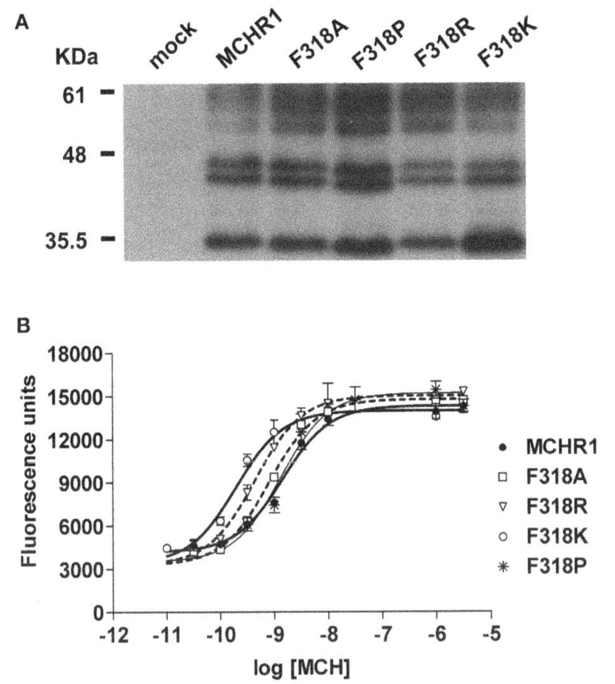

FIGURE 2 | Analysis of the effects of substitution mutations of the highly conserved Phe318 in the MCHR1 NPxxY(x)$_{5,6}$F motif on receptor function in HEK293T cells. (A) Protein expression of Flag-MCHR1 and mutant receptors. After lysis of transfected cells with SDS-sample buffer, 15 μg total protein were separated by 15% SDS-PAGE, transferred to a polyvinyl difluoride membrane, and immunoblotted with an anti-Flag M2 antibody. Four major immunoreactive bands of 35, 44, 45, and 60 kDa are present in Flag-MCHR1 and individual mutant receptors. **(B)** Dose-response relationship of MCH-stimulated calcium influx in HEK293T cells expressing Flag-MCHR1 or mutant receptors. Cells transfected with Flag-MCHR1 or the substitution mutant receptors were stimulated with the indicated concentrations of MCH, and the subsequent changes in cytoplasmic free Ca^{2+} levels were measured using a FlexStation. Results shown are representative of at least three-independent experiments.

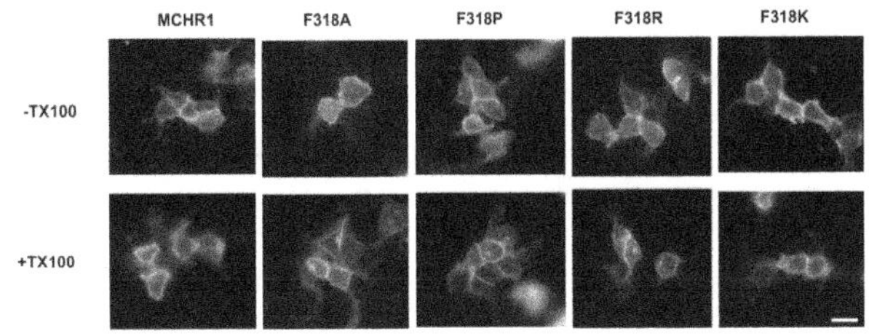

FIGURE 3 | Confocal immunolocalization of Flag-MCHR1 and the mutant receptors using an anti-Flag M2 antibody in HEK293T cells. Cell surface expression was compared using transfected non-permeabilized cells (-TX100, without Triton X-100; upper row) and permeabilized cells (+TX100, with Triton X-100; lower row). Vector-transfected cells incubated with the anti-Flag M2 antibody showed no significant staining (data not shown). Bar, 10 μm.

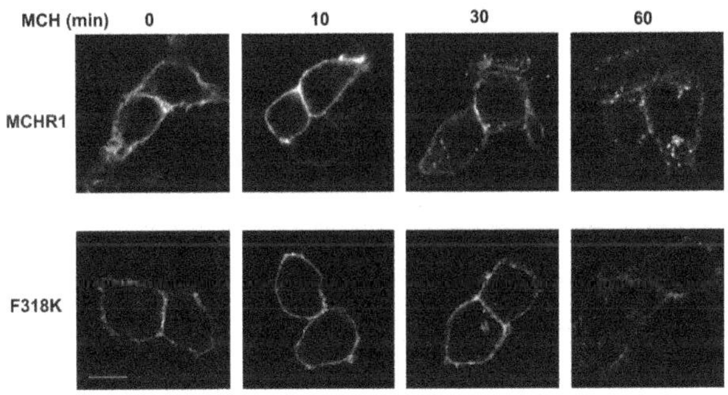

FIGURE 4 | MCH-mediated receptor internalization in HEK293T cells. Cells expressing MCHR1 or the F318K mutant were stimulated with 1 μM MCH for the time shown, fixed and imaged by confocal fluorescence microscopy. *Prior* to MCH addition, cells were incubated with serum-free DMEM for 3 h. Bar, 10 μm.

contrast with similar mutants of other GPCRs including the α2B-AR (Delos Santos et al., 2006; Duvernay et al., 2009; Málaga-Diéguez et al., 2010), in which membrane translocation was dramatically impaired by mutation of the conserved Phe residue in the NPxxY(x)$_{5,6}$F motif. Using fluorescence microscopy, we also examined the features of receptor internalization following exposure to MCH, because rat MCHR1 undergoes rapid MCH-induced internalization during the 30 min after stimulation (Saito et al., 2004). Consistent with this previous study, treatment with MCH for 30 min caused a loss of membrane localization and the appearance of MCHR1-containing vesicles. This distribution was also observed following 60 min of incubation. A similar time-course of MCH-induced receptor internalization was obtained for the F318K mutant (**Figure 4**).

The effects of Phe318 mutations on MCHR1 responsiveness to MCH in calcium mobilization are shown in **Table 3** and **Figure 2B**. In cells expressing single-substitution mutants, the MCH EC_{50} was 7.8 nM and 0.8 nM for F318P and F318R, respectively, with identical maximal responses. Importantly, MCH had increased potency in releasing calcium *via* the F318K mutant receptor ($EC_{50} = 0.4 \pm 0.1$ nM, compared with 2.5 ± 0.8 nM for Flag-MCHR1, **Table 3**), although the maximal response was unchanged. We also mutated the uncharged hydrophobic Phe to other uncharged polar amino acid residues (Gly, Ser, and Cys), a different hydrophobic residue (Trp) and a different basic residue (His) and measured the responsiveness of the resultant mutant receptors in the calcium mobilization assay (**Table 3**). Among the mutants, F318K and F318R exhibited significantly enhanced cellular signaling, but F318K caused a higher responsiveness than F318R. In addition to using MCH itself, we also tested the activity of the mammalian MCH analog, Compound 15, which efficiently binds with high affinity to MCHR1 (Bednarek et al., 2002). The potency of Compound 15 was also enhanced in cells expressing F318K compared to Flag-MCHR1 (0.15 ± 0.10 nM vs. 1.3 ± 0.4 nM, respectively; mean ± S.E.M. from three-independent experiments). This enhanced response to MCH was also observed when F318K was transiently transfected into CHO cells and COS7 cells (data not shown).

To elucidate further the effect of Lys mutation, mutagenesis of single or multiple residues around Phe318 was performed, as shown in **Figure 5**. The E316K, T317K, and R319K/R321K

Table 3 | Calcium mobilization by MCH *via* Flag-MCHR1 and variants [containing single point mutations at F318 in the NPxxY(x)$_{5,6}$F motif] expressed in HEK293T cells.

Receptor	EC_{50} of MCH (nM)	Maximum Response (%)
Flag-MCHR1	2.5 ± 0.8	100
F318A	1.2 ± 0.2	92.4 ± 7.2
F318P	7.8 ± 3.2^a	93.7 ± 11.4
F318R	0.8 ± 0.3^b	99.4 ± 3.0
F318K	0.4 ± 0.1^b	102.0 ± 8.0
F318G	2.3 ± 0.9	99.6 ± 9.8
F318S	2.4 ± 0.7	104.7 ± 18.7
F318C	9.7 ± 1.2^b	101.3 ± 17.7
F318W	3.1 ± 1.3	102.6 ± 9.2
F318H	3.6 ± 0.7	92.3 ± 16.7
E316K	2.2 ± 0.5	99.7 ± 10.9
T317K	3.8 ± 0.9	82.6 ± 6.4^a
R319K/R321K	2.6 ± 0.5	84.8 ± 9.5^a

Results represent the mean ± S.E.M. of at least three-independent experiments performed in duplicate.

[a] *$P < 0.05$, significantly different from Flag-MCHR1 by Student's t-test.*

[b] *$P < 0.01$, significantly different from Flag-MCHR1 by Student's t-test.*

mutations resulted in no higher potency or efficacy of MCH in the calcium mobilization assay. Instead, the T317K and R319K/R321K mutants had a significantly depressed maximal response relative to Flag-MCHR1 (**Table 3**, **Figure 5**). Taken together, the activity of MCHR1 in calcium mobilization is enhanced by the introduction of a positively charged Lys residue at the 318 position, but not at the adjacent amino acid residues, indicating that the 318 position seems to be critical for receptor conformation and/or receptor interaction with the Gα proteins that mediate calcium signaling. We then investigated the effects of a similar mutation in human MCHR2, the human ortholog of rat MCHR1. The corresponding Phe in MCHR2 was mutated to Lys (F313K) and tested for MCH responsiveness in calcium mobilization, since MCHR2 is known to couple exclusively to $G\alpha_q$ (An et al., 2001). As shown in **Table 4**, however, F313K was no more responsive than the non-mutated receptor, and rather showed a 22% reduced maximal response. These results imply that the effect of the Phe-to-Lys substitution on receptor signaling seems to be a specific and intrinsic feature of MCHR1.

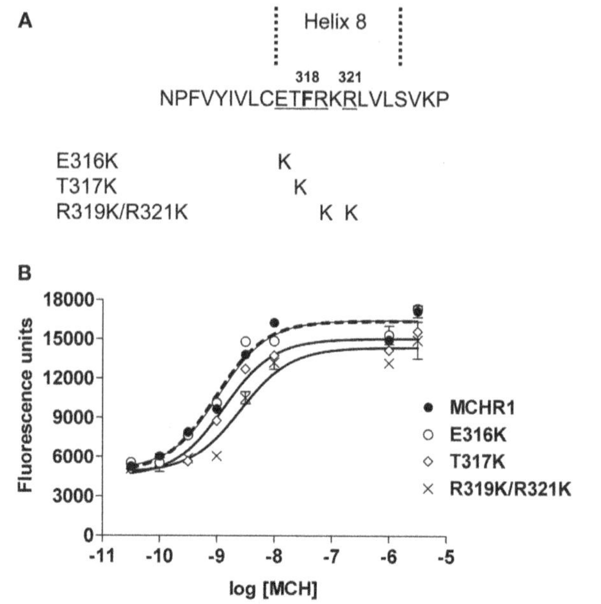

FIGURE 5 | Effects on receptor activity of substitution mutations of the residues adjacent to Phe318 in HEK293T cells. (A) Sequences of Flag-MCHR1 and three mutants for which native residues were replaced with Lys (E316K, T317K and R319K/R321K). **(B)** Dose-response relationship of MCH-stimulated calcium influx in HEK293T cells expressing Flag-MCHR1 or substitution mutant receptors. Cells transfected with Flag-MCHR1 or substitution mutant receptors were stimulated with the indicated concentrations of MCH, and the subsequent changes in cytoplasmic free Ca^{2+} levels were measured using a FlexStation. Results shown are representative of at least three-independent experiments.

Table 4 | Signaling of human MCHR2 and its single-substitution (F313K) mutant after transfection into HEK293T cells.

Receptor	EC_{50} of MCH (nM)	Maximum response (%)
MCHR2	5.2 ± 2.5	100
F313K/MCHR2	5.4 ± 2.4	78.7 ± 7.7

Since the F313 residue corresponds to F318 in rat MCHR1, the F313K mutant of human MCH2R was analyzed for its effect on receptor signaling to calcium mobilization. The data represent the mean ± S.E.M of three-independent experiments performed in duplicate.

SELECTIVITY OF F318K FOR G PROTEINS IN MCHR1

MCHR1-stimulated calcium signaling is mediated through both $G\alpha_q$- and $G\alpha_{i/o}$-dependent pathways (Hawes et al., 2000; Tetsuka et al., 2004). To confirm which G protein was primarily responsible for the enhancement of calcium signaling by the F318K receptor, we used pertussis-toxin (PTX) to uncouple $G\alpha_{i/o}$ from MCHR1. In cells expressing Flag-MCHR1, PTX pretreatment increased the EC_{50} value to 3.6 ± 0.6 nM (compared to 1.1 ± 0.3 nM in untreated cells), which equates to a +PTX (PTX-insensitive, $G\alpha_q$-dependent response)/-PTX (combined $G\alpha_{i/o}$ and $G\alpha_q$-dependent response) ratio of 3.30 (i.e., 3.6/1.1 nM). Following PTX pretreatment, the EC_{50} of MCH in cells expressing F318K was 0.48 ± 0.08 nM (compared to 0.13 ± 0.03 nM in untreated cells), giving a +PTX/−PTX ratio of 3.70. The maximal calcium response to MCH at either receptor was not affected by the addition of PTX. Because PTX reduced the potency of MCH but did not abolish its effect, it is clear that F318K and Flag-MCHR1 both drive calcium influx by a combination of $G\alpha_q$- and $G\alpha_{i/o}$-dependent pathways. Because MCH still stimulated calcium influx at a lower agonist concentration in F318K after treatment of PTX ($EC_{50} = 3.6$ nM at Flag-MCHR1 vs. 0.48 nM at F318K), it is clear that PTX-insensitive $G\alpha_q$ protein is involved in mediating calcium responses in both receptors. However, the ratio of MCH potency in the presence and absence of PTX was remarkably similar in both mutated and non-mutated receptors, suggesting that the selectivity of the mutant receptor is likely to be the same as in the wild-type receptor (i.e., that the mutation has not introduced a strong preference for $G\alpha_q$). However, calcium signals by $G\alpha_q$ tend to dwarf those induced by $G\alpha_{i/o}$ in HEK293T cells (Tetsuka et al., 2004), so it is difficult to judge what effect the mutation has on the ability of the receptor to couple to $G\alpha_{i/o}$. Thus, it was necessary to analyze other signal transduction events related to MCHR1-$G\alpha_{i/o}$ protein interactions.

It has been shown previously that MCH stimulation of cells expressing MCHR1 can activate a $G\alpha_{i/o}$-mediated pathway to cause a decrease in adenylyl cyclase activity, thus reducing cAMP production (Chambers et al., 1999; Saito et al., 1999; Hawes et al., 2000). We therefore tried to measure the interaction between MCHR1 and $G\alpha_{i/o}$ in cells where cAMP accumulation had been induced by forskolin. Although stable clones for F318K were established, their signaling profiles were very different to transiently transfected cells. For instance, F318K clones were unable to inhibit forskolin-stimulated cAMP accumulation, even at MCH concentrations up to 100 nM MCH (data not shown). These results suggest that the F318K stable clones have lost the ability to couple to $G\alpha_{i/o}$ protein. Because the amount of total protein and the glycosylation pattern of these proteins in cells were equivalent to that of Flag-MCHR1 (as determined by western blotting), the uncoupling from $G\alpha_{i/o}$ in stably-transfected cells may be due to some aberration in structure and/or functionality when cultured long-term in the presence of antibiotic selection.

Given the difficulties in measuring $G\alpha_{i/o}$ protein activation using cAMP assays in stable clones, we employed an alternative technique. It is well-established that the key step in GPCR activation is the induction of guanine nucleotide exchange (GDP-GTP) on the G protein α-subunit. The nucleotide exchange process can be monitored by measuring the binding of non-hydrolyzable GTPγS analog, [^{35}S]GTPγS. Because the $G\alpha_i$ family of G proteins has a substantially higher basal rate of guanine nucleotide exchange than other G proteins, this assay is ostensibly a measure of GPCR-mediated activation of $G\alpha_{i/o}$ proteins (Milligan, 2003). Indeed, the GTPγS binding assay has been widely used to measure the activation of $G\alpha_i$ proteins by various GPCRs. Therefore, we examined both basal and MCH-stimulated [^{35}S]GTPγS binding using the membrane fraction of HEK293T cells transiently expressing Flag-MCHR1 and the F318K mutant (**Figure 6**). In cells expressing Flag-MCHR1, MCH dose-dependently stimulated binding of GTPγS with an EC_{50} value of 0.23 ± 0.07 nM, while the value for F318K was 0.47 ± 0.25 nM (mean ± S.E.M. from three-independent experiments). The values for F318K were slightly higher, but a significant difference was not observed. The maximal amount of binding for Flag-MCHR1 with 1 μM MCH was $208.3 \pm 25.2\%$ of basal, while that for F318K was $190.6 \pm 20.3\%$ of basal. Overall, there was no difference in the amount of GTPγS binding between cells expressing Flag-MCHR1 and the F318K mutant, in contrast to the clear influence of the F318K mutation on $G\alpha_q$-mediated signaling. There was no significant difference in basal GTPγS binding (100% for Flag-MCHR1 vs. $97.6 \pm 0.4\%$ for F318K), suggesting that the F318K mutation does not affect constitutive receptor activation.

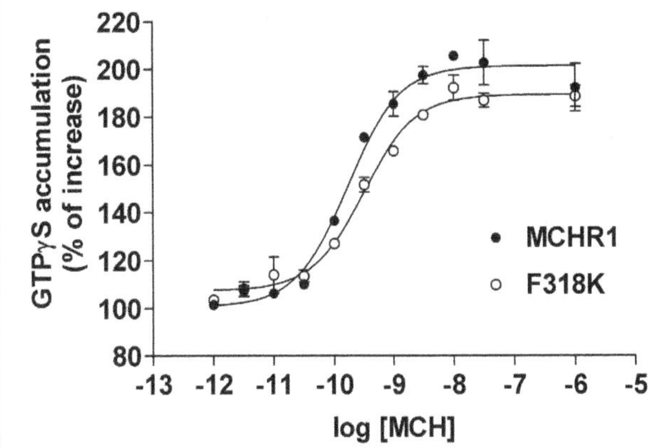

FIGURE 6 | MCH-induced [^{35}S]GTPγS binding to Flag-MCHR1 and F318K. HEK293T cells were transfected with Flag-MCHR1 or F318K. After 48 h, the cells were harvested and the membrane fractions recovered. Membrane proteins (10 μg) were subsequently incubated with 0.2 nM [^{35}S]GTPγS and 0.001–1000 nM MCH in GTPγS binding buffer for 30 min at 30°C. The amounts of radioactivity bound to the membrane preparations are shown for Flag-MCHR1 (filled circles) and F318K (open circles). Results shown are representative of three-independent experiments.

INTERPRETATION OF THE FUNCTIONAL IMPORTANCE OF F318K IN MCHR1

To understand better how the signaling dynamics of F318K are related to its interaction with (and activation of) $G\alpha_q$, we constructed a molecular model of F318K activation of G protein based on that for the active structure of rhodopsin in complex with a transducin peptide as a reference (Kleinau et al., 2010). Because MCHR1 belongs to the same GPCR subfamily as rhodopsin, the existing rhodopsin sequence alignment allowed us to construct a preliminary model of MCHR1 conformation. We refined this model to account for the specific properties of MCHR1 using software for protein model building and a molecular dynamics software package. Our model highlighted several putative amino acid contacts between the receptor and $G\alpha_q$ protein, notably at intracellular loop 1 (i1) and helix 8 (**Figure 7**, left). Lys318 is predicted to interact efficiently with Asp79 (located in i1) *via* a distinct hydrogen-bonding pattern, and these two residues create an accessible intracellular interface for the Asn357 residue in the $G\alpha_q$ protein. However, Asp79 in i1 also exists in human MCHR2, in which F313K had no effect on MCH potency in calcium signaling, as shown in **Table 4**. We therefore searched for alternative candidate residues that may be involved in the interaction with Asn357 by comparing sequences between rat MCHR1 and other GPCRs, including human MCHR2. The sequences we used are for GPCRs in which mutation at the position corresponding to Phe318 of MCHR1 did not produce increased signaling potency (Fritze et al., 2003; Delos Santos et al., 2006; Anavi-Goffer et al., 2007; Duvernay et al., 2009; Málaga-Diéguez et al., 2010; Kaye et al., 2011). By making multiple alignments of these sequences, we found several amino acid insertions in i1 that occurred only in rat MCHR1, and were absent in other GPCRs (**Table 5**). Notably, a sequence in i1 includes Trp73, which possesses a bulky, aromatic side chain. Hydrophobic

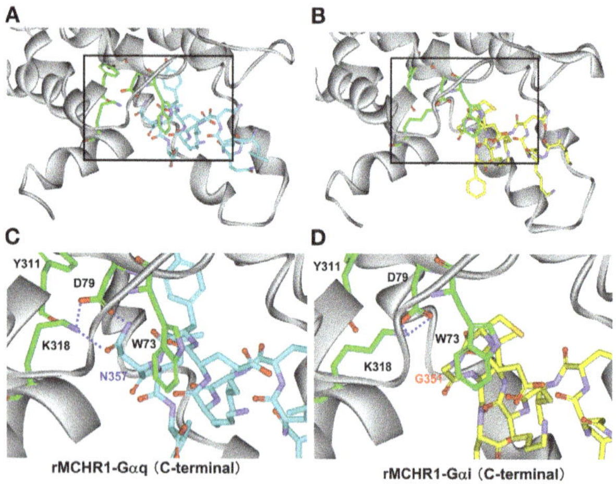

FIGURE 7 | Structural analysis of critical amino acids in a proposed model of rat MCHR1 mutant F318K with $G\alpha_q$ or $G\alpha_i$ proteins. Homology model of rat MCHR1 mutant F318K was constructed using the crystal structure of rhodopsin E113Q mutant in complex with the C-terminal tail of transducin (PDB ID 2X72). Amino acid residues involved in coupling to $G\alpha_q$ or $G\alpha_i$ proteins in intracellular loop 1 (i1) and K318 in helix 8 are shown. **(A)** The model structure of MCHR1(F318K)-$G\alpha_q$ C-terminal tail. The area demarcated by the square is magnified below in panel **(C)**. **(B)** The model structure of MCHR1(F318K)-$G\alpha_i$ C-terminal tail. The area demarcated by the square is magnified below in panel **(D)**. **(C)** Positions of Lys318, Tyr311, Trp73, and Asp79 residues and their position relative to Asn357 of $G\alpha_q$. This model depicts the hydrogen bond network between Lys318 and Asp79 in the receptor and Asn357 in $G\alpha_q$ C-terminal tail. Note that interactions between Trp73 in i1 loop and Asn357 in the G protein C-terminal tail. Green, red, and blue areas indicate carbon, oxygen and nitrogen atoms, respectively, within the key residues of the receptor. Carbon atoms in the $G\alpha_q$ protein are colored cyan. **(D)** Magnified view of Lys318, Tyr311, Trp73, and Asp79 residues in the receptor and their position relative to Gly351 of $G\alpha_i$. Intramolecular hydrogen interactions predicted between Lys318 and Asp79 in the receptor are shown. Carbon atoms in the $G\alpha_i$ protein are colored yellow.

interaction of Trp73 with Asn357 in the $G\alpha_q$ C-terminal tail is predicted to stabilize the intracellular interaction between MCHR1 and $G\alpha_q$. Conversely, the Gly351 residue in $G\alpha_i$ has no side chain to interact with Lys318 (**Figure 7**, right), which may explain the lack of enhancing effect of the F318K mutation on $G\alpha_i$-mediated signaling. Collectively, a predicted model of F318K combined with sequence alignments suggests that the key residues of the MCHR1-$G\alpha_q$ interface are Trp73 and Asp79 in the receptor and Asn357 in the $G\alpha_q$ protein. We speculate that the F318K mutation somehow enhances this interface, either by promoting heightened interaction or by facilitating G protein activation, possibly by changing the binding affinity (see section "Discussion").

DISCUSSION

Recent studies have underscored that, the Phe residue is a key position in the conserved $NPxxY(x)_{5,6}F$ motif, which connects TM7 and helix 8 (Palczewski et al., 2000; Fritze et al., 2003). Indeed, of 180 class A GPCRs, this Phe residue is the most highly conserved in 135 of these receptors (Okuno et al., 2005). Mutation of the conserved Phe to Ala in rhodopsin and the M1 muscarinic acetylcholine receptor considerably reduced the potency in $G\alpha_t$- and $G\alpha_q$-mediated signaling, respectively (Fritze et al., 2003; Kaye et al., 2011). Furthermore, Phe-to-Ala substitution in this motif dramatically reduced cell surface expression of α2B-AR, resulting in extensive ER arrest (Duvernay et al., 2009). These data suggest that the highly hydrophobic Phe residue in the conserved $NPxxY(x)_{5,6}F$ motif of many GPCRs is necessary for the maintenance of proper receptor conformation, and is often involved in receptor export from the ER. In the present study, we showed that Phe-to-Ala substitution (F318A) in rat MCHR1 did not significantly affect either the level of cell surface expression or MCH-induced calcium mobilization. However, by analyzing a series of substitution mutants, Phe-to-Lys substitution led to the most increased MCH potency in stimulating calcium mobilization, a pathway largely mediated *via* $G\alpha_q$. In contrast, F318K had no significant effect in the GTPγS-binding assay that measures receptor interaction with $G\alpha_i$ protein. These findings are surprising considering that they contradict findings in Phe substitutions of other GPCRs. Therefore, our study provides new insight into the role of the $NPxxY(x)_{5,6}F$ motif Phe residue in term of G protein activation. Although the consensus is that this residue is a key determinant of receptor structure and function, its effect may be dependent on the specific sequence of the receptor and the presence or absence of other residues that make up the receptor-G protein binding/activation interface.

We showed that MCH was the most potent in stimulating calcium mobilization in cells expressing F318K among our mutants. To date, many mutations or truncations in MCHR1 have been designed to study the roles of certain residues and sequences in the diverse functionality of the receptor (Macdonald et al., 2000; Saito et al., 2003, 2004, 2005; Tetsuka et al., 2004; Fan et al., 2005). Some caused a slight or moderate decrease in calcium mobilization (Saito et al., 2003, 2004) and the others resulted in more severe impairment or loss of function (Macdonald et al., 2000; Tetsuka et al., 2004; Fan et al., 2005; Saito et al., 2005; Aizaki et al., 2009). F318K is, therefore, the first mutation characterized by an active variant with more efficient signaling properties. We conclude that substitution of Phe318 with the moderately positively charged Lys is most responsible, at least in part, for producing increased MCH potency in stimulating calcium mobilization *via* MCHR1. Replacement with another positively charged amino acid, His, at the 318 position had no effect for signaling enhancement. Furthermore, the highly positively charged Arg could not induce equivalent effects to F318K (**Figure 2**, **Table 3**). These findings suggest that unique and strict physicochemical characteristics, including the extent of positive charge, polarity and the size of the side chain, may be required for this phenomenon to occur.

GPCRs that bind promiscuously to several Gα protein subtypes are useful tools for clarifying the determinants of G protein selectivity. To date, most studies of rhodopsin family GPCRs have emphasized the role of membrane-proximal regions in the i2 and i3 loops and/or the cytoplasmic loop of the receptor (Anavi-Goffer et al., 2007; Kunieda et al., 2007; Kleinau et al., 2010). Our present data suggest that MCHR1 couples to both $G\alpha_i$ and

Table 5 | Amino acid sequence alignment from the transmembrane 1 (TM1) to TM3 of rat MCHR1 and other GPCRs.

```
                      TM1                       i1            TM2                  extracellular loop 1          TM3
rMCHR1      38:---YINIIMPSVFGTICLLGIVGNSTVIFAVVKKSKLHWCSNVPDIFIINLSVVDLLF-LLGMPFMIHQLMGNGVWHFGETMCTLITAMDANSQFTSTYILTAMTIDRYL 143
hMCHR2      35:------VILPSMIGIICSTGLVGNILIVFTIIRSRKK----TVPDIYICNLAVADLVH-IVGMPFLIHQWARGGEWVFGGPLCTIITSLDTCNQFACSAIMTVMSVDRYF 133
rmAChR1     30:----------ITTGLLSLATVTGNLLVLISFKVNTELK---TVNNYFLLSLACADLIIGTFSMNLYTTYLLMG-HWALGTLACDLWLALDYVASNASVMNLLLISFDRYF 125
rA1AR       15:-----------IEVLIALVSVPGNVLVIWAVKVNQALR---DATFCFIVSLAVADVAVGALVIPLAILINIGPQTYFH---TCLMVACPVLILTQSSILALLAIAVDRYL 107
ra(2B)-AR   23:-----------AITFLILFTIFGNALVILAVLTSRSLR---APQNLFLVSLAAADILVATLIIPFSLANELLG-YWYFWRAWCEVYLALDVLFCTSSIVHLCAISLDRYW 117
hb1AR       56:---QWTAGMGLLMALIVLLIVAGNVLVIVAIAKTPRLQ---TLTNLFIMSLASADLVMGLLVVPFGATIVVWG-RWEYGSFFCELWTSVDVLCVTASIETLCVIALDRYL 158
bovineRho   35:---WQFSMLAAYMFLLIMLGFPINFLTLYVTVQHKKLR---TPLNYILLNLAVADLFMVFGGFTTTLYTSLHG-YFVFGPTGCNLEGFFATLGGEIALWSLVVLAIERYV 137
hCB1       111:LNPSQQLAIAVLSLTLGTFTVLENLLVLCVILHSRSLR--CRPSYHFIGSLAVADLLGSVIFVYSFIDFHVFHRKDSRNVFLFKLGG--VTASFTASVGSLFLTAIDRYI 216
                             .      .* ..      .          ..  *. .*.   .  .         . ..  .         .   .    .**
```

Stars beneath sequence indicate sequence identity across the alignment, and single dot indicates conserved substitutions.

hMCHR2, human MCHR2; rmAChR1, rat muscarinic acetylcholine receptor M1; rA1AR, rat adenosine 1A receptor; ra(2B)-AR, rat α2B adrenergic receptor; hb1AR, human β1 adrenergic receptor, bovineRho, bovine rhodopsin; hCB1, human cannobinoid receptor 1.

$G\alpha_q$ proteins *via* overlapping intracellular regions but that Lys mutation of the 318 position in the NPxxY$(x)_{5,6}$F motif appears to affect only the coupling of the receptor to $G\alpha_q$. Phe318 is located in the juxtamembrane helix 8 in the C-terminal tail. The role of helix 8 is believed to be in regulating G protein activation by GPCRs, yet few studies have established the pivotal role of helix 8 in G protein selectivity. The position in cannabinoid receptor 1 that corresponds to the MCHR1 Phe318 residue is not a Phe but is a hydrophobic residue (Leu404), and the L404I mutation led to impaired activation of $G\alpha_{i3}$ but not $G\alpha_{oA}$ among the $G\alpha_{i/o}$ protein subgroup (Anavi-Goffer et al., 2007). Furthermore, the positively charged Arg687 in helix 8 of the thyrotropin receptor is important for selective interaction with $G\alpha_q$ (Kleinau et al., 2010). In helix 8 of MCHR1, three basic amino acid residues (Arg319, Lys320, and Arg321) are juxtaposed with Phe318. This basic region in helix 8 seems not to be involved in Gα protein coupling specificity, since alteration of the positive charge of these residues (R319Q/K320Q/R321Q) caused an equally strong inhibition of both $G\alpha_q$ and $G\alpha_i$ (Tetsuka et al., 2004). Taken together, we might conclude that each amino acid residue in helix 8 of MCHR1 may have different roles in determining receptor activity and G protein selectivity. Our clarification here of the significance of the Phe position will hopefully allow additional understanding of dual G protein coupling in other GPCRs.

Upon stimulation, GPCRs undergo a conformational change that results in G protein activation. Light-induced conformational changes in rhodopsin were elucidated by a series of biophysical studies. Evidence indicates that an important hydrophobic pairing between Tyr306 and Phe313 in the NPxxY$(x)_{5,6}$F motif stabilizes the ground state of rhodopsin (Palczewski et al., 2000; Nygaard et al., 2009). Comparative molecular dynamics simulations of MCHR1 have also suggested that the release of intramolecular interactions between the Tyr and Phe residues in the motif is an important step in transitioning from an inactive to an active form (Vitale et al., 2004). We initially hypothesized that the Tyr311-Phe318-based switch in MCHR1, which is the homolog of a crucial relay point in rhodopsin, would be modified by substituting Phe with Lys, with disruption of an aromatic stacking interaction in the resultant ternary complex somehow affecting the efficacy of signaling. However, the activated F318K structure bound with $G\alpha_q$ protein (**Figure 7**) has suggested that an additional and distinct interface may exist between Phe318 and Asp79 in the i1 loop. Further analysis with multiple alignment data for other GPCRs showed that close proximity of Phe318, Asp79, and Asn357 is insufficient to induce such signaling changes and that Trp73 in the i1 loop may be important in stabilizing/maintaining the efficient binding/activation of the $G\alpha_q$ protein by the activated receptor. A series of combinational mutations involving F318K and several amino acid residues in the i1 loop (Trp, Cys, and Ser, as described in **Table 5**) may clarify the importance and role of each residue. A precise three-dimensional crystal structure of the MCHR1-G protein complex would also facilitate our understanding, but our present model helps to understand how a single amino acid substitution, F318K, can alter the intra-/inter-molecular interactions of the receptor-G protein complex to modulate G protein signaling *via* this receptor. At this time, we cannot exclude the possibility that F318K has an increased binding affinity, although the EC_{50} value of MCH in the GTPγS-binding assay showed no change between Flag-MCHR1 and F318K. The concept of modes in agonism of GPCRs has recently been expanding (Smith et al., 2011), implying that receptors can convey different signals through different pathways with varying degrees of potency or efficacy depending on the ligand used. Therefore, it may be possible that the functional selectivity observed in F318K results from enhancement of the binding affinity that favors $G\alpha_q$-binding but not $G\alpha_i$-binding. Overall, based on our data, we favor an interpretation that F318 is involved in receptor dynamics.

In conclusion, by analyzing a series of mutants, we report for the first time that F318K, a point mutation in the NPxxY$(x)_{5,6}$F motif of MCHR1, most efficiently enhances the potency of MCH in stimulating calcium mobilization *via* MCHR1 without showing any increase in cell surface expression. We speculate that Phe318 might be involved in the interface between the receptor and G protein, and may regulate which G proteins the receptor can bind and activate. Because there are a limited number of GPCR mutant that significantly enhanced the signaling (Reinscheid et al., 2005; Kato et al., 2008), F318K may provide useful clues in understanding the process of intrinsic receptor dynamics. However, further research is required to demonstrate whether the role of Phe318 described here is of physiological and functional significance.

ACKNOWLEDGMENTS

We thank Yuki Kobayashi, Akiko Kojo, Yui Funakoshi and Saori Utsuda for expert technical assistance and helpful support. Source of funding: This work was supported by research grants from the Ministry of Education, Culture, Sports, Science and Technology of Japan (Kakenhi 20500337, 00215568 to Yumiko Saito).

REFERENCES

Acharya, S., and Karnik, S. S. (1996). Modulation of GDP release from transducin by the conserved Glu134-Arg135 sequence in rhodopsin. *J. Biol. Chem.* 271, 25406–25411.

Aizaki, Y., Maruyama, K., Nakano-Tetsuka, M., and Saito, Y. (2009). Distinct roles of the DRY motif in rat melanin-concentrating hormone receptor 1 in signaling control. *Peptides* 30, 974–981.

Anavi-Goffer, S., Fleischer, D., Hurst, D. P., Lynch, D. L., Barnett-Norris, J., Shi, S., et al. (2007). Helix 8 Leu in the CB1 cannabinoid receptor contributes to selective signal transduction mechanisms. *J. Biol. Chem.* 282, 25100–25113.

An, S., Cutler, G., Zhao, J. J., Huang, S. G., Tian, H., Li, W., et al. (2001). Identification and characterization of a melanin-concentrating hormone receptor. *Proc. Natl. Acad. Sci. U.S.A.* 98, 7576–7581.

Bednarek, M. A., Tan, C., Hreniuk, D. L., Palyha, O. C., MacNeil, D. J., van der Ploeg, L. H., et al. (2002). Synthesis and biological evaluation *in vitro* of a selective, high potency peptide agonist of human melanin-concentrating hormone action at human melanin-concentrating hormone receptor 1. *J. Biol. Chem.* 277, 13821–13826.

Bittencourt, J. C., Presse, F., Arias, C., Peto, C., Vaughan, J., Nahon, J. L., et al. (1992). The melanin-concentrating hormone system of the rat brain: an immuno- and hybridization histochemical characterization. *J. Comp. Neurol.* 319, 218–245.

Borowsky, B., Durkin, M. M., Ogozalek, K., Marzabadi, M. R., DeLeon, J., Lagu, B., et al. (2002). Antidepressant, anxiolytic and anorectic effects of a melanin-concentrating hormone-1 receptor antagonist. *Nat. Med.* 8, 825–830.

Chambers, J., Ames, R. S., Bergsma, D., Muir, A., Fitzgerald, L. R., Hervieu, G., et al. (1999). Melanin-concentrating hormone is the cognate ligand for the orphan G-protein-coupled receptor SLC-1. *Nature* 400, 261–265.

Chen, Y., Hu, C., Hsu, C. K., Zhang, Q., Bi, C., Asnicar, M., et al. (2002). Targeted disruption of the melanin-concentrating hormone receptor-1 results in hyperphagia and resistance to diet-induced obesity. *Endocrinology* 143, 2469–2477.

Delos Santos, N. M., Gardner, L. A., White, S. W., and Bahouth, S. W. (2006). Characterization of the residues in helix 8 of the human beta1-adrenergic receptor that are involved in coupling the receptor to G proteins. *J. Biol. Chem.* 281, 12896–12907.

Duvernay, M. T., Dong, C., Zhang, X., Zhou, F., Nichols, C. D., and Wu, G. (2009). Anterograde trafficking of G protein-coupled receptors: function of the C-terminal F(X)6LL motif in export from the endoplasmic reticulum. *Mol. Pharmacol.* 75, 751–761.

Fan, J., Perry, S. J., Gao, Y., Schwarz, D. A., and Maki, R. A. (2005). A point mutation in the human melanin concentrating hormone receptor 1 reveals an important domain for cellular trafficking. *Mol. Endocrinol.* 19, 2579–2590.

Fritze, O., Filipek, S., Kuksa, V., Palczewski, K., Hofmann, K. P., and Emst, O. P. (2003). Role of the conserved NPxxY(x)5, 6F motif in the rhodopsin ground state and during activation. *Proc. Natl. Acad. Sci. U.S.A.* 100, 2290–2295.

Georgescu, D., Sears, R. M., Hommel, J. D., Barrot, M., Bolaños, C. A., Marsh, D. J., et al. (2005). The hypothalamic neuropeptide melanin-concentrating hormone acts in the nucleus accumbens to modulate feeding behavior and forced-swim performance. *J. Neurosci.* 25, 2933–2940.

Gether, U. (2000). Uncovering molecular mechanisms involved in activation of G protein-coupled receptors. *Endocr. Rev.* 21, 90–113.

Hawes, B. E., Kil, E., Green, B., O'Neill, K., Fried, S., and Graziano, M. P. (2000). The melanin-concentrating hormone couples to multiple G proteins to activate diverse intracellular signaling pathways. *Endocrinology* 141, 4524–4532.

Huynh, J., Thomas, W. G., Aquilar, M. I., and Pattenden, L. K. (2009). Role of helix 8 in G protein-coupled receptors based on structure-function studies on the type 1 angiotensin receptor. *Mol. Cell. Endocrinol.* 302, 118–127.

Kato, A., Katada, S., and Touhara, K. (2008). Amino acids involved in conformational dynamics and G protein coupling of an odorant receptor: targeting gain-of-function mutation. *J. Neurochem.* 107, 1261–1270.

Kaye, R. G., Saldanha, J. W., Lu, Z. L., and Hulme, E. C. (2011). Helix 8 of the M1 muscarinic acetylcholine receptor: scanning mutagenesis delineates a G protein recognition site. *Mol. Pharamacol.* 79, 701–709.

Kleinau, G., Jaeschke, H., Worth, C. L., Mueller, S., Gonzalez, J., Paschke, R., et al. (2010). Principles and determinants of G-protein coupling by the rhodopsin-like thyrotropin receptor. *PLoS ONE* 5:e9745. doi: 10.1371/journal.pone.0009745

Kunieda, K., Okuno, T., Terawaki, K., Miyano, M., Yokomizo, T., and Shimizu, T. (2007). Identification of the intracellular region of the leukotriene B4 receptor type 1 that is specifically involved in Gi activation. *J. Biol. Chem.* 282, 3998–4006.

Macdonald, D., Murgolo, N., Zhang, R., Durkin, J. P., Yao, X., Strader, C. D., et al. (2000). Molecular characterization of the melanin-concentrating hormone/receptor complex: identification of critical residues involved in binding and activation. *Mol. Pharmacol.* 58, 217–225.

Málaga-Diéguez, L., Yang, Q., Bauer, J., Pankevych, H., Freissmuth, M., and Nanoff, C. (2010). Pharmacochaperoning of the A1 adenosine receptor is contingent on the endoplasmic reticulum. *Mol. Pharmacol.* 77, 940–952.

Marsh, D. J., Weingarth, D. T., Novi, D. E., Chen, H. Y., Trumbauer, M. E., Chen, A. S., et al. (2002). Melanin-concentrating hormone 1 receptor-deficient mice are lean, hyperactive, and hyperphagic and have altered metabolism. *Proc. Natl. Acad. Sci. U.S.A.* 99, 3240–3245.

Milligan, G. (2003). Principles: extending the utility of [^{35}S]GTP gamma S binding assays. *Trends Pharmacol. Sci.* 24, 87–90.

Nygaard, R., Frimurer, T. M., Holst, B., Rosenkilde, M. M., and Schwartz, T. W. (2009). Ligand binding and micro-switches in 7TM receptor structures. *Trends Pharmacol. Sci.* 30, 249–259.

Okuno, T., Yokomizo, T., Hori, T., Miyano, M., and Shimizu, T. (2005). Leukotriene B4 receptor and the function of its helix 8. *J. Bio. Chem.* 280, 32049–32052.

Palczewski, K., Kumasaka, T., Hori, T., Behnke, C. A., Motoshima, H., Fox, B. A., et al. (2000). Crystal structure of rhodopsin: a G protein-coupled receptor. *Science* 289, 739–745.

Reinscheid, R. K., Xu, Y. L., Okamura, N., Zeng, J., Chung, S., Pai, R., et al. (2005). Pharmacological characterization of human and murine neuropeptide s receptor variants. *J. Pharmacol. Exp. Ther.* 315, 1338–1345.

Rossi, M., Choi, S. J., O'Shea, D., Miyoshi, T., Ghatei, M. A., and Bloom, S. R. (1997). Melanin-concentrating hormone acutely stimulates feeding, but chronic administration has no effect on body weight. *Endocrinology* 138, 351–355.

Saito, Y., Cheng, M., Leslie, F. M., and Civelli, O. (2001). Expression of the melanin-concentrating hormone (MCH) receptor mRNA in the rat brain. *J. Comp. Neurol.* 435, 26–40.

Saito, Y., Nothacker, H. P., Wang, Z., Lin, S. H., Leslie, F., and Civelli, O. (1999). Molecular characterization of the melanin-concentrating-hormone receptor. *Nature* 400, 265–269.

Saito, Y., Tetsuka, M., Li, Y., Kurose, H., and Maruyama, K. (2004). Properties of rat melanin-concentrating hormone receptor 1 internalization. *Peptides* 25, 1597–1604.

Saito, Y., Tetsuka, M., Saito, S., Imai, K., Yoshikawa, A., Doi, H., et al. (2005). Arginine residue 155 in the second intracellular loop plays a critical role in rat melanin-concentrating hormone receptor 1. *Endocrinology* 146, 3452–3462.

Saito, Y., Tetsuka, M., Yue, L., Kawamura, Y., and Maruyama,

K. (2003). Functional role of *N*-linked glycosylation on the rat melanin-concentrating hormone receptor 1. *FEBS Lett.* 533, 29–34.

Shearman, L. P., Camacho, R. E., Sloan Stribling, D., Zhou, D., Bednarek, M. A., Hreniuk, D. L., et al. (2003). Chronic MCHR1eceptor modulation alters appetite, body weight and adiposity in rats. *Eur. J. Pharmacol.* 475, 37–47.

Shimada, M., Tritos, N. A., Lowell, B. B., Flier, J. S., and Maratos-Flier, E. (1998). Mice lacking melanin-concentrating hormone are hypophagic and lean. *Nature* 396, 670–674.

Smith, N. J., Bennett, K. A., and Milligan, G. (2011). When simple agonism is not enough: emerging modalities of GPCR ligands. *Mol. Cell. Endocrinol.* 331, 241–247.

Takekawa, S., Asami, A., Ishihara, Y., Terauchi, J., Kato, K., Shimomura, Y., et al. (2002). T-226296: a novel, orally active and selective melanin-concentrating hormone receptor antagonist. *Eur. J. Pharmacol.* 438, 129–135.

Tan, C. P., Sano, H., Iwaasa, H., Pan, J., Sailer, A. W., Hreniuk, D. L., et al. (2002). Melanin-concentrating hormone receptor subtypes 1 and 2: species-specific gene expression. *Genomics* 79, 785–792.

Tetsuka, M., Saito, Y., Imai, K., Doi, H., and Maruyama, K. (2004). The basic residues in the membrane-proximal C-terminal tail of the rat melanin-concentrating hormone receptor 1 are required for receptor function. *Endocrinology* 145, 3712–3723.

Vitale, R. M., Pedone, C., de Benedetti, P. G., and Fanelli, F. (2004). Structural features of the inactive and active states of the melanin-concentrating hormone receptors: insights from molecular simulations. *Proteins* 56, 430–448.

2

The melanocortin receptors and their accessory proteins

Shwetha Ramachandrappa, Rebecca J. Gorrigan, Adrian J. L. Clark and Li F. Chan*

Centre for Endocrinology, William Harvey Research Institute, Queen Mary University of London, Barts and The London School of Medicine and Dentistry, London, UK

Edited by:
Jae Young Seong, Korea University, South Korea

Reviewed by:
Akiyoshi Takahashi, Kitasato University, Japan
Robert Dores, University of Minnesota, USA

Correspondence:
Li F. Chan, Centre for Endocrinology, William Harvey Research Institute, Queen Mary University of London, Barts and The London School of Medicine and Dentistry, Charterhouse Square, London EC1M 6BQ, UK.
e-mail: l.chan@qmul.ac.uk

The five melanocortin receptors (MCRs) named MC1R–MC5R have diverse physiological roles encompassing pigmentation, steroidogenesis, energy homeostasis and feeding behavior as well as exocrine function. Since their identification almost 20 years ago much has been learnt about these receptors. As well as interacting with their endogenous ligands the melanocortin peptides, there is now a growing list of important peptides that can modulate the way these receptors signal, acting as agonists, antagonists, and inverse agonists. The discovery of melanocortin 2 receptor accessory proteins as a novel accessory factor to the MCRs provides further insight into the regulation of these important G protein-coupled receptor.

Keywords: melanocortin receptors, accessory proteins, adrenal cortex, familial glucocorticoid deficiency, obesity

THE MELANOCORTIN SYSTEM

The melanocortin receptors (MCRs) are a family of five G protein-coupled receptors (GPCRs; MC1R–MC5R) expressed in diverse tissues, which serve discrete physiological functions. Early studies delineated a preliminary model where the receptors were activated by melanocortin peptides, derived from post-translational processing and proteolytic cleavage of the precursor protein proopiomelanocortin (Eipper and Mains, 1980). Receptor activation increased intracellular cyclic adenosine monophosphate (cAMP) levels triggering several downstream signaling pathways. Subsequent research into melanocortin signaling has added several additional tiers of complexity to this basic schema. It has emerged that many of the MCRs bind to endogenous peptides beyond the melanocortin peptides, which can act as agonists, antagonists, partial agonists, and even inverse agonists at these receptors (Cone, 2006). Furthermore, although the cAMP pathway continues to serve as the predominant readout of MCR function in many studies, numerous other intracellular signaling cascades for example the mitogen-activated protein kinase pathway have also been implicated in melanocortin signaling (Vongs et al., 2004; Sutton et al., 2005; Patten et al., 2007; Rodrigues et al., 2009). An additional feature of MCR signaling which has come to light over recent years is the presence of accessory proteins which regulate receptor function. These observations have broadened our understanding of MCR signaling, unveiling a highly specialized system, which on a cellular level enables individual cells to generate a complex co-ordinated response to the unique complement of ligands in their microenvironment (**Table 1**).

MC1R

MC1R is expressed in the melanocytes of the skin and hair follicles. Activation of MC1R results in a switch from red/yellow pheomelanin pigment production to the production of brown/black eumelanin pigment; it also promotes cell proliferation, DNA repair, and cell survival. Variants in MC1R are associated with red hair color, fair skin, and increased skin cancer risk (Valverde et al., 1995). Many of these variant receptors have been studied *in vitro* and their function, as measured by cAMP production in response to [Nle4,D-Phe7]-α-MSH (NDP-MSH), has been shown to be impaired compared to wild-type. Until recently MC1R was thought to be exclusively activated by alpha-MSH endogenously produced by keratinocytes in response to ultraviolet radiation. Human β-defensin 3 has since emerged as a novel endogenous MC1R ligand whose binding appears to initiate a discrete complement of intracellular signaling pathways *in vitro* (Beaumont et al., 2012; Swope et al., 2012). The physiological importance of this interaction remains to be seen. MC1R is also expressed in macrophages and in adipocytes where its role is less clearly defined. At extremely high plasma adrenocorticotropin hormone (ACTH) concentrations, ACTH activation of MC1R leads to hyperpigmentation observed in patients with familial glucocorticoid deficiency (FGD) (Turan et al., 2012). The study of the genetic determinants of coat color in animal models led to the discovery of agouti (also known as agouti signaling peptide), a high-affinity antagonist of the MC1R (Lu et al., 1994). The identification of an endogenous, physiologically relevant GPCR antagonist marked the beginning of a paradigm shift in our understanding of GPCR signaling. Later work demonstrated the complexity of this molecule by exploring its ability to act as an inverse agonist (Vage et al., 1997), inhibiting constitutively active MC1R.

MC2R

MC2R is predominantly expressed in the adrenal gland where it promotes the expression of steroidogenic enzymes in response to binding plasma ACTH. Mutations in MC2R result in FGD (Clark et al., 1993; Tsigos et al., 1993). This is a rare, life-threatening autosomal recessive disorder of adrenal resistance to ACTH wherein affected individuals have low serum levels of cortisol despite the presence of extremely high circulating levels of plasma ACTH. Patients typically present within a few months

Table 1 | The members of the melanocortin receptor family, expression, action, and phenotype of individuals with mutations.

Receptor	Main sites of expression	Physiological functions	Disease phenotype of patients with loss-of-function mutations	OMIM
MC1R	Melanocytes, macrophage	Pigmentation, inflammation	Increased risk of skin cancers	155555
MC2R	Adrenal cortex	Adrenal steroidogenesis	Familial glucocorticoid deficiency	202200
MC3R	Central nervous system (CNS), gastrointestinal (GI) tract, Kidney	Energy homeostasis, inflammation	Obesity	155540
MC4R	CNS, spinal cord	Energy homeostasis, appetite regulation, erectile function	Obesity	155541
MC5R	Lymphocytes, exocrine cells	Exocrine function, regulation of sebaceous glands	Decreased production of sebaceous lipids in mice	600042

of life with symptoms of cortisol deficiency including recurrent infections, hypoglycemia, convulsions, failure to thrive, and shock. Milder forms of the disease have been observed to present later in life (Metherell et al., 2009; Hughes et al., 2010; Meimaridou et al., 2012). The classical presentation of FGD comprises isolated perturbation of the glucocorticoid axis; however, a small number of cases have been described where this is accompanied by a disorder of mineralocorticoid secretion (Lin et al., 2007; Chan et al., 2009a).

Mutations in MC2R account for 25% of cases of FGD. The remaining 75% of patients with FGD in whom mutations in MC2R have been excluded have formed the subject of genetic approaches to elucidate other causative loci. To date, mutations in three further genes have been associated with FGD. Mutations in the melanocortin 2 receptor accessory protein (MRAP), a single pass transmembrane protein implicated in MC2R function account for approximately 15–20% of cases of FGD (Metherell et al., 2005). Mutations in steroidogenic acute regulatory (STAR) protein are known to give rise to lipoid congenital adrenal hyperplasia, a severe form of adrenal insufficiency characterized by both glucocorticoid and mineralocorticoid deficiency together with gonadal deficiency; however, STAR mutations have also been identified in a number of patients with FGD suggesting that mutations in this gene can give rise to a spectrum of clinical phenotypes encompassing FGD (Metherell et al., 2009). Recently, mutations in nicotinamide nucleotide transhydrogenase (NNT) a mitochondrial membrane constituent which is involved in detoxification of reactive oxygen species were also associated with FGD (Meimaridou et al., 2012). Notably, mutations in minichromosome maintenance-deficient 4 (MCM4) which forms part of a protein complex which is essential for DNA replication and genome stability are associated with a variant of FGD found in the Irish Traveller population where adrenal failure is accompanied by short stature, chromosome instability, and natural killer cell dysfunction (O'Riordan et al., 2008; Gineau et al., 2012; Hughes et al., 2012).

MC3R

MC3R is primarily expressed in the central nervous system where it is found in the hypothalamus and the limbic regions (Roselli-Rehfuss et al., 1993). Targeted deletion of MC3R in murine models results in animals with increased fat mass, reduced lean mass, and reduced physical activity in the absence of hyperphagia (Butler et al., 2000; Chen et al., 2000). Additionally, these animals exhibit accelerated weight gain when placed on a high fat diet which is independent of hyperphagia implying that MC3R may be involved in nutrient partitioning. An emerging aspect of the MC3R deficient phenotype is that when these animals are subjected to food restriction regimes they exhibit impaired synchronized oscillation of the transcription factors which regulate liver clock activity and metabolism, utilize carbohydrates inappropriately, and fail to demonstrate the food anticipatory behaviors which are seen in wild-type mice (Sutton et al., 2008, 2010). These observations have led to the suggestion that MC3R is involved in coordinating appropriate homeostatic metabolic and behavioral responses to nutrient cues. Interestingly, despite focused investigation, rare variants at the MC3R locus have not been definitively associated with monogenic obesity in humans (Seng Lee et al., 2007; Mencarelli et al., 2011).

MC4R

MC4R is widely expressed in the central nervous system where it is abundant in several regions including the paraventricular nucleus (PVN) of the hypothalamus (Mountjoy et al., 1994). Targeted deletion of MC4R in a mouse model results in animals which are severely obese, with hyperphagia and reduced energy expenditure (Huszar et al., 1997). In an informative study, Cre-lox technology was used to selectively re-express MC4R at endogenous levels in the PVN and the amygdale of MC4R knockout animals (Balthasar et al., 2005). This was able to partially rescue their obese phenotype by normalizing their food intake suggesting that MC4Rs in these regions are responsible for regulating eating behavior while MC4Rs in anatomically distinct neuronal populations are relevant to its control of energy expenditure.

The PVN is a key integration center for diverse signals which impact upon energy balance and is densely innervated by the arcuate nucleus of the hypothalamus. The release of proopiomelanocortin (POMC)-derived peptides from neurons in the arcuate nucleus, which are stimulated by leptin results in the activation of MC4R signaling in the PVN (Cheung et al., 1997; Schwartz et al., 1997). Uniquely for a biological system, a physiologically relevant endogenous antagonist and inverse agonist of MC4R (as well as MC3R) signaling is also produced in the hypothalamus, agouti-related peptide (AGRP; Nijenhuis et al., 2001; Breit et al., 2006). ARGP is produced by leptin responsive neurons in the arcuate nucleus that are inhibited by leptin. The presence of endogenous agonists and antagonists for this receptor enables MC4R signaling in the PVN to be delicately balanced.

Mutations in the MC4R are the most prevalent form of monogenic obesity identified to date accounting for up to 6% of patients with severe obesity (Vaisse et al., 1998; Yeo et al., 1998). The signaling capacities of specific mutant receptors studied *in vitro* correlates with the severity of the phenotype of corresponding MC4R deficient individuals (Farooqi et al., 2003). This demonstrates that the system is sensitive to degrees of loss in function at the level of the receptor. In addition to rare variants which cause highly penetrant forms of monogenic obesity, common variants in MC4R have been associated with body mass index (BMI) in genome wide association scans suggesting that variation at this locus also contributes to obesity in the general population (Willer et al., 2009).

MC5R

The MC5R is widely expressed in peripheral tissues. Mice lacking MC5R are unable to produce the full complement of sebaceous lipids which constitute the water repellent component of their coats (Chen et al., 1997). As a result they demonstrate impaired water repulsion and thermoregulation. Studies in these mice have also suggested that MC5Rs play a role in the generation of pheromones which in turn influences aspects of behavior (Morgan et al., 2004; Morgan and Cone, 2006). High levels of MC5R are found in multiple exocrine tissues where they are thought to regulate the synthesis and secretion of a diverse range of exocrine products.

THE MELANOCORTIN RECEPTOR ACCESSORY PROTEINS

THE DISCOVERY OF MRAP

The functional properties of the MCRs have been extensively examined in *in vitro* expression systems. Comparable studies of MC2R function were initially impeded by difficulties in expressing functional receptor in conventionally used cell lines. It became apparent that unlike other MCRs functional MC2R could only be expressed in cell lines of adrenal origin, suggesting that its expression was contingent upon the presence of a tissue-specific protein. This factor was identified in a study of genetic loci associated with FGD. Mutations in MC2R were known to lead to this inherited syndrome of ACTH resistance, but were only able to account for approximately 25% of cases. Whole genome single nucleotide polymorphism (SNP) analysis in two affected consanguineous families in whom mutations in MC2R had been excluded identified a region of interest encompassing a novel protein, which was highly expressed in the adrenal gland. *In vitro* studies confirmed that expression of this protein alongside MC2R enabled functional MC2R receptor expression in heterologous cell types and it was subsequently named MRAP (Metherell et al., 2005). Fifteen to twenty percent of cases of FGD are now known to be caused by mutations in MRAP.

MRAP STRUCTURE

Human MRAP is a single pass transmembrane protein which exists as two isoforms which differ in their C-termini. Both isoforms have been shown by reverse transcription polymerase chain reaction (RT-PCR) in a cDNA panel derived from human tissues to be expressed at high levels in the adrenal gland (Metherell et al., 2005). MRAP expression has also been demonstrated in a variety of other human tissues including testis, breast, thyroid, lymph nodes, ovary, and skin (Metherell et al., 2005). Immunofluorescence microscopy staining of cultured cells which endogenously express MRAP, using antibodies raised against N-terminal and C-terminal MRAP peptides, have shown that both regions of MRAP are present at the cell surface (Sebag and Hinkle, 2007). *In vitro* studies where differentially epitope-tagged forms of the protein were co-expressed in cells and their interaction and orientation were studied show that MRAP monomers form unique anti-parallel homodimeric structures (Sebag and Hinkle, 2007; Cooray et al., 2008). These dimers can be visualized in the endoplasmic reticulum and at the plasma membrane in live cells using biomolecular fluorescence complementation techniques (Sebag and Hinkle, 2009b, 2010). The deletion of amino acids 31–37 in mouse MRAP which directly precede the transmembrane portion of the protein abolishes its ability to homodimerize suggesting that this region of the protein constitutes a critical component of the interface between the two monomers (Sebag and Hinkle, 2009b). This mutant is unable to assist trafficking of the MC2R to the cell surface, suggesting that this unique conformation is essential to certain aspects of MRAP function (**Figure 1**).

MRAP AND MC2R

Cell lines derived from adrenocortical tissue express both MC2R and MRAP and generate cAMP in response to treatment with ACTH. This response is abrogated by MRAP knockdown in these cells (Cooray et al., 2008). MRAP expression is necessary and sufficient for the functional expression of MC2R constructs in heterologous cell lines such as chinese hamster ovary (CHO) cells and SK-N-SH cells which are derived from ovarian and neuroblastoma tissue, respectively and do not endogenously express measurable levels of MRAP (Metherell et al., 2005; Sebag and Hinkle, 2007).

MRAP FACILITATES TRAFFICKING OF THE MC2R TO THE CELL SURFACE

When epitope-tagged MC2R is expressed in CHO cells it is visualized in the endoplasmic reticulum, however, when it is expressed alongside MRAP it is predominantly localized to the plasma membrane (Metherell et al., 2005; Sebag and Hinkle, 2007; Webb et al., 2009). Consistent with this finding, in cells of adrenal origin with endogenously expression of MRAP, MC2R can be demonstrated at the cell surface. Western blotting of cell lysates yields a different complement of MC2R species in the presence and absence of MRAP, suggesting that MRAP may enhance receptor trafficking to the cell surface by promoting post-translational modification (Sebag and Hinkle, 2007). Deletion mutants of the N-terminal region of human MRAP which lack amino acids 1–24 or 1–35 are unable to promote MC2R trafficking to the cell surface suggesting that the N-terminal region plays a prominent role in receptor trafficking (Webb et al., 2009).

MRAP FACILITATES MC2R SIGNALING

In vitro experiments examining MC2R signaling in the presence of various MRAP mutants suggest that the ability of MRAP to

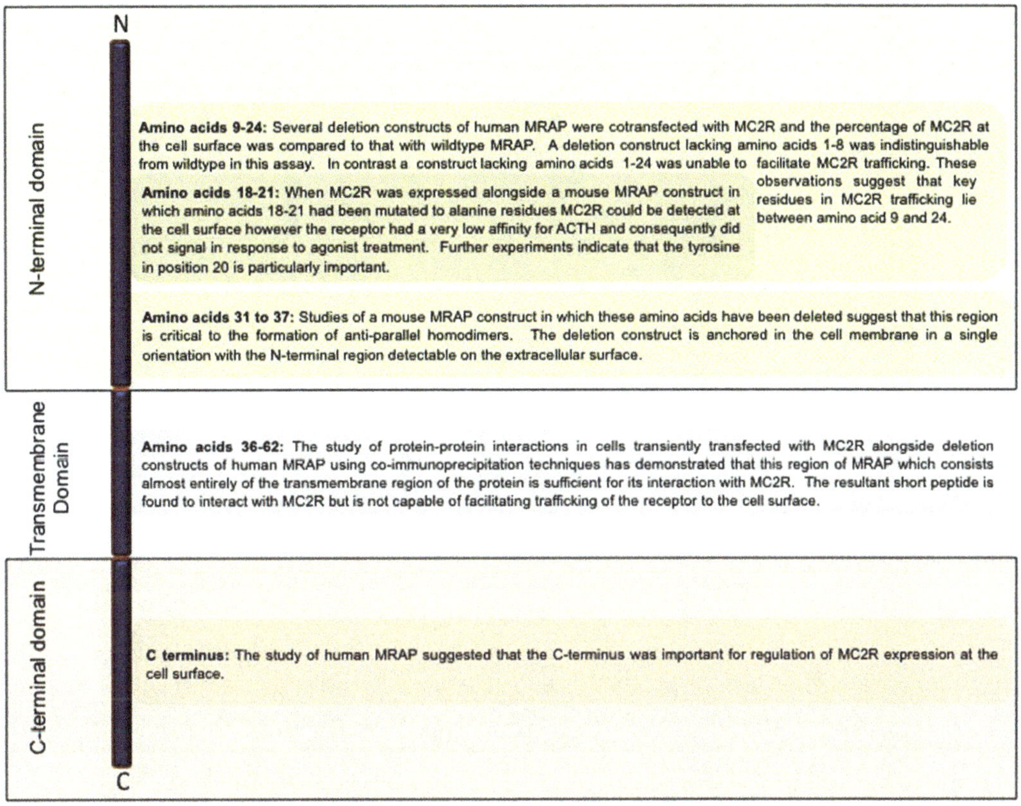

FIGURE 1 | Schematic representation of the domain structure of MRAP highlighting regions of functional significance in MRAP dimerization and in its interaction with MC2R (Sebag and Hinkle, 2009b; Webb et al., 2009).

promote MC2R trafficking to the cell surface does not wholly account for its role in facilitating MC2R signaling. Amino acids within the N-terminal region of MRAP appear to influence MC2R signaling independently of enhancing receptor trafficking. Specifically, MC2R receptor is able to traffic to the cell surface but is unable to bind to ACTH in the presence of a deletion mutant of mouse MRAP in which amino acids 18–21 have been mutated to alanine residues (Sebag and Hinkle, 2009b).

MRAP AND MC2R COMPLEXES

Protein complexes containing both MRAP and MC2R can be reciprocally isolated using co-immunoprecipitation techniques in transiently transfected cells (Metherell et al., 2005; Webb et al., 2009). Analogous experiments using MRAP deletion mutations indicate that the transmembrane region of MRAP interacts with MC2R (Webb et al., 2009). A model has emerged wherein MRAP–MC2R complexes interact with one another to form higher order complexes which facilitate MC2R function. BRET techniques have been used to explore some of the interactions within these complexes in more detail in live cultured cells with specific reference to the effect of the MC2R agonist ACTH. These experiments have shown that ACTH enhances the interaction between MC2R homodimers and MRAP–MC2R heterodimers (Cooray et al., 2011). Schematic representation of the role of MRAP in MC2R signaling is shown in **Figure 2**.

MRAP INTERACTIONS WITH OTHER MEMBERS OF THE MELANOCORTIN RECEPTOR FAMILY

MRAP can be demonstrated to form protein complexes with all five members of the MCR family using co-immunoprecipitation techniques in cultured cells (Chan et al., 2009b). Aside from MC2R, the remaining members of the MCR family are capable of efficiently trafficking to the cell surface when expressed in CHO cells. In a series of experiments using human constructs, co-expression of MRAP alongside either MC1R or MC3R in CHO cells was not found to alter cell surface expression of the receptors or influence their ability to generate cAMP in response to agonist treatment. In contrast, the cell surface expression and signaling capacities of both MC4R and MC5R were found to be significantly reduced in the presence of MRAP in these cells (**Table 2**). Signaling in these experiments was assessed by measuring cAMP generation using a competitive protein binding assay in response to treatment with a single concentration of agonist (Chan et al., 2009b). When the signaling properties of MC4R in the presence of MRAP were studied by measuring cAMP generation with a luciferase assay across a range of agonist concentrations using mouse constructs, co-expression of MRAP was not found to influence MC4R signaling (Sebag and Hinkle, 2010). Further examination of this interaction is needed to definitively understand whether MRAP interacts with MC4R *in vivo* and to determine the impact of this interaction on MC4R signaling. The *in vitro* interaction of

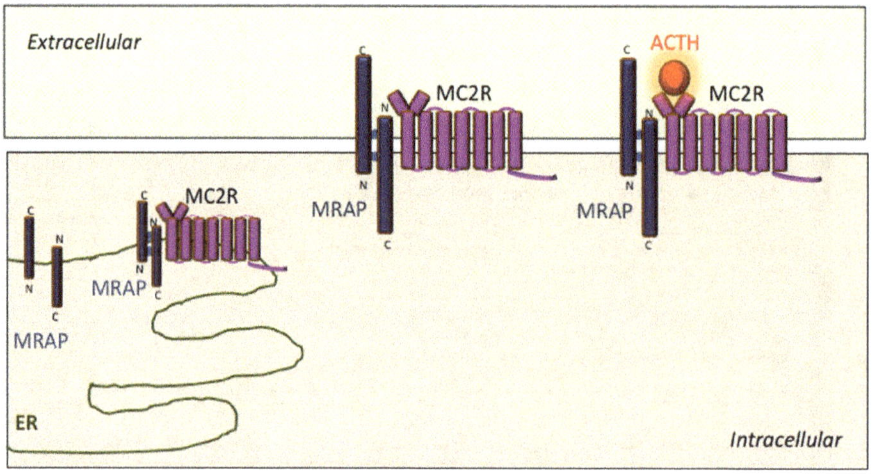

FIGURE 2 | Schematic representation of the role of MRAP in MC2R signaling. MRAP monomers form unique anti-parallel homodimeric complexes in the endoplasmic reticulum which interact with MC2R and assist its trafficking to the cell surface. The MRAP/MC2R structure is capable of binding ACTH at the cell surface and initiating intracellular signaling.

MRAP and MC5R has been explored more fully using bimolecular fluorescence complementation techniques (Sebag and Hinkle, 2009a). When MC5R constructs are expressed in CHO cells MC5R monomers interact to from homodimers or oligomers. When MRAP is expressed alongside MC5R fewer multimeric complexes are formed and fewer receptors are expressed at the cell surface. This data suggests that MRAP is capable of interacting with members of the MCR family beyond MC2R and may differentially regulate aspects of their function. However, patients with MRAP mutations present with isolated glucocorticoid deficiency apparently without any other additional symptoms (Chung et al., 2010). One patient with FGD caused by a mutation in MRAP was described as being concomitantly obese, although the significance of this is unclear as the rest of the family had similarly high BMIs (Rumie et al., 2007).

MRAP IN ADIPOCYTES

Prior to its advent as an accessory factor for MC2R in the adrenal gland, MRAP was identified as a novel protein expressed in mouse adipocytes (Xu et al., 2002). Both isoforms of MRAP have subsequently been shown by RT-PCR to be expressed in human adipocyte tissue (Metherell et al., 2005). The function of MRAP in these cells is not known. Given its established role in facilitating MC2R function in the adrenal gland it is likely that its function is related to the melanocortin system. The distribution of epitope-tagged MRAP within cultured adipocytes is responsive to insulin treatment suggesting that its role is contingent upon metabolic cues. Notably, gross metabolic dysfunctions have not been reported in patients with mutations in MRAP; however, this may reflect functional redundancy with the related protein MRAP2 in this tissue whose expression in adipocytes has not yet been investigated. The components of the melanocortin system which are expressed in adipocyte tissue show species-specific differences. 3T3L1 cells which are cells of murine origin that are commonly used in the study of adipocyte function express both MC2R and MC5R. Human adipose tissue samples have been shown to express MC1R and low levels of MC4R and MC5R (Hoch et al., 2007). Treatment of 3T3L1 cells with melanocortin ligands promotes lipolysis and cytokine production *in vitro*, however, this observation has not been replicated in human mesenchymal cell derived adipocytes (Hoch et al., 2008; Jun et al., 2010; Moller et al., 2011).

IDENTIFICATION OF MRAP2

Following the discovery of MRAP a related gene of unknown function with a comparable structure and a high degree of N-terminal and C-terminal sequence similarity was identified on

Table 2 | *In vitro* effects of MRAP on melanocortin receptors, based on data derived from Metherell et al. (2005) Sebag and Hinkle (2007, 2009a, 2010), Chan et al. (2009b) and Cooray et al. (2011).

Receptor	Effect of MRAP on trafficking	Effect of MRAP on signaling (cAMP generation)
MC1R	No change in cell surface expression	No effect in response to NDP-MSH
MC2R	Required for surface expression and receptor maturation	Required of receptor signaling in response to ACTH
MC3R	No change in cell surface expression	No effect in response to NDP-MSH
MC4R	Reduction in the surface expression	Reduction in response to NDP-MSH (No change was seen in another study)
MC5R	Reduction in the surface expression	Reduction in response to NDP-MSH

chromosome 6 and was named MRAP2 (Metherell et al., 2005; Chan et al., 2009b). MRAP2 is a single pass transmembrane protein, in humans it has been shown by RT-PCR to be expressed in the brain and the adrenal gland (Chan et al., 2009b). Western blotting of mouse tissues resolves a single band of MRAP2 reactive species whose molecular weight corresponds to a dimer suggesting that endogenous MRAP2 exists in dimeric complexes (Chan et al., 2009b). MRAP2 undergoes N-linked glycosylation at its N-terminus and is thought to form anti-parallel homodimeric complexes analogous to those formed by MRAP (Chan et al., 2009b; Sebag and Hinkle, 2009a, 2010). MRAP2 constructs can be visualized in the endoplasmic reticulum and the plasma membrane of transiently transfected CHO cells (Chan et al., 2009b).

MRAP2 AND MC2R SIGNALING

The physiological role of MRAP2 is not yet known. In view of the structural similarities between MRAP and MRAP2 and its concurrent expression in the adrenal gland, the interaction between MRAP2 and MC2R has been explored in detail. As discussed previously, when MC2R constructs are expressed in CHO cells in isolation the receptors are unable to reach the cell surface. Concurrent expression of MRAP facilitates MC2R trafficking to the cell surface. At the cell surface MC2Rs are activated by ACTH binding and generate a cAMP response, the magnitude of which is dependent on the ambient ligand concentration. Expression of MRAP2 alongside MC2R promotes MC2R trafficking to the cell surface to a similar extent as MRAP; however, the resultant complex has an extremely low affinity for ACTH binding. As a result the response curve of cAMP generated plotted against ligand concentration is significantly shifted to the right when MC2R is co-expressed with MRAP2 compared to when MC2R is expressed with MRAP (Sebag and Hinkle, 2009a, 2010; Gorrigan et al., 2011). It was suggested that this difference was due to lack of the leucine, aspartic acid, tyrosine, isoleucine (LDYI) motif in MRAP2, which was present in MRAP, and insertion of the LDYI residues enabled the MRAP2/MC2R complex to respond to lower concentrations of ACTH (Sebag and Hinkle, 2009b). MRAP and MRAP2 are able to form heterodimeric complexes *in vitro*, however, whether such a complex is physiologically relevant is not known (Chan et al., 2009b; Sebag and Hinkle, 2010). In one study MC2R was expressed alongside both MRAP and MRAP2, the resulting dose response curve appeared sensitive to the ratio of MRAP to MRAP2, with increasing proportions of MRAP2 shifting the curve further to the right (Sebag and Hinkle, 2010). Importantly, this effect has not been observed in other studies (Chan et al., 2009b; Agulleiro et al., 2010). Interestingly, Y1 cells which are of murine adrenocortical origin and endogenously expresses MRAP, MRAP2 and MC2R generate cAMP in response to ACTH treatment and this effect can be abrogated by transient expression of MRAP2 within these cells (Sebag and Hinkle, 2010). Taken together, further work is required to determine if the expression levels of MRAP and MRAP2 in the adrenal gland could act as a physiological mechanism dictating ACTH responsiveness.

Mutations in MC2R and MRAP lead to the inherited condition FGD. In contrast, mutations in the MRAP2 gene have not been linked with this condition suggesting that it may not be involved in MC2R signaling *in vivo* and that any degree of functional redundancy between MRAP and MRAP2 is unable to completely compensate for MRAP dysfunction. In-keeping with this observation *in situ* hybridization studies and quantitative RT-PCR using rat tissue have demonstrated that MRAP is expressed at much higher levels than MRAP2 in adult adrenal glands (Gorrigan et al., 2011).

MRAP2 BEYOND MC2R SIGNALING

Consistent with the findings discussed above, exploring the interaction of MRAP with other members of the MCR family, MRAP2 has also been shown to interact with all five members of the MCR family by co-immunoprecipitation assays in transiently transfected cultured cells (Chan et al., 2009b). In one series of experiments when cell surface expression of individual MCRs was quantified in the presence or absence of MRAP2, expression levels of MC1R and MC3R were not affected by MRAP2 expression, however, expression levels of MC4R and MC5R were significantly reduced when they were co-expressed with MRAP2. Furthermore, when MCR signaling was examined in the presence of MRAP2, its expression was detrimental to MC3R, MC4R, and MC5R signaling but had no effect on MC1R signaling. In these experiments signaling was studied by quantifying cAMP generation in response to treatment with a single concentration of ligand. The effect of MRAP2 on MC4R signaling has been explored using a luciferase reporter assay to measure cAMP production across a range of ligand concentrations. In this study the authors concluded that although MC4R surface expression was reduced in the presence of MRAP2 that MC4R signaling did not appear to be affected (Sebag and Hinkle, 2010). The experiments discussed here have been conducted in CHO cells which do not endogenously express any of the components of the melanocortin system, further research will address whether MRAP2 interacts with MCRs beyond this experimental system and will further delineate the nature of these interactions. As the main site of MRAP2 expression is in brain and specifically in the hypothalamus it is likely that the main physiological function of MRAP2 is in the central nervous system, perhaps involving MC4R and/or MC3R.

THE FUTURE OF MRAPs

Numerous lines of genetic evidence suggest that subtle perturbations of signaling capacity at the level of MCRs can have pathological consequences. As our appreciation of the complex nature of the melanocortin system grows, a large family of molecules is emerging which impact upon signaling and confer the ability to integrate extracellular and intracellular cues into a co-ordinated biological signal. The discovery of two proteins which may interact with multiple members of the MCR family in distinct ways represents a significant advance in our understanding of melanocortin signaling and paves the way for further lines of research to explore the physiological roles of these proteins.

ACKNOWLEDGMENTS

Li F. Chan holds an MRC/Academy of Medical Sciences Clinician Scientist Fellowship [G0802796] and Rebecca J. Gorrigan is supported by a WellcomeTrust Research Training Fellowship [092024/Z/10/Z].

REFERENCES

Agulleiro, M. J., Roy, S., Sanchez, E., Puchol, S., Gallo-Payet, N., and Cerda-Reverter, J. M. (2010). Role of melanocortin receptor accessory proteins in the function of *zebrafish* melanocortin receptor type 2. *Mol. Cell. Endocrinol.* 320, 145–152.

Balthasar, N., Dalgaard, L. T., Lee, C. E., Yu, J., Funahashi, H., Williams, T., et al. (2005). Divergence of melanocortin pathways in the control of food intake and energy expenditure. *Cell* 123, 493–505.

Beaumont, K. A., Smit, D. J., Liu, Y. Y., Chai, E., Patel, M. P., Millhauser, G. L., et al. (2012). Melanocortin-1 receptor-mediated signalling pathways activated by NDP-MSH and HBD3 ligands. *Pigment Cell Melanoma Res.* 25, 370–374.

Breit, A., Wolff, K., Kalwa, H., Jarry, H., Buch, T., and Gudermann, T. (2006). The natural inverse agonist agouti-related protein induces arrestin-mediated endocytosis of melanocortin-3 and -4 receptors. *J. Biol. Chem.* 281, 37447–37456.

Butler, A. A., Kesterson, R. A., Khong, K., Cullen, M. J., Pelleymounter, M. A., Dekoning, J., et al. (2000). A unique metabolic syndrome causes obesity in the melanocortin-3 receptor-deficient mouse. *Endocrinology* 141, 3518–3521.

Chan, L. F., Metherell, L. A., Krude, H., Ball, C., O'Riordan, S. M., Costigan, C., et al. (2009a). Homozygous nonsense and frameshift mutations of the ACTH receptor in children with familial glucocorticoid deficiency (FGD) are not associated with long-term mineralocorticoid deficiency. *Clin. Endocrinol.* 71, 171–175.

Chan, L. F., Webb, T. R., Chung, T.-T., Meimaridou, E., Cooray, S. N., Guasti, L., et al. (2009b). MRAP and MRAP2 are bidirectional regulators of the melanocortin receptor family. *Proc. Natl. Acad. Sci. U.S.A.* 106, 6146–6151.

Chen, A. S., Marsh, D. J., Trumbauer, M. E., Frazier, E. G., Guan, X. M., Yu, H., et al. (2000). Inactivation of the mouse melanocortin-3 receptor results in increased fat mass and reduced lean body mass. *Nat. Genet.* 26, 97–102.

Chen, W., Kelly, M. A., Opitz-Araya, X., Thomas, R. E., Low, M. J., and Cone, R. D. (1997). Exocrine gland dysfunction in MC5-R-deficient mice: evidence for coordinated regulation of exocrine gland function by melanocortin peptides. *Cell* 91, 789–798.

Cheung, C. C., Clifton, D. K., and Steiner, R. A. (1997). Proopiomelanocortin neurons are direct targets for leptin in the hypothalamus. *Endocrinology* 138, 4489–4492.

Chung, T. T., Chan, L. F., Metherell, L. A., and Clark, A. J. (2010). Phenotypic characteristics of familial glucocorticoid deficiency (FGD) type 1 and 2. *Clin. Endocrinol.* 72, 589–594.

Clark, A. J., Mcloughlin, L., and Grossman, A. (1993). Familial glucocorticoid deficiency associated with point mutation in the adrenocorticotropin receptor. *Lancet* 341, 461–462.

Cone, R. D. (2006). Studies on the physiological functions of the melanocortin system. *Endocr. Rev.* 27, 736–749.

Cooray, S. N., Almiro Do Vale, I., Leung, K.-Y., Webb, T. R., Chapple, J. P., Egertova, M., et al. (2008). The melanocortin 2 receptor accessory protein exists as a homodimer and is essential for the function of the melanocortin 2 receptor in the mouse Y1 cell line. *Endocrinology* 149, 1935–1941.

Cooray, S. N., Chung, T. T., Mazhar, K., Szidonya, L., and Clark, A. J. (2011). Bioluminescence resonance energy transfer reveals the adrenocorticotropin (ACTH)-induced conformational change of the activated ACTH receptor complex in living cells. *Endocrinology* 152, 495–502.

Eipper, B. A., and Mains, R. E. (1980). Structure and biosynthesis of pro-adrenocorticotropin/endorphin and related peptides. *Endocr. Rev.* 1, 1–27.

Farooqi, I. S., Keogh, J. M., Yeo, G. S., Lank, E. J., Cheetham, T., and O'Rahilly, S. (2003). Clinical spectrum of obesity and mutations in the melanocortin 4 receptor gene. *N. Engl. J. Med.* 348, 1085–1095.

Gineau, L., Cognet, C., Kara, N., Lach, F. P., Dunne, J., Veturi, U., et al. (2012). Partial MCM4 deficiency in patients with growth retardation, adrenal insufficiency, and natural killer cell deficiency. *J. Clin. Invest.* 122, 821–832.

Gorrigan, R. J., Guasti, L., King, P., Clark, A. J. L., and Chan, L. F. (2011). Localisation of the melanocortin-2-receptor and its accessory proteins in the developing and adult adrenal gland. *J. Mol. Endocrinol.* 46, 227–232.

Hoch, M., Eberle, A. N., Wagner, U., Bussmann, C., Peters, T., and Peterli, R. (2007). Expression and localization of melanocortin-1 receptor in human adipose tissues of severely obese patients. *Obesity (Silver Spring)* 15, 40–49.

Hoch, M., Hirzel, E., Lindinger, P., Eberle, A. N., Linscheid, P., Martin, I., et al. (2008). Weak functional coupling of the melanocortin-1 receptor expressed in human adipocytes. *J. Recept. Signal Transduct. Res.* 28, 485–504.

Hughes, C. R., Chung, T. T., Habeb, A. M., Kelestimur, F., Clark, A. J., and Metherell, L. A. (2010). Missense mutations in the melanocortin 2 receptor accessory protein that lead to late onset familial glucocorticoid deficiency type 2. *J. Clin. Endocrinol. Metab.* 95, 3497–3501.

Hughes, C. R., Guasti, L., Meimaridou, E., Chuang, C. H., Schimenti, J. C., King, P. J., et al. (2012). MCM4 mutation causes adrenal failure, short stature, and natural killer cell deficiency in humans. *J. Clin. Invest.* 122, 814–820.

Huszar, D., Lynch, C. A., Fairchild-Huntress, V., Dunmore, J. H., Fang, Q., Berkemeier, L. R., et al. (1997). Targeted disruption of the melanocortin-4 receptor results in obesity in mice. *Cell* 88, 131–141.

Jun, D. J., Na, K. Y., Kim, W., Kwak, D., Kwon, E. J., Yoon, J. H., et al. (2010). Melanocortins induce interleukin 6 gene expression and secretion through melanocortin receptors 2 and 5 in 3T3-L1 adipocytes. *J. Mol. Endocrinol.* 44, 225–236.

Lin, L., Hindmarsh, P. C., Metherell, L. A., Alzyoud, M., Al-Ali, M., Brain, C. E., et al. (2007). Severe loss-of-function mutations in the adrenocorticotropin receptor (ACTHR, MC2R) can be found in patients diagnosed with salt-losing adrenal hypoplasia. *Clin. Endocrinol.* 66, 205–210.

Lu, D., Willard, D., Patel, I. R., Kadwell, S., Overton, L., Kost, T., et al. (1994). Agouti protein is an antagonist of the melanocyte-stimulating-hormone receptor. *Nature* 371, 799–802.

Meimaridou, E., Kowalczyk, J., Guasti, L., Hughes, C. R., Wagner, F., Frommolt, P., et al. (2012). Mutations in NNT encoding nicotinamide nucleotide transhydrogenase cause familial glucocorticoid deficiency. *Nat. Genet.* 44, 740–742.

Mencarelli, M., Dubern, B., Alili, R., Maestrini, S., Benajiba, L., Tagliaferri, M., et al. (2011). Rare melanocortin-3 receptor mutations with in vitro functional consequences are associated with human obesity. *Hum. Mol. Genet.* 20, 392–399.

Metherell, L. A., Chapple, J. P., Cooray, S., David, A., Becker, C., Ruschendorf, F., et al. (2005). Mutations in MRAP, encoding a new interacting partner of the ACTH receptor, cause familial glucocorticoid deficiency type 2. *Nat. Genet.* 37, 166–170.

Metherell, L. A., Naville, D., Halaby, G., Begeot, M., Huebner, A., Nurnberg, G., et al. (2009). Nonclassic lipoid congenital adrenal hyperplasia masquerading as familial glucocorticoid deficiency. *J. Clin. Endocrinol. Metab.* 94, 3865–3871.

Moller, C. L., Raun, K., Jacobsen, M. L., Pedersen, T. A., Holst, B., Conde-Frieboes, K. W., et al. (2011). Characterization of murine melanocortin receptors mediating adipocyte lipolysis and examination of signalling pathways involved. *Mol. Cell. Endocrinol.* 341, 9–17.

Morgan, C., and Cone, R. D. (2006). Melanocortin-5 receptor deficiency in mice blocks a novel pathway influencing pheromone-induced aggression. *Behav. Genet.* 36, 291–300.

Morgan, C., Thomas, R. E., and Cone, R. D. (2004). Melanocortin-5 receptor deficiency promotes defensive behavior in male mice. *Horm. Behav.* 45, 58–63.

Mountjoy, K. G., Mortrud, M. T., Low, M. J., Simerly, R. B., and Cone, R. D. (1994). Localization of the melanocortin-4 receptor (MC4-R) in neuroendocrine and autonomic control circuits in the brain. *Mol. Endocrinol.* 8, 1298–1308.

Nijenhuis, W. A., Oosterom, J., and Adan, R. A. (2001). AgRP(83–132) acts as an inverse agonist on the human-melanocortin-4 receptor. *Mol. Endocrinol.* 15, 164–171.

O'Riordan, S. M., Lynch, S. A., Hindmarsh, P. C., Chan, L. F., Clark, A. J., and Costigan, C. (2008). A novel variant of familial glucocorticoid deficiency prevalent among the Irish Traveler population. *J. Clin. Endocrinol. Metab.* 93, 2896–2899.

Patten, C. S., Daniels, D., Suzuki, A., Fluharty, S. J., and Yee, D. K. (2007). Structural and signaling requirements of the human melanocortin 4 receptor for MAP kinase activation. *Regul. Pept.* 142, 111–122.

Rodrigues, A. R., Pignatelli, D., Almeida, H., and Gouveia, A. M. (2009). Melanocortin 5 receptor activates ERK1/2 through a PI3K-regulated signaling mechanism. *Mol. Cell. Endocrinol.* 303, 74–81.

Roselli-Rehfuss, L., Mountjoy, K. G., Robbins, L. S., Mortrud, M. T., Low, M. J., Tatro, J. B., et al. (1993). Identification of a receptor for gamma melanotropin and other proopiomelanocortin peptides in the hypothalamus and limbic system. *Proc. Natl. Acad. Sci. U.S.A.* 90, 8856–8860.

Rumie, H., Metherell, L. A., Clark, A. J., Beauloye, V., and Maes, M. (2007).

Clinical and biological phenotype of a patient with familial glucocorticoid deficiency type 2 caused by a mutation of melanocortin 2 receptor accessory protein. *Eur. J. Endocrinol.* 157, 539–542.

Schwartz, M. W., Seeley, R. J., Woods, S. C., Weigle, D. S., Campfield, L. A., Burn, P., et al. (1997). Leptin increases hypothalamic pro-opiomelanocortin mRNA expression in the rostral arcuate nucleus. *Diabetes* 46, 2119–2123.

Sebag, J. A., and Hinkle, P. M. (2007). Melanocortin-2 receptor accessory protein MRAP forms antiparallel homodimers. *Proc. Natl. Acad. Sci. U.S.A.* 104, 20244–20249.

Sebag, J. A., and Hinkle, P. M. (2009a). Opposite effects of the melanocortin-2 (MC2) receptor accessory protein MRAP on MC2 and MC5 receptor dimerization and trafficking. *J. Biol. Chem.* 284, 22641–22648.

Sebag, J. A., and Hinkle, P. M. (2009b). Regions of melanocortin 2 (MC2) receptor accessory protein necessary for dual topology and MC2 receptor trafficking and signaling. *J. Biol. Chem.* 284, 610–618.

Sebag, J. A., and Hinkle, P. M. (2010). Regulation of G protein-coupled receptor signaling: specific dominant-negative effects of melanocortin 2 receptor accessory protein 2. *Sci. Signal.* 3, ra28.

Seng Lee, Y., Kok Seng Poh, L., Lay Kee Kek, B., and Yin Loke, K. (2007). The role of melanocortin 3 receptor gene in childhood obesity. *Diabetes* 56, 2622–2630.

Sutton, G. M., Begriche, K., Kumar, K. G., Gimble, J. M., Perez-Tilve, D., Nogueiras, R., et al. (2010). Central nervous system melanocortin-3 receptors are required for synchronizing metabolism during entrainment to restricted feeding during the light cycle. *FASEB J.* 24, 862–872.

Sutton, G. M., Duos, B., Patterson, L. M., and Berthoud, H. R. (2005). Melanocortinergic modulation of cholecystokinin-induced suppression of feeding through extracellular signal-regulated kinase signaling in rat solitary nucleus. *Endocrinology* 146, 3739–3747.

Sutton, G. M., Perez-Tilve, D., Nogueiras, R., Fang, J., Kim, J. K., Cone, R. D., et al. (2008). The melanocortin-3 receptor is required for entrainment to meal intake. *J. Neurosci.* 28, 12946–12955.

Swope, V. B., Jameson, J. A., Mcfarland, K. L., Supp, D. M., Miller, W. E., Mcgraw, D. W., et al. (2012). Defining MC1R regulation in human melanocytes by its agonist alpha-melanocortin and antagonists agouti signaling protein and beta-defensin 3. *J. Invest. Dermatol.* 132, 2255–2262.

Tsigos, C., Arai, K., Hung, W., and Chrousos, G. P. (1993). Hereditary isolated glucocorticoid deficiency is associated with abnormalities of the adrenocorticotropin receptor gene. *J. Clin. Invest.* 92, 2458–2461.

Turan, S., Hughes, C., Atay, Z., Guran, T., Haliloglu, B., Clark, A. J., et al. (2012). An atypical case of familial glucocorticoid deficiency without pigmentation caused by coexistent homozygous mutations in MC2R (T152K) and MC1R (R160W). *J. Clin. Endocrinol. Metab.* 97, E771–E774.

Vage, D. I., Lu, D., Klungland, H., Lien, S., Adalsteinsson, S., and Cone, R. D. (1997). A non-epistatic interaction of agouti and extension in the fox, Vulpes vulpes. *Nat. Genet.* 15, 311–315.

Vaisse, C., Clement, K., Guy-Grand, B., and Froguel, P. (1998). A frameshift mutation in human MC4R is associated with a dominant form of obesity. *Nat. Genet.* 20, 113–114.

Valverde, P., Healy, E., Jackson, I., Rees, J. L., and Thody, A. J. (1995). Variants of the melanocyte-stimulating hormone receptor gene are associated with red hair and fair skin in humans. *Nat. Genet.* 11, 328–330.

Vongs, A., Lynn, N. M., and Rosenblum, C. I. (2004). Activation of MAP kinase by MC4-R through PI3 kinase. *Regul. Pept.* 120, 113–118.

Webb, T. R., Chan, L., Cooray, S. N., Cheetham, M. E., Chapple, J. P., and Clark, A. J. L. (2009). Distinct melanocortin 2 receptor accessory protein domains are required for melanocortin 2 receptor interaction and promotion of receptor trafficking. *Endocrinology* 150, 720–726.

Willer, C. J., Speliotes, E. K., Loos, R. J., Li, S., Lindgren, C. M., Heid, I. M., et al. (2009). Six new loci associated with body mass index highlight a neuronal influence on body weight regulation. *Nat. Genet.* 41, 25–34.

Xu, A., Choi, K. L., Wang, Y., Permana, P. A., Xu, L. Y., Bogardus, C., et al. (2002). Identification of novel putative membrane proteins selectively expressed during adipose conversion of 3T3-L1 cells. *Biochem. Biophys. Res. Commun.* 293, 1161–1167.

Yeo, G. S., Farooqi, I. S., Aminian, S., Halsall, D. J., Stanhope, R. G., and O'Rahilly, S. (1998). A frameshift mutation in MC4R associated with dominantly inherited human obesity. *Nat. Genet.* 20, 111–112.

3

Neurotensin and its high affinity receptor 1 as a potential pharmacological target in cancer therapy

Zherui Wu[1], Daniel Martinez-Fong[2], Jean Trédaniel[1,3] and Patricia Forgez[1]*

[1] INSERM-UPMC UMR_S938, Hôpital Saint-Antoine, Paris, France
[2] Departamento de Fisiología, Biofísica y Neurociencias, Centro de Investigación y de Estudios Avanzados del Instituto Politécnico Nacional, Mexico City, Mexico
[3] Unité de Cancérologie Thoracique, Groupe Hospitalier Paris Saint-Joseph/Université Paris Descartes, Paris, France

Edited by:
Jae Young Seong, Korea University, South Korea

Reviewed by:
Jean Mazella, Centre National de la Recherche Scientifique, France
Aixa R. Bello, University of La Laguna, Spain

***Correspondence:**
Patricia Forgez, INSERM-UPMC UMR_S938, Hôpital Saint-Antoine, Bâtiment Raoul Kourilsky, 184 rue du Faubourg St-Antoine, 75571 Paris Cedex 12, France.
e-mail: patricia.forgez@inserm.fr

Cancer is a worldwide health problem. Personalized treatment represents a future advancement for cancer treatment, in part due to the development of targeted therapeutic drugs. These molecules are expected to be more effective than current treatments and less harmful to normal cells. The discovery and validation of new targets are the foundation and the source of these new therapies. The neurotensinergic system has been shown to enhance cancer progression in various cancers such as pancreatic, prostate, lung, breast, and colon cancer. It also triggers multiple oncogenic signaling pathways, such as the PKC/ERK and AKT pathways. In this review, we discuss the contribution of the neurotensinergic system to cancer progression, as well as the regulation and mechanisms of the system in order to highlight its potential as a therapeutic target, and its prospect for its use as a treatment in certain cancers.

Keywords: cancer therapy, cancer progression, carcinogenesis, neurotensin, neurotensin receptor

INTRODUCTION

Cancer is one of the first, if not the first cause, of death in the world. Conventional treatment methods include surgery, radiotherapy, and chemotherapy. In many cases, only a supportive treatment can be offered to the patient. The last few decades have been marked by the accumulation of knowledge about the inner workings of the normal and cancer cell. Thus arose the therapeutic arsenal against cancer, and the so-called targeted biological therapies. Due to these new drugs, great progress has recently been achieved in the treatment of cancers considered refractory to previous therapies, including cancers of the liver, kidney, and melanoma skin. But other tumors, such as breast and lung cancer, have also greatly benefited from these advances. However, remissions are often transient and do not yet provide definitive cures of the patient. In this context the neurotensin system is proposed to be a candidate for therapeutical development.

Neurotensin (NTS) is a tridecapeptide originally isolated from calf hypothalamus (Carraway and Leeman, 1973). It acts as neurotransmitter or neuromodulator in the central nervous system and as a local hormone in the periphery, mainly the gastrointestinal tract (Vincent et al., 1999). In the brain, NTS modulates dopaminergic transmission in the nigrostriatal and mesocorticolimbic pathways as well as hormone secretion from the anterior pituitary (Vincent et al., 1999). It also exerts potent hypothermic and analgesic effects when injected into the central nervous system (Popp et al., 2007). NTS has also been related to central nervous system pathology such as Parkinson disease and schizophrenia (St-Gelais et al., 2006; Mustain et al., 2011). In the periphery, NTS is released by endocrine-like N cells predominantly in the small intestine (Reinecke, 1985). NTS has a dual function, as a paracrine and endocrine modulator of the digestive tract and as a growth factor on a variety of normal or cancer cells (Vincent et al., 1999; Carraway and Plona, 2006). The NTS/NTSR1 complex has been proposed to contribute to cancer progression because of the various oncogenic effects induced by NTS in tumors and in cancer cells from diverse origins (Thomas et al., 2003; Dupouy et al., 2011). In this review, we elaborate on how the NTS/NTSR1 complex could be developed as a possible target for cancer therapy.

NEUROTENSIN/NEUROTENSIN RECEPTOR COMPLEX

NEUROTENSINERGIC SYSTEM

The biological effects of NTS are known to be mediated through three receptors, two G protein-coupled receptors, NTSR1 and NTSR2, and a single transmembrane domain sorting receptor, the NTSR3 (Vincent et al., 1999; Mazella and Vincent, 2006). NTSR3 is a member of the receptor family related to the yeast sorting receptor Vps10p (Petersen et al., 1997).

Neurotensin receptor 1, NTSR1

The effects of NTS are primarily transmitted through its high affinity receptor, the NTSR1 which has a sub-nanomolar affinity for NTS. This 424 amino acid receptor has been identified in the brain and in various cancer cells (Tanaka et al., 1990). The signaling pathways induced by the NTS/NTSR1 complex have been studied in different cellular types, such as N1E-115, HT-29, and NTSR1-transfected CHO overexpressing NTSR1. The stimulation of NTSR1 by its ligand (NTS) leads to activation of phospholipase C (PLC) via its coupling to the prime $G\alpha q/11$ subunit (Wang and Wu, 1996; Najimi et al., 2002). The activation of PLC leads to the production of inositol triphosphate (IP3) and diacylglycerol from membrane phospholipids (PIP2). These two second messengers induce the activation of PKC and the mobilization of intracellular calcium which are key oncogenic effectors (Bozou et al., 1986; Snider et al., 1986; Turner et al., 1990).

Several signaling pathways potentially involved in cell proliferation, survival, migration, and invasion are described after NTSR1 stimulation. The signaling mechanisms mediating the effects of neurotensinergic system involve multiple pathways and are cell-dependent. The NTS-induced PKC/ERK signaling pathway is the most well studied. The PKC activation stimulated by NTS/NTSR1 was demonstrated by using broad isotype inhibitors, such as Gö6976 which specifically inhibit the conventional PKCs α and $\beta 1$ in CHO-NTSR1-transfected cells and in endogenously NTSR1-expressing cells from colon, lung, and pancreatic cells (Poinot-Chazel et al., 1996; Seufferlein and Rozengurt, 1996; Ehlers et al., 2000; Muller et al., 2011). The NTSR1 contribution in this activation was confirmed by its inhibition by a specific NTSR1 antagonist, the SR 489692 (Gully et al., 1993). PKC activation induce mitogen-activated protein kinase (MAPK) via direct stimulation of Raf-1, independently of Ras, or by transactivation of the epidermal growth factor receptor (EGFR) (Guha et al., 2003). EGFR transactivation by NTS/NTSR1 complex has been observed in several cell lines. In prostatic cancer PC3 cell line, NTS activates mitogenesis through EGFR transactivation in a PKC-dependent pathway, and the stimulation of the Raf–MEK–ERK. This effect was also PI3 kinase (PI3K)-dependent (Hassan et al., 2004). NTS also induces a time-dependent increase in Tyr_{845} EGFR phosphorylation, c-Src phosphorylation and signal transducer. NTS is also an activator of transcription 5b (Stat5b), a downstream effector of Tyr_{845} EGFR phosphorylated (Amorino et al., 2007). In colonic HT-29 cells, the EGFR tyrosine kinase inhibitor, gefitinib, blocks NTS-stimulated phosphorylation of both MAPK and Akt, indicating the transactivation of EGFR independently of PKC activation. However, in the colonic HCT116 cells, NTS/NTSR1 induces a PKC-dependent MAPK phosphorylation and an EGFR metalloproteinase-mediated transactivation, that is associated with a gefitinib sensitive phosphorylation of the downstream adaptor protein Shc. The activation of Akt is only partly inhibited by gefitinib, suggesting an additional mechanism to EGFR transactivation (Muller et al., 2011). The mechanism of NTS-induced EGFR transactivation is still not clearly elucidated. The release of EGFR ligands-like (TGF-α, Hb-EGF, or amphiregulin), pre-existing at the plasma membrane, as proligand, by NTS has been proposed. These ligands are released by proteolytic cleavage involving enzymes of the metalloproteinase family, including ADAMS (disintegrin and metalloprotease) and MMP (matrix metalloproteinase; Sanderson et al., 2006; Zhao et al., 2007; Kataoka, 2009). Once released, these ligands bind to EGFR and activate the downstream signaling cascades of EGFR activation (Hassan et al., 2004). These results suggest a cooperative relationship between the neurotensinergic system and EGFR pathway.

Activation of MAPK pathway by NTS results in gene transcription stimulation, due to transcription factor activation, such as the induction of the early growth response gene-1 (Egr-1), the Ets family factors ELK1, and the AP-1 transcription factor family (Poinot-Chazel et al., 1996; Portier et al., 1998; Ehlers et al., 2000; Zhao et al., 2007). In colonic HCT166 cells, inhibition of PKC was shown to block NTS-induced DNA synthesis (Muller et al., 2011). In a tumor-initiating cell line derived from hepatocellular carcinoma (HCC) which is characterized by membrane expression of CD133, addition of exogenous NTS resulted in concomitant upregulation of IL-8 and CXCL1 with simultaneous activation of MAPK and Raf-1, and promotion of angiogenesis, tumorigenesis, and self-renewal (Tang et al., 2012). The activation of MAPK via NTSR1 is mainly associated with uncontrolled cell growth, which can aggravate the growth of tumors (Harikumar et al., 2010; Kisfalvi et al., 2010).

Neurotensin also induces RhoGTPases and the non-receptor kinases focal adhesion kinase (FAK) and Src. Neurotensinergic system stimulation can modulate the activity of small RhoGTPases Rac1, Cdc42, and RhoA, which are partly responsible for the dynamics of the cytoskeleton. This modulation has an effect on cell migration. In the cell line U373 glioblastoma, the NTS has been associated with the stimulation of the activity of protein Rac1, RhoA, and Cdc42 (Zhao et al., 2003; Servotte et al., 2006). In addition, in small cell lung and prostate cancer cell lines, it has been shown that NTS can enhance the activity of focal adhesion kinase (FAK) (Tallett et al., 1996; Lee et al., 2001).

Neurotensin receptor 2, NTSR2

The low affinity receptor of NTS, NTSR2, is a protein of 410 amino acids, with a high homology to NTSR1 (64%) (Chalon et al., 1996). NTSR2 exhibits a low binding property for NTS and this binding can be inhibited by levocabastine, a non-peptide histamine H1 receptor antagonist (Schotte et al., 1986). SR48692, which has a lower affinity for NTSR2 than for NTSR1, can stimulate the activity of this receptor (Yamada et al., 1998). When the cloned mouse NTSR2 coding sequence is expressed in *Xenopus laevis* ovocytes, NTS, neuromedin N, levocabastine, and SR48692, are capable of triggering an inward current which is calcium-dependent (Mazella et al., 1996). Using CHO cells transfected with the cloned rat or human NTSR2 cDNA, levocabastine and SR 48692 can mobilize intracellular Ca^{2+} more intensively than NTS agonists and phosphorylate Erk1/2, suggesting that NTSR1 and NTSR2 receptors present distinct functional characteristics (Botto et al., 1997; Yamada et al., 1998; Gendron et al., 2004). In CHO cells transfected with human NTSR2 cDNA, both NTSR1 antagonists, SR48692 and SR142948A, enhance inositol phosphate (IP) formation with subsequent $[Ca^{2+}]$ immobilization, induce arachidonic acid release, and stimulate MAPK activity. Interestingly, these activities were inhibited by NTS and levocabastine in a dose-dependent manner. In summary, the signaling pathway triggered by NTSR2 is cell-dependent, and mainly based on its overexpression. This response is far different from that of the physiological endogenous expression.

Neurotensin receptor 3, gp85/sortilin, NTSR3

NTSR3 functions as a modulator of neurotensinergic signaling when it is co-expressed with another receptor of NTS, and as a functional receptor involved in the migration when expressed alone. This receptor is not NTS-specific. It can bind other ligands such as lipoprotein lipase, proneurotrophins, protein RAP (receptor-associated protein), or protein SAP (sphingolipid activator protein) (Nielsen et al., 1999; Lefrancois et al., 2003). NTSR3 may act as a co-receptor to participate in true NTS/NTSR1 signaling. The study by immunoprecipitation using the adenocarcinoma cell line HT29, demonstrated that the NTSR3 forms heterodimers with the NTSR1. Additionally, upon NTS stimulation, the NTSR1/NTSR3 complex is internalized and the interaction between the two receptors modulates both the NTS-induced phosphorylation of MAPK and the phosphoinositide (PI) turnover mediated by NTSR1 (Martin et al., 2002).

In the human microglial cell line C13NJ, NTSR3 is the only known endogenous NTS receptor. In these cells, NTS elicited cell migration by a mechanism dependent on both PI3K and MAPK pathways (Martin et al., 2003). The NTS/NTSR3 complex has been shown to phosphorylate both Erk1/2 and Akt kinases in a murine microglial cell line (Dicou, 2008).

NEUROTENSIN/NEUROTENSIN RECEPTOR COMPLEX AND CANCER BIOLOGY

Few years after its discovery, high-level expression of NTS was found in the plasma of pancreatic tumor patients (Gutniak et al., 1980). This discovery inspired investigations on the relationship between NTS and cancer. Many studies have since been performed to clarify the role of NTS in carcinogenesis in diverse cancer cells.

PANCREATIC CANCER

Pancreatic cancer is the eighth leading cause of cancer death in the world (Yabushita et al., 2012). It has the poorest prognosis amongst all human malignant solid tumors, mainly due to its high rate of metastasis (Cheng et al., 2012). The growth promoting action of NTS has been observed in pancreatic cancer cell lines both *in vitro* and *in vivo*. In both cases, the NTSR1 antagonist, SR48692, inhibited the NTS-induced effects (Sumi et al., 1993; Iwase et al., 1997). Recently, NTS was shown to protect insulin producing cells (b-TC3, INS-1E) against apoptosis induced by IL-1b and staurosporine (STS) (Coppola et al., 2008). NTSR2 and NTSR3 have been shown to be essential for the NTS mediated survival of these cells (Beraud-Dufour et al., 2009). NTS also influenced the migratory ability of pancreatic cancer cells, while NTS significantly reduced the migration levels of collectively migrating cells on vitronectin, NTS significantly increased the levels of individually migrating cells (Mijatovic et al., 2007). Thus, NTS-induced migration is dependent on the extracellular matrix environment and their respective migratory mode.

COLORECTAL CANCER

Colorectal cancer is the third most common cancer worldwide and the fourth most common cause of death (Jemal et al., 2011). NTS stimulates the growth of mouse and human colon cancer cell lines in tissue culture and after being xenografted into nude mice (Maoret et al., 1999). *In vivo*, systemic NTS administration stimulates tumor size and weight, DNA, RNA, and the protein contents of the murine colon cancer, MC26 (Yoshinaga et al., 1992). Recently, the expression of NTSR1 was significantly correlated to an increase in the number of tumors when sporadic cancer was generated in mouse models by inflammation. However, no effect of NTSR1 expression was noticed on the number of aberrant crypt foci or tumor size, suggesting that the NTS/NTSR1 signaling complex has a major role in tumor progression (Bugni et al., 2012). NTS is also known to enhance colon cancer cell migration by increasing IL-8 expression and secretion. These effects are blocked by NTSR1 antagonists and curcumin, a diet-derived chemopreventive and/or chemotherapeutic agent which blocks AP-1 and NF-κB induction (Wang et al., 2006a). The role of IL-8 identified as an integral part of the metastasis process, was shown due to its triggering of the release of enzymes [MMPs, and uroplasminogen activator (uPA)], responsible for extracellular matrix degradation (Xie, 2001).

PROSTATE CANCER

Prostate cancer is the most common male malignancy in Western countries and the second most common cause of male cancer-related death in the UK and USA (Jemal et al., 2011). The androgen-dependent human prostate cancer LNCaP cell line has been shown to exhibit an autocrine growth response to NTS in androgen-deprived only conditions (Sehgal et al., 1994). Vias et al. (2007) found that long-term anti-androgen treatment of LNCaP cells produced a sub-line exhibiting upregulated expression of NTS and NTS receptors, which increased the proliferation rate, accelerated cell cycle progression, and increased invasiveness through Matrigel. These effects are sensitive to NTS siRNA. NTSR1 expression was found at very high levels in the human androgen-independent PC3 cell line, derived from prostate cancer metastasized to bone. The growth responses of these cells to NTS were found at concentrations close to human postprandial blood levels (Seethalakshmi et al., 1997). These studies proposed that NTS is a potential autocrine, paracrine, and endocrine regulator of prostate cancer growth in humans, after androgen ablation therapy and during the devastating final stages of the disease.

LUNG CANCER

Lung cancer is the most common cause of cancer-related deaths throughout the world (Jemal et al., 2011). High concentration of NTS is present in and secreted from half classic small cell lung cancer cells (SCLC; Moody et al., 1985). NTS is one of the 73 genes overexpressed in the highly metastatic human lung cell line, H460-M, as compared to control cells (de Lange et al., 2003). In lung cancer cell lines, NCI-H209 and H345, SR48692 inhibited NTS-mediated calcium mobilization cells and c-fos mRNA induction and proliferation in a dose-dependent manner (Moody et al., 1985). SR48692 also inhibited tumor growth of NCI-H209 xenografts.

BREAST CANCER

Breast cancer is the most common cancer in women, and the second leading cause of cancer deaths in women worldwide (Jemal et al., 2011). NTS immunoreactivity has been observed in breast cancers *in vivo*. NTSR1 expression has also been demonstrated in several breast cancer cell lines (Elek et al., 2000). The NTS anti-apoptotic effect has been described in the cell line MCF-7 originating from breast adenocarcinoma. Prolonged exposure to JMV449, a NTS-specific agonist, protected MCF-7 cells from serum deprivation-induced death, and reduced the number of apoptotic cells by two to three times. These effects have been predicted to be due, in part, to NTS-mediated induction of Bcl-2 mRNA and protein levels which depends on stimulation of MAPK (Somaï et al., 2002). By using NTSR1 Sh-RNA and SR 48692, tumor growth was significantly decreased when NTSR1 expression was abolished or blocked in experimental tumors of the breast (Souaze et al., 2006a).

REGULATION OF THE NEUROTENSINERGIC SYSTEM

REGULATION OF NTS

Neurotensin deregulation has been observed in many cancers such as in colonic adenocarcinomas, small cell lung carcinomas, non-small cell lung adenocarcinomas, medullary thyroid carcinomas, and in fibrolamellar HCCs (Baca and Schmidt-Gayk, 1981; Ulich et al., 1983; Moody et al., 1985; Dammrich et al., 1988; Ehrenfried et al., 1994). DNA methylation has been shown to play a crucial role in the expression of the gut endocrine gene neurotensin/neuromedin N (NT/N). In the human hepatoma cell line Hep G2 cells, methylation of a NT/N promoter construct resulted in a severe reduction of the promoter activity, whereas treatment with the demethylating agent 5-azacytidine-induced NT/N expression (Dong et al., 1998). These observations have been confirmed in different human colon cancer cell lines, either expressing or not the gene coding for NTS (Dong et al., 2000). Interestingly, NTS gene can be regulated by Ras while expressed. Both wild-type and activated Ras enhances expression of NTS in the gut-derived CaCo-2 cell line, by activating the proximal AP-1/CRE motif (Evers et al., 1995). More recently, the PI3K catalytic subunit, p110alfa, was demonstrated to negatively regulate NTS secretion *in vitro* and *in vivo*. This process involves several regulatory proteins such as α-tubulin deacetylase, small GTPase, and kinase D-interacting substrate (Li et al., 2012).

REGULATION OF NTSR1

The mechanisms involved in NTSR1 deregulation in cancer cells have been studied in the context of colorectal carcinogenesis. These studies implicate an important role of the Wnt/β-catenin pathway deregulation. The mutation or loss of the protein APC (adenomatous polyposis coli) causes a dysfunction in the degradation of β-catenin. The accumulation of the latter in the cytoplasm, and its subsequent translocation to the nucleus induces NTSR1 gene expression via its association with transcription factors Tcf/Lef (T cell factor/lymphoid enhancing factor) (Souaze et al., 2006b). The NTSR1 promoter can be activated by the complex β-catenin/Tcf because it contains a consensus site for the transcription factors Tcf. In agreement with this result, it has been demonstrated that inhibitors of GSK-3β (protein kinase involved in the phosphorylation of β-catenin and its degradation) which cause the significant accumulation of β-catenin, upregulates the level of NTSR1 transcription (Wang et al., 2010). Similar results have been obtained in other cancers such as lung, prostate, and breast cancers (Chesire et al., 2002; Turashvili et al., 2006).

REGULATION OF NTSR1 BY ITS OWN LIGAND

Upon acute agonist exposure, and under physiological conditions, initiated by β-arrestin-1 (βARR1), and β-arrestin-2 (βARR2), the NTS/NTSR1 complex is internalized and degraded in lysosomes through clathrin-coated vesicles. Cell resensitization occurs from *de novo* receptor synthesis a few hours after agonist removal (Souaze and Forgez, 2006; Law et al., 2012). However, some studies on cellular models such as the murine neuroblastoma cell line N1E-115 and human colon cancer cell line HT-29, showed a change in the traffic situation when the cell had a prolonged exposure to saturating doses of agonist (Souaze et al., 1997; Najimi et al., 1998). Instead of being degraded in the lysosome, NTSR1 accumulated transiently with NTS in the perinuclear recycling compartment (PNRC) where it was latter recycled to the plasma membrane (Toy-Miou-Leong et al., 2004). More recent research has shown the activity of endothelin-converting enzyme-1 (ECE-1) and βARRs being crucial for NTSR1 recycling and enhance NTS degradation (Law et al., 2012). Thus, NTS stimulation induces cellular adaptation by altering the degradation process of NTSR1. This phenomenon leads to permanently sensitizing cells to the neurotensinergic signal. The implementation of this mechanism could lead to deregulation of multiple signaling pathways involved in the cancer progression such as MAPK and its target genes.

NEUROTENSIN/NEUROTENSIN RECEPTORS AND THERAPY

The implications of the previous sections suggest a more direct role for NTS/NTSR1 in cancer growth and progression, than has been previously attributed. Nevertheless, the ability to develop therapeutic strategies, around this complex, remain a challenge. Yet, despite them, the characteristics and qualities associated with this system should provide new pharmaceutical approaches as the system becomes further studied.

In the periphery and in the central nervous system, NTS mainly modulates the action of other molecules which are the principal effectors. Support for this view was confirmed by experiments with NTS- or NTSRs-deficient mice. These mice do not present any physiological disorder, are viable, and show normal growth and overt behavior. The deficient mice were also useful to implicate the NTS system in body temperature control (Pettibone et al., 2002), feeding regulation, weight control, and locomotion (Remaury et al., 2002). Mice were also less responsive or sensitive to exogenous agents or conditions. NTSR1 ko mice were less sensitive to the anorectic effects caused by leptin (Kim et al., 2008), and less responsive to morphine-induced analgesia (Roussy et al., 2010). Experiments with NTSR1- and NTSR2-deficient mice indicate a role in the regulation of ethanol consumption. However, NTSR1 regulates ethanol intoxication while NTSR2 is involved in ethanol-induced hypnosis (Lee et al., 2010, 2011). This suggests that the disruption of NTS system in the periphery is unlikely to generate side effects superior to the benefits expected in cancer treatment. On the other hand, the quasi exclusive alteration of the NTS system in tumors would confer an advantage in its use as a therapeutic target.

BIOLOGICAL TOOLS USED TO INTERACT WITH THE NTS/NSTR SYSTEMS

Few biological tools have been developed to specifically target NTS system. The two most studied ones are the NTSR1 antagonists, SR 48692, and SR142948A (Gully et al., 1996, 1997). These molecules were developed to counteract NTS effects in central and peripheral nervous system. For this purpose, both molecules are specific and efficient. These compounds have been extensively used to successfully counteract exogenous NTS oncogenic actions. Nevertheless, these molecules remain weak and problematic to use to counteract intense autocrine regulation. For example, at high concentrations, SR48692 is toxic for the cells, and as no significant information exists on the biodegradability of these molecules, the dosage levels are unknown. In addition, SR 48692 acts as a low affinity agonist with NTSR2 (Yamada et al., 1998). NTRS2 expression also occurs in the gastric mucosa, in neuroendocrine cells of the stomach, and the small and large intestine, and in cells of the exocrine pancreas. NTSR2 is rarely detected in human-derived tumors (Schulz et al., 2006). Recently, NTSR2 was found overexpressed in B cell leukemia patient's cells (Saada et al., 2012), and upregulated in prostate cancer cells luminal phenotype (Swift et al., 2010). It will be difficult to estimate NTSR2 impact on tumorigenesis until more information on its expression in human tumors becomes available.

In contrast, NTSR3 exhibits an ubiquitous expression in normal and tumoral cells. Its contribution on neoplastic progression is not known. The exact impact of SR48692 on NTSR3 remains complex. The most advanced hypothesis is that SR 48692 inhibits the oncogenic effects through NTSR1, when NTSR1 is expressed and in conjunction or not with NTSR3. In this context it was shown that SR 48692 inhibited the tumor growth of colon, breast, pancreas, and small lung cancer cells xenografted in mice (Iwase et al., 1997; Maoret et al., 1999; Moody et al., 2001; Souaze et al., 2006a). SR 48692 counteracts exogenously treated NTS in pancreas cells MIA PaCa-2 cells, bearing high and low affinity sites (Iwase et al., 1997), or circulating NTS as in the case of SW480, MDA-MB 231, and NCI-H209 cells (Maoret et al., 1999; Moody et al., 2001; Souaze et al., 2006a). It has to be noted that the use of SR 48692 does not stop tumor growth, but delays the growth rate by two to three times. The creation of the experimental tumor in mice results in tumors having an abnormal ratio (up to 10×) between the tumor size and body size, an observation uncommon and not seen in human tumors. Summarizing the effects induced by NTS, at the onset of cancer, NTS acts on the progression rather than on cellular transformation. Those actions, mediated by NTS include proliferation, survival, and metastatic effects. It is, therefore, not surprising to observe that the abolition of NTS/NTSR1 expression or signaling enhances the effect of several anti-tumoral treatments. For example, NTSR1 inhibition efficiently sensitized prostate regulation in orthotopic human tumor xenografts in mice to radiotherapy by significantly reducing tumor size, and in prostate cancer cells bearing NTS autocrine regulation (Valerie et al., 2011).

Another approach employed in the development of specific biological tools, uses Sh-RNA or Si RNA targeting NSTR1. The total or partial abolition of the target results in a decrease in cellular invasion, migration in HNSCC (Shimizu et al., 2008), or tumor growth of the human breast cancer cells (Souaze et al., 2006a). The two experimental designs demonstrate a contribution of NTS in these oncologic processes, through its interaction with NTRS1. At present, more knowledge is needed on the distribution and the coupling of NTSR2 in tumoral cells, as well as on the pharmaceutical tools specifically inhibiting NTSR2, to determine if NTSR2 is implicated in any oncogenic process.

TARGETED APPROACHES FOR NTS/NTSR1

A recent approach under investigation is to use NTSR1-specific overexpression as a means to target the delivery of therapeutic or visualizing molecules in tumoral cells. This approach is made possible since NTSR1 endocytosis permits the introduction of molecules of interest inside the targeted cell and several strategies have been developed. In the first case, a non-viral gene transfer particle bearing six NTS molecules covalently bound to poly-lysine, enabled the transfer of a reporter and therapeutic gene to those tumor cells expressing NTSR1 when injected in the tumor or into the blood circulation of xenografted nude mice (Arango-Rodriguez et al., 2006). Interestingly, both injection sites showed a high proportion of transfected cells. In a second case, a therapeutic effect was also detected on experimental neuroblastoma tumors transfected with a thymidine kinase gene associated with ganciclovir. A severe reduction of tumor growth was also observed (Rubio-Zapata et al., 2009). In the same vein, a protein interfering with the cell synthesis machinery by inducing irreversible ADP-ribosylation of elongation factor 2, exotoxin A, was fused with NTS. This recombinant protein was able to specifically recognize NTSR1 positive cells and to exert a real *in vitro* cytotoxicity (Wick and Groner, 1997). In another strategy, oligo-branched peptides were used because of their proteolysis resistant nature. Tetra-branched NTS, armed with 5-FdU, increased *in vitro* and *in vivo* tumoral cell cytotoxicity as compared to the free drug (Falciani et al., 2010a,b). The same idea was applied to carry the *cis,cis,trans*-diamminedichloridodisuccinatoplatinum(IV)–neurotensin bioconjugate specifically to tumor cells. The cytotoxicity of this molecule was tested on cell proliferation and found efficient when compared to the non-targeted platinum (Gaviglio et al., 2012).

Neurotensin-based radiopharmaceuticals have also been developed for tumor localization and therapy. Several strategies using different NTSR1 ligands were constructed whose main objectives were to limit the degradation of the molecule while maintaining the ligand specificity and a good affinity for NTSRs. Thus, the analog NT-XIX, with the three enzymatic cleavage sites stabilized showed a high specificity for NTSR1. A low accumulation of activity in the kidneys and a proper tumor-to-tissue ratio radioactivity clearance was observed *in vivo*, as well as a decrease in xenograft tumor growth (Garcia-Garayoa et al., 2009). More recently, new NTS analogs, DOTA-NT-20.3, and DOTA-NT-20.4 showed promising characteristics for imaging of NTS receptor-positive tumors and therapy (Alshoukr et al., 2009, 2011).

NTSR1/NTS COMPLEX EXPRESSION IN HUMAN TUMORS

Several experiments have investigated the expression of NTSR1 in human tumors, but most of these studies remain too small or local. In normal colonic tissue, NTSR1 was not detected by immunohistochemistry, whereas in human colonic adenomas expression, NTSR1 was associated with cytoplasmic beta-catenin localization. This was one of the first suggestions that NTSR1 expression was an early event in colon carcinogenesis (Souaze et al., 2006b). NTSR1 mRNA expression studied by *in situ* hybridization showed a higher level of expression in adenocarcinoma as compared to adenomas. In addition, a higher intensity of NTSR1 expression was observed in filtrated adenocarcinomas into and beyond the muscularis propria as compared with tumors that were localized to the mucosa or submucosa, suggesting a contribution of NTS/NTSR1 complex in tumor expansion (Gui et al., 2008).

In pancreas, NTS binding sites were first studied by autoradiography, and found specifically in pancreatic cancer but not in normal pancreas and chronic pancreatitis. Nevertheless, northern blots showed NTSR1 mRNA in normal pancreatic cells, but an increase of transcript level in chronic pancreatitis and pancreatic cancer. Within the tumors, NTSR1 expression was higher in advanced stages as compared to early stages (Wang et al., 2000). NTSR1 and NTS protein expression was confirmed by immunohistochemistry in normal and tumoral tissue. In this latter case 80% expressed both NSTR1 and NTS (Wang et al., 2011).

More recently, a correlation between NTSR1 or NTS expression with outcome of the disease was evoked. In non-small lung cancer cells, NTS and NTSR1 expression were not detectable, whereas 60% of patients with stage 1 adenocarcinoma expressed either NTS or NTSR1 and 40% expressed both markers. Patients treated only by surgery did not receive adjuvant therapy and, in this cohort, NTRS1 expression was correlated with a worse prognosis of the disease (Alifano et al., 2010b). In contrast, NTS was found to be expressed in normal epithelial cells of breast tissue, whereas NTSR1 was absent. In breast invasive carcinomas high expression of NTSR1 was correlated with pejorative clinical parameters and disease outcome (Dupouy et al., 2009). In head and neck squamous cell carcinomas, NTS and NTSR1 mRNA high levels were significantly correlated with higher rates of distant metastasis as well as with the survival rate (Shimizu et al., 2008). In normal pleura, NTS and NTSR1 were found in 30 and 77%, respectively. In malignant pleural mesothelioma, expression increased to 71.1 and 90.4%, respectively. Interestingly in benign tissue, NTSR1 was located at the cell membrane whereas in tumoral cells, NTSR1 expression was granular and mainly restricted to the cytoplasm. The lack of presence at the cell surface suggested a state of permanent activation. In these cases, NTS high expression was associated with poor disease outcome (Alifano et al., 2010a).

CONCLUSION

Cancer is more often regarded as a generalized disease and its treatment is mainly based on chemotherapy. In openly metastatic cancers, healing the sick is rarely achieved. In these cases only a prolongation of survival associated with a better quality of life can be expected. Therefore, it is necessary to improve our strategies. Recent treatment developments include the customization and selection of drugs specifically directed against biological and genetic abnormalities expressed by the tumor. However, as with conventional chemotherapy, these treatments are still insufficiently targeted and are often accompanied by serious side effects.

Two potential approaches (amongst others) to improve this situation include the highlighting of abnormalities specific to cancer cells, or the delivery of specific drugs against these pathological processes. This latter avenue would allow for effective treatment without side effects or benefit from a metabolic pathway in which it would be possible to connect conventional medicines and transfer them inside the cancer cells.

The neurotensin and neurotensin 1 receptor system have provided insights for certain oncological situations. As seen above, NTS/NTSR1 is overactive in many tumors (**Figure 1**). The development of active antagonists, and those well tolerated by the patient, in human clinical trials will be a necessary step. NTS/NTSR1 may also be considered to become a carrier of chemotherapy drugs for tumor cells. In this regard, platinum salts, such as cisplatin, whose digestive and renal toxicity is well documented, are a prime target for the development of such tests. In all cases, the effectiveness of treatment can only be improved if the selection of patients is likely to benefit from such treatment. The last 45 years of work on the NTS/NTSR1 system have allowed for a better understanding of normal and cancer cells. This system can be further exploited for therapeutic purposes and for improving the management of cancer.

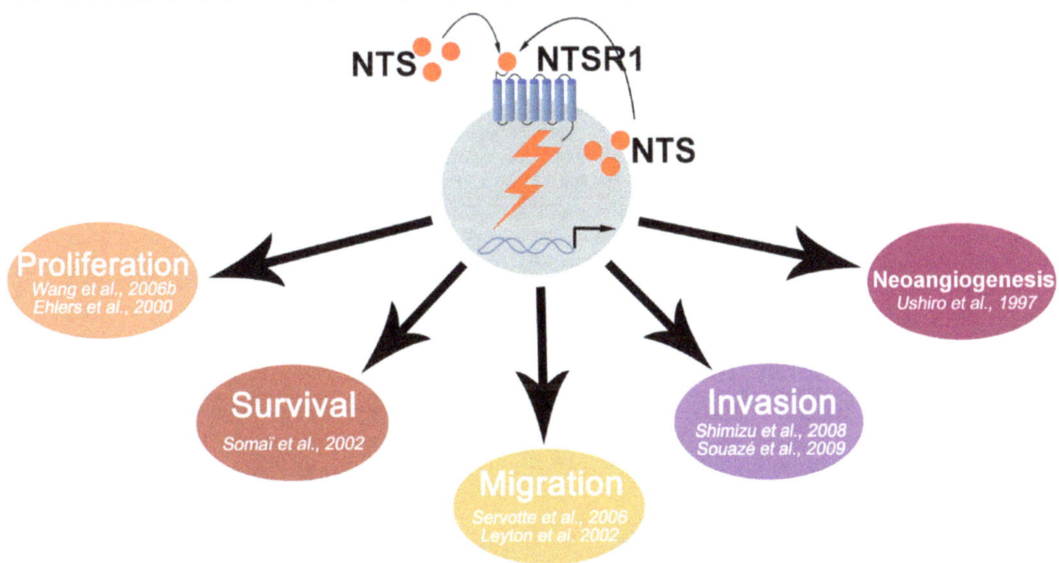

FIGURE 1 | Schematic representation of NTS oncogenic effects.

REFERENCES

Alifano, M., Loi, M., Camilleri-Broet, S., Dupouy, S., Regnard, J. F., and Forgez, P. (2010a). Neurotensin expression and outcome of malignant pleural mesothelioma. *Biochimie* 92, 164–170.

Alifano, M., Souaze, F., Dupouy, S., Camilleri-Broet, S., Younes, M., Ahmed-Zaïd, S. M., et al. (2010b). Neurotensin receptor 1 determines the outcome of non-small cell lung cancer. *Clin. Cancer Res.* 16, 4401-4410.

Alshoukr, F., Prignon, A., Brans, L., Jallane, A., Mendes, S., Talbot, J. N., et al. (2011). Novel DOTA-neurotensin analogues for 111In scintigraphy and 68Ga PET imaging of neurotensin receptor-positive tumors. *Bioconjug. Chem.* 22, 1374–1385.

Alshoukr, F., Rosant, C., Maes, V., Abdelhak, J., Raguin, O., Burg, S., et al. (2009). Novel neurotensin analogues for radioisotope targeting to neurotensin receptor-positive tumors. *Bioconjug. Chem.* 20, 1602-1610.

Amorino, G. P., Deeble, P. D., and Parsons, S. J. (2007). Neurotensin stimulates mitogenesis of prostate cancer cells through a novel c-Src/Stat5b pathway. *Oncogene* 26, 745–756.

Arango-Rodriguez, M. L, Navarro-Quiroga, I., Gonzalez-Barrios, J. A., Martinez-Arguelles, D. B., Bannon, M. J., Kouri, J., et al. (2006). Biophysical characteristics of neurotensin polyplex for *in vitro* and *in vivo* gene transfection. *Biochim. Biophys. Acta* 1760, 1009–1020.

Baca, I., and Schmidt-Gayk, H. (1981). Neurotensin and medullary carcinoma of the thyroid gland. *J. Cancer Res. Clin. Oncol.* 100, 229–230.

Beraud-Dufour, S., Coppola, T., Massa, F., and Mazella, J. (2009). Neurotensin receptor-2 and -3 are crucial for the anti-apoptotic effect of neurotensin on pancreatic beta-TC3 cells. *Int. J. Biochem. Cell Biol.* 41, 2398–2402.

Botto, J. M., Guillemare, E., Vincent, J. P., and Mazella, J. (1997). Effects of SR 48692 on neurotensin-induced calcium-activated chloride currents in the *Xenopus* oocyte expression system: agonist-like activity on the levocabastine-sensitive neurotensin receptor and absence of antagonist effect on the levocabastine insensitive neurotensin receptor. *Neurosci. Lett.* 223, 193–196.

Bozou, J. C., Amar, S., Vincent, J. P., and Kitabgi, P. (1986). Neurotensin-mediated inhibition of cyclic AMP formation in neuroblastoma N1E115 cells: involvement of the inhibitory GTP-binding component of adenylate cyclase. *Mol. Pharmacol.* 29, 489–496.

Bugni, J. M., Rabadi, L. A., Jubbal, K., Karagiannides, I., Lawson, G., and Pothoulakis, C. (2012). The neurotensin receptor-1 promotes tumor development in a sporadic but not an inflammation-associated mouse model of colon cancer. *Int. J. Cancer* 130, 1798–1805.

Carraway, R., and Leeman, S. E. (1973). The isolation of a new hypotensive peptide, neurotensin, from bovine hypothalami. *J. Biol. Chem.* 248, 6854–6861.

Carraway, R. E., and Plona, A. M. (2006). Involvement of neurotensin in cancer growth: evidence, mechanisms and development of diagnostic tools. *Peptides* 27, 2445–2460.

Chalon, P., Vita, N., Kaghad, M., Guillemot, M., Bonnin, J., Delpech, B., et al. (1996). Molecular cloning of a levocabastine-sensitive neurotensin binding site. *FEBS Lett.* 386, 91–94.

Cheng, H., Shi, S., Cai, X., Long, J., Xu, J., Liu, C., et al. (2012). microRNA signature for human pancreatic cancer invasion and metastasis. *Exp. Ther. Med.* 4, 181–187.

Chesire, D. R., Ewing, C. M., Gage, W. R., and Isaacs, W. B. (2002). In vitro evidence for complex modes of nuclear beta-catenin signaling during prostate growth and tumorigenesis. *Oncogene* 21, 2679–2694.

Coppola, T., Beraud-Dufour, S., Antoine, A., Vincent, J. P., and Mazella, J. (2008). Neurotensin protects pancreatic beta cells from apoptosis. *Int. J. Biochem. Cell Biol.* 40, 2296–2302.

Dammrich, J., Ormanns, W., Kahaly, G., and Schrezenmeir, J. (1988). Multiple peptide hormone producing adenocarcinoma of lung with neurotensin and CRF-like immunoreactivity. *Pathol. Res. Pract.* 183, 670–674.

de Lange, R., Dimoudis, N., and Weidle, U. H. (2003). Identification of genes associated with enhanced metastasis of a large cell lung carcinoma cell line. *Anticancer Res.* 23, 187–194.

Dicou, E. (2008). Neurotensin protects pancreatic beta cells from serum deprivation. *Arch. Physiol. Biochem.* 114, 299–300.

Dong, Z., Wang, X., and Evers, B. M. (2000). Site-specific DNA methylation contributes to neurotensin/neuromedin N expression in colon cancers. *Am. J. Physiol. Gastrointest. Liver Physiol.* 279, G1139–G1147.

Dong, Z., Wang, X., Zhao, Q., Townsend, C. M. Jr., and Evers, B. M. (1998). DNA methylation contributes to expression of the human neurotensin/neuromedin N gene. *Am. J. Physiol.* 274, G535–G543.

Dupouy, S., Mourra, N., Doan, V. K., Gompel, A., Alifano, M., and Forgez, P. (2011). The potential use of the neurotensin high affinity receptor 1 as a biomarker for cancer progression and as a component of personalized medicine in selective cancers. *Biochimie* 93, 1369–1378.

Dupouy, S., Viardot-Foucault, V., Alifano, M., Souazé, F., Plu-Bureau, G., Chaouat, M., et al. (2009). The neurotensin receptor-1 pathway contributes to human ductal breast cancer progression. *PLoS ONE.* 4:e4223. doi: 10.1371/journal.pone.0004223

Ehlers, R. A., Zhang, Y., Hellmich, M. R., and Evers, B. M. (2000). Neurotensin-mediated activation of MAPK pathways and AP-1 binding in the human pancreatic cancer cell line, MIA PaCa-2. *Biochem. Biophys. Res. Commun.* 269, 704–708.

Ehrenfried, J. A., Zhou, Z., Thompson, J. C., and Evers, B. M. (1994). Expression of the neurotensin gene in fetal human liver and fibrolamellar carcinoma. *Ann. Surg.* 220, 484–489.

Elek, J., Pinzon, W., Park, K. H., and Narayanan, R. (2000). Relevant genomics of neurotensin receptor in cancer. *Anticancer Res.* 20, 53–58.

Evers, B. M., Zhou, Z., Celano, P., and Li, J. (1995). The neurotensin gene is a downstream target for Ras activation. *J. Clin. Invest.* 95, 2822–2830.

Falciani, C., Brunetti, J., Pagliuca, C., Menichetti, S., Vitellozzi, L., Lelli, B., et al. (2010a). Design and in vitro evaluation of branched peptide conjugates: turning nonspecific cytotoxic drugs into tumor-selective agents. *ChemMedChem* 5, 567–574.

Falciani, C., Lelli, B., Brunetti, J., Pileri, S., Cappelli, A., Pini, A., et al. (2010b). Modular branched neurotensin peptides for tumor target tracing and receptor-mediated therapy: a proof-of-concept. *Curr. Cancer Drug Targets* 10, 695–704.

Garcia-Garayoa, E., Blauenstein, P., Blanc, A., Maes, V., Tourwe, D., and Schubiger, P. A. (2009). A stable neurotensin-based radiopharmaceutical for targeted imaging and therapy of neurotensin receptor-positive tumours. *Eur. J. Nucl. Med. Mol. Imaging* 36, 37–47.

Gaviglio, L., Gross, A., Metzler-Nolte, N., and Ravera, M. (2012). Synthesis and in vitro cytotoxicity of cis,cis,trans-diamminedichloridodisuccinatoplatinum(IV)-peptide bioconjugates. *Metallomics* 4, 260–266.

Gendron, L., Perron, A., Payet, M. D., Gallo-Payet, N., Sarret, P., and Beaudet, A. (2004). Low-affinity neurotensin receptor (NTS2) signaling: internalization-dependent activation of extracellular signal-regulated kinases 1/2. *Mol. Pharmacol.* 66, 1421–1430.

Guha, S., Lunn, J. A., Santiskulvong, C., and Rozengurt, E. (2003). Neurotensin stimulates protein kinase C-dependent mitogenic signaling in human pancreatic carcinoma cell line PANC-1. *Cancer Res.* 63, 2379–2387.

Gui, X., Guzman, G., Dobner, P. R., and Kadkol, S. S. (2008). Increased neurotensin receptor-1 expression during progression of colonic adenocarcinoma. *Peptides* 29, 1609–1615.

Gully, D., Canton, M., Boigegrain, R., Jeanjean, F., Molimard, J. C., Poncelet, M., et al. (1993). Biochemical and pharmacological profile of a potent and selective nonpeptide antagonist of the neurotensin receptor. *Proc. Natl. Acad. Sci. U.S.A.* 90, 65–69.

Gully, D., Labeeuw, B., Boigegrain, R., Oury-Donat, F., Bachy, A., Poncelet, M., et al. (1997). Biochemical and pharmacological activities of SR 142948A, a new potent neurotensin receptor antagonist. *J. Pharmacol. Exp. Ther.* 280, 802–812.

Gully, D., Lespy, L., Canton, M., Rostene, W., Kitabgi, P., Le, F. G., et al. (1996). Effect of the neurotensin receptor antagonist SR48692 on rat blood pressure modulation by neurotensin. *Life Sci.* 58, 665–674.

Gutniak, M., Rosenqvist, U., Grimelius, L., Lundberg, J. M., Hokfelt, T., Rokaeus, A., et al. (1980). Report on a patient with watery diarrhoea syndrome caused by a pancreatic tumour containing neurotensin, enkephalin and calcitonin. *Acta Med. Scand.* 208, 95–100.

Harikumar, K. B., Kunnumakkara, A. B., Ochi, N., Tong, Z., Deorukhkar, A., Sung, B., et al. (2010). A novel small-molecule inhibitor of protein kinase D blocks pancreatic cancer growth in vitro and in vivo. *Mol. Cancer Ther.* 9, 1136–1146.

Hassan, S., Dobner, P. R., and Carraway, R. E. (2004). Involvement of MAP-kinase, PI3-kinase and EGF-receptor in the stimulatory effect of neurotensin on DNA synthesis in PC3 cells. *Regul. Pept.* 120, 155–166.

Iwase, K., Evers, B. M., Hellmich, M. R., Kim, H. J., Higashide, S.,

Gully, D., et al. (1997). Inhibition of neurotensin-induced pancreatic carcinoma growth by a nonpeptide neurotensin receptor antagonist, SR48692. *Cancer* 79, 1787–1793.

Jemal, A., Bray, F., Center, M. M., Ferlay, J., Ward, E., and Forman, D. (2011). Global cancer statistics. *CA Cancer J. Clin.* 61, 69–90.

Kataoka, H. (2009). EGFR ligands and their signaling scissors, ADAMs, as new molecular targets for anticancer treatments. *J. Dermatol. Sci.* 56, 148–153.

Kim, E. R., Leckstrom, A., and Mizuno, T. M. (2008). Impaired anorectic effect of leptin in neurotensin receptor 1-deficient mice. *Behav. Brain Res.* 194, 66–71.

Kisfalvi, K., Hurd, C., Guha, S., and Rozengurt, E. (2010). Induced overexpression of protein kinase D1 stimulates mitogenic signaling in human pancreatic carcinoma PANC-1 cells. *J. Cell. Physiol.* 223, 309–316.

Law, I. K., Murphy, J. E., Bakirtzi, K., Bunnett, N. W., and Pothoulakis, C. (2012). Neurotensin-induced proinflammatory signaling in human colonocytes is regulated by beta-arrestins and endothelin-converting enzyme-1-dependent endocytosis and resensitization of neurotensin receptor 1. *J. Biol. Chem.* 287, 15066–15075.

Lee, L. F., Guan, J., Qiu, Y., and Kung, H. J. (2001). Neuropeptide-induced androgen independence in prostate cancer cells: roles of nonreceptor tyrosine kinases Etk/Bmx, Src, and focal adhesion kinase. *Mol. Cell. Biol.* 21, 8385–8397.

Lee, M. R., Hinton, D. J., Song, J. Y., Lee, K. W., Choo, C., Johng, H., et al. (2010). Neurotensin receptor type 1 regulates ethanol intoxication and consumption in mice. *Pharmacol. Biochem. Behav.* 95, 235–241.

Lee, M. R., Hinton, D. J., Unal, S. S., Richelson, E., and Choi, D. S. (2011). Increased ethanol consumption and preference in mice lacking neurotensin receptor type 2. *Alcohol Clin. Exp. Res.* 35, 99–107.

Lefrancois, S., Zeng, J., Hassan, A. J., Canuel, M., and Morales, C. R. (2003). The lysosomal trafficking of sphingolipid activator proteins (SAPs) is mediated by sortilin. *EMBO J.* 22, 6430–6437.

Leyton, J., Garcia-Marin, L., Jensen, R. T., and Moody, T. W. (2002). Neurotensin causes tyrosine phosphorylation of focal adhesion kinase in lung cancer cells. *Eur. J. Pharmacol.* 442, 179–186.

Li, J., Song, J., Cassidy, M. G., Rychahou, P., Starr, M. E., Liu, J., et al. (2012). PI3K p110alpha/Akt signaling negatively regulates secretion of the intestinal peptide neurotensin through interference of granule transport. *Mol. Endocrinol.* 26, 1380–1393.

Maoret, J. J., Anini, Y., Rouyer-Fessard, C., Gully, D., and Laburthe, M. (1999). Neurotensin and a non-peptide neurotensin receptor antagonist control human colon cancer cell growth in cell culture and in cells xenografted into nude mice. *Int. J. Cancer* 80, 448–454.

Martin, S., Navarro, V., Vincent, J. P., and Mazella, J. (2002). Neurotensin receptor-1 and -3 complex modulates the cellular signaling of neurotensin in the HT29 cell line. *Gastroenterology* 123, 1135–1143.

Martin, S., Vincent, J. P., and Mazella, J. (2003). Involvement of the neurotensin receptor-3 in the neurotensin-induced migration of human microglia. *J. Neurosci.* 23, 1198–1205.

Mazella, J., Botto, J. M., Guillemare, E., Coppola, T., Sarret, P., and Vincent, J. P. (1996). Structure, functional expression, and cerebral localization of the levocabastine-sensitive neurotensin/neuromedin N receptor from mouse brain. *J. Neurosci.* 16, 5613–5620.

Mazella, J., and Vincent, J. P. (2006). Functional roles of the NTS2 and NTS3 receptors. *Peptides* 27, 2469–2475.

Mijatovic, T., Gailly, P., Mathieu, V., De, N. N., Yeaton, P., Kiss, R., et al. (2007). Neurotensin is a versatile modulator of in vitro human pancreatic ductal adenocarcinoma cell (PDAC) migration. *Cell. Oncol.* 29, 315–326.

Moody, T. W., Carney, D. N., Korman, L. Y., Gazdar, A. F., and Minna, J. D. (1985). Neurotensin is produced by and secreted from classic small cell lung cancer cells. *Life Sci.* 36, 1727–1732.

Moody, T. W., Chiles, J., Casibang, M., Moody, E., Chan, D., and Davis, T. P. (2001). SR48692 is a neurotensin receptor antagonist which inhibits the growth of small cell lung cancer cells. *Peptides* 22, 109–115.

Muller, K. M., Tveteraas, I. H., Aasrum, M., Odegard, J., Dawood, M., Dajani, O., et al. (2011). Role of protein kinase C and epidermal growth factor receptor signalling in growth stimulation by neurotensin in colon carcinoma cells. *BMC Cancer* 11:421. doi: 10.1186/1471-2407-11-421

Mustain, W. C., Rychahou, P. G., and Evers, B. M. (2011). The role of neurotensin in physiologic and pathologic processes. *Curr. Opin. Endocrinol. Diabetes Obes.* 18, 75–82.

Najimi, M., Maloteaux, J. M., and Hermans, E. (2002). Cytoskeleton-related trafficking of the EAAC1 glutamate transporter after activation of the G(q/11)-coupled neurotensin receptor NTS1. *FEBS Lett.* 523, 224–228.

Najimi, M., Souaze, F., Mendez, M., Hermans, E., Berbar, T., Rostene, W., et al. (1998). Activation of receptor gene transcription is required to maintain cell sensitization after agonist exposure. Study on neurotensin receptor. *J. Biol. Chem.* 273, 21634–21641.

Nielsen, M. S., Jacobsen, C., Olivecrona, G., Gliemann, J., and Petersen, C. M. (1999). Sortilin/neurotensin receptor-3 binds and mediates degradation of lipoprotein lipase. *J. Biol. Chem.* 274, 8832–8836.

Petersen, C. M., Nielsen, M. S., Nykjaer, A., Jacobsen, L., Tommerup, N., Rasmussen, H. H., et al. (1997). Molecular identification of a novel candidate sorting receptor purified from human brain by receptor-associated protein affinity chromatography. *J. Biol. Chem.* 272, 3599–3605.

Pettibone, D. J., Hess, J. F., Hey, P. J., Jacobson, M. A., Leviten, M., Lis, E. V., et al. (2002). The effects of deleting the mouse neurotensin receptor NTR1 on central and peripheral responses to neurotensin. *J. Pharmacol. Exp. Ther.* 300, 305–313.

Poinot-Chazel, C., Portier, M., Bouaboula, M., Vita, N., Pecceu, F., Gully, D., et al. (1996). Activation of mitogen-activated protein kinase couples neurotensin receptor stimulation to induction of the primary response gene Krox-24. *Biochem. J.* 320(Pt 1), 145–151.

Popp, E., Schneider, A., Vogel, P., Teschendorf, P., and Bottiger, B. W. (2007). Time course of the hypothermic response to continuously administered neurotensin. *Neuropeptides* 41, 349–354.

Portier, M., Combes, T., Gully, D., Maffrand, J. P., and Casellas, P. (1998). Neurotensin type 1 receptor-mediated activation of krox24, c-fos and Elk-1: preventing effect of the neurotensin antagonists SR 48692 and SR 142948. *FEBS Lett.* 432, 88–93.

Reinecke, M. (1985). Neurotensin. Immunohistochemical localization in central and peripheral nervous system and in endocrine cells and its functional role as neurotransmitter and endocrine hormone. *Prog. Histochem. Cytochem.* 16, 1–172.

Remaury, A., Vita, N., Gendreau, S., Jung, M., Arnone, M., Poncelet, M., et al. (2002). Targeted inactivation of the neurotensin type 1 receptor reveals its role in body temperature control and feeding behavior but not in analgesia. *Brain Res.* 953, 63–72.

Roussy, G., Beaudry, H., Lafrance, M., Belleville, K., Beaudet, N., Wada, K., et al. (2010). Altered morphine-induced analgesia in neurotensin type 1 receptor null mice. *Neuroscience* 170, 1286–1294.

Rubio-Zapata, H. A., Rembao-Bojorquez, J. D., Arango-Rodriguez, M. L., Dupouy, S., Forgez, P., and Martinez-Fong, D. (2009). NT-polyplex: a new tool for therapeutic gene delivery to neuroblastoma tumors. *Cancer Gene Ther.* 16, 573–584.

Saada, S., Marget, P., Fauchais, A. L., Lise, M. C., Chemin, G., Sindou, P., et al. (2012). Differential expression of neurotensin and specific receptors, NTSR1 and NTSR2, in normal and malignant human B lymphocytes. *J. Immunol.* 189, 5293–5303.

Sanderson, M. P., Dempsey, P. J., and Dunbar, A. J. (2006). Control of ErbB signaling through metalloprotease mediated ectodomain shedding of EGF-like factors. *Growth Factors* 24, 121–136.

Schotte, A., Leysen, J. E., and Laduron, P. M. (1986). Evidence for a displaceable non-specific [3H]neurotensin binding site in rat brain. *Naunyn Schmiedebergs Arch. Pharmacol.* 333, 400–405.

Schulz, S., Rocken, C., Ebert, M. P., and Schulz, S. (2006). Immunocytochemical identification of low-affinity NTS2 neurotensin receptors in parietal cells of human gastric mucosa. *J. Endocrinol.* 191, 121–128.

Seethalakshmi, L., Mitra, S. P., Dobner, P. R., Menon, M., and Carraway, R. E. (1997). Neurotensin receptor expression in prostate cancer cell line and growth effect of NT at physiological concentrations. *Prostate* 31, 183–192.

Sehgal, I., Powers, S., Huntley, B., Powis, G., Pittelkow, M., and Maihle, N. J. (1994). Neurotensin is an autocrine trophic factor stimulated by androgen withdrawal in human prostate cancer. *Proc. Natl. Acad. Sci. U.S.A.* 91, 4673–4677.

Servotte, S., Camby, I., Debeir, O., Deroanne, C., Lambert, C. A., Lapiere, C. M., et al. (2006). The in vitro influences of neurotensin on the motility characteristics of human U373 glioblastoma cells.

Neuropathol. Appl. Neurobiol. 32, 575–584.

Seufferlein, T., and Rozengurt, E. (1996). Galanin, neurotensin, and phorbol esters rapidly stimulate activation of mitogen-activated protein kinase in small cell lung cancer cells. *Cancer Res.* 56, 5758–5764.

Shimizu, S., Tsukada, J., Sugimoto, T., Kikkawa, N., Sasaki, K., Chazono, H., et al. (2008). Identification of a novel therapeutic target for head and neck squamous cell carcinomas: a role for the neurotensin-neurotensin receptor 1 oncogenic signaling pathway. *Int. J. Cancer* 123, 1816–1823.

Snider, R. M., Forray, C., Pfenning, M., and Richelson, E. (1986). Neurotensin stimulates inositol phospholipid metabolism and calcium mobilization in murine neuroblastoma clone N1E-115. *J. Neurochem.* 47, 1214–1218.

Somaï, S., Gompel, A., Rostene, W., and Forgez, P. (2002). Neurotensin counteracts apoptosis in breast cancer cells. *Biochem. Biophys. Res. Commun.* 295, 482–488.

Souaze, F., Dupouy, S., Viardot-Foucault, V., Bruyneel, E., Attoub, S., Gespach, C., et al. (2006a). Expression of neurotensin and NT1 receptor in human breast cancer: a potential role in tumor progression. *Cancer Res.* 66, 6243–6249.

Souaze, F., Viardot-Foucault, V., Roullet, N., Toy-Miou-Leong, M., Gompel, A., Bruyneel, E., et al. (2006b). Neurotensin receptor 1 gene activation by the Tcf/beta-catenin pathway is an early event in human colonic adenomas. *Carcinogenesis* 27, 708–716.

Souaze, F., and Forgez, P. (2006). Molecular and cellular regulation of neurotensin receptor under acute and chronic agonist stimulation. *Peptides* 27, 2493–2501.

Souaze, F., Rostene, W., and Forgez, P. (1997). Neurotensin agonist induces differential regulation of neurotensin receptor mRNA. Identification of distinct transcriptional and post-transcriptional mechanisms. *J. Biol. Chem.* 272, 10087–10094.

St-Gelais, F., Jomphe, C., and Trudeau, L. E. (2006). The role of neurotensin in central nervous system pathophysiology. what is the evidence? *J. Psychiatry Neurosci.* 31, 229–245.

Sumi, S., Evers, B. M., Townsend, C. M. Jr., Yoshinaga, K., Uchida, T., Murakami, M., et al. (1993). Comparative effects of neurotensin and neuromedin N on growth of human pancreatic cancer, MIA PaCa-2. *Surg. Oncol.* 2, 267–272.

Swift, S. L., Burns, J. E., and Maitland, N. J. (2010). Altered expression of neurotensin receptors is associated with the differentiation state of prostate cancer. *Cancer Res.* 70, 347–356.

Tallett, A., Chilvers, E. R., MacKinnon, A. C., Haslett, C., and Sethi, T. (1996). Neuropeptides stimulate tyrosine phosphorylation and tyrosine kinase activity in small cell lung cancer cell lines. *Peptides* 17, 665–673.

Tanaka, K., Masu, M., and Nakanishi, S. (1990). Structure and functional expression of the cloned rat neurotensin receptor. *Neuron* 4, 847–854.

Tang, K. H., Ma, S., Lee, T. K., Chan, Y. P., Kwan, P. S., Tong, C. M., et al. (2012). CD133(+) liver tumor-initiating cells promote tumor angiogenesis, growth, and self-renewal through neurotensin/interleukin-8/CXCL1 signaling. *Hepatology* 55, 807–820.

Thomas, R. P., Hellmich, M. R., Townsend, C. M. Jr., and Evers, B. M. (2003). Role of gastrointestinal hormones in the proliferation of normal and neoplastic tissues. *Endocr. Rev.* 24, 571–599.

Toy-Miou-Leong, M., Bachelet, C. M., Pelaprat, D., Rostene, W., and Forgez, P. (2004). NT agonist regulates expression of nuclear high-affinity neurotensin receptors. *J. Histochem. Cytochem.* 52, 335–345.

Turashvili, G., Bouchal, J., Burkadze, G., and Kolar, Z. (2006). Wnt signaling pathway in mammary gland development and carcinogenesis. *Pathobiology* 73, 213–223.

Turner, J. T., James-Kracke, M. R., and Camden, J. M. (1990). Regulation of the neurotensin receptor and intracellular calcium mobilization in HT29 cells. *J. Pharmacol. Exp. Ther.* 253, 1049–1056.

Ulich, T. R., Cheng, L., Glover, H., Yang, K., and Lewin, K. J. (1983). A colonic adenocarcinoma with argentaffin cells. An immunoperoxidase study demonstrating the presence of numerous neuroendocrine products. *Cancer* 51, 1483–1489.

Ushiro, S., Mizoguchi, K., Yoshida, S., Jimi, S., Fujiwara, T., Yoshida, M., et al. (1997). Stimulation of cell-surface urokinase-type plasminogen activator activity and cell migration in vascular endothelial cells by a novel hexapeptide analogue of neurotensin. *FEBS Lett.* 418, 341–345.

Valerie, N. C., Casarez, E. V., Dasilva, J. O., Dunlap-Brown, M. E., Parsons, S. J., Amorino, G. P., et al. (2011). Inhibition of neurotensin receptor 1 selectively sensitizes prostate cancer to ionizing radiation. *Cancer Res.* 71, 6817–6826.

Vias, M., Burtt, G., Culig, Z., Veerakumarasivam, A., Neal, D. E., and Mills, I. G. (2007). A role for neurotensin in bicalutamide resistant prostate cancer cells. *Prostate* 67, 190–202.

Vincent, J. P., Mazella, J., and Kitabgi, P. (1999). Neurotensin and neurotensin receptors. *Trends Pharmacol. Sci.* 20, 302–309.

Wang, H. L., and Wu, T. (1996). G alpha q/11 mediates neurotensin excitation of substantia nigra dopaminergic neurons. *Brain Res. Mol. Brain Res.* 36, 29–36.

Wang, J. G., Li, N. N., Li, H. N., Cui, L., and Wang, P. (2011). Pancreatic cancer bears overexpression of neurotensin and neurotensin receptor subtype-1 and SR 48692 counteracts neurotensin induced cell proliferation in human pancreatic ductal carcinoma cell line PANC-1. *Neuropeptides* 45, 151–156.

Wang, L., Friess, H., Zhu, Z., Graber, H., Zimmermann, A., Korc, M., et al. (2000). Neurotensin receptor-1 mRNA analysis in normal pancreas and pancreatic disease. *Clin. Cancer Res.* 6, 566–571.

Wang, X., Jackson, L. N., Johnson, S. M., Wang, Q., and Evers, B. M. (2010). Suppression of neurotensin receptor type 1 expression and function by histone deacetylase inhibitors in human colorectal cancers. *Mol. Cancer Ther.* 9, 2389–2398.

Wang, X., Wang, Q., Ives, K. L., and Evers, B. M. (2006a). Curcumin inhibits neurotensin-mediated interleukin-8 production and migration of HCT116 human colon cancer cells. *Clin. Cancer Res.* 12, 5346–5355.

Wang, Q., Zhou, Y., and Evers, B. M. (2006b). Neurotensin phosphorylates GSK-3alpha/beta through the activation of PKC in human colon cancer cells. *Neoplasia* 8, 781–787.

Wick, B., and Groner, B. (1997). Evaluation of cell surface antigens as potential targets for recombinant tumor toxins. *Cancer Lett.* 118, 161–172.

Xie, K. (2001). Interleukin-8 and human cancer biology. *Cytokine Growth Factor Rev.* 12, 375–391.

Yabushita, S., Fukamachi, K., Tanaka, H., Sumida, K., Deguchi, Y., Sukata, T., et al. (2012). Circulating microRNAs in serum of human K-ras oncogene transgenic rats with pancreatic ductal adenocarcinomas. *Pancreas* 41, 1013–1018.

Yamada, M., Yamada, M., Lombet, A., Forgez, P., and Rostene, W. (1998). Distinct functional characteristics of levocabastine sensitive rat neurotensin NT2 receptor expressed in Chinese hamster ovary cells. *Life Sci.* 62, PL375–PL380.

Yoshinaga, K., Evers, B. M., Izukura, M., Parekh, D., Uchida, T., Townsend, C. M. Jr., et al. (1992). Neurotensin stimulates growth of colon cancer. *Surg. Oncol.* 1, 127–134.

Zhao, D., Kuhnt-Moore, S., Zeng, H., Wu, J. S., Moyer, M. P., and Pothoulakis, C. (2003). Neurotensin stimulates IL-8 expression in human colonic epithelial cells through Rho GTPase-mediated NF-kappa B pathways. *Am. J. Physiol. Cell Physiol.* 284, C1397–C1404.

Zhao, D., Zhan, Y., Zeng, H., Koon, H. W., Moyer, M. P., and Pothoulakis, C. (2007). Neurotensin stimulates expression of early growth response gene-1 and EGF receptor through MAP kinase activation in human colonic epithelial cells. *Int. J. Cancer* 120, 1652–1656.

4

Neuropeptide Y receptors: How to get subtype selectivity

Xavier Pedragosa-Badia, Jan Stichel and Annette G. Beck-Sickinger*

Institute of Biochemistry, Faculty of Biosciences, Pharmacy and Psychology, Universität Leipzig, Leipzig, Germany

Edited by:
Hubert Vaudry, University of Rouen, France

Reviewed by:
Janine A. Danks, Royal Melbourne Institute of Technology-University, Australia
William Colmers, University of Alberta, Canada

***Correspondence:**
Annette G. Beck-Sickinger, Institute of Biochemistry, Faculty of Biosciences, Pharmacy and Psychology, Universität Leipzig, Brüderstraße 34, 04103 Leipzig, Germany.
e-mail: beck-sickinger@uni-leipzig.de

The neuropeptide Y (NPY) system is a multireceptor/multiligand system consisting of four receptors in humans (hY_1, hY_2, hY_4, hY_5) and three agonists (NPY, PYY, PP) that activate these receptors with different potency. The relevance of this system in diseases like obesity or cancer, and the different role that each receptor plays influencing different biological processes makes this system suitable for the design of subtype selectivity studies. In this review we focus on the latest findings within the NPY system, we summarize recent mutagenesis studies, structure activity relationship studies, receptor chimera, and selective ligands focusing also on the binding mode of the native agonists.

Keywords: GPCR, NPY, YR, subtype selectivity, ligand side, receptor side

INTRODUCTION TO THE NEUROPEPTIDE Y FAMILY

The neuropeptide Y (NPY) family is a multireceptor/multiligand system consisting of four receptors in humans and three polypeptides that bind and activate them with different affinity and potency. The NPY receptors belong to the class A or rhodopsin-like G-protein coupled receptors (GPCR). Five receptors have been cloned from mammals so far, Y_1, Y_2, Y_4, Y_5, and y_6 but only four of the members are functional in humans (hY_1, hY_2, hY_4, hY_5; **Table 1**). The y6 receptor however is active in rabbit and mouse (Starback et al., 2000). The existence of an additional receptor subtype (Y_3) was suggested by pharmacological studies of several human, rat, and rabbit tissues including the human adrenal medulla. This receptor subtype is characterized by a much lower affinity for PYY, compared to NPY (Gehlert, 1998; Lee and Miller, 1998). However, since all attempts to clone this receptor subtype were unsuccessful so far, the existence of Y_3 is not very likely.

Neuropeptide Y receptors (NPYR) generally couple to G_i or G_0 proteins, which leads to the inhibition of adenylate cyclase and finally to the inhibition of cAMP accumulation (Cabrele and Beck-Sickinger, 2000) and modulation of Ca^{2+} and K^+ channels (Holliday et al., 2004). Besides this, it has been described that Y_2 and Y_4 receptors also couple to the G_q protein increasing inositol 1,4,5-phosphate (IP_3) production via the activation of the phospholipase C-β (PLC) in rabbit smooth muscle cells (Misra et al., 2004).

Neuropeptide Y, peptide YY (PYY), and pancreatic polypeptide (PP) are the native ligands of the NPY family. NPY is the most abundant peptide in the mammalian brain and has been suggested to adopt a largely open structure. In surface association with phospholipid micelles a flexible N-terminus and a C-terminal alpha helix were identified (Lerch et al., 2004; Parker et al., 2011). However, PYY and PP are suggested to form the typical hairpin-like structure also called PP-fold, a suggestion for pPYY supported by NMR (Keire et al., 2000a; Neumoin et al., 2007), and for PP by the X-ray structure of the peptide (Blundell et al., 1981). Despite some structural differences between the ligands, these polypeptides have a common length of 36 amino acids (**Table 2**) and an amidated C-terminus. Furthermore, these polypeptides share high sequence identity. Whereas NPY and PYY show the highest percentage of common residues with 70%, NPY and PP share only 50% identity (Blomqvist et al., 1992; Zhang et al., 2011). Seven positions in NPY, PYY, and PP are strongly conserved throughout all species: Pro^5, Pro^8, Gly^9, Ala^{12}, Tyr^{27}, Arg^{33}, and Arg^{35}. Apart from these, highly conserved positions are: Pro^2, Tyr^{20}, Thr^{32}, and Tyr^{36} (Cabrele and Beck-Sickinger, 2000). Regarding its pharmacological properties, NPY acts as a neurotransmitter whereas PYY and PP act as neuroendocrine hormones.

The first identified member of the family PP, was isolated from avian pancreas in 1975 (Kimmel et al., 1975). This polypeptide is secreted in the pancreas by PP cells in the Langerhans islets after food ingestion in proportion to the caloric content (Boguszewski et al., 2010; Suzuki et al., 2010). It is thought to act mainly in brain stem and vagal nerve where it promotes appetite suppression, inhibition of gastric emptying and increases in energy expenditure (Asakawa et al., 2003) in addition to direct responses in the gut.

The second member of the ligand family PYY, was isolated from porcine intestinal extracts in 1980 (Tatemoto and Mutt, 1980) and is expressed by entero-endocrine L cells of the distal gut (Lundberg et al., 1982). PYY_{1-36} is released in proportion to nutrient intake along the gut and cleaved to PYY_{3-36} by the dipeptidyl aminopeptidase VI. The ligand PYY_{3-36}, the predominant form released in the circulation, is selective for Y_2 and produces anorexigenic effects (Pittner et al., 2004). This polypeptide acts on peripheral receptors but also on those located in the CNS (Hankir et al., 2011; Schloegl et al., 2011). The last family member, NPY, was isolated from porcine brain in 1982 (Tatemoto, 1982) and is one of the most broadly distributed peptides of the central and peripheral nervous system. This peptide is well conserved among different species. It stimulates food intake in response to negative energy balance (Stanley et al., 1986). Additional roles of NPY are decreased bone

Table 1 | Amino acid sequence of the NPY ligands.

Peptides	Amino acid sequence																																			
	1				5					10					15					20					25					30					35	
pNPY	Y	P	S	K	P	D	N	P	G	E	D	A	P	A	E	D	L	A	R	Y	Y	S	A	L	R	H	Y	I	N	L	I	T	R	Q	R	Y
hPYY	Y	P	I	K	P	E	A	P	G	E	D	A	S	P	E	E	L	N	R	Y	Y	A	S	L	R	H	Y	L	N	L	V	T	R	Q	R	Y
hPP	A	P	L	E	P	V	Y	P	G	D	N	A	T	P	E	Q	M	A	Q	Y	A	A	D	L	R	R	Y	I	N	M	L	T	R	P	R	Y

Table 2 | NPYR: sequence length and ligand preference.

Receptor	hY_1	hY_2	hY_4	hY_5
Amino acids number	384	381	375	445–455
Native ligand	NPY	NPY	PP	NPY
	PYY	PYY		PYY

formation (Baldock et al., 2009; Sousa et al., 2012), regulation of mood and anxiety disorders, the modulation of stress responses (Heilig, 2004), and ethanol intake (Thiele et al., 1998).

Neuropeptide Y family peptides mediate their activity in humans via four receptors. Structurally, these receptors contain two Cys residues in the extracellular regions that form a disulfide bond between extracellular loop I and II. This disulfide bond is a common feature of class A GPCRs and has been confirmed by X-ray crystallography for several members including bovine rhodopsin and the human β2 adrenergic receptor (Palczewski et al., 2000; Cherezov et al., 2007).

The evolution of this system shows that vertebrate ancestors probably had three receptor genes. These genes, possibly located in close proximity in the same chromosomal segment, would be the precursors of the receptor subfamilies. The Y_1 subfamily includes the Y_1, Y_4, and y_6 receptors, the Y_2 subfamily comprises Y_2 and Y_7 (in zebrafish and frogs), and the Y_5 subfamily consists of only the Y_5 due to lack of close relatives of this receptor (Larhammar and Salaneck, 2004). Although the Y_1 and Y_2 receptor subtypes have a common pharmacological profile, they only share 27% of sequence identity. Y_1 and y_6 receptors share the highest sequence identity (51%), whereas Y_1 and Y_4 receptors share 44% identity, increasing to 56% identity in transmembrane regions (Larhammar et al., 2001). The Y_4 receptor conserves 75% of overall identity between human and rat suggesting this protein may be the most rapidly evolving member of the family and the only member that has a selective agonist, the pancreatic polypeptide (Larhammar, 1996; Blomqvist and Herzog, 1997). The Y_5 receptor displays low sequence identity, around 30%, with all members of the family. Compared with other GPCRs, neuropeptide Y receptors share a high sequence identity with $NPFF_1$ and $NPFF_2$ receptors, which are members of the RFamide receptor family (Bonini et al., 2000).

The Y_1 receptor has 384 amino acids and its main agonists are NPY and PYY. It can be also activated by PP with a minor potency (**Table 2**). The receptor is expressed in the hypothalamus, hippocampus, neocortex, and thalamus (Caberlotto et al., 1997), but is also present in adipose tissue (Castan et al., 1993; Hausman et al., 2008), blood vessels (Cabrele and Beck-Sickinger, 2000), colon, kidney, adrenal gland, heart, and placenta (Wharton et al., 1993). It plays a role in the regulation of food intake (Kanatani et al., 2000b), vasoconstriction of blood vessels (Cabrele and Beck-Sickinger, 2000), heart rate, anxiety (Balasubramaniam, 2002), and bone homeostasis (Sousa et al., 2012).

The Y_2 receptor is predominantly expressed in hippocampal neurons, in the thalamus, hypothalamus, and parts of the peripheral nervous system (Widdowson, 1993; Cabrele and Beck-Sickinger, 2000). It is mainly found in pre-synaptic neurons and exerts its action through the regulation of neurotransmitter release (Wahlestedt et al., 1986; Potter et al., 1989). Typical effects correlated with activation of this receptor include enhanced memory retention, the regulation of the circadian rhythm, angiogenesis (Flood and Morley, 1989; Golombek et al., 1996; Gribkoff et al., 1998; Zukowska-Grojec et al., 1998) and bone formation (Baldock et al., 2002). This receptor consists of 381 amino acids and its preferred agonists are NPY and PYY (**Table 2**).

The Y_4 receptor subtype is the only member of the family with the endogenous agonist PP, while PYY and NPY can still activate this receptor with minor potency (**Table 2**). It consists of 375 amino acids and is mainly expressed in the gastrointestinal tract (Lundell et al., 1995; Ferrier et al., 2002) but also in the brain (Bard et al., 1995), as well as pancreas and prostate (Lundell et al., 1995). It plays a role in the regulation of feeding (Asakawa et al., 1999; Sainsbury et al., 2010), circadian ingestion and energy homeostasis (Edelsbrunner et al., 2009), colonic transit (Moriya et al., 2010), and stimulation of the luteinizing hormone release (Jain et al., 1999).

The Y_5 receptor subtype is expressed in two different splice variants, composed of 445 and 455 amino acids, respectively (**Table 1**). The N-terminus of the longer isoform is extended by 10 amino acids. However, these differences in the sequence of the receptor isoforms do not result in differences in their pharmacological profile (Rodriguez et al., 2003). Both receptor isoforms bind NPY and PYY with comparable affinities. The affinity for PP is slightly lower, but still in the nanomolar range (Gerald et al., 1996). Y_5 receptors are mainly expressed in the central nervous system. Tissues with high receptor density include the hippocampus and hypothalamus. The Y_5 receptor subtype has been shown to be strongly involved in food intake (Gerald et al., 1996). Other possible roles of the Y_5 receptor are the regulation of the circadian rhythm (Matsumoto et al., 1996b; Gribkoff et al., 1998) and reproduction through inhibition of LH release (Raposinho et al., 2001).

The y6 receptor encodes a 371 amino acid protein that has been cloned from rabbit, mouse, and chicken among others (Bromee et al., 2006). However, the sequence in humans and monkeys contains a frame shift mutation in the third intracellular loop, resulting in a non-functional truncated receptor protein (Matsumoto et al., 1996a; Michel et al., 1998).

Taken together, this multireceptor/multiligand system mediates many relevant physiological and pathological processes. This makes the NPY family truly attractive for the design of subtype selective analogs and receptors. Even if selective ligands are pharmacologically the most attractive approach to tackle subtype selectivity, development of receptor chimeras or receptor mutants will also help to understand how the receptors refined their binding pockets during evolution and, as a result, will show how the ligands tend to have distinct affinities for one or the other receptor subtype.

DEVELOPING SELECTIVE LIGANDS FOR NPY RECEPTORS

As it has been previously described, the binding affinity of each peptide differs from receptor to receptor and the role that each receptor plays in regulating physiological processes is different. In light of this, the NPY system is a perfect candidate in which to develop selective ligands and selective receptors to modulate these characteristics.

GENERAL STRATEGIES

The most conventional way of investigating subtype selectivity is the synthesis of selective ligands. Consequently, to obtain subtype selective ligands, the peptides have to be modified in key positions allowing the investigator to modulate the ligand preference for a receptor. Although the peptides of the NPY family share high sequence homology, they do not necessarily have the same binding mode. The truncation of certain fragments can direct the selectivity to a certain receptor subtype providing information about essential fragments of the peptide. Therefore, one of the approaches to investigate important positions on the peptides are N- or C- terminal truncations.

Another approach to investigate subtype selectivity is the alanine-scan or Ala-scan: this means that each residue in the sequence is one by one individually substituted with Ala. When an Ala occurs naturally in a certain position, this residue is then changed to Gly. In this scan, only the functional groups are substituted permitting the investigation of ionic interactions as well as dipole-dipole and hydrophobic interactions. Once all the analogs are synthesized they must be tested at all the receptor subtypes to determine how the substitution of the native amino acid affects the binding or the activation. In case a residue shows a great loss in binding or activation for a certain receptor, further exchanges in this position can be done. For example the exchange of a certain residue of NPY by the residue present in PP can achieve Y_4 receptor binding with the analog. The use of D-amino acids in a scan can provide information about the side chain orientation and steric information concerning ligand binding too, Pro-scans reveal favorable turn-structures and Phe-scans hydrophobic interactions (Lindner et al., 2008a).

As small peptides can adopt several active conformations and these conformations can be recognized by different receptor subtypes in structure-activity relationships, the knowledge of these binding subtypes is of great interest. Furthermore, to investigate the binding mode and receptor preference of small antagonists or non-peptidic drugs, knowledge of the bioactive conformation is of major importance. Constraining the ligand conformation and testing the peptide on several receptor subtypes, can provide information about its bioactive conformation and receptor selectivity. Several strategies can be used to investigate structure activity relationships constraining the conformation of small peptides (Beck-Sickinger, 1997). First of all, non-proteinogenic amino acids can be incorporated, reducing the number of angle combinations that a natural amino acid could adopt, and thereby decreasing the flexibility of the peptide. One example of a non-proteinogenic amino acid is Aib (aminoisobutyric acid). This residue is one the most commonly used in this kind of study. Secondly, the use of several templates and amino acid linkers to induce a desired conformation might be also a good strategy, although this does not always lead to the desired effect because of other amino acids within the sequence. The use of more flexible linkers such as Ahx (6-aminohexanoic acid) or ω-amino alkanoic acids might be a better method to determine the distance between two segments. Finally, the use of cyclization can significantly constrain the conformation of a ligand. Several cyclization techniques can be applied, the most commonly used are: cyclization by disulfide formation between two Cys residues, cyclization by lactamization of N- and/or C-terminus or by the N- and C-group-containing side chains Lys, Orn, Dab, Asp, and Glu and backbone to side-chain cyclization. Recent studies also use click reactions to cyclize peptides using triazoles to mimic disulfide bridges (Holland-Nell and Meldal, 2011) and peptide stapling to increase the propensity to form α-helices, therefore improving pharmacological properties (Verdine and Walensky, 2007).

Y_1 RECEPTOR

N-/C-terminal truncations of NPY confirm the importance of these two segments for Y_1 receptor binding. N-terminally truncated analogs are not well accepted by the Y_1 receptor as can be seen in studies using the shortened sequences NPY(3–36), (13–36), and (18–36). These show only micromolar affinities for this receptor and even the truncation of the first amino acid NPY(2–36), results in a loss of affinity (Beck-Sickinger and Jung, 1995). C-terminal truncations show the importance of the amide group in the binding with the receptor (Hoffmann et al., 1996). Centrally truncated analogs containing the spacer Ahx and structurally constrained analogs showed that the N- and C-terminal fragments must have a certain length to bind with a good affinity to the receptor (Kirby et al., 1993b). Furthermore, using an Ala-scan it was found that, Pro^2, Pro^5, Arg^{19}, and Tyr^{20} are important for ligand affinity. Also the amino acids from positions 27 to 36 were found to be crucial for the peptide, especially position 27. Moreover, positions 33 and 35 showed to be extremely important, as Ala analogs at these positions produced a dramatic loss in binding of >5000-fold over wt (**Figure 3**; Beck-Sickinger et al., 1994; Cabrele and Beck-Sickinger, 2000; Lindner et al., 2008b). The importance of Arg^{35} was further confirmed as this residue was found to form a subtype-specific ionic interaction with $Asp^{6.59}$ of the receptor (Merten et al., 2007). The Tyr on position 36 was also found to be relevant for the ligand binding; this position does however tolerate the exchange to Phe, but not Ala, Bpa, or His. Similar results were obtained using a D-amino acid scan (Kirby et al., 1993a).

Positions 7, 25, 26, 31, and 34 were revealed to be important for subtype selectivity (**Figure 1A**). Modifications in positions 25 and 26 showed that [D-Arg^{25}]NPY and [D-His^{26}]NPY bind selectively to the Y_1 receptor (Mullins et al., 2001). Also the introduction of Pro in position 34, present in pancreatic polypeptide, redirected the affinity of the peptide to Y_1/Y_5 receptors. Apart from Gln^{34}, an additional exchange in Asn^{7} introducing Phe at this position, a similar residue like the Tyr present on the hPP, yielded [Phe^{7}, Pro^{34}]pNPY. This is a selective Y_1 receptor binder and illustrated the importance of an aromatic residue in this position (Soll et al., 2001). Also the combination of Pro^{34} with an exchange in position 31 by Leu contributes to a$Y_1/Y_4/Y_5$receptor selective profile (Fuhlendorff et al., 1990; Cabrele et al., 2000). All this strongly indicates the importance of N- and C-terminal fragments for the Y_1 receptor subtype.

The synthesis of small selective ligands has also been a topic of interest in the past years and many peptides have been synthesized and characterized. Although the first experiments with short- or medium-sized pNPY truncations showed low binding affinity at the hY_1 receptor, in recent years several short antagonists, mimicking the NPY C-terminus have been synthesized such as, GR231118 (1229U91 or GW1229), T-241, and T-190. Unfortunately, these ligands also have Y_4 agonistic properties (**Figure 2**; Parker et al., 1998). Taking the short NPY analog NPY (28–36) and the antagonist GR231118, Zwanziger et al. (2009) designed a set of 19 short peptide analogs. Only [Pro^{30}, Nle^{31}, Bpa^{32}, Leu^{34}]NPY(28–36) displayed hY_1 receptor selectivity and was able to activate the receptor (**Figure 1B**). Follow-up investigations were made by Hofmann and colleagues (Neuropeptides, accepted) on position 32. The authors could further stabilize the peptide by replacing Bpa by Bip (biphenylalanine) and could switch the activity from hY_1 receptor to hY_2/hY_4 receptors by introducing an ortho-carbaboranyl moiety. Other small peptide antagonists are BW1911U90 and [$^{32-34}$βACC]-NPY(25–36)]; **Figure 2**; Koglin et al., 2003), and examples of known non-peptidic antagonists are BIBP3226, BIBO3304, LY357897, J-104870 (**Figure 4A**; Rudolf et al., 1994; Hipskind et al., 1997; Wieland et al., 1998; Sjodin et al., 2006; Antal-Zimanyi et al., 2008).

Y_2 RECEPTOR

As with the human Y_1 receptor, the Y_2 receptor binds NPY and PYY with comparable affinities. Beside these two native high-affinity ligands, a number of Y_2-selective NPY-derived peptide

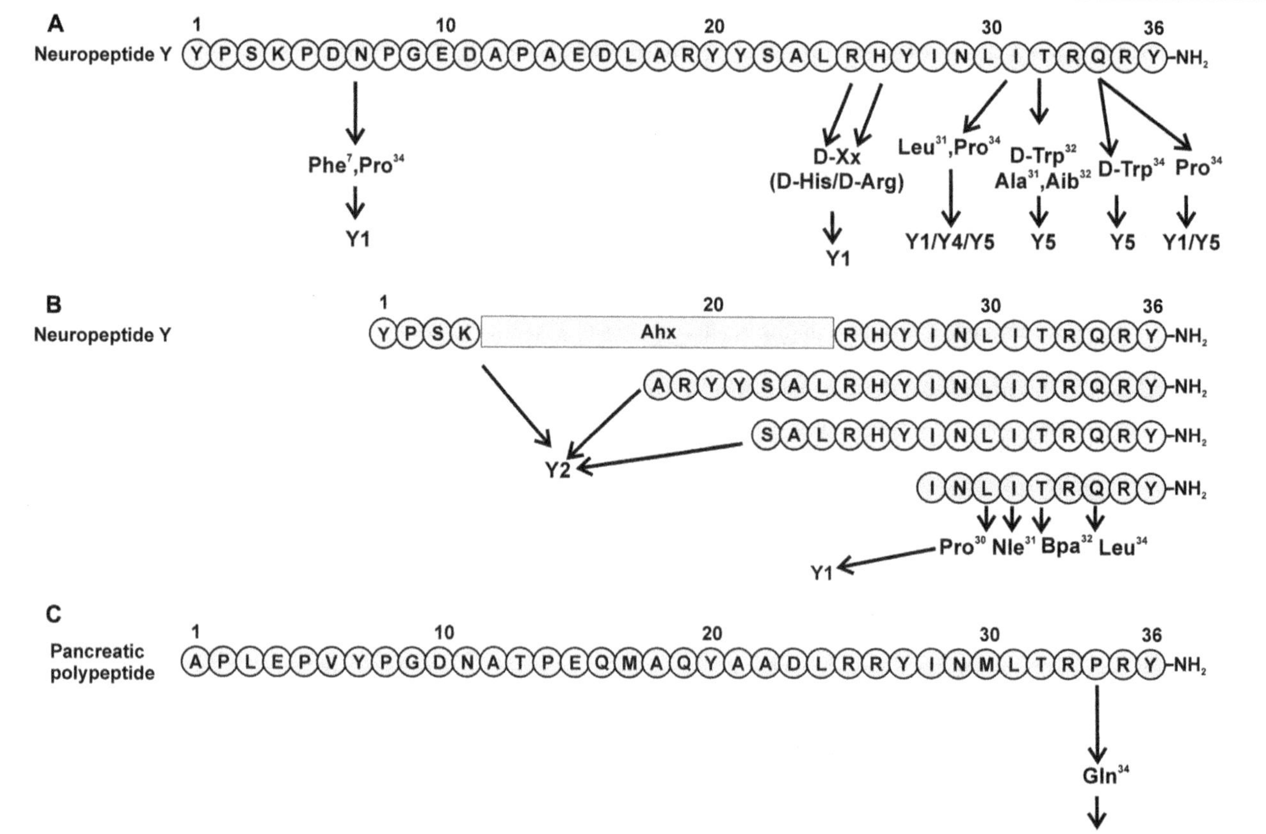

FIGURE 1 | Important amino acid positions and truncated peptides to introduce selectivity to NPY receptors. (A) Important positions in pNPY (Fuhlendorff et al., 1990; Cabrele et al., 2000, 2002; Parker et al., 2000; Mullins et al., 2001; Soll et al., 2001); **(B)** Truncations of pNPY (Beck et al., 1989; Fournier et al., 1994; Beck-Sickinger and Jung, 1995; Keire et al., 2000b; Zwanziger et al., 2009). **(C)** Important positions in hPP (Schwartz, 2006).

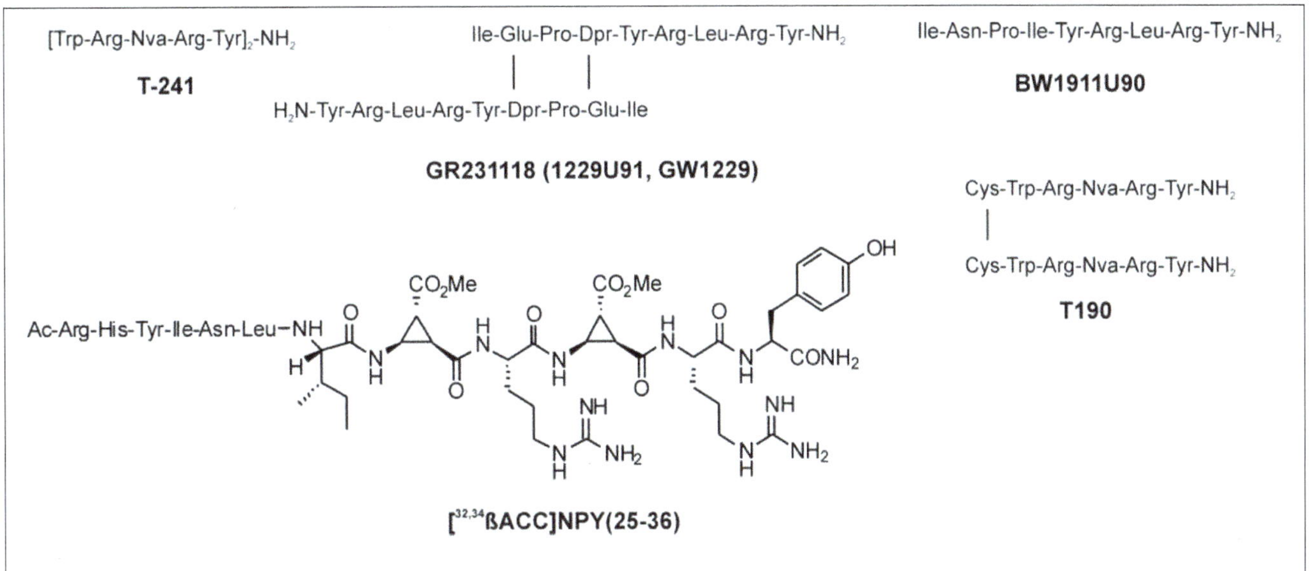

FIGURE 2 | Peptidic antagonists of the Y_1 receptor (Parker et al., 1998; Koglin et al., 2003).

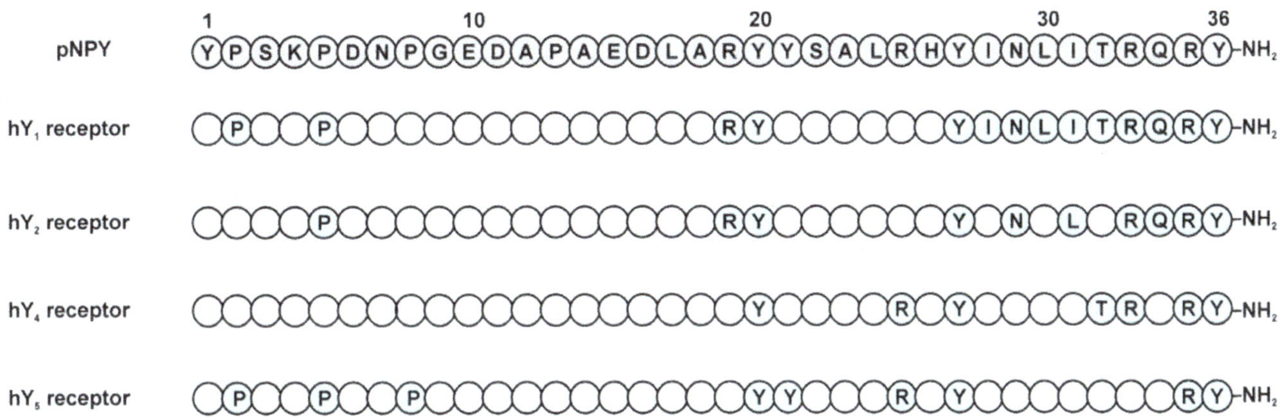

FIGURE 3 | Relevant amino acids in pNPY Ala-scan at NPY receptors. Positions in blue represent the amino acids showing a high impact when exchanged to Ala (Beck-Sickinger et al., 1994).

agonists have been synthesized in the past. Interestingly, in contrast to all other Y receptors, Y_2 receptors allow large truncations of the peptidic ligands without loss of affinity (Beck-Sickinger and Jung, 1995) and also cyclizations between N- and C-terminally located residues are tolerated (Kirby et al., 1993b). Most commonly used Y_2 receptor selective NPY-analogs are the N-terminally truncated NPY(3–36) and NPY(13–36). Even larger N-terminal truncations and centrally truncated analogs can bind to the Y_2 receptor with nanomolar affinity [e.g., NPY(18–36), NPY(22–36), [Ahx$^{5-24}$]NPY; **Figure 1B**; Beck et al., 1989; Fournier et al., 1994; Beck-Sickinger and Jung, 1995; Keire et al., 2000b]. An Ala-scan of the complete NPY peptide revealed only few positions to be highly important (**Figure 3**).

The substitution of Pro^5 to Ala led to a 600-fold loss of affinity. Accordingly, all other important residues except Pro^5 are located in the C-terminal part of NPY. The individual substitution of Arg^{19}, Tyr^{20}, Tyr^{27}, and Asn^{29} in the NPY peptide showed a 30- to 40-fold lower affinity. A more dramatic effect could be observed for the residues Leu^{31} (1000-fold lower affinity), Arg^{33} (1350-fold), Gln^{34} (150-fold), Arg^{35} (75000-fold), and Tyr^{36} (17500-fold; **Figure 3**; Cabrele and Beck-Sickinger, 2000; Eckard et al., 2001). Interestingly, the introduction of a Pro residue at position 34 is not tolerated at the Y_2 receptor, which is in contrast to the effect observed on the other Y receptor subtypes (Beck-Sickinger et al., 1994; Keire et al., 2000b; Eckard et al., 2001). Although Tyr^{36} may not be substituted by Ala, the introduction of Hty (homotyrosine) or p-substituted Phe in PYY(3–36) is well tolerated at the Y_2 receptor, but almost completely abolishes binding of the modified NPY analogs at Y_1 or Y_4 receptors (Pedersen et al., 2009). Taken together, these data underline the importance of the C-terminal part of the peptide ligand for high-affinity binding to the Y_2 receptor, despite the fact that the binding pocket for NPY at the Y_2 receptor seems to be less narrow than the ones of Y_1 or Y_4 receptors.

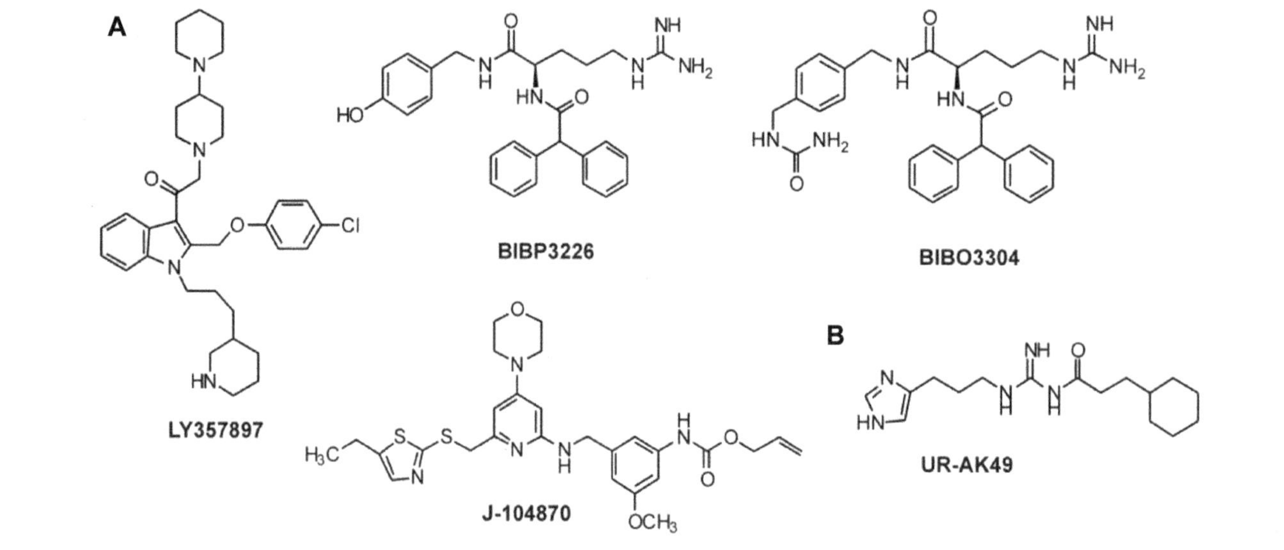

FIGURE 4 | Non-peptidic antagonists for Y_1 and Y_4 receptors. (A) Antagonists for the Y_1 receptor (Rudolf et al., 1994; Hipskind et al., 1997; Wieland et al., 1998; Balasubramaniam et al., 2001; Sjodin et al., 2006; Antal-Zimanyi et al., 2008); **(B)** Antagonists for the Y_4 receptor (Ziemek et al., 2007).

A number of selective high-affinity antagonists at the Y_2 receptor have been published so far. The most widely used compound in pharmacological studies is BIIE0246 (**Figure 5A**; Doods et al., 1999). In order to identify compounds with improved biostability, bioavailability, and brain permeability, further studies have been conducted. A number of molecules and scaffolds have been reported as highly selective and affine small molecule Y_2 receptor antagonists (**Figure 5A**) including JNJ-527787 (Bonaventure et al., 2004; Jablonowski et al., 2004), SF-11, SF-21, SF-22, SF-31, SF-41 (Brothers et al., 2010), ML072 to ML075 (Saldanha et al., 2009), JNJ-31020028 (Shoblock et al., 2010; Swanson et al., 2011), a series of substituted 3-chloranilides (Lunniss et al., 2009, 2010), CYM 9484, and CYM 9552 (Mittapalli et al., 2012).

Y_4 RECEPTOR

The Ala-scan of the NPY (Eckard et al., 2001) revealed that again Arg[33] and Arg[35] are crucial for receptor affinity. Ala substitutions in these positions led to a dramatic loss in binding. Positions

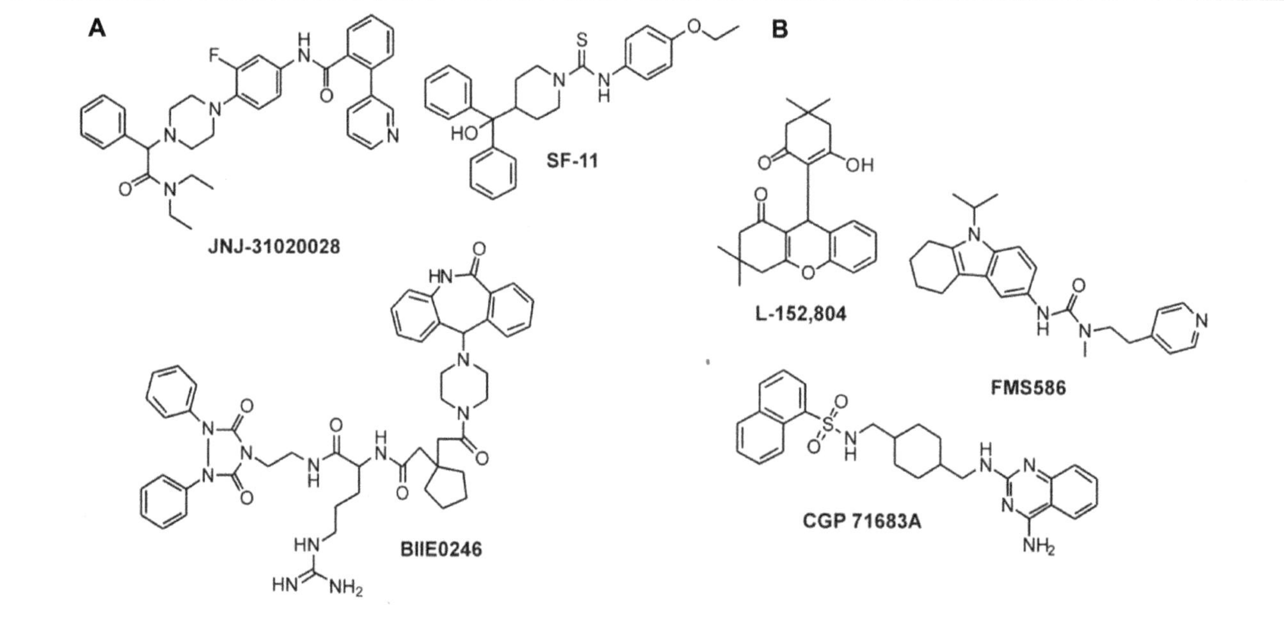

FIGURE 5 | Non-peptidic antagonists of Y_2 and Y_5 receptors. (A) Y_2 receptor antagonists (Doods et al., 1999; Saldanha et al., 2009; Shoblock et al., 2010; Swanson et al., 2011); **(B)** Y_5 receptor antagonists (Criscione et al., 1998; Kanatani et al., 2000a; Rueeger et al., 2000; Kakui et al., 2006).

Tyr^{20}, Tyr^{27}, Arg^{25}, Thr^{32}, and Tyr^{36} are also important residues in the ligand and showed a loss in binding affinity (30- to 60-fold), whereas Pro^{5}, Pro^{8}, and Tyr^{21} proved to be less relevant, causing only a slight loss in affinity (5- to 10-fold) when changed to Ala (**Figure 3**).

In a follow-up study using hPP (Merten et al., 2007), Arg residues 33 and 35 were confirmed to be essential for receptor activation, showing a dramatic effect when exchanged to Ala in position 33. Position Arg^{35} was found to interact with $Asp^{6.59}$ of the receptor.

Because this receptor subtype has its own selective ligand, peptide research is more focused on improving proteolytic stability and increasing bioavailability of the peptide. However, a number of specific ligands have been published in the past years for this receptor. As previously described, position 34 of NPY peptides is a key residue to introduce Y_4 receptor selectivity to NPY and PYY, whereas in PP when exchanging Pro^{34} for Gln the peptide acquires Y_2 agonistic properties without losing Y_4 receptor activity. Some of the analogs published like $[Gln^{34}]$-hPP, the so called Obinepitide (Schwartz, 2006), which is selective for Y_2 and Y_4 receptors, contains this exchange (**Figure 1C**). Other small peptide agonists described also as Y_1 receptor antagonists are: GR23-1118 (1229U91 or GW1229), T-241, and T-190 (**Figure 2**; Schober et al., 1998).

To our knowledge, only one ligand with antagonistic properties at the hY_4 receptor has been published up to now. UR-AK49 (**Figure 4B**) is a weak hY_4 receptor antagonist but unselective, because it can also bind to hY_1 and hY_5 receptors (Ziemek et al., 2007).

Y_5 RECEPTOR

The hY_5 receptor subtype does not tolerate large truncations of NPY. While the deletion of the first amino acid is accepted by the hY_5 receptor, further N-terminal truncation of NPY results in a decreased affinity of the peptides. Similarly, larger central truncations of NPY are not tolerated by Y_5 receptors. The only centrally truncated analog of NPY with high Y_5 receptor affinity is $[Ahx^{9-17}]$pNPY with a ~15-fold decreased affinity compared to pNPY (Cabrele and Beck-Sickinger, 2000).

An Ala scan of the complete peptide revealed the Pro residues 2, 5, and 8 to be important for the affinity of NPY at the Y_5 (**Figure 3**). Haack et al. (2008) could confirm the importance of the peptide N-terminus for high-affinity binding at the Y_5 receptor by a pyridone dipeptide scan. In addition to these findings, the individual substitution of Tyr residues 20, 21, 27, and 36 to Ala led to a loss of affinity; Arg^{25} was also shown to be important for the ligand affinity. The highest impact could be observed for Tyr^{27} (~400-fold) and Arg^{35} (1000-fold; Cabrele and Beck-Sickinger, 2000), these findings fit with the fact that these two positions are involved in interactions with the receptor.

A number of selective high-affinity analogs of NPY and PYY have been developed in the past. It has been shown that especially the substitution of position 32 of the peptide ligands is critical for Y_5 selectivity (**Figure 1A**). $[D\text{-}Trp^{32}]$NPY and $[Ala^{31}, Aib^{32}]$NPY have been reported to be highly selective and potent agonists of Y_5 receptor (Parker et al., 2000; Cabrele et al., 2002). However, the most potent and selective activator of the Y_5 receptor subtype is a chimeric peptide derived from chicken PP, human NPY, and human PP ($[cPP^{1-7}, NPY^{19-23}, His^{34}]$hPP; Cabrele and Beck-Sickinger, 2000). In addition, Y_5 receptors display high-affinity to some NPY analogs which also have a considerable affinity for other Y receptor subtypes. $[Leu^{31}, Pro^{34}]$pNPY is a $Y_1/Y_4/Y_5$ selective agonist (Fuhlendorff et al., 1990; Widdowson et al., 1997), whereas the deletion of the first Tyr residue results in the Y_2/Y_5 selective agonist NPY (2–36) (Gerald et al., 1996).

Since NPY has been shown to stimulate feeding via the Y_5 receptor, intensive research has been performed to identify small molecule antagonists of the human Y_5 receptor as potential feeding suppressors. The first compound that was published as an antagonist of Y_5 receptor was CGP71683A (**Figure 5B**), which displayed high-affinity and selectivity at the rY_5 receptor (Criscione et al., 1998). Later studies confirmed the high-affinity and selectivity also for the hY_5 receptor subtype (Rueeger et al., 2000). Other selective small antagonists at the human Y_5 receptor include L152,804 (Kanatani et al., 2000a), FMS586 (Kakui et al., 2006), MK-0557 (Erondu et al., 2007), and SCH 500946 (Mullins et al., 2008). In the last 5 years, more than 10 studies have been published presenting newly identified or improved small molecule antagonists of the Y_5 receptor. This clearly shows the importance of the Y_5 receptor as an anti-obesity target.

HOW TO IDENTIFY RELEVANT RESIDUES ON THE RECEPTOR FOR BINDING AND SUBTYPE SELECTIVITY

GENERAL STRATEGIES

As these receptors consist of 350–450 residues it is impossible to perform a single mutagenesis approach to investigate each amino acid. In order to overcome this problem chimeric receptors can be used, in which fragments of a receptor (e.g., extracellular loops or transmembrane helices) can be exchanged between receptor subtypes. Testing these new constructs with the main agonist from both receptor subtypes can provide information about the importance of one or the other segment, in terms of interaction with the ligand. As soon as an important area in a receptor has been identified, a more detailed study can be carried out using single and multiple mutants, where certain residues of a receptor subtype are exchanged by the ones present on the other receptor subtype of investigation. This strategy allows to find amino acids that may play a role in selectivity to a certain agonist.

When investigating the relevance of the N-terminus, successive truncations or substitutions using tags or spacers can be an elegant method. Furthermore, C-terminal truncations can provide information about segments relevant for internalization. It is known that this receptor part is involved in arrestin-dependent internalization processes of Y_1, Y_2, and Y_5 receptors (Walther et al., 2011). However, single mutagenesis techniques can be used to investigate important residues for the structure or for ligand receptor interactions. Using this approach, certain residues located in extracellular areas of the protein are mutated to Ala or other amino acids in single substitutions. The residues can be chosen according to its location, charge, aromaticity, hydrophobicity. Moreover, 3-D models are also a good tool to select new targets, although mutagenesis data are needed to refine the models and make them more reliable. Once a relevant residue has been identified, double cycle mutagenesis can be used to find the type of interaction that includes both positions. In this technique, peptide analogs containing modifications in positions of interest are investigated with receptor mutants. The aim is to form artificial bonds to proof a native interaction. The introduction of charged residues in the peptide and receptor positions to create a repulsion/attraction, or aromatic residues and hydrophobic residues are feasible ways to prove a ligand receptor interaction. In order to finally prove a ligand-receptor interaction, a reciprocal mutation approach can be followed, where the residue of interest on the peptide side is exchanged by the residue present on the receptor side and *vice versa.* In the case of a critical position or segment, the binding affinity of the native ligand should significantly decrease, whereas in signal transduction assays the EC_{50} or half maximal activation value should increase. Despite all the advantages that these approaches provide, it has to be taken into account that they also present some disadvantages. Thus, when constructing receptor chimeras or receptor mutants, alterations in the receptor structure may arise due to misfolding and therefore may lead to impaired receptor export. Moreover, these modifications might result in a reduced receptor retention time at the cell surface and an enhanced degradation. All together, this might lead to a loss in binding or receptor activity. In order to analyze such phenomena, fluorescence microscopy, cell surface ELISA or radioligand binding studies are a good tool to ensure cell surface expression.

Y_1 RECEPTOR

In the past years, much effort has been made to characterize this receptor. Using N-terminal truncations and receptor chimera, it could be elucidated that the N-terminal part of NPY receptors does not participate in the binding pocket. N-terminal truncation in the hY_1 receptor disrupts the membrane expression; however any eight residues are enough to recover the membrane expression (Lindner et al., 2009).

From all these studies, a number of residues emerged as important for the receptor. First of all, two negatively charged residues are able to establish electrostatic interaction. $Asp^{2.68}$ and $Asp^{6.59}$ were found to be important for the receptor as the peptide loses affinity when mutated to Ala (Sautel et al., 1995, 1996; Kannoa et al., 2001; Sjodin et al., 2006). Furthermore $Asp^{6.59}$ was shown to bind Arg^{35} of pNPY being the first and only proved interaction for this receptor (Merten et al., 2007). Other residues that appeared to be important in several studies are $Tyr^{2.64}$, $Phe^{6.58}$, and $His^{7.31}$ (Sautel et al., 1995, 1996; Kannoa et al., 2001; Sjodin et al., 2006), although a direct interaction was never established for any of the amino acids of the ligand. It was suggested that these residues form a hydrophobic pocket in the receptor. Further investigations using the Y_1 receptor antagonist BIBP 3226 showed that $Tyr^{2.64}$ and $His^{7.31}$ did not affect the conformation of the receptor in a major way (Sautel et al., 1996) as the antagonist was perfectly bound. Taken together, it is very likely that position 6.58 and 7.31 interact with a C-terminally located amino acid, on the other hand it is unlikely that $Tyr^{2.64}$ interacts with the C-terminus as it seems to be too far from the other two residues.

Other relevant residues of the receptor are $Trp^{6.60}$, $Asn^{6.55}$, and $Asn^{7.32}$ (Kannoa et al., 2001). Although position 6.55 is in a slightly deeper position, $Asn^{6.55}$ and $Asn^{7.32}$ showed a loss in PYY binding and also in antagonist binding suggesting that they could play a role in ligand binding (**Figure 6A**).

Studies with antagonists indicate that the binding of these compounds differs depending on the ligand between transmembrane helices 3 and 7. Taking all the data into consideration, it can be assumed that the binding pattern of the native ligands and the small antagonists overlaps in TM6 because several residues have been found to be relevant in both cases.

Y_2 RECEPTOR

In this receptor subtype, the N-terminus does not play a role in membrane expression and it does not participate in a subtype specific binding pocket. However, it does play a role in agonist induced internalization processes since the complete truncation slowed down the process, although it could be seen that the exchange of the N-terminal fragment by the hY_1 receptor or hY_5 receptor fragment did not affect ligand dependent internalization (Lindner et al., 2009).

Mutagenesis studies to identify residues that contribute to ligand binding in the Y_2 receptor were initially motivated by the finding that human and chicken Y_2 receptors show a significantly different pharmacological profile. The chicken Y_2 receptor is able to bind [Leu^{31},Pro^{34}]-NPY, a peptide agonist selective for mammalian $Y_1/Y_4/Y_5$ receptors, but was unable to bind BIIE0246, a small molecule antagonist for mammalian Y_2 receptors (Salaneck et al., 2000). Sequence comparison and reciprocal mutagenesis revealed three residues in transmembrane helices 3, 5, and 6 that contribute to the binding of BIIE0246. Individual and combined substitution of $Gln^{3.37}$, $Leu^{5.51}$, and $Leu^{6.51}$ in the hY_2 receptor decreased the affinity for BIIE0246 to a chY_2-like level, whereas substitution of the corresponding residues in the chY_2 by the human residues increased the affinity for BIIE0246 (Berglund et al., 2002). Further mutagenesis studies on the human Y_2 receptor revealed interaction partners for the native peptidic ligand NPY. Several acidic residues have been tested for their importance for NPY binding. $Glu^{5.27}$ and $Asp^{6.59}$ turned out to be highly important for the binding of NPY (**Figure 6C**). While $Asp^{6.59}$ is important for all Y receptor subtypes, $Glu^{5.27}$ only plays a role in the Y_2 receptor. Both receptor mutants were tested in a signal transduction assay using pNPY, [Ala^{25}]pNPY, [Ala^{33}]pNPY, and [Ala^{35}]pNPY to identify the interaction partner of the two acidic residues in the peptide. It could be shown that $Asp^{6.59}$ interacts with Arg^{33} of the peptidic ligand in the Y_2 and Y_5 receptors, whereas the interaction partner in Y_1 and Y_4 receptors is Arg^{35}. However, no direct interaction partner could be identified for $Glu^{5.27}$ (Merten et al., 2007). More recent studies investigated additional residues in the Y_2 receptor for their impact on the binding of pPYY, pNPY, hPYY (3–36), pNPY(13–36), and the non-peptidic antagonist BIIE0246 (Akerberg et al., 2010; Fallmar et al., 2011). The residues tested, namely $Tyr^{2.64}$, $Gly^{2.68}$, $Thr^{3.40}$, $Leu^{4.60}$, $Gln^{6.55}$, $Val^{6.58}$, and $Tyr^{7.31}$, were chosen by similarity to residues in the Y_1 receptor subtype, which were proven to be important for ligand binding in this receptor subtype. It could be shown, that of the tested residues, only $Tyr^{2.64}$ participates in the binding of all tested peptidic ligands and

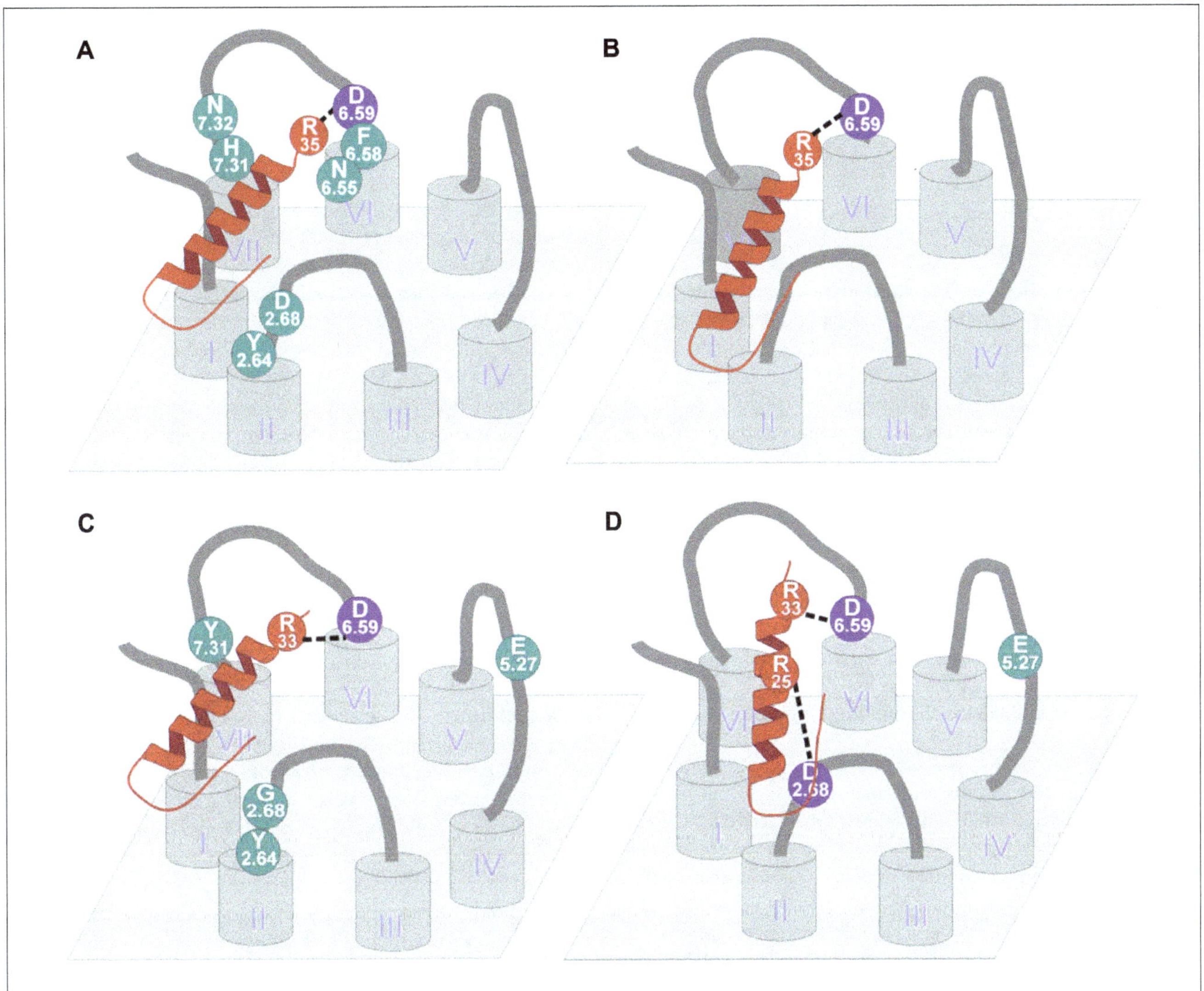

FIGURE 6 | Binding mode of NPY receptors. **(A)** hY_1 receptor binding mode (Sautel et al., 1995, 1996; Kannoa et al., 2001; Sjodin et al., 2006; Merten et al., 2007); **(B)** hY_4 receptor binding mode (Merten et al., 2007); **(C)** hY_2 receptor binding mode (Merten et al., 2007; Akerberg et al., 2010); **(D)** hY_5 receptor binding mode (Merten et al., 2007; Lindner et al., 2008b).

the non-peptidic antagonist BIIE0246. The substitution of this residue to Ala resulted in a five- to ninefold reduction in affinity (Akerberg et al., 2010).

The individual substitution of $Tyr^{7.31}$ by Ala and $Gly^{2.68}$ by the bigger and more polar residue Asn revealed a lower affinity only for the truncated peptide agonists. The authors hypothesize that $Tyr^{7.31}$ does not play a role in binding of the full-length peptide, but may contribute to a compensatory interaction for ligands that lack the N-terminal residues. Furthermore, the authors could show that an introduction of a His residue in position 7.31 (the corresponding residue in Y_1 receptor) completely abolished the binding of $[^{125}I]$-pPYY (Akerberg et al., 2010). These findings are somewhat unexpected, since this His residue was shown to be involved in ligand binding in the Y_1 receptor (Sjodin et al., 2006). This indicates that position 7.31 is important in both receptor subtypes, but may have different modes of action (Akerberg et al., 2010). For position 2.68, a mode of binding is proposed in which the lack of Asp (a residue common to all other Y receptor subtypes at this position) contributes to the selectivity of truncated peptides [e.g., NPY(3–36)] for the Y_2 receptor (Fallmar et al., 2011). The $Leu^{4.60}$Ala mutant showed a slightly decreased affinity for hPYY(3–36) and a strong loss of affinity for BIIE0246, which may be caused by a weakened or lost hydrophobic interaction. This indicates that this residue is highly important for antagonist binding. The corresponding position in Y_1 receptor ($Phe^{4.60}$) has been shown to be involved in the binding of $[^{125}I]$NPY, $[^{3}H]$BIBP3226 (Sautel et al., 1996) as well as $[^{3}H]$J-104870 (Kannoa et al., 2001). This indicates that position 4.60 is involved in the binding of small molecule antagonists at both receptor subtypes, Y_1 and Y_2.

The Y_2 receptor mutants $Thr^{3.40}$Ile and $Gln^{6.55}$Ala showed increased affinity for pNPY and hPYY(3–36), but decreased affinity for the non-peptidic antagonist BIIE0246. Taken into account that these positions are located deeper in the transmembrane part of the receptor, an indirect effect on the binding of peptidic ligands would be the most likely explanation. However, the decreased binding of BIIE0246 may be also explained by a different binding pocket for small molecule antagonists, located more deeply in the transmembrane (Fallmar et al., 2011) and surrounded not only by $Thr^{3.40}$ and $Gln^{6.55}$, but also by the nearby residue $Gln^{3.37}$, which was earlier shown to participate in the binding of BIIE0246 earlier (Berglund et al., 2002).

Y_4 RECEPTOR

N-terminal truncations and substitutions revealed the importance of this fragment for membrane expression and indicated that the N-terminus is not involved in forming a specific binding pocket. It is likely that this part could stabilize the TM1 to ensure the correct receptor structure (Lindner et al., 2009).

Two positions were investigated to find the binding partners on the ligand side (Merten et al., 2007). $Glu^{5.24}$ was mutated to Ala in order to test the influence of the side chain, $Glu^{5.24}$Ala showed a threefold loss in potency. On the other hand, $Asp^{6.59}$ was mutated to Ala, Glu, Asn, and Arg to test the influence of charge and length of the side chain. The mutation to Ala showed a complete loss of both binding and activity, the exchange to Glu displayed wild-type-like binding and activation. In addition, the mutation to Asn showed indeterminate binding and a 200-fold loss in activation. Finally the exchange to Arg resulted in a dramatic loss in potency (>600-fold) and in no detectable binding (**Figure 6B**).

Y_5 RECEPTOR

The Y_5 subtype N-terminus could play a role in ligand binding, since the partial truncation of the segment produced a loss in activation. Interestingly, the receptor remains on the membrane even when the complete N-terminus is removed (Lindner et al., 2009).

Only few mutagenesis studies have been published so far for the human Y_5 receptor. Merten et al. (2007) exchanged three acidic residues in the extracellular domains of Y_5 receptor. While the $Asp^{6.62}$Ala mutant showed wild-type-like pharmacological properties, $Asp^{6.59}$Ala and $Glu^{5.27}$Ala displayed a dramatically reduced affinity for NPY. Additional residues were investigated by Lindner et al. (2008b), resulting in identification of a third acidic residue ($Asp^{2.68}$) which is important for ligand binding at the Y_5 receptor. These Ala-mutants have also been tested with NPY analogs in which theTyr^{27}, Tyr^{36}, and the Arg residues at position 25, 33, and 35 were individually substituted by Ala (**Figure 6D**). This approach revealed no further loss of affinity for [Ala^{33}]pNPY on the $Asp^{6.59}$Ala mutant of the receptor, indicating a direct interaction between Ala^{33} of the peptide and $Asp^{6.59}$ of the receptor. Similarly, Arg^{25} of the NPY peptide could be identified as the interaction partner for $Asp^{2.68}$ of the receptor (Lindner et al., 2008b).

CONCLUSION AND PERSPECTIVES

The NPY system has been extensively characterized in the last years. The modulation of actions mediated by the distinct receptors like, e.g., its involvement in obesity, cancer, and epilepsy are of great importance. Therefore, the development of receptor subtype-selective ligands and structure-activity relationship studies have been a major objective in the past years. Primarily, amino acid scans and truncations have identified the important residues and areas of the ligand with respect to binding at each receptor. The Y receptors have been extensively studied, several important residues have been characterized and some of the binding pockets have been partially characterized. Two subtype-selective interactions have been elucidated so far. A similar binding mode has been identified on NPY receptors, where a common residue $Asp^{6.59}$ binds to one of the two C-terminally located Arg of the peptide depending on the receptor subtype. Moreover, a second binding interaction has been found on the Y_5 receptor where $Asp^{2.68}$ located at the top of TM2 interacts with Arg^{25} of the peptide (Merten et al., 2007; Lindner et al., 2008b). This finding would suggest that probably a second interaction could take place in other receptor subtypes. Nevertheless, further investigations have to be performed. It is likely that more interactions between the receptors and the peptides could occur, therefore structure activity relationship studies are still a focus of interest.

The design of short analogs and antagonists have confirmed these findings, indicating that this is a great tool to modulate and study the receptors. Some promising progresses have been achieved in cancer diagnosis using Y_1 receptor selective short ligands. However the development of short analogs for treatment of this pathology still remains challenging. Also in anti-obesity drugs, Y_2/Y_4receptor selective agonists are in progress and currently in clinical trials of Phase I/II. On the basis of well studied characteristics accounting for receptor subtype selectivity, it is likely that subsequent investigations could be focused on the improvement of pharmacological properties such as stability and half-life. In addition the development of more potent selective ligands might be a focus of interest.

ACKNOWLEDGMENT

The financial contribution of the German Research Foundation (DFG) for SFB 610/3, project A1 is kindly acknowledged.

REFERENCES

Akerberg, H., Fallmar, H., Sjodin, P., Boukharta, L., Gutierrez-De-Teran, H., Lundell, I., et al. (2010). Mutagenesis of human neuropeptide Y/peptide YY receptor Y2 reveals additional differences to Y1 in interactions with highly conserved ligand positions. *Regul. Pept.* 163, 120–129.

Antal-Zimanyi, I., Bruce, M. A., Leboulluec, K. L., Iben, L. G., Mattson, G. K., Mcgovern, R. T., et al. (2008). Pharmacological characterization and appetite suppressive properties of BMS-193885, a novel and selective neuropeptide Y(1) receptor antagonist. *Eur. J. Pharmacol.* 590, 224–232.

Asakawa, A., Inui, A., Ueno, N., Fujimiya, M., Fujino, M. A., and Kasuga, M. (1999). Mouse pancreatic polypeptide modulates food intake, while not influencing anxiety in mice. *Peptides* 20, 1445–1448.

Asakawa, A., Inui, A., Yuzuriha, H., Ueno, N., Katsuura, G., Fujimiya, M., et al. (2003). Characterization of the effects of pancreatic polypeptide in the regulation of energy balance. *Gastroenterology* 124, 1325–1336.

Balasubramaniam, A. (2002). Clinical potentials of neuropeptide Y family of hormones. *Am. J. Surg.* 183, 430–434.

Balasubramaniam, A., Dhawan, V. C., Mullins, D. E., Chance, W. T., Sheriff, S., Guzzi, M., et al. (2001). Highly selective and potent neuropeptide Y (NPY) Y1 receptor antagonists based on [Pro(30), Tyr(32), Leu(34)]NPY(28–36)-NH2 (BW1911U90). *J. Med. Chem.* 44, 1479–1482.

Baldock, P. A., Lee, N. J., Driessler, F., Lin, S., Allison, S., Stehrer, B., et al. (2009). Neuropeptide Y knockout mice reveal a central role of NPY in the coordination of bone mass to body weight. *PLoS ONE* 4:e8415. doi: 10.1371/journal.pone.0008415

Baldock, P. A., Sainsbury, A., Couzens, M., Enriquez, R. F., Thomas, G.

P., Gardiner, E. M., et al. (2002). Hypothalamic Y2 receptors regulate bone formation. *J. Clin. Invest.* 109, 915–921.

Bard, J. A., Walker, M. W., Branchek, T. A., and Weinshank, R. L. (1995). Cloning and functional expression of a human Y4 subtype receptor for pancreatic polypeptide, neuropeptide Y, and peptide YY. *J. Biol. Chem.* 270, 26762–26765.

Beck-Sickinger, A. G. (1997). "Synthesis of conformationally restricted peptides," in *Neuropeptide Protocols*, eds G. Brent Irvine and Carvell H. Williams (Totowa, NJ: Humana Press), 61–74.

Beck-Sickinger, A. G., and Jung, G. (1995). Structure-activity relationships of neuropeptide Y analogues with respect to Y1 and Y2 receptors. *Biopolymers* 37, 123–142.

Beck-Sickinger, A. G., Wieland, H. A., Wittneben, H., Willim, K. D., Rudolf, K., and Jung, G. (1994). Complete L-alanine scan of neuropeptide Y reveals ligands binding to Y1 and Y2 receptors with distinguished conformations. *Eur. J. Biochem.* 225, 947–958.

Beck, A., Jung, G., Gaida, W., Koppen, H., Lang, R., and Schnorrenberg, G. (1989). Highly potent and small neuropeptide Y agonist obtained by linking NPY 1–4 via spacer to alpha-helical NPY 25–36. *FEBS Lett.* 244, 119–122.

Berglund, M. M., Fredriksson, R., Salaneck, E., and Larhammar, D. (2002). Reciprocal mutations of neuropeptide Y receptor Y2 in human and chicken identify amino acids important for antagonist binding. *FEBS Lett.* 518, 5–9.

Blomqvist, A. G., and Herzog, H. (1997). Y-receptor subtypes – how many more? *Trends Neurosci.* 20, 294–298.

Blomqvist, A. G., Soderberg, C., Lundell, I., Milner, R. J., and Larhammar, D. (1992). Strong evolutionary conservation of neuropeptide Y: sequences of chicken, goldfish, and Torpedo marmorata DNA clones. *Proc. Natl. Acad. Sci. U.S.A.* 89, 2350–2354.

Blundell, T. L., Pitts, J. E., Tickle, I. J., Wood, S. P., and Wu, C. W. (1981). X-ray analysis (1. 4-A resolution) of avian pancreatic polypeptide: small globular protein hormone. *Proc. Natl. Acad. Sci. U.S.A.* 78, 4175–4179.

Boguszewski, C. L., Paz, G., and Velloso, L. A. (2010). Neuroendocrine body weight regulation: integration between fat tissue, gastrointestinal tract, and the brain. *Endokrynol. Pol.* 61, 194–206.

Bonaventure, P., Nepomuceno, D., Mazur, C., Lord, B., Rudolph, D. A., Jablonowski, J. A., et al. (2004). Characterization of *N*-(1-Acetyl-2,3-dihydro-1H-indol-6-yl)-3-(3-cyano-phenyl)-*N*-[1-(2-cyclopentyl-ethyl)-piperidin-4yl]acrylamide (JNJ-5207787), a small molecule antagonist of the neuropeptide Y Y2 receptor. *J. Pharmacol. Exp. Ther.* 308, 1130–1137.

Bonini, J. A., Jones, K. A., Adham, N., Forray, C., Artymyshyn, R., Durkin, M. M., et al. (2000). Identification and characterization of two G protein-coupled receptors for neuropeptide FF. *J. Biol. Chem.* 275, 39324–39331.

Bromee, T., Sjodin, P., Fredriksson, R., Boswell, T., Larsson, T. A., Salaneck, E., et al. (2006). Neuropeptide Y-family receptors Y6 and Y7 in chicken. Cloning, pharmacological characterization, tissue distribution and conserved synteny with human chromosome region. *FEBS J.* 273, 2048–2063.

Brothers, S. P., Saldanha, S. A., Spicer, T. P., Cameron, M., Mercer, B. A., Chase, P., et al. (2010). Selective and brain penetrant neuropeptide y y2 receptor antagonists discovered by whole-cell high-throughput screening. *Mol. Pharmacol.* 77, 46–57.

Caberlotto, L., Fuxe, K., Sedvall, G., and Hurd, Y. L. (1997). Localization of neuropeptide Y Y1 mRNA in the human brain: abundant expression in cerebral cortex and striatum. *Eur. J. Neurosci.* 9, 1212–1225.

Cabrele, C., and Beck-Sickinger, A. G. (2000). Molecular characterization of the ligand-receptor interaction of the neuropeptide Y family. *J. Pept. Sci.* 6, 97–122.

Cabrele, C., Langer, M., Bader, R., Wieland, H. A., Doods, H. N., Zerbe, O., et al. (2000). The first selective agonist for the neuropeptide YY5 receptor increases food intake in rats. *J. Biol. Chem.* 275, 36043–36048.

Cabrele, C., Wieland, H. A., Koglin, N., Stidsen, C., and Beck-Sickinger, A. G. (2002). Ala31-Aib32: identification of the key motif for high affinity and selectivity of neuropeptide Y at the Y5-receptor. *Biochemistry* 41, 8043–8049.

Castan, I., Valet, P., Larrouy, D., Voisin, T., Remaury, A., Daviaud, D., et al. (1993). Distribution of PYY receptors in human fat cells: an antilipolytic system alongside the alpha 2-adrenergic system. *Am. J. Physiol.* 265, E74–E80.

Cherezov, V., Rosenbaum, D. M., Hanson, M. A., Rasmussen, S. G., Thian, F. S., Kobilka, T. S., et al. (2007). High-resolution crystal structure of an engineered human beta2-adrenergic G protein-coupled receptor. *Science* 318, 1258–1265.

Criscione, L., Rigollier, P., Batzl-Hartmann, C., Rueger, H., Stricker-Krongrad, A., Wyss, P., et al. (1998). Food intake in free-feeding and energy-deprived lean rats is mediated by the neuropeptide Y5 receptor. *J. Clin. Invest.* 102, 2136–2145.

Doods, H., Gaida, W., Wieland, H. A., Dollinger, H., Schnorrenberg, G., Esser, F., et al. (1999). BIIE0246: a selective and high affinity neuropeptide Y Y(2) receptor antagonist. *Eur. J. Pharmacol.* 384, R3–R5.

Eckard, C. P., Cabrele, C., Wieland, H. A., and Beck-Sickinger, A. G. (2001). Characterisation of neuropeptide Y receptor subtypes by synthetic NPY analogues and by anti-receptor antibodies. *Molecules* 6, 448–467.

Edelsbrunner, M. E., Painsipp, E., Herzog, H., and Holzer, P. (2009). Evidence from knockout mice for distinct implications of neuropeptide-Y Y2 and Y4 receptors in the circadian control of locomotion, exploration, water and food intake. *Neuropeptides* 43, 491–497.

Erondu, N., Wadden, T., Gantz, I., Musser, B., Nguyen, A. M., Bays, H., et al. (2007). Effect of NPY5R antagonist MK-0557 on weight regain after very-low-calorie diet-induced weight loss. *Obesity (Silver Spring)* 15, 895–905.

Fallmar, H., Akerberg, H., Gutierrez-De-Teran, H., Lundell, I., Mohell, N., and Larhammar, D. (2011). Identification of positions in the human neuropeptide Y/peptide YY receptor Y2 that contribute to pharmacological differences between receptor subtypes. *Neuropeptides* 45, 293–300.

Ferrier, L., Segain, J. P., Bonnet, C., Cherbut, C., Lehur, P. A., Jarry, A., et al. (2002). Functional mapping of NPY/PYY receptors in rat and human gastro-intestinal tract. *Peptides* 23, 1765–1771.

Flood, J. F., and Morley, J. E. (1989). Dissociation of the effects of neuropeptide Y on feeding and memory: evidence for pre- and postsynaptic mediation. *Peptides* 10, 963–966.

Fournier, A., Gagnon, D., Quirion, R., Cadieux, A., Dumont, Y., Pheng, L. H., et al. (1994). Conformational and biological studies of neuropeptide-Y analogs containing structural alterations. *Mol. Pharmacol.* 45, 93–101.

Fuhlendorff, J., Gether, U., Aakerlund, L., Langeland-Johansen, N., Thogersen, H., Melberg, S. G., et al. (1990). [Leu31, Pro34]neuropeptide Y: a specific Y1 receptor agonist. *Proc. Natl. Acad. Sci. U.S.A.* 87, 182–186.

Gehlert, D. R. (1998). Multiple receptors for the pancreatic polypeptide (PP-fold) family: physiological implications. *Proc. Soc. Exp. Biol. Med.* 218, 7–22.

Gerald, C., Walker, M. W., Criscione, L., Gustafson, E. L., Batzl-Hartmann, C., Smith, K. E., et al. (1996). A receptor subtype involved in neuropeptide-Y-induced food intake. *Nature* 382, 168–171.

Golombek, D. A., Biello, S. M., Rendon, R. A., and Harrington, M. E. (1996). Neuropeptide Y phase shifts the circadian clock *in vitro* via a Y2 receptor. *Neuroreport* 7, 1315–1319.

Gribkoff, V. K., Pieschl, R. L., Wisialowski, T. A., Van Den Pol, A. N., and Yocca, F. D. (1998). Phase shifting of circadian rhythms and depression of neuronal activity in the rat suprachiasmatic nucleus by neuropeptide Y: mediation by different receptor subtypes. *J. Neurosci.* 18, 3014–3022.

Haack, M., Enck, S., Seger, H., Geyer, A., and Beck-Sickinger, A. G. (2008). Pyridone dipeptide backbone scan to elucidate structural properties of a flexible peptide segment. *J. Am. Chem. Soc.* 130, 8326–8336.

Hankir, M. K., Parkinson, J. R., Minnion, J. S., Addison, M. L., Bloom, S. R., and Bell, J. D. (2011). Peptide YY 3-36 and pancreatic polypeptide differentially regulate hypothalamic neuronal activity in mice *in vivo* as measured by manganese-enhanced magnetic resonance imaging. *J. Neuroendocrinol.* 23, 371–380.

Hausman, G. J., Barb, C. R., and Dean, R. G. (2008). Patterns of gene expression in pig adipose tissue: insulin-like growth factor system proteins, neuropeptide Y (NPY), NPY receptors, neurotrophic factors and other secreted factors. *Domest. Anim. Endocrinol.* 35, 24–34.

Heilig, M. (2004). The NPY system in stress, anxiety and depression. *Neuropeptides* 38, 213–224.

Hipskind, P. A., Lobb, K. L., Nixon, J. A., Britton, T. C., Bruns, R. F., Catlow, J., et al. (1997). Potent and selective 1,2,3-trisubstituted indole NPY Y-1 antagonists. *J. Med. Chem.* 40, 3712–3714.

Hoffmann, S., Rist, B., Videnov, G., Jung, G., and Beck-Sickinger, A. G. (1996). Structure-affinity studies of C-terminally modified analogs of neuropeptide Y led to a novel class of peptidic Y1 receptor antagonist. *Regul. Pept.* 65, 61 70.

Holland-Nell, K., and Meldal, M. (2011). Maintaining biological activity by using triazoles as disulfide bond mimetics. *Angew. Chem. Int. Ed. Engl.* 50, 5204–5206.

Holliday, N. D., Michel, M. C., and Cox, H. M. (2004). "NPY receptor subtypes and their signal transduction" in *Neuropeptide Y and Related Peptides*, ed. M. C. Michel (Berlin: Springer), 45–73.

Jablonowski, J. A., Chai, W., Li, X., Rudolph, D. A., Murray, W. V., Youngman, M. A., et al. (2004). Novel non-peptidic neuropeptide Y Y2 receptor antagonists. *Bioorg. Med. Chem. Lett.* 14, 1239–1242.

Jain, M. R., Pu, S., Kalra, P. S., and Kalra, S. P. (1999). Evidence that stimulation of two modalities of pituitary luteinizing hormone release in ovarian steroid-primed ovariectomized rats may involve neuropeptide Y Y1 and Y4 receptors. *Endocrinology* 140, 5171–5177.

Kakui, N., Tanaka, J., Tabata, Y., Asai, K., Masuda, N., Miyara, T., et al. (2006). Pharmacological characterization and feeding-suppressive property of FMS586 [3-(5,6,7,8-tetrahydro-9-isopropyl-carbazol-3-yl)-1-methyl-1-(2-pyridin-4-yl-ethy l)-urea hydrochloride], a novel, selective, and orally active antagonist for neuropeptide Y Y5 receptor. *J. Pharmacol. Exp. Ther.* 317, 562–570.

Kanatani, A., Ishihara, A., Iwaasa, H., Nakamura, K., Okamoto, O., Hidaka, M., et al. (2000a). L-152,804: orally active and selective neuropeptide Y Y5 receptor antagonist. *Biochem. Biophys. Res. Commun.* 272, 169–173.

Kanatani, A., Mashiko, S., Murai, N., Sugimoto, N., Ito, J., Fukuroda, T., et al. (2000b). Role of the Y1 receptor in the regulation of neuropeptide Y-mediated feeding: comparison of wild-type, Y1 receptor-deficient, and Y5 receptor-deficient mice. *Endocrinology* 141, 1011–1016.

Kannoa, T., Kanatani, A., Keen, S. L., Arai-Otsuki, S., Haga, Y., Iwama, T., et al. (2001). Different binding sites for the neuropeptide Y Y1 antagonists 1229U91 and J-104870 on human Y1 receptors. *Peptides* 22, 405–413.

Keire, D. A., Kobayashi, M., Solomon, T. E., and Reeve, J. R. Jr. (2000a). Solution structure of monomeric peptide YY supports the functional significance of the PP-fold. *Biochemistry* 39, 9935–9942.

Keire, D. A., Mannon, P., Kobayashi, M., Walsh, J. H., Solomon, T. E., and Reeve, J. R. Jr. (2000b). Primary structures of PYY, [Pro(34)]PYY, and PYY-(3-36) confer different conformations and receptor selectivity. *Am. J. Physiol. Gastrointest. Liver Physiol.* 279, G126-G131.

Kimmel, J. R., Hayden, L. J., and Pollock, H. G. (1975). Isolation and characterization of a new pancreatic polypeptide hormone. *J. Biol. Chem.* 250, 9369–9376.

Kirby, D. A., Boublik, J. H., and Rivier, J. E. (1993a). Neuropeptide Y: Y1 and Y2 affinities of the complete series of analogues with single D-residue substitutions. *J. Med. Chem.* 36, 3802–3808.

Kirby, D. A., Koerber, S. C., Craig, A. G., Feinstein, R. D., Delmas, L., Brown, M. R., et al. (1993b). Defining structural requirements for neuropeptide Y receptors using truncated and conformationally restricted analogues. *J. Med. Chem.* 36, 385–393.

Koglin, N., Zorn, C., Beumer, R., Cabrele, C., Bubert, C., Sewald, N., et al. (2003). Analogues of neuropeptide Y containing beta-aminocyclopropane carboxylic acids are the shortest linear peptides that are selective for the Y1 receptor. *Angew. Chem. Int. Ed. Engl.* 42, 202–205.

Larhammar, D. (1996). Structural diversity of receptors for neuropeptide Y, peptide YY and pancreatic polypeptide. *Regul. Pept.* 65, 165–174.

Larhammar, D., and Salaneck, E. (2004). Molecular evolution of NPY receptor subtypes. *Neuropeptides* 38, 141–151.

Larhammar, D., Wraith, A., Berglund, M. M., Holmberg, S. K., and Lundell, I. (2001). Origins of the many NPY-family receptors in mammals. *Peptides* 22, 295–307.

Lee, C. C., and Miller, R. J. (1998). Is there really an NPY Y3 receptor? *Regul. Pept.* 75–76, 71–78.

Lerch, M., Mayrhofer, M., and Zerbe, O. (2004). Structural similarities of micelle-bound peptide YY (PYY) and neuropeptide Y (NPY) are related to their affinity profiles at the Y receptors. *J. Mol. Biol.* 339, 1153–1168.

Lindner, D., Stichel, J., and Beck-Sickinger, A. G. (2008a). Molecular recognition of the NPY hormone family by their receptors. *Nutrition* 24, 907–917.

Lindner, D., Van Dieck, J., Merten, N., Morl, K., Gunther, R., Hofmann, H. J., et al. (2008b). GPC receptors and not ligands decide the binding mode in neuropeptide Y multireceptor/multiligand system. *Biochemistry* 47, 5905–5914.

Lindner, D., Walther, C., Tennemann, A., and Beck-Sickinger, A. G. (2009). Functional role of the extracellular N-terminal domain of neuropeptide Y subfamily receptors in membrane integration and agonist-stimulated internalization. *Cell. Signal.* 21, 61–68.

Lundberg, J. M., Tatemoto, K., Terenius, L., Hellstrom, P. M., Mutt, V., Hokfelt, T., et al. (1982). Localization of peptide YY (PYY) in gastrointestinal endocrine cells and effects on intestinal blood flow and motility. *Proc. Natl. Acad. Sci. U.S.A.* 79, 4471–4475.

Lundell, I., Blomqvist, A. G., Berglund, M. M., Schober, D. A., Johnson, D., Statnick, M. A., et al. (1995). Cloning of a human receptor of the NPY receptor family with high affinity for pancreatic polypeptide and peptide YY. *J. Biol. Chem.* 270, 29123–29128.

Lunniss, G. E., Barnes, A. A., Barton, N., Biagetti, M., Bianchi, F., Blowers, S. M., et al. (2009). The identification and optimisation of novel and selective diamide neuropeptide Y Y2 receptor antagonists. *Bioorg. Med. Chem. Lett.* 19, 4022–4025.

Lunniss, G. E., Barnes, A. A., Barton, N., Biagetti, M., Bianchi, F., Blowers, S. M., et al. (2010). The identification of a series of novel, soluble non-peptidic neuropeptide Y Y2 receptor antagonists. *Bioorg. Med. Chem. Lett.* 20, 7341–7344.

Matsumoto, M., Nomura, T., Momose, K., Ikeda, Y., Kondou, Y., Akiho, H., et al. (1996a). Inactivation of a novel neuropeptide Y/peptide YY receptor gene in primate species. *J. Biol. Chem.* 271, 27217–27220.

Matsumoto, S., Basil, J., Jetton, A. E., Lehman, M. N., and Bittman, E. L. (1996b). Regulation of the phase and period of circadian rhythms restored by suprachiasmatic transplants. *J. Biol. Rhythms* 11, 145–162.

Merten, N., Lindner, D., Rabe, N., Rompler, H., Morl, K., Schoneberg, T., et al. (2007). Receptor subtype-specific docking of Asp6.59 with C-terminal arginine residues in Y receptor ligands. *J. Biol. Chem.* 282, 7543–7551.

Michel, M. C., Beck-Sickinger, A., Cox, H., Doods, H. N., Herzog, H., Larhammar, D., et al. (1998). XVI. International Union of Pharmacology recommendations for the nomenclature of neuropeptide Y, peptide YY, and pancreatic polypeptide receptors. *Pharmacol. Rev.* 50, 143–150.

Misra, S., Murthy, K. S., Zhou, H., and Grider, J. R. (2004). Coexpression of Y1, Y2, and Y4 receptors in smooth muscle coupled to distinct signaling pathways. *J. Pharmacol. Exp. Ther.* 311, 1154–1162.

Mittapalli, G. K., Vellucci, D., Yang, J., Toussaint, M., Brothers, S. P., Wahlestedt, C., et al. (2012). Synthesis and SAR of selective small molecule neuropeptide Y Y2 receptor antagonists. *Bioorg. Med. Chem. Lett.* 22, 3916–3920.

Moriya, R., Fujikawa, T., Ito, J., Shirakura, T., Hirose, H., Suzuki, J., et al. (2010). Pancreatic polypeptide enhances colonic muscle contraction and fecal output through neuropeptide Y Y4 receptor in mice. *Eur. J. Pharmacol.* 627, 258–264.

Mullins, D., Adham, N., Hesk, D., Wu, Y., Kelly, J., Huang, Y., et al. (2008). Identification and characterization of pseudoirreversible nonpeptide antagonists of the neuropeptide Y Y5 receptor and development of a novel Y5-selective radioligand. *Eur. J. Pharmacol.* 601, 1–7.

Mullins, D., Kirby, D., Hwa, J., Guzzi, M., Rivier, J., and Parker, E. (2001). Identification of potent and selective neuropeptide Y Y(1) receptor agonists with orexigenic activity *in vivo*. *Mol. Pharmacol.* 60, 534–540.

Neumoin, A., Mares, J., Lerch-Bader, M., Bader, R., and Zerbe, O. (2007). Probing the formation of stable tertiary structure in a model miniprotein at atomic resolution: determinants of stability of a helical hairpin. *J. Am. Chem. Soc.* 129, 8811–8817.

Palczewski, K., Kumasaka, T., Hori, T., Behnke, C. A., Motoshima, H., Fox, B. A., et al. (2000). Crystal structure of rhodopsin: a G protein-coupled receptor. *Science* 289, 739–745.

Parker, E. M., Babij, C. K., Balasubramaniam, A., Burrier, R. E., Guzzi, M., Hamud, F., et al. (1998). GR231118 (1229U91) and other analogues of the C-terminus of neuropeptide Y are potent neuropeptide Y Y1 receptor antagonists and neuropeptide Y Y4 receptor agonists. *Eur. J. Pharmacol.* 349, 97–105.

Parker, E. M., Balasubramaniam, A., Guzzi, M., Mullins, D. E., Salisbury, B. G., Sheriff, S., et al. (2000). [D-Trp(34)] neuropeptide Y is a potent and selective neuropeptide Y Y(5) receptor agonist with dramatic effects on food intake. *Peptides* 21, 393–399.

Parker, M. S., Sah, R., Balasubramaniam, A., Sallee, F. R., Zerbe, O., and Parker, S. L. (2011). Non-specific binding and general cross-reactivity of Y receptor agonists are correlated and should importantly depend on their acidic sectors. *Peptides* 32, 258–265.

Pedersen, S. L., Holst, B., Vrang, N., and Jensen, K. J. (2009). Modifying the conserved C-terminal tyrosine of the peptide hormone PYY3-36 to improve Y2 receptor selectivity. *J. Pept. Sci.* 15, 753–759.

Pittner, R. A., Moore, C. X., Bhavsar, S. P., Gedulin, B. R., Smith, P. A.,

Jodka, C. M., et al. (2004). Effects of PYY[3-36] in rodent models of diabetes and obesity. *Int. J. Obes. Relat. Metab. Disord.* 28, 963–971.

Potter, E. K., Mitchell, L., Mccloskey, M. J., Tseng, A., Goodman, A. E., Shine, J., et al. (1989). Pre- and postjunctional actions of neuropeptide Y and related peptides. *Regul. Pept.* 25, 167–177.

Raposinho, P. D., Pierroz, D. D., Broqua, P., White, R. B., Pedrazzini, T., and Aubert, M. L. (2001). Chronic administration of neuropeptide Y into the lateral ventricle of C57BL/6J male mice produces an obesity syndrome including hyperphagia, hyperleptinemia, insulin resistance, and hypogonadism. *Mol. Cell. Endocrinol.* 185, 195–204.

Rodriguez, M., Audinot, V., Dromaint, S., Macia, C., Lamamy, V., Beauverger, P., et al. (2003). Molecular identification of the long isoform of the human neuropeptide Y Y5 receptor and pharmacological comparison with the short Y5 receptor isoform. *Biochem. J.* 369, 667–673.

Rudolf, K., Eberlein, W., Engel, W., Wieland, H. A., Willim, K. D., Entzeroth, M., et al. (1994). The first highly potent and selective nonpeptide neuropeptide Y Y1 receptor antagonist: BIBP3226. *Eur. J. Pharmacol.* 271, R11–R13.

Rueeger, H., Rigollier, P., Yamaguchi, Y., Schmidlin, T., Schilling, W., Criscione, L., et al. (2000). Design, synthesis and SAR of a series of 2-substituted 4-aminoquinazoline neuropeptide Y Y5 receptor antagonists. *Bioorg. Med. Chem. Lett.* 10, 1175–1179.

Sainsbury, A., Shi, Y. C., Zhang, L., Aljanova, A., Lin, Z., Nguyen, A. D., et al. (2010). Y4 receptors and pancreatic polypeptide regulate food intake via hypothalamic orexin and brain-derived neurotropic factor dependent pathways. *Neuropeptides* 44, 261–268.

Salaneck, E., Holmberg, S. K., Berglund, M. M., Boswell, T., and Larhammar, D. (2000). Chicken neuropeptide Y receptor Y2: structural and pharmacological differences to mammalian Y2(1). *FEBS Lett.* 484, 229–234.

Saldanha, S. A., Brothers, S. P., Spicer, T., Cameron, M., Mercer, B. A., Chase, P., et al. (2009). "Probe report for NPY-Y2 receptor antagonists," in *Probe Reports from the NIH Molecular Libraries Program [Internet]* (Bethesda, MD: National Center for Biotechnology Information). Available at: http://www.ncbi.nlm.nih.gov/books/NBK47354/ [updated August 6, 2010].

Sautel, M., Martinez, R., Munoz, M., Peitsch, M. C., Beck-Sickinger, A. G., and Walker, P. (1995). Role of a hydrophobic pocket of the human Y1 neuropeptide Y receptor in ligand binding. *Mol. Cell. Endocrinol.* 112, 215–222.

Sautel, M., Rudolf, K., Wittneben, H., Herzog, H., Martinez, R., Munoz, M., et al. (1996). Neuropeptide Y and the nonpeptide antagonist BIBP 3226 share an overlapping binding site at the human Y1 receptor. *Mol. Pharmacol.* 50, 285–292.

Schloegl, H., Percik, R., Horstmann, A., Villringer, A., and Stumvoll, M. (2011). Peptide hormones regulating appetite – focus on neuroimaging studies in humans. *Diabetes Metab. Res. Rev.* 27, 104–112.

Schober, D. A., Van Abbema, A. M., Smiley, D. L., Bruns, R. F., and Gehlert, D. R. (1998). The neuropeptide Y Y1 antagonist, 1229U91, a potent agonist for the human pancreatic polypeptide-preferring (NPY Y4) receptor. *Peptides* 19, 537–542.

Schwartz, T. W. (2006). *Y2/Y4 Selective Receptor Agonists for Therapeutic Intervention.* Patent GB20060018812.2.

Shoblock, J. R., Welty, N., Nepomuceno, D., Lord, B., Aluisio, L., Fraser, I., et al. (2010). *In vitro* and *in vivo* characterization of JNJ-31020028 (*N*-(4-{4-[2-(diethylamino)-2-oxo-1-phenylethyl]piperazin-1-yl}-3-fluorophenyl)-2- pyridin-3-ylbenzamide), a selective brain penetrant small molecule antagonist of the neuropeptide Y Y(2) receptor. *Psychopharmacology (Berl)* 208, 265–277.

Sjodin, P., Holmberg, S. K., Akerberg, H., Berglund, M. M., Mohell, N., and Larhammar, D. (2006). Re-evaluation of receptor-ligand interactions of the human neuropeptide Y receptor Y1: a site-directed mutagenesis study. *Biochem. J.* 393, 161–169.

Soll, R. M., Dinger, M. C., Lundell, I., Larhammer, D., and Beck-Sickinger, A. G. (2001). Novel analogues of neuropeptide Y with a preference for the Y1-receptor. *Eur. J. Biochem.* 268, 2828–2837.

Sousa, D. M., Baldock, P. A., Enriquez, R. F., Zhang, L., Sainsbury, A., Lamghari, M., et al. (2012). Neuropeptide Y Y1 receptor antagonism increases bone mass in mice. *Bone* 51, 8–16.

Stanley, B. G., Kyrkouli, S. E., Lampert, S., and Leibowitz, S. F. (1986). Neuropeptide Y chronically injected into the hypothalamus: a powerful neurochemical inducer of hyperphagia and obesity. *Peptides* 7, 1189–1192.

Starback, P., Wraith, A., Eriksson, H., and Larhammar, D. (2000). Neuropeptide Y receptor gene y6: multiple deaths or resurrections? *Biochem. Biophys. Res. Commun.* 277, 264–269.

Suzuki, K., Simpson, K. A., Minnion, J. S., Shillito, J. C., and Bloom, S. R. (2010). The role of gut hormones and the hypothalamus in appetite regulation. *Endocr. J.* 57, 359–372.

Swanson, D. M., Wong, V. D., Jablonowski, J. A., Shah, C., Rudolph, D. A., Dvorak, C. A., et al. (2011). The discovery and synthesis of JNJ 31020028, a small molecule antagonist of the Neuropeptide Y Y(2) receptor. *Bioorg. Med. Chem. Lett.* 21, 5552–5556.

Tatemoto, K. (1982). Neuropeptide Y: complete amino acid sequence of the brain peptide. *Proc. Natl. Acad. Sci. U.S.A.* 79, 5485–5489.

Tatemoto, K., and Mutt, V. (1980). Isolation of two novel candidate hormones using a chemical method for finding naturally occurring polypeptides. *Nature* 285, 417–418.

Thiele, T. E., Marsh, D. J., Ste Marie, L., Bernstein, I. L., and Palmiter, R. D. (1998). Ethanol consumption and resistance are inversely related to neuropeptide Y levels. *Nature* 396, 366–369.

Verdine, G. L., and Walensky, L. D. (2007). The challenge of drugging undruggable targets in cancer: lessons learned from targeting BCL-2 family members. *Clin. Cancer Res.* 13, 7264–7270.

Wahlestedt, C., Yanaihara, N., and Hakanson, R. (1986). Evidence for different pre-and post-junctional receptors for neuropeptide Y and related peptides. *Regul. Pept.* 13, 307–318.

Walther, C., Morl, K., and Beck-Sickinger, A. G. (2011). Neuropeptide Y receptors: ligand binding and trafficking suggest novel approaches in drug development. *J. Pept. Sci.* 17, 233–246.

Wharton, J., Gordon, L., Byrne, J., Herzog, H., Selbie, L. A., Moore, K., et al. (1993). Expression of the human neuropeptide tyrosine Y1 receptor. *Proc. Natl. Acad. Sci. U.S.A.* 90, 687–691.

Widdowson, P. S. (1993). Quantitative receptor autoradiography demonstrates a differential distribution of neuropeptide-Y Y1 and Y2 receptor subtypes in human and rat brain. *Brain Res.* 631, 27–38.

Widdowson, P. S., Buckingham, R., and Williams, G. (1997). Distribution of [Leu31,Pro34]NPY-sensitive, BIBP3226-insensitive [125I]PYY(3–36) binding sites in rat brain: possible relationship to Y5 NPY receptors. *Brain Res.* 778, 242–250.

Wieland, H. A., Engel, W., Eberlein, W., Rudolf, K., and Doods, H. N. (1998). Subtype selectivity of the novel nonpeptide neuropeptide Y Y1 receptor antagonist BIBO 3304 and its effect on feeding in rodents. *Br. J. Pharmacol.* 125, 549–555.

Zhang, L., Bijker, M. S., and Herzog, H. (2011). The neuropeptide Y system: pathophysiological and therapeutic implications in obesity and cancer. *Pharmacol. Ther.* 131, 91–113.

Ziemek, R., Schneider, E., Kraus, A., Cabrele, C., Beck-Sickinger, A. G., Bernhardt, G., et al. (2007). Determination of affinity and activity of ligands at the human neuropeptide Y Y4 receptor by flow cytometry and aequorin luminescence. *J. Recept. Signal Transduct. Res.* 27, 217–233.

Zukowska-Grojec, Z., Karwatowska-Prokopczuk, E., Rose, W., Rone, J., Movafagh, S., Ji, H., et al. (1998). Neuropeptide Y: a novel angiogenic factor from the sympathetic nerves and endothelium. *Circ. Res.* 83, 187–195.

Zwanziger, D., Bohme, I., Lindner, D., and Beck-Sickinger, A. G. (2009). First selective agonist of the neuropeptide Y1-receptor with reduced size. *J. Pept. Sci.* 15, 856–866.

5

Update on the urotensinergic system: New trends in receptor localization, activation, and drug design

David Chatenet[1,2]*, Thi-Tuyet M. Nguyen[1,2], Myriam Létourneau[1,2] and Alain Fournier[1,2]*

[1] Laboratoire d'études moléculaires et pharmacologiques des peptides, INRS – Institut Armand-Frappier, Université du Québec, Ville de Laval, QC, Canada
[2] Laboratoire International Associé Samuel de Champlain (INSERM/INRS-Université de Rouen), France

Edited by:
Hubert Vaudry, University of Rouen, France

Reviewed by:
Stacia A. Sower, University of New Hampshire, USA
Ishwar S. Parhar, Monash University, Malaysia

***Correspondence:**
David Chatenet and Alain Fournier, Laboratoire d'études moléculaires et pharmacologiques des peptides, INRS – Institut Armand-Frappier, Université du Québec, 531 Boulevard des Prairies, Ville de Laval, QC H7V 1B7, Canada.
e-mail: david.chatenet@iaf.inrs.ca; alain.fournier@iaf.inrs.ca

The urotensinergic system plays central roles in the physiological regulation of major mammalian organ systems, including the cardiovascular system. As a matter of fact, this system has been linked to numerous pathophysiological states including atherosclerosis, heart failure, hypertension, diabetes as well as psychological, and neurological disorders. The delineation of the (patho)physiological roles of the urotensinergic system has been hampered by the absence of potent and selective antagonists for the urotensin II-receptor (UT). Thus, a more precise definition of the molecular functioning of the urotensinergic system, in normal conditions as well as in a pathological state is still critically needed. The recent discovery of nuclear UT within cardiomyocytes has highlighted the cellular complexity of this system and suggested that UT-associated biological responses are not only initiated at the cell surface but may result from the integration of extracellular and intracellular signaling pathways. Thus, such nuclear-localized receptors, regulating distinct signaling pathways, may represent new therapeutic targets. With the recent observation that urotensin II (UII) and urotensin II-related peptide (URP) exert different biological effects and the postulate that they could also have distinct pathophysiological roles in hypertension, it appears crucial to reassess the recognition process involving UII and URP with UT, and to push forward the development of new analogs of the UT system aimed at discriminating UII- and URP-mediated biological activities. The recent development of such compounds, *i.e.* urocontrin A and rUII(1–7), is certainly useful to decipher the specific roles of UII and URP *in vitro* and *in vivo*. Altogether, these studies, which provide important information regarding the pharmacology of the urotensinergic system and the conformational requirements for binding and activation, will ultimately lead to the development of potent and selective drugs.

Keywords: urotensin II, urotensin II-related peptide, allosteric modulation, biased agonist, nuclear receptors

THE UROTENSINERGIC SYSTEM

During the last decade, the urotensinergic system has drawn the attention of the scientific community due to its marked involvement in various pathological states including cardiovascular diseases. Initially isolated from the caudal neurosecretory system of the teleostean fish *Gillichthys mirabilis*, urotensin II (UII), a somatostatin-like peptide, was first characterized as a spasmogenic agent (Pearson et al., 1980). During more than 15 years, this peptide and its unknown receptors were thought to be restricted to fishes until it was demonstrated that UII was able to induce the relaxation of the mouse anococcygeus muscle (Gibson et al., 1984) and provoke the contraction of rat aortic strips (Gibson, 1987). These results, suggesting the presence of an homologous peptide in higher vertebrates, led to the isolation and characterization of UII in the frog *Rana ridibunda* (Conlon et al., 1992). Following this discovery, UII isoforms were either characterized or isolated in various vertebrate species including humans (Vaudry et al., 2010). A few years later, a peptide paralog, termed urotensin II-related peptide (URP), was isolated in rat brain extracts and subsequently identified in other mammalian species (Vaudry et al., 2010). Sequence comparison of all UII and URP isoforms revealed a striking conservation of the C-terminal cyclic hexapeptide (Vaudry et al., 2010). Conversely, the N-terminal region is highly variable both in length, ranging from 11 residues in humans to 17 residues in mice, and sequence composition (**Figure 1**) (Vaudry et al., 2010). In the human genome, UII and URP genes are respectively found at position 1p36 and 3q29 (Sugo et al., 2003). Those two genes are primarily expressed in motoneurons located in discrete brainstem nuclei and in the ventral horn of the spinal cord (Vaudry et al., 2010). However, UII and URP mRNAs have also been detected, although at a much lower level, in various peripheral tissues including the pituitary, heart, spleen, lung, liver, thymus, pancreas, kidney, small intestine, adrenal, and prostate (**Figure 2**) (Vaudry et al., 2010).

Both peptides are endogenous ligands of a G protein-coupled receptor initially identified as the orphan GPR14 receptor (Ames et al., 1999; Liu et al., 1999; Mori et al., 1999; Nothacker et al., 1999). Structural studies of this urotensin II receptor (UT) showed that, in addition to the common features found in the 1A GPCR family, such as the existence of a disulfide bridge between extracellular loops 1 and 2, N-linked glycosylation sites in the N-terminus portion, and phosphorylation sites in intracellular

Species	Sequence
Urotensin II	
Mouse	<Gln-His-Lys-Gln-His-Gly-Ala-Ala-Pro-Glu-Cys-Phe-Trp-Lys-Tyr-Cys-Ile-OH
Rat	<Gln-His-Gly-Thr-Ala-Pro-Glu-Cys-Phe-Trp-Lys-Tyr-Cys-Ile-OH
Chimpanzee	H-Glu-Thr-Pro-Asp-Cys-Phe-Trp-Lys-Tyr-Cys-Val-OH
Human	H-Glu-Thr-Pro-Asp-Cys-Phe-Trp-Lys-Tyr-Cys-Val-OH
URP	
Mouse	H-Ala-Cys-Phe-Trp-Lys-Tyr-Cys-Val-OH
Rat	H-Ala-Cys-Phe-Trp-Lys-Tyr-Cys-Val-OH
Chimpanzee	H-Ala-Cys-Phe-Trp-Lys-Tyr-Cys-Val-OH
Human	H-Ala-Cys-Phe-Trp-Lys-Tyr-Cys-Val-OH

FIGURE 1 | Amino acid sequences of UII and URP in mammalian species; <Gln, pyroglumatic acid. Modified from Vaudry et al. (2010).

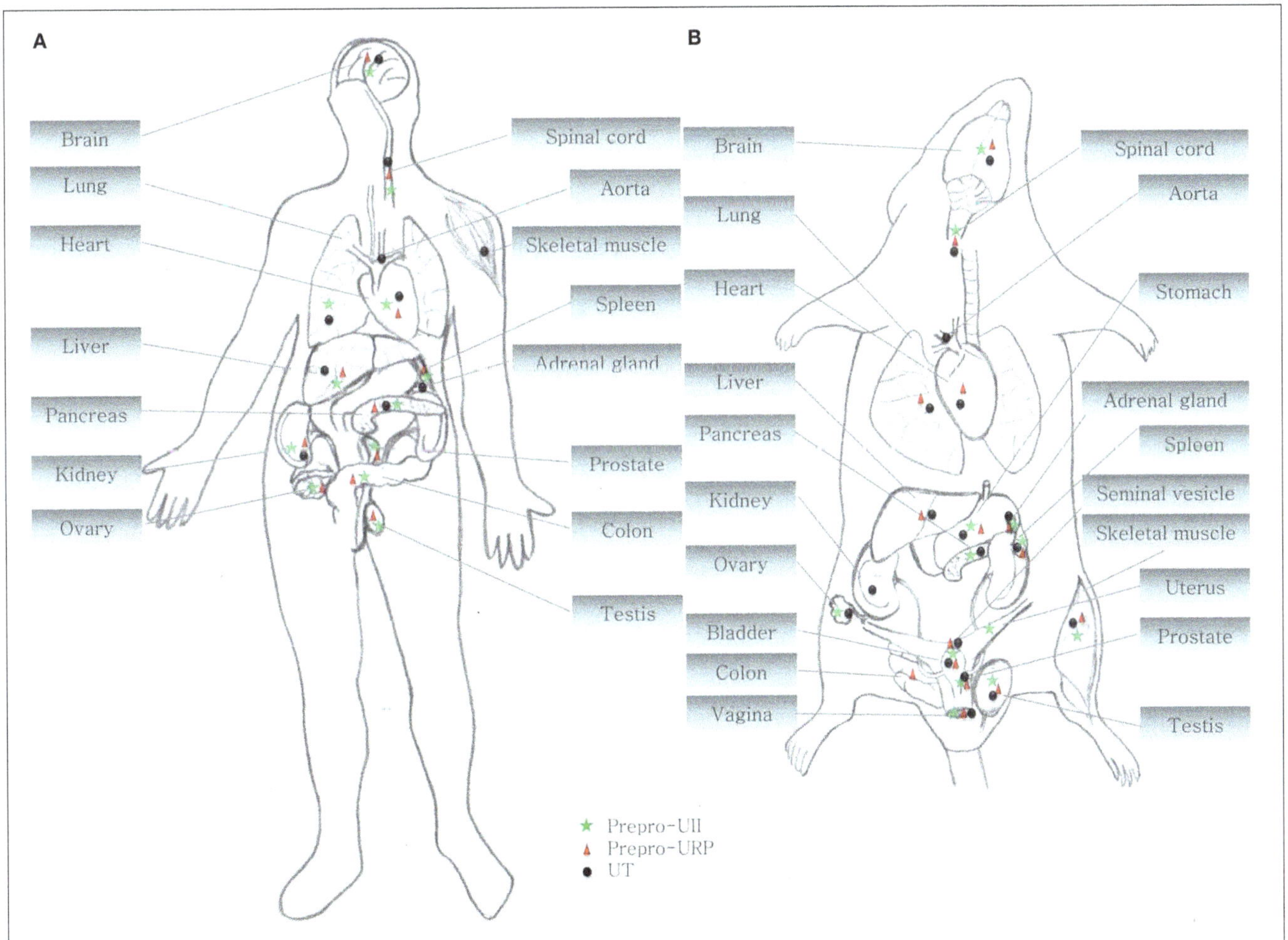

FIGURE 2 | Central and peripheral distribution of prepro-UII, prepro-URP, and UT in (A) primates (human and cynomolgus monkey) and (B) rodents (rat and mouse) (Ames et al., 1999; Sugo et al., 2003; Dubessy et al., 2008; Maguire et al., 2008; Doan et al., 2012; Nguyen et al., 2012).

loops (Douglas et al., 2000), this protein also possesses a palmitoylation site located in the C-terminal segment of the rodent isoform that is not present in the human isoform (**Figure 3**). Worth to mention, the rat UT, consisting of 386 amino acids, shows only 75% homology with the human protein while sequences of human and monkey receptors, comprising 389 residues, are almost identical (Elshourbagy et al., 2002). Like UII and URP, UT is widely expressed in the central nervous system as well as

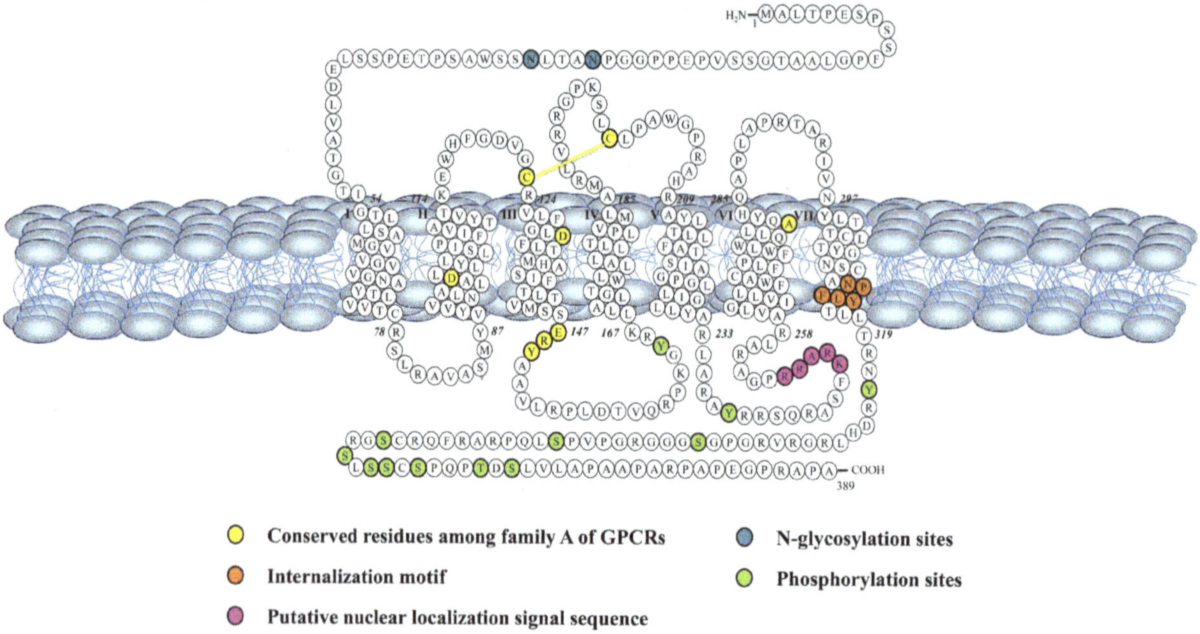

FIGURE 3 | Schematic representation of the human urotensin II (hUT) receptor. Adapted from Douglas et al. (2000).

in various peripheral organs including the cardiovascular system, kidneys, bladder, pancreas, and adrenal gland (**Figure 2**) (Vaudry et al., 2010).

The urotensinergic system plays a seminal role in the physiological regulation of major mammalian organ systems, including the cardiovascular system (Vaudry et al., 2010). As a matter of fact, UII exerts potent haemodynamic effects (Krum and Kemp, 2007), positive inotropic and chronotropic responses (Watson et al., 2003), and osmoregulatory actions (Song et al., 2006), induces collagen and fibronectin accumulation (Dai et al., 2007; Zhang et al., 2008), modulates the inflammatory response (Shiraishi et al., 2008), plays a role in the induction of cardiac and vascular hypertrophy (Papadopoulos et al., 2008), causes a strong angiogenic effect (Guidolin et al., 2010) and inhibits the glucose-induced insulin release (Silvestre et al., 2004). Thus, the urotensinergic system was linked to numerous pathophysiological states including atherosclerosis, heart failure, hypertension, pre-eclampsia, diabetes, renal and liver diseases, variceal bleeding, ulcers, as well as psychological, and neurological disorders (Ross et al., 2010).

The present review focuses on the latest findings about the urotensinergic system in terms of receptor localization and pharmacology as well as receptor activation with the conception of new urotensinergic ligands aimed at discriminating UII- and/or URP-mediated biological actions.

DISCOVERY OF AN INTRACRINE PHARMACOLOGY OF THE UROTENSINERGIC SYSTEM

PRESENCE OF NUCLEAR UT IN THE HEART AND IN THE CENTRAL NERVOUS SYSTEM

In many ways, UII exhibits actions similar to other key neurohormonal factors, *i.e.* angiotensin II (Ang-II) and endothelin-1 (ET-1), in driving a variety of cardiac and vascular disease processes (Maguire and Davenport, 2002). These include vasoconstriction as well as mitogenic, trophic and pro-fibrotic effects (Vaudry et al., 2010). A clear interaction of the urotensinergic system with the renin-angiotensin-aldosterone and endothelin systems is acknowledged in terms of regulation of systolic and diastolic functions (Fontes-Sousa et al., 2009). However, key differences were observed between these systems. In particular, UII induces a rather weak or absent vasoconstriction in a variety of human vascular beds (Maguire et al., 2000; Hillier et al., 2001) while it can also acts as a vasodilator in some vascular beds, such as those in the pulmonary vasculature (Stirrat et al., 2001). The recent discovery of specific intracellular receptors associated with the physiological and pathophysiological actions of Ang-II and ET-1 highlighted a high level of complexity for these peptidergic systems in the regulation of cardiovascular homeostasis. Traditionally, GPCRs are located at the plasma membrane where they modulate the activity of membrane-associated second messengers. As such, GPCRs can exert their effects through the regulation of ion channels, second messenger production, and protein kinase cascades in order to control cellular activity, gene expression, plasticity, differentiation, morphogenesis, and migration. However, in the recent years, the presence of functional intracellular receptors has almost become "a classic GPCR paradigm" (Boivin et al., 2008). These intracellular GPCRs could be involved in the control of several cellular processes including regulation of gene transcription, ionic homeostasis, cellular proliferation, and remodeling (Boivin et al., 2008). Intracellular GPCRs may be constitutively active, or may be activated by ligands internalized from the extracellular space or synthesized within the cell (**Figure 4**). Besides, they can regulate signaling pathways distinct from those activated by the

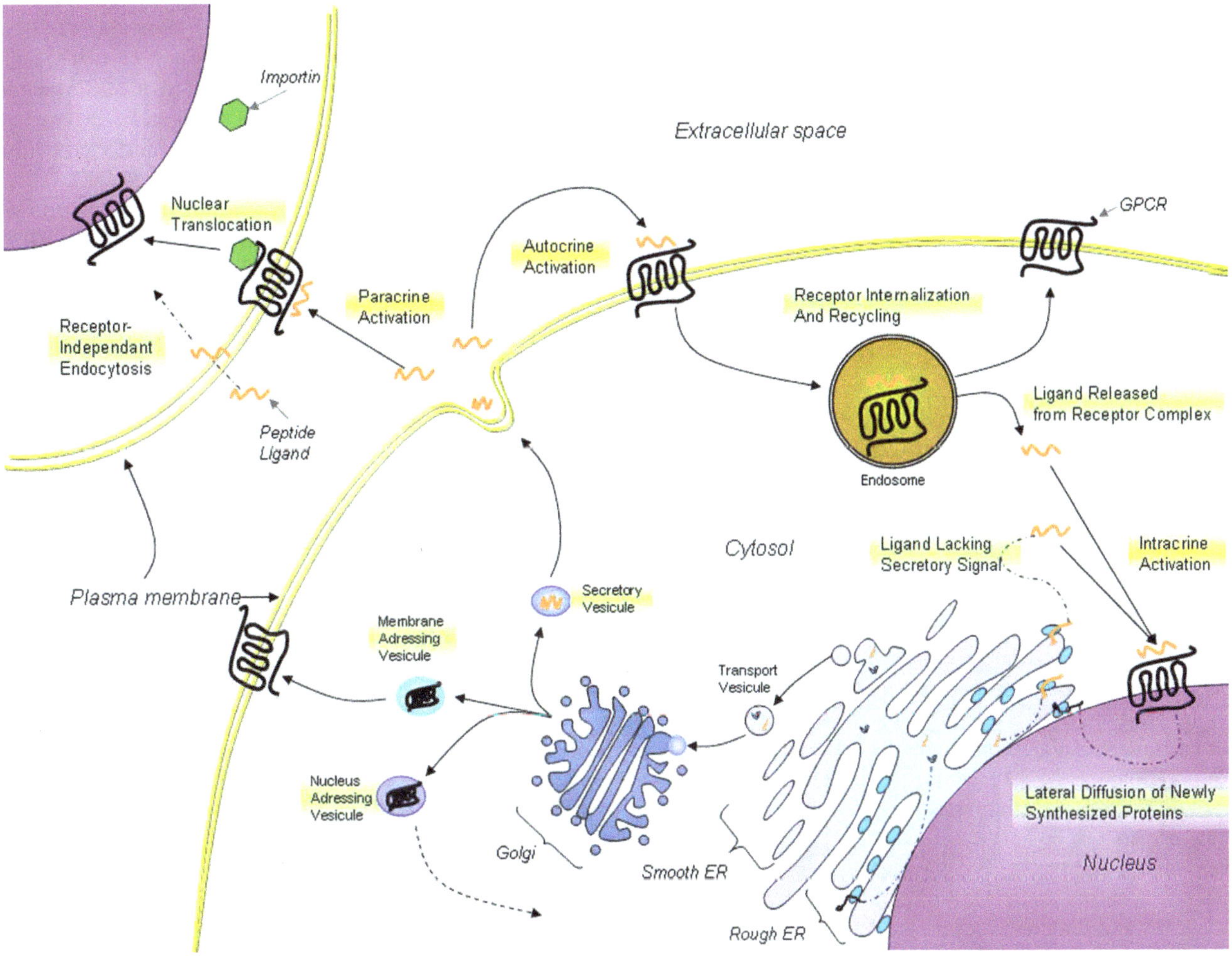

FIGURE 4 | Proposed trafficking of UT and endogenous ligands. UT receptors are located either at the plasma membrane or at the nucleus. The presence of nuclear UTs can be attributed to lateral diffusion of newly synthesized proteins from the rough endoplasmic reticulum surface, which is contiguous with the nuclear shell, to specific nuclear addressing following modification in the Golgi apparatus or importin-assisted nuclear translocation after ligand stimulation. UII or URP binds to UT receptors at the cell surface but can also cross the plasma membrane to stimulate intracellular receptors. From Lee et al. (2004); Giebing et al. (2005); Gobeil et al. (2006); Doan et al. (2012); Tadevosyan et al. (2012).

same receptor at the cell surface (Re, 1999). As such, biological outcomes might result from the integration of extracellular and intracellular signaling events (Terrillon and Bouvier, 2004; Hanyaloglu and von Zastrow, 2008; Sorkin and von Zastrow, 2009). This new paradigm for cellular signaling provides more complexity to study the function and physiological roles of GPCRs.

In a recent report, specific UII binding sites were observed on heart and brain cell nuclei from rat and monkey tissues (Doan et al., 2012; Nguyen et al., 2012). Except those two tissues and the spinal cord, none of the tested tissues including kidneys, lung, and skeletal muscle, all expressing UT at the cell surface, presented a subcellular localization of UT (Doan et al., 2012; Nguyen et al., 2012). Supporting the presence of such nuclear expression also in humans, the presence of nuclear UT was also observed in two human cell lines, *i.e.* SH-SY5Y neuroblastoma and U87 astrocytoma cell lines (Nguyen et al., 2012).

NUCLEAR UT ACTIVATION CAN MODULATE TRANSCRIPTION INITIATION

As previously reported for nuclear Ang-II (Eggena et al., 1993), β3-adrenergic (Boivin et al., 2006; Vaniotis et al., 2011), and ET-1 receptors (Boivin et al., 2003), nuclear UT receptors can initiate transcription (Doan et al., 2012; Nguyen et al., 2012). Although UII and URP stimulated the transcription in isolated brain cell nuclei (Nguyen et al., 2012), only UII was able to trigger a similar effect in rat cardiac nuclei (Doan et al., 2012). Two-dimensional gel electrophoresis clearly indicated the occurrence of different immunoreactive species in both brain and heart membrane and nuclear fractions (Doan et al., 2012; Nguyen et al., 2012). Nuclear and membrane proteins extracted from heart tissues expressed three major UT-immunoreactive spots with an apparent molecular weight of 60 kDa at a pI value of 6–7 (Doan et al., 2012). Interestingly, a different pattern was observed in brain tissue (Nguyen et al., 2012). Since the UT gene is intronless, the various immunoreactive species were principally ascribed to post-translational modifications (Doan et al., 2012; Nguyen et al., 2012). Whether or not these UT species are involved in distinct UII-associated biological activities will require further investigation. However, it is well-known that glycosylation can modulate the cellular compartmentalization and functionality of the receptor, thereby influencing its intracellular trafficking and biological activity (**Figure 4**) (Duverger et al., 1995; Rondanino et al., 2003; Gobeil et al., 2006).

A growing body of evidence supports the presence of GPCRs at the surface of the nuclear membrane, their orientation within this membrane, however, remains controversial. If they maintain the topology adopted in the endoplasmic reticulum during protein synthesis, the ligand binding site would be located in the lumen of the nuclear envelop (perinuclear space) with the C-terminal of the protein being localized either within or outside the nucleus. In fact, the topology of the nuclear membrane lumen is very similar to the extracellular space, which makes it a favorable environment for a binding site (Jong et al., 2005; Bootman et al., 2009). Since signaling starts with the recruitment of specific proteins to the C-terminal portion of the receptor, signals would be sent toward the cytosol or into the nucleus in accordance with the adopted GPCR orientation within the nuclear shell (**Figure 5**). Hence, the orientation of those nuclear GPCRs would determine the direction in which the signal is transmitted. As recently reported, nuclear UT receptors are able to regulate gene transcription (Doan et al., 2012; Nguyen et al., 2012). Furthermore, it is well-known that calcium ions play an important role in the control of gene expression (Bootman et al., 2009). In isolated nuclei, nuclear calcium levels can regulate gene transcription by interacting with the cyclic AMP response element-binding protein (CREB) and the downstream regulatory element antagonist modulator (DREAM), which are constitutively present in the nucleus. Changes in nucleoplasmic calcium can be achieved by triggering inositol(1,4,5)-triphosphate receptors (IP_3Rs) located on the inner nuclear membrane (Bootman et al., 2009). Because it is generally accepted that UT activation is associated with the recruitment of Gαq/11 proteins to its C-terminal tail resulting in an IP_3 increase (Proulx et al., 2008), it is highly probable that this portion of the receptor is located into the nucleoplasm (**Figure 5**). Interestingly, IP3Rs are concentrated in the nuclear membrane of heart ventricular cells and their activation was shown to initiate a pro-hypertrophic pathway (Arantes et al., 2012). These findings are well-correlated with the UII-induced cardiomyocyte hypertrophy and the presence of nuclear UT receptors in cardiac tissues (Gruson et al., 2010; Doan et al., 2012). Nevertheless, these intracellular UT receptors may have the capacity to regulate signaling pathways that differ from those of their plasma membrane counterparts, as recently demonstrated for the metabotropic glutamate receptor 5 (Jong et al., 2009), and the renin–angiotensin system (De Mello, 2008). As such, this intracrine pharmacology of the urotensinergic system represents a complementary system that could potentially involve the regulation of physiological functions.

INTRACELLULAR TRAFFICKING OF UT

This new intracrine pharmacology clearly highlights the complexity of this peptidergic system where UII and URP can trigger not only common but also different biological activities (Prosser et al., 2008; Jarry et al., 2010; Doan et al., 2012). Previous studies have detected the presence of GPCRs, such as Ang-II receptors, at the nucleus in an agonist-independent manner (Lee et al., 2004). Confocal microscopy of heart and brain tissue sections as well as various non-transfected cell lines clearly revealed a constitutive nuclear localization for UT (Doan et al., 2012; Nguyen et al., 2012). However, it is also possible that following their agonist-stimulated internalization, GPCRs relocate at the nuclear membrane (Lee et al., 2004). In such a case, the translocation is initiated by the presence of a nuclear localization signal (NLS), a short stretch of basic amino acid residues often localized within the intracellular loops that is recognized by importins α and/or β (**Figure 4**). For example, a NLS was observed in the seventh transmembrane domain and the carboxy-terminal segment of the Ang-II receptor subtype1 (Lys-Lys-Phe-Lys-Arg) and the third intracellular loop of the apelin receptors (Arg-Lys-Arg-Arg-Arg) (Lee et al., 2004). Interestingly, a similar sequence, *i.e.* Lys-Arg-Ala-Arg-Arg, is also observed in the third intracellular loop of human and monkey UT isoforms (**Figure 3**) while a Lys-Gln-Thr-Arg-Arg segment is observed in rat and mouse UT. However, it is important to note that many NLS signals are still unknown and that the presence of an obvious NLS motif may mask the existence of still uncharacterized NLS sequences. Specific post-translational modifications such as palmitoylation were reported to be involved in the addressing of the receptor either to the membrane or the nuclei. For instance, it was demonstrated that de-palmitoylation of GRK6A promoted its translocation from the plasma membrane to both the cytoplasm and nucleus (Jiang et al., 2007). Such a putative palmitoylation site is also found within the seventh transmembrane domain (Cys^{339}) of rat and mouse UT isoforms but is absent in the primate (human and monkey) receptor (Marchese et al., 1995; Tal et al., 1995; Ames et al., 1999). Under chemically mediated hypoxic conditions, an increase of total UT expression, was observed suggesting that hypoxia might induce *de novo* synthesis of the peptide receptor. However, a significant decrease in nuclear UT expression was reported that could be interpreted as an increase in translocation of the protein to the membrane or a decrease of internalization with concomitant nuclear translocation (Nguyen et al., 2012). Altogether, it could be noted that the subcellular UT localization could be either attributed to translocation from the cell surface and/or *de novo* synthesis (**Figure 4**).

UII AND URP AS INTRACRINE LIGANDS

UII, and by extension URP, were originally thought to act as autocrine and paracrine modulators rather than as hormones (Yoshimoto et al., 2004). The term "intracrine" ligand relates to intracellular molecules binding to and activating intracellular receptors (**Figure 4**). Such ligands can be synthesized and targeted to the Golgi apparatus for secretion or act intracellularly either before secretion or following reuptake. The intracrine gene product might also arise from an alternative transcription initiation site, differences in mRNA maturation or translation leading to a gene product lacking secretory signals and consequently active only in the intracellular space (**Figure 4**) (Kiefer et al., 1994; Lee-Kirsch et al., 1999; Xu et al., 2009). To this extent, it is interesting

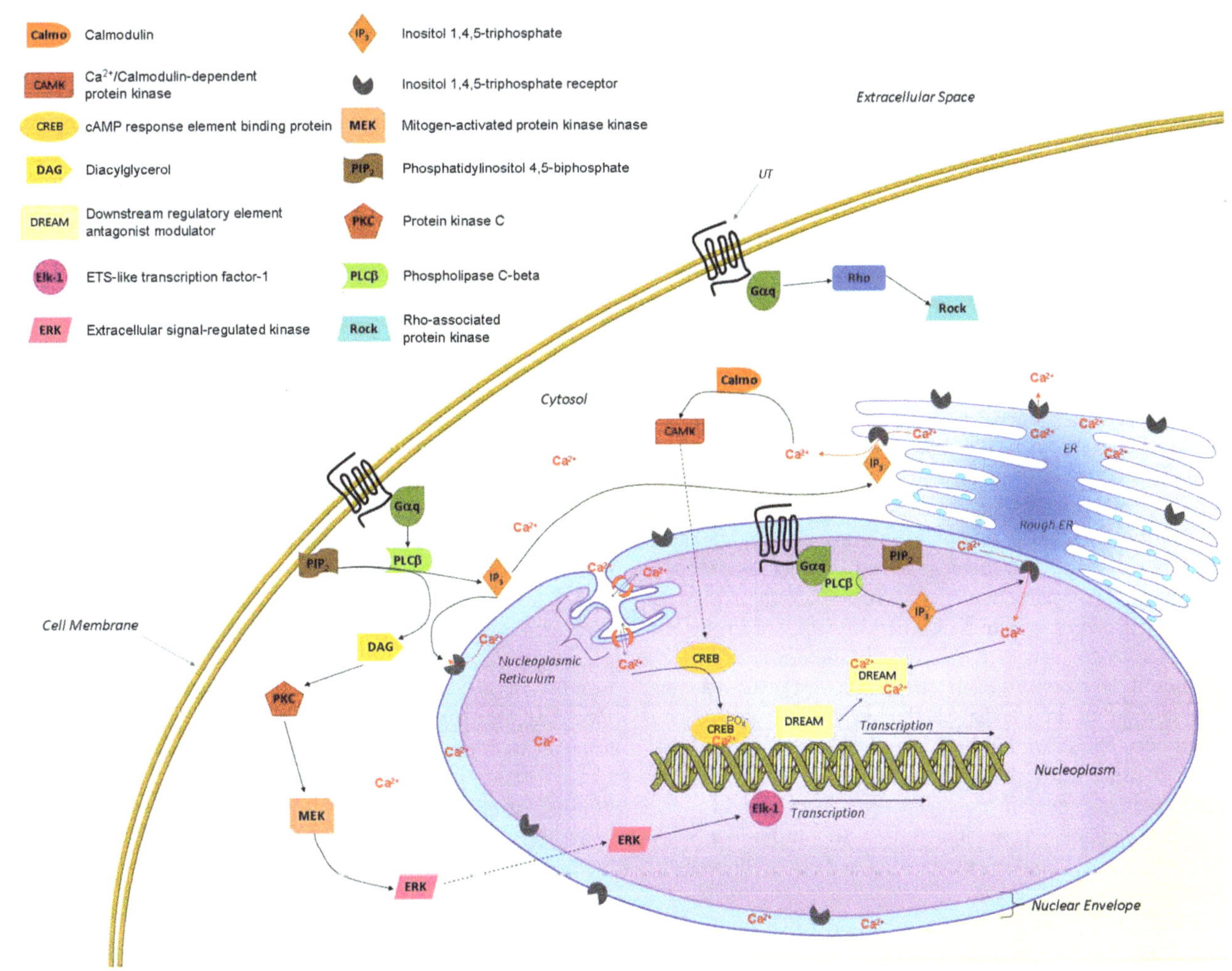

FIGURE 5 | Proposed UT-associated signaling pathways. Activated UTs are known to recruit Gαq/11 proteins and to signal through different pathways associated with an elevation of intracellular calcium and gene transcription. Nuclear UTs could induce transcription through a pathway involving the production of IP_3 that would trigger IP_3Rs at the inner nuclear envelop, releasing calcium in the nucleoplasm. This latter event is crucial to initiate transcription through transcription factors such as CREB and DREAM. From Proulx et al. (2008); Bootman et al. (2009); Vaudry et al. (2010); Roskoski (2012); Tadevosyan et al. (2012).

to note that two isoforms of the human UII precursor, differing mostly by their peptide signal, were discovered (Coulouarn et al., 1998; Ames et al., 1999).

A recent study demonstrated that FITC-conjugated hUII and URP were both internalized in non-expressing UT cell lines through receptor-independent mediated endocytosis (Doan et al., 2012) (**Figure 4**). This receptor-independent endocytic mechanism brought a new perception of the pseudo-irreversible binding characteristics often described for the urotensinergic system. Indeed, the lack of rapid UT desensitization through classic mechanisms (acid wash or trypsin treatments) was thought to reflect a strong, pseudo-irreversible binding of the ligands (Douglas and Ohlstein, 2000). However, this pseudo-irreversible character could also be due to the ability of both endogenous peptides to reach the internal compartment of the cell. Moreover, it is yet possible that following the internalization of ligand-receptor complexes, ligands are subsequently released from internalized endosomes within the cell. As such, internalized peptide-receptor complexes can be dissociated under the acidic environment found in endosomes, giving rise to receptor recycling at the plasma membrane (**Figure 4**) (Giebing et al., 2005). At this point, the fate of the peptide is unknown but based on the results published by Doan et al. (2012), it is conceivable that UII, and to a lesser extend URP, could leak from the vesicle and ultimately activate intracellular receptors.

PROSPECTIVE ROLES OF NUCLEAR UT

The precise role of this new intracrine urotensinergic system has yet to be elucidated both in physiological and pathological conditions. However, as for other GPCRs including Ang-II and ET-1 receptors, these intracellular receptors are important regulators of physiological and pathological functions and could therefore represent new targets for therapeutic interventions (Boivin et al., 2008; Tadevosyan et al., 2012).

Elevated UII plasma levels were observed in numerous disease conditions, including hypertension, atherosclerosis, heart failure, pulmonary hypertension, diabetes, renal failure, and metabolic syndrome (Ross et al., 2010). As demonstrated, the cellular uptake of UII but not URP is increased at lower pH (Doan et al., 2012). Pathological conditions such as cancer, ischemic stroke, inflammation, and atherosclerotic plaques often induce an increase in metabolic activity and hypoxia associated with an elevated extracellular acidity (Andreev et al., 2010). In these conditions, UII would enter more easily than URP inside the cell triggering transcription of UII-associated genes by activating the nuclear receptor. Thus, the elevated concentration of UII observed during the etiology of various diseases could sustain specific cellular responses while an intracellular feedback loop could maintain a particular cellular state (Petersen et al., 2006). Interestingly, known intracrines do not present any structural or chemical similarities but are generally growth regulators that can directly or indirectly modulate angiogenic or anti-angiogenic actions. Therefore, the angiogenic actions of the urotensinergic system, reported both *in vivo* and *in vitro* (Spinazzi et al., 2006), could thus involve the activation of nuclear UT.

The urotensinergic system is also highly expressed in the central nervous system, but its physiological function is still poorly understood. UT was observed in cortical astrocytes (Castel et al., 2006), a ubiquitous type of glial cell that greatly outnumbers neurons and occupies 25% to 50% of brain volume (Bignami et al., 1991). It is noteworthy that glioblastoma multiform (GBM) is characterized by exuberant angiogenesis, a key event in tumor growth and progression and that UII, URP, and UT mRNAs were systematically found to be expressed in different glioma and glioblastoma tumors (Diallo et al., 2007). These results support a role for the urotensinergic system, and in particular nuclear UT, in human brain tumorogenesis possibly via angiogenesis regulation. Finally, in the CNS, UII is able to induce norepinephrine, dopamine, and serotonin release in noradrenergic neurons (Ono et al., 2008). Intracerebroventricular UII administration modulates cardiac homeostasis via β-adrenoreceptor activation (Hood et al., 2005). These observations bring up the idea that the presence of nuclear UT receptors could also be associated to excitatory neurotransmission. In accordance with this hypothesis, various intracrines were reported to act as neurotransmitters within the CNS (Re, 2004).

Whether specific UII or URP biological actions on the CNS and the cardiovascular system are mediated totally or in part by the nuclear UT will need further studies as well as the development of specific nuclear UT probes. Although still poorly understood, the diverse functions exerted by agonists and hormones acting on intracellular GPCRs suggest that intracrine signaling might activate cellular responses distinct from those at the cell surface for a given receptor. In the last decade, biological actions of intracrines in heart and vasculature, including those of the renin–angiotensin-system in cardiac pathology, dynorphin B in cardiac development, as well as endothelin, highlighted the importance of intracrine physiology in pathological processes such as left ventricular hypertrophy, diabetic cardiomyopathy, and arrythmogenesis. So, the presence of functional UT receptors at the cell membrane and at the nucleus will probably be a new aspect to take into account during the development of therapeutic compounds for the treatment of pathologies associated with the urotensinergic system.

NEW INSIGHTS INTO UT ACTIVATION

The precise definition of the (patho) physiological roles of the urotensinergic system *in vivo* was hampered by the absence of potent and selective UT antagonists. Indeed, the lack of efficacy observed with Palosuran (ACT-058362) (Clozel et al., 2004, 2006), the only UT antagonist that reached a phase II clinical trial in patients with diabetic nephropathy, was clouded by its low antagonist potency (Behm et al., 2008). Therefore, drug discovery programs continued to focus on the identification of potent and selective UT antagonists suitable for assessment in both preclinical species and man (Maryanoff and Kinney, 2010). As reported earlier this year, Sanofi launched a phase I clinical trial regarding a long acting UT antagonist, derived from a 5,6-bisaryl-2-pyridine-carboxamide scaffold (European patent application *EP2439193*), for the treatment of diabetic nephropathy. Similarly, GlaxoSmithKline started a phase I clinical trial for the use of an UT antagonist, *i.e.* SB1440115 (United States Patent application *12,373,901*), for the treatment of asthma. Finally, over the past few years, Boehringer-Ingelheim (European patent application *EP2155748*) as well as Janssen Pharmaceutical (United States Patent application *8,193,191*) filled several patents regarding UT antagonists but no phase I clinical trial was yet reported. With the recent discovery that UII and URP could exert common as well as different biological activities (Prosser et al., 2008; Hirose et al., 2009; Jarry et al., 2010), development of selective UT antagonists has become a more complex task.

UT AS SHAPESHIFTING PROTEINS

GPCRs represent the largest and most diverse family of cell surface receptors. These plasma membrane proteins bind their endogenous ligands in order to activate an intracellular signaling cascade that will result in a biological action. Conventional views of ligand-receptor activation considered all components of the signaling cascade to be linearly related, *i.e.* to emanate from the initial activation of the receptor. However, multiple studies pointed out the ability of some ligands to selectively trigger specific signaling pathways, therefore having collateral and not linear efficacy (Roettger et al., 1997; Kohout et al., 2004). As such, GPCRs cannot be considered as pharmacological on/off switches anymore. Their intrinsic nature rather suggests that dynamic changes in the receptor conformation, resulting from ligand binding, are a mean of information transfer (Kenakin and Miller, 2010). Hence, the propensity of GPCRs to assume multiple conformations make them allosteric proteins that are able to select specific subsets of secondary messengers depending on the ligand-induced adopted conformation. As such, various ligands were reported to possess differential functional profiles for a given receptor, as it was initially described for the CCR7 receptor (Kohout et al., 2004).

The URP sequence, strictly conserved throughout species, supports the concept that specific receptor interactions were maintained despite variation in the receptor amino acid sequence (Elshourbagy et al., 2002). Based on the specific expression of

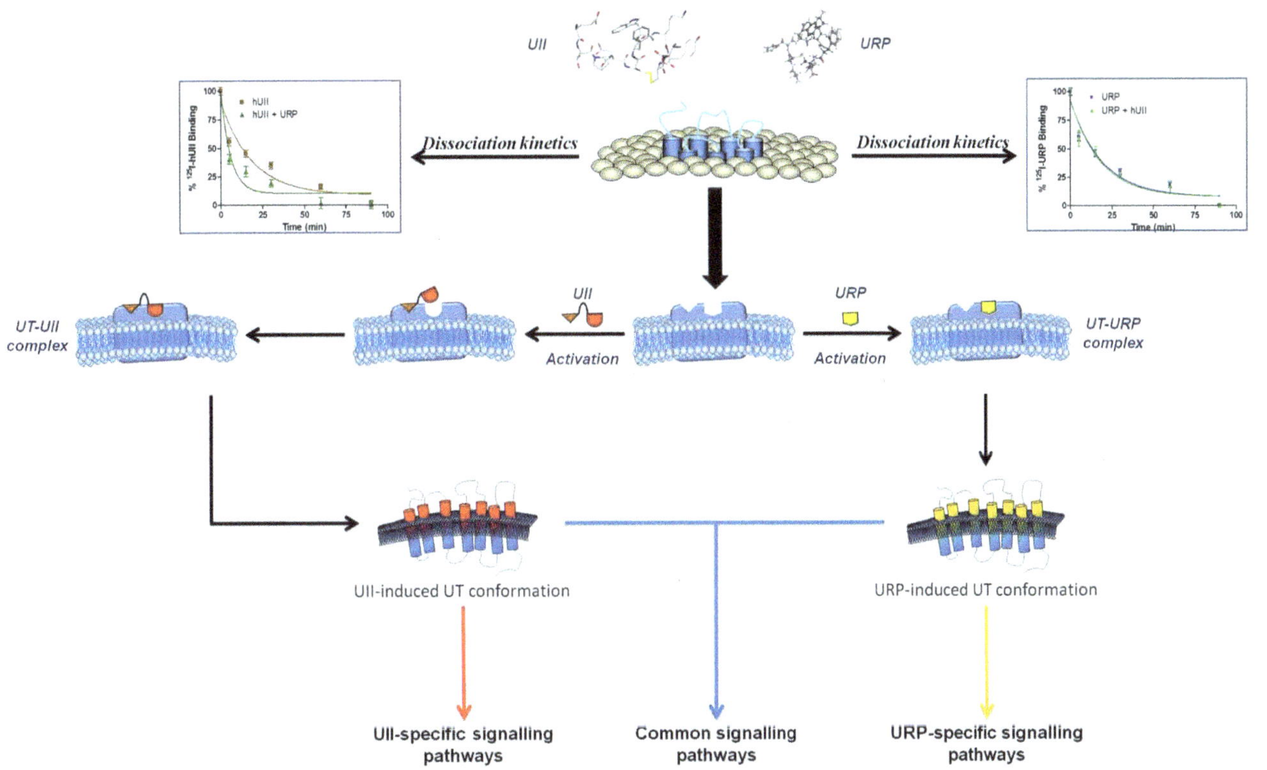

FIGURE 6 | Schematic representation of a proposed binding mode for UII and URP. Following the initial interaction between the N-terminal domain of UII and its receptor, UT undergoes a conformational change aimed at welcoming the C-terminal domain of UII, characterized by an intracyclic β-turn, in a specific binding pocket. However, URP, lacking this N-terminal portion and characterized by the presence of an intracyclic γ-turn, is also able to bind UT but in a slightly different manner, probably characterized by the activation of a different subset of signaling pathways. Modified from Chatenet et al. (2012a).

URP mRNA in several cerebral structures (rostroventrolateral medulla) and tissues (heart, seminal vesicle), it was suggested that URP rather than UII would be the biologically active peptide in the UT-associated regulation of autonomic, cardiovascular and reproductive functions (Dubessy et al., 2008). Moreover, distinct pathophysiological roles for UII and URP in hypertension have been suggested (Hirose et al., 2009). Indeed, mRNA expression of both UII and URP was up-regulated in the atrium of spontaneously hypertensive rats (SHR) when compared with age-matched Wistar Kyoto (WKY) rats. However, the specific up-regulation of URP but not UII mRNA in aorta and kidney of SHR rats supported the idea that these peptides might act individually in various biological systems (Hirose et al., 2009). Accordingly, it was demonstrated that UII and URP were able to exert not only common but also divergent physiological actions clearly suggesting the propensity of these two endogenous ligands to select a specific UT conformation (Prosser et al., 2008; Jarry et al., 2010; Doan et al., 2012). The concept of biased agonism has recently emerged from various studies, putting forward the notion that specific ligand-induced conformational changes can lead to particular signaling (Patel et al., 2010). In isolated ischaemic heart experiments, UII and URP were both able to reduce myocardial damages through creatine kinase reduction but only UII was able to reduce atrial natriuretic peptide (ANP) production (Prosser et al., 2008). Supporting the idea that UII and URP interact with UT in a distinct manner, it was recently demonstrated that URP, an equipotent UII paralog, was able to accelerate the dissociation rate of membrane bound ^{125}I-hUII while hUII had no noticeable effect on URP dissociation kinetics (Chatenet et al., 2012a). Altogether, these results suggest that each ligand is able to select a specific UT conformation that triggers definite biological activities for each of these two peptides.

The peptide N-terminal region was initially pointed out as potentially involved in the observed biological activity differences between UII and URP (Prosser et al., 2008). However, it is only recently that this region was clearly associated with a putative differential binding mode of hUII and URP (Chatenet et al., 2012a). Using exocyclic Ala-derivatives of hUII, acting as very potent ligands of the UT receptor (Brkovic et al., 2003), dissociation kinetics experiments revealed a putative interaction between UT and the glutamic residue at position 1 of hUII. Indeed, it was observed that the replacement of this residue by an alanine moiety, *i.e.* [Ala^1]hUII, provoked an increase of the dissociation rate of hUII but not URP (Chatenet et al., 2012a). In agreement with this view, an important electrostatic interaction between Glu^1 of hUII and its receptor was previously reported in docking studies (Lescot et al., 2008). No other substitution was able to induce such pharmacological changes. Because this compound was reported to exert almost equipotent contractile activity compared to hUII and URP, the lost of a putative specific interaction with UT was thought to have generated an analog behaving as an URP derivative therefore acting at the URP-associated orthosteric binding site. Supporting this hypothesis, hUII(4–11), considered as the minimal hUII fragment to exert full biological activity, was also able to alter hUII but not URP dissociation rate (Chatenet et al., 2012a). This N-terminal segment could thus be crucial for signaling pathway selection upon activation and its deletion could lead to signaling mechanism misinterpretation, all UII truncated analogs potentially acting as URP derivatives.

Overall, these results support the presence of specific pockets/interactions within UT, aimed at selecting distinct UT conformations that can differentiate UII and URP biological activities (**Figure 6**). Briefly, it is hypothesized that upon the initial UII-UT interaction, involving the N-terminal region of UII, UT undergoes conformational changes aimed at welcoming the C-terminal domain of UII, characterized by an intracyclic β-turn (Carotenuto et al., 2004). To the opposite, URP, lacking this N-terminal portion and characterized by the presence of an intracyclic γ-turn (Chatenet et al., 2004), would bind UT in a slightly different manner; ultimately triggering a slightly different subset of signaling pathways. These observations have clearly highlighted the crucial need to reassess the development of pan UT antagonists, *i.e.* blocking UII- and URP-mediated receptor activation, and to develop new analogs of the urotensinergic system aimed at discriminating UII- or URP-mediated biological activities. Such compounds would allow a better understanding of the pathophysiological roles of the urotensinergic system and also expand our knowledge on allosteric modulation of class A GPCRs.

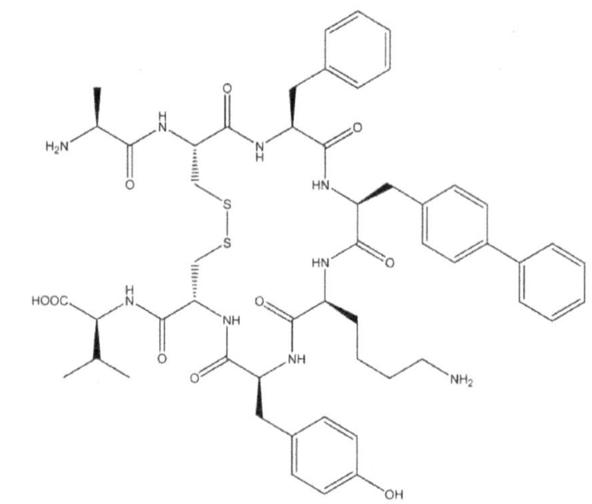

[Bip⁴]URP
Urocontrin

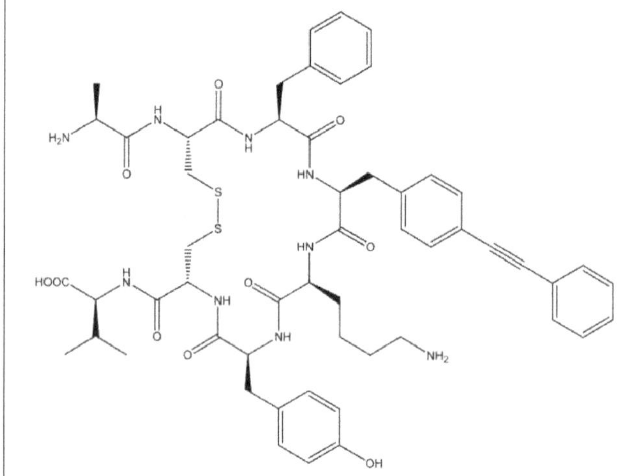

[Pep⁴]URP
Urocontrin A

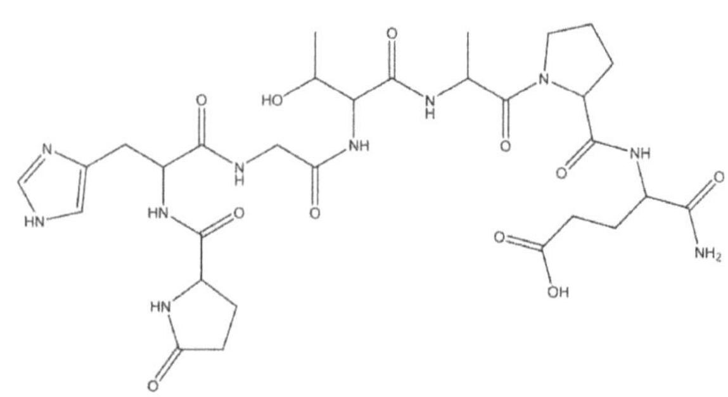

rUII(1-7)

FIGURE 7 | Structure of the novel UT allosteric modulators of the urotensinergic system, *i.e.* [Bip[4]]URP (urocontrin), [Pep[4]]URP (urocontrin A; UCA), and rUII(1–7). Modified from Chatenet et al. (2012a,b).

Allosteric modulation of the urotensinergic system

As demonstrated, the urotensinergic system is far more complex than previously thought with the presence of nuclear receptors and UII/URP specific as well as common actions. For the past two decades, identification of peptidic and non-peptidic agonists and antagonists of the urotensinergic system has gathered much interest for the treatment of various cardiovascular pathologies. An extensive review regarding the various peptidic and non-peptidic ligands of the urotensinergic system, all acting as competitive compounds, is beyond the scope of this review but more details can be found elsewhere (Maryanoff and Kinney, 2010).

Additional biological complexity, but also novel opportunities for drug discovery, has arisen from the fact that many GPCRs possess allosteric binding sites (Christopoulos and Kenakin, 2002). Similar to the initial concept of agonism, *i.e.* linear efficacy, antagonism has been historically viewed as a simple "turning off" of the receptor. As such, this non-accommodating mechanism does not allow any agonist to impart information to the receptor, the orthosteric binding site being occupied by the competitive antagonist. However, an allosteric modulator binds to its own site, different from the orthosteric site, forming a complex characterized by the concomitant presence of the endogenous agonist and the allosteric modulator. Such modulators can alter the biological properties of the endogenous orthosteric ligand either via changing its affinity, its efficacy, or both (Leach et al., 2007; May et al., 2007). This type of antagonism, termed permissive, can modify the reactivity of the receptor toward the agonist probably through conformation selection and stabilization of one or part of the receptor states. Targeting receptor allosteric sites can offer the possibility of greater selectivity due to a lower sequence conservation within allosteric pockets across subtypes of a given GPCR, as well as the potential to fine-tune physiological signaling in a more spatial and temporally-selective manner (Kenakin, 2011).

The urotensinergic system, encompassing two endogenous peptides, provides potential for allosteric compounds to differentially modulate individual peptide responses, a behavior termed "probe dependence" (Kenakin, 2008). During the course of structure-activity relationship studies on URP derivatives, two compounds, *i.e.* [Bip^4]URP and [Pep^4]URP, termed urocontrin and urocontrin A (UCA) respectively, showed a specific behavior that has set them apart from known UT antagonists (**Figure 7**) (Chatenet et al., 2012a,b). Indeed, these compounds were able to selectively and significantly reduce hUII-induced contraction without altering URP-mediated vasoconstriction (Chatenet et al., 2012a,b). For instance, the efficacy of hUII-induced rat aortic ring vasoconstriction was significantly reduced (~31%) by a pretreatment with a nanomolar concentration of UCA (**Figure 8**). Interestingly, this ability to selectively and significantly reduce UII-induced contraction was not specie-dependent since a similar effect was observed on cynomolgus monkey aortic rings. To the best of our knowledge, only two other UT ligands exerted insurmountable activity (Herold et al., 2003; Behm et al., 2010). However, none of them could differentially alter hUII and URP biological activity. The insurmountable nature of urocontrin and UCA antagonism was attributed to an allosteric modulation of UT. Indeed, an excess of UCA accelerated the ^{125}I-hUII dissociation rate, thus suggesting that the binding of the antagonist changes the receptor conformation in such a way that the radioligand is released from the receptor. Accordingly, no difference in ^{125}I-URP dissociation kinetics was observed in similar conditions (**Figure 8**). The apparent absence of effect on the URP pharmacological profile by UCA was attributed to its ability to select a receptor conformation through functional allosteric modulation that impairs hUII-associated actions but not URP-mediated biological activities.

As stated above, for a given receptor, an allosteric modulation that depends on the type of orthosteric ligand used is referred to as "probe dependence" (Kenakin, 2005; Keov et al., 2011). This probe dependence phenomenon supports the idea that the two endogenous ligands, despite depicting a high structure homology and recognizing a similar binding pocket, represent chemically distinct entities interacting in different structural environments within the orthosteric pocket. Because hUII and URP differ only by the length and composition of their N-terminal domain (Vaudry et al., 2010), it was postulated that this region could be involved in their putative different binding modes. Corroborating this hypothesis, the hUII counterpart of UCA, *i.e.* [Pep^7]hUII,

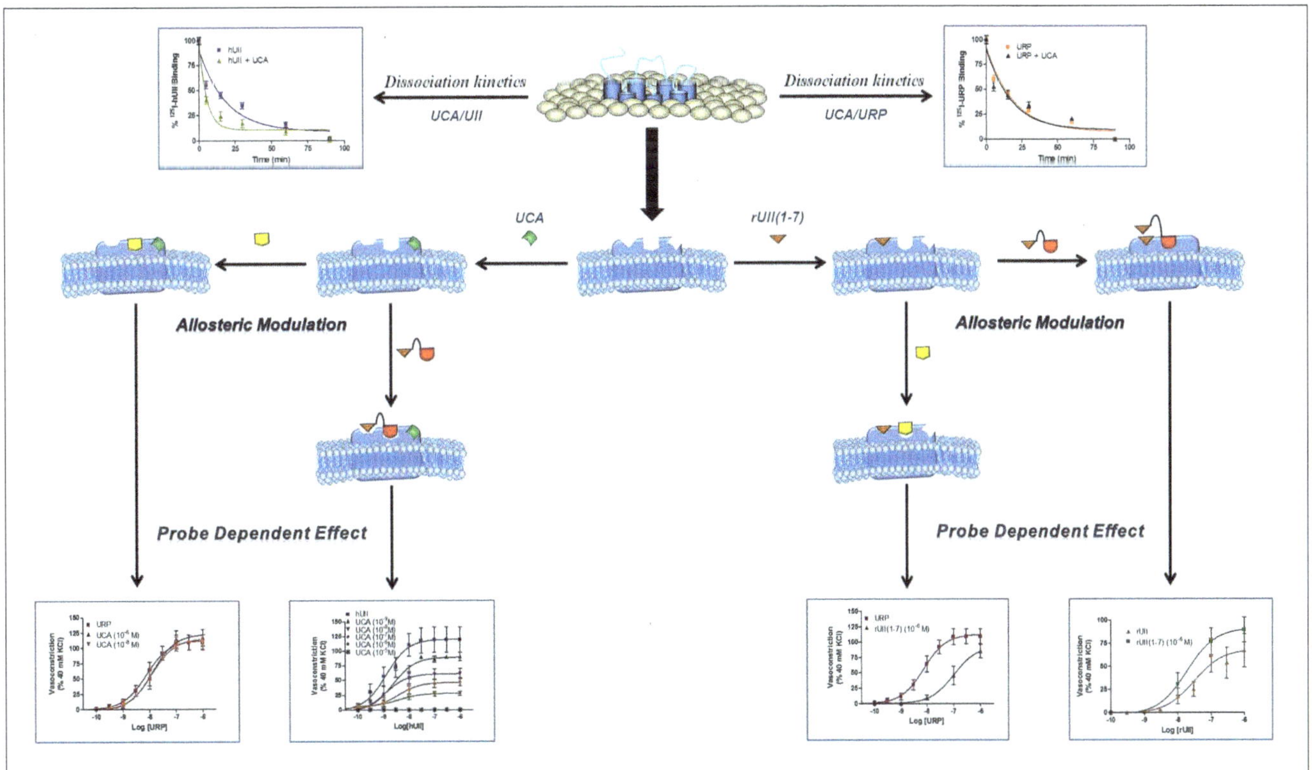

FIGURE 8 | Schematic representation of a proposed allosteric modulation of the urotensinergic system by urocontrin A and rUII(1–7). By acting at an allosteric binding site, UCA is able to modify the receptor topography preventing the proper interaction of UT with the linear UII N-terminal region ultimately leading to an inefficient activation characterized by a reduced efficacy. On the opposite, such a receptor conformational change has no effect on URP-mediated action. Conversely, binding of the rUII(1–7) N-terminal segment, initiates a topographical change that antagonizes the effect of URP, but not UII. Modified from Chatenet et al. (2012a).

acted as a weak but full agonist of the UT receptor (Chatenet et al., 2012a). This N-terminal domain is thus able to modulate the topology of the receptor in such a manner that the C-terminal domain of UII is able to trigger receptor activation. However, could this N-terminal segment be biologically active? As an agonist, the N-terminal domain of rat UII [rUII(1–7)], *i.e.* Pyr-His-Gly-Thr-Ala-Pro-Glu-amide (**Figure 7**), was unable to induce the contraction of rat aortic rings (Chatenet et al., 2012a). Amazingly, pre-treatment of rat aortic rings with rUII(1–7) induced an apparent increase in rUII contractile efficacy while reducing the potency and the efficacy of URP-mediated vasoconstriction (Chatenet et al., 2012a). These results clearly suggested that rUII(1–7) acted as a probe dependant allosteric modulator on rUII- and URP-mediated vasoconstriction (**Figure 8**) (Chatenet et al., 2012a). Since all UII isoforms possess different N-terminal domains, it is hypothesized that these regions could act as specie-selective specific URP modulators but there is currently no clue regarding an endogenous production of those N-terminal UII domains *in vivo*.

CONCLUSIONS

These latest findings about the urotensinergic system will probably generate a considerable interest within the scientific community. First, the discovery of UT on the nuclear membrane and the presence of intracellular ligands open up new avenues in UT signaling physiology. In general, nuclear-localized receptors may regulate distinct signaling pathways, suggesting that biological responses mediated by GPCRs are not only initiated at the cell surface but might result from the integration of extracellular and intracellular signaling pathways. These receptors are therefore well-positioned to play major roles in the physiological and pathophysiological responses associated with their endogenous ligands. Finally, the discovery of allosteric modulators of the urotensinergic systems such as urocontrin, UCA, and rUII(1–7), will surely enable a better understanding of the urotensinergic system by allowing to discriminate *in vitro* and *in vivo* specific biological actions mediated by UII and/or URP. Therefore, these unique derivatives will be useful as chemical templates for the rational design of novel UT receptor ligands, as well as pharmacological tools for *in vitro* and particularly *in vivo* studies aimed at clarifying the role(s) played by the UII/URP/UT receptor system in physiology and pathology.

ACKNOWLEDGMENTS

This work was supported by the Canadian Institutes for Health Research (awarded to Alain Fournier).

REFERENCES

Ames, R. S., Sarau, H. M., Chambers, J. K., Willette, R. N., Aiyar, N. V., Romanic, A. M., et al. (1999). Human urotensin-II is a potent vasoconstrictor and agonist for the orphan receptor GPR14. *Nature* 401, 282–286.

Andreev, O. A., Karabadzhak, A. G., Weerakkody, D., Andreev, G. O., Engelman, D. M., and Reshetnyak, Y. K. (2010). pH (low) insertion peptide (pHLIP) inserts across a lipid bilayer as a helix and exits by a different path. *Proc. Natl. Acad. Sci. U.S.A.* 107, 4081–4086.

Arantes, L. A., Aguiar, C. J., Amaya, M. J., Figueiro, N. C., Andrade, L. M., Rocha-Resende, C., et al. (2012). Nuclear inositol 1, 4, 5-trisphosphate is a necessary and conserved signal for the induction of both pathological and physiological cardiomyocyte hypertrophy. *J. Mol. Cell. Cardiol.* 53, 475–486.

Behm, D. J., Aiyar, N. V., Olzinski, A. R., McAtee, J. J., Hilfiker, M. A., Dodson, J. W., et al. (2010). GSK1562590, a slowly dissociating urotensin-II receptor antagonist, exhibits prolonged pharmacodynamic activity *ex vivo*. *Br. J. Pharmacol.* 161, 207–228.

Behm, D. J., McAtee, J. J., Dodson, J. W., Neeb, M. J., Fries, H. E., Evans, C. A., et al. (2008). Palosuran inhibits binding to primate UT receptors in cell membranes but demonstrates differential activity in intact cells and vascular tissues. *Br. J. Pharmacol.* 155, 374–386.

Bignami, A., Asher, R., and Perides, G. (1991). Brain extracellular matrix and nerve regeneration. *Adv. Exp. Med. Biol.* 296, 197–206.

Boivin, B., Chevalier, D., Villeneuve, L. R., Rousseau, E., and Allen, B. G. (2003). Functional endothelin receptors are present on nuclei in cardiac ventricular myocytes. *J. Biol. Chem.* 278, 29153–29163.

Boivin, B., Lavoie, C., Vaniotis, G., Baragli, A., Villeneuve, L. R., Ethier, N., et al. (2006). Functional beta-adrenergic receptor signalling on nuclear membranes in adult rat and mouse ventricular cardiomyocytes. *Cardiovasc. Res.* 71, 69–78.

Boivin, B., Vaniotis, G., Allen, B. G., and Hebert, T. E. (2008). G protein-coupled receptors in and on the cell nucleus: a new signaling paradigm? *J. Recept. Signal Transduct. Res.* 28, 15–28.

Bootman, M. D., Fearnley, C., Smyrnias, I., Macdonald, F., and Roderick, H. L. (2009). An update on nuclear calcium signalling. *J. Cell Sci.* 122, 2337–2350.

Brkovic, A., Hattenberger, A., Kostenis, E., Klabunde, T., Flohr, S., Kurz, M., et al. (2003). Functional and binding characterizations of urotensin II-related peptides in human and rat urotensin II-receptor assay. *J. Pharmacol. Exp. Ther.* 306, 1200–1209.

Carotenuto, A., Grieco, P., Campiglia, P., Novellino, E., and Rovero, P. (2004). Unraveling the active conformation of urotensin II. *J. Med. Chem.* 47, 1652–1661.

Castel, H., Diallo, M., Chatenet, D., Leprince, J., Desrues, L., Schouft, M. T., et al. (2006). Biochemical and functional characterization of high-affinity urotensin II receptors in rat cortical astrocytes. *J. Neurochem.* 99, 582–595.

Chatenet, D., Dubessy, C., Leprince, J., Boularan, C., Carlier, L., Segalas-Milazzo, I., et al. (2004). Structure-activity relationships and structural conformation of a novel urotensin II-related peptide. *Peptides* 25, 1819–1830.

Chatenet, D., Nguyen, Q. T., Letourneau, M., Doan, N. D., Dupuis, J., and Fournier, A. (2012a). Discovery of new antagonists aimed at discriminating UII and URP-mediated biological activities: insight into UII and URP receptor activation. *Br. J. Pharmacol.* doi: 10.1111/j.1476-5381.2012.02217.x. [Epub ahead of print].

Chatenet, D., Nguyen, Q. T., Letourneau, M., Dupuis, J., and Fournier, A. (2012b). Urocontrin, a novel UT receptor ligand with a unique pharmacological profile. *Biochem. Pharmacol.* 83, 608–615.

Christopoulos, A., and Kenakin, T. (2002). G protein-coupled receptor allosterism and complexing. *Pharmacol. Rev.* 54, 323–374.

Clozel, M., Binkert, C., Birker-Robaczewska, M., Boukhadra, C., Ding, S. S., Fischli, W., et al. (2004). Pharmacology of the urotensin-II receptor antagonist palosuran (ACT-058362; 1-[2-(4-benzyl-4-hydroxy-piperidin-1-yl)-ethyl]-3-(2-methyl-quinolin-4-yl)-urea sulfate salt): first demonstration of a pathophysiological role of the urotensin System. *J. Pharmacol. Exp. Ther.* 311, 204–212.

Clozel, M., Hess, P., Qiu, C., Ding, S. S., and Rey, M. (2006). The urotensin-II receptor antagonist palosuran improves pancreatic and renal function in diabetic rats. *J. Pharmacol. Exp. Ther.* 316, 1115–1121.

Conlon, J. M., O'Harte, F., Smith, D. D., Tonon, M. C., and Vaudry, H. (1992). Isolation and primary structure of urotensin II from the brain of a tetrapod, the frog Rana ridibunda. *Biochem. Biophys. Res. Commun.* 188, 578–583.

Coulouarn, Y., Lihrmann, I., Jegou, S., Anouar, Y., Tostivint, H., Beauvillain, J. C., et al. (1998). Cloning of the cDNA encoding the urotensin II precursor in frog and human reveals intense expression of the urotensin II gene in motoneurons of the spinal cord. *Proc. Natl. Acad. Sci. U.S.A.* 95, 15803–15808.

Dai, H. Y., Kang, W. Q., Wang, X., Yu, X. J., Li, Z. H., Tang, M. X., et al. (2007). The involvement of transforming growth factor-beta1 secretion in urotensin II-induced collagen synthesis in neonatal cardiac fibroblasts. *Regul. Pept.* 140, 88–93.

De Mello, W. C. (2008). Intracellular and extracellular renin have opposite effects on the regulation of heart cell volume. Implications for myocardial ischaemia. *J. Renin Angiotensin Aldosterone Syst.* 9, 112–118.

Diallo, M., Castel, H., Jarry, M., Desrues, L., Lefebvre, T., Leprince, J., et al. (2007). Urotensin II and urotensin II-related peptide regulate normal astrocyte activity. Potential involvement in glioma proliferation. *Neuron Glia Biol.* 3, S161.

Doan, N. D., Nguyen, T. T., Letourneau, M., Turcotte, K., Fournier, A., and Chatenet, D. (2012). Biochemical and pharmacological characterization of nuclear urotensin-II binding sites in rat heart. *Br. J. Pharmacol.* 166, 243–257.

Douglas, S. A., Ashton, D. J., Sauermelch, C. F., Coatney, R. W., Ohlstein, D. H., Ruffolo, M. R., et al. (2000). Human urotensin-II is a potent vasoactive peptide: pharmacological characterization in the rat, mouse, dog and primate. *J. Cardiovasc. Pharmacol.* 36, S163–S166.

Douglas, S. A., and Ohlstein, E. H. (2000). Human urotensin-II, the most potent mammalian vasoconstrictor identified to date, as a therapeutic target for the management of cardiovascular disease. *Trends Cardiovasc. Med.* 10, 229–237.

Dubessy, C., Cartier, D., Lectez, B., Bucharles, C., Chartrel, N., Montero-Hadjadje, M., et al. (2008). Characterization of urotensin II, distribution of urotensin II, urotensin II-related peptide and UT receptor mRNAs in mouse: evidence of urotensin II at the neuromuscular junction. *J. Neurochem.* 107, 361–374.

Duverger, E., Pellerin-Mendes, C., Mayer, R., Roche, A. C., and Monsigny, M. (1995). Nuclear import of glycoconjugates is distinct from the classical NLS pathway. *J. Cell Sci.* 108(Pt 4), 1325–1332.

Eggena, P., Zhu, J. H., Clegg, K., and Barrett, J. D. (1993). Nuclear angiotensin receptors induce transcription of renin and angiotensinogen mRNA. *Hypertension* 22, 496–501.

Elshourbagy, N. A., Douglas, S. A., Shabon, U., Harrison, S., Duddy, G., Sechler, J. L., et al. (2002). Molecular and pharmacological characterization of genes encoding urotensin-II peptides and their cognate G-protein-coupled receptors from the mouse and monkey. *Br. J. Pharmacol.* 136, 9–22.

Fontes-Sousa, A. P., Pires, A. L., Monteiro-Cardoso, V. F., and Leite-Moreira, A. F. (2009). Urotensin II-induced increase in myocardial distensibility is modulated by angiotensin II and endothelin-1. *Physiol. Res.* 58, 653–660.

Gibson, A. (1987). Complex effects of Gillichthys urotensin II on rat aortic strips. *Br. J. Pharmacol.* 91, 205–212.

Gibson, A., Bern, H. A., Ginsburg, M., and Botting, J. H. (1984). Neuropeptide-induced contraction and relaxation of the mouse anococcygeus muscle. *Proc. Natl. Acad. Sci. U.S.A.* 81, 625–629.

Giebing, G., Tolle, M., Jurgensen, J., Eichhorst, J., Furkert, J., Beyermann, M., et al. (2005). Arrestin-independent internalization and recycling of the urotensin receptor contribute to long-lasting urotensin II-mediated vasoconstriction. *Circ. Res.* 97, 707–715.

Gobeil, F., Fortier, A., Zhu, T., Bossolasco, M., Leduc, M., Grandbois, M., et al. (2006). G-protein-coupled receptors signalling at the cell nucleus: an emerging paradigm. *Can. J. Physiol. Pharmacol.* 84, 287–297.

Gruson, D., Ginion, A., Decroly, N., Lause, P., Vanoverschelde, J. L., Ketelslegers, J. M., et al. (2010). Urotensin II induction of adult cardiomyocytes hypertrophy involves the Akt/GSK-3beta signaling pathway. *Peptides* 31, 1326–1333.

Guidolin, D., Albertin, G., and Ribatti, D. (2010). Urotensin-II as an angiogenic factor. *Peptides* 31, 1219–1224.

Hanyaloglu, A. C., and von Zastrow, M. (2008). Regulation of GPCRs by endocytic membrane trafficking and its potential implications. *Annu. Rev. Pharmacol. Toxicol.* 48, 537–568.

Herold, C. L., Behm, D. J., Buckley, P. T., Foley, J. J., Wixted, W. E., Sarau, H. M., et al. (2003). The neuromedin B receptor antagonist, BIM-23127, is a potent antagonist at human and rat urotensin-II receptors. *Br. J. Pharmacol.* 139, 203–207.

Hillier, C., Berry, C., Petrie, M. C., O'Dwyer, P. J., Hamilton, C., Brown, A., et al. (2001). Effects of urotensin II in human arteries and veins of varying caliber. *Circulation* 103, 1378–1381.

Hirose, T., Takahashi, K., Mori, N., Nakayama, T., Kikuya, M., Ohkubo, T., et al. (2009). Increased expression of urotensin II, urotensin II-related peptide and urotensin II receptor mRNAs in the cardiovascular organs of hypertensive rats: comparison with endothelin-1. *Peptides* 30, 1124–1129.

Hood, S. G., Watson, A. M., and May, C. N. (2005). Cardiac actions of central but not peripheral urotensin II are prevented by beta-adrenoceptor blockade. *Peptides* 26, 1248–1256.

Jarry, M., Diallo, M., Lecointre, C., Desrues, L., Tokay, T., Chatenet, D., et al. (2010). The vasoactive peptides urotensin II and urotensin II-related peptide regulate astrocyte activity through common and distinct mechanisms: involvement in cell proliferation. *Biochem. J.* 428, 113–124.

Jiang, X., Benovic, J. L., and Wedegaertner, P. B. (2007). Plasma membrane and nuclear localization of G protein coupled receptor kinase 6A. *Mol. Biol. Cell* 18, 2960–2969.

Jong, Y. J., Kumar, V., Kingston, A. E., Romano, C., and O'Malley, K. L. (2005). Functional metabotropic glutamate receptors on nuclei from brain and primary cultured striatal neurons. Role of transporters in delivering ligand. *J. Biol. Chem.* 280, 30469–30480.

Jong, Y. J., Kumar, V., and O'Malley, K. L. (2009). Intracellular metabotropic glutamate receptor 5 (mGluR5) activates signaling cascades distinct from cell surface counterparts. *J. Biol. Chem.* 284, 35827–35838.

Kenakin, T. (2005). New concepts in drug discovery: collateral efficacy and permissive antagonism. *Nat. Rev. Drug Discov.* 4, 919–927.

Kenakin, T. (2008). Functional selectivity in GPCR modulator screening. *Comb. Chem. High Throughput Screen.* 11, 337–343.

Kenakin, T. (2011). Functional selectivity and biased receptor signaling. *J. Pharmacol. Exp. Ther.* 336, 296–302.

Kenakin, T., and Miller, L. J. (2010). Seven transmembrane receptors as shapeshifting proteins: the impact of allosteric modulation and functional selectivity on new drug discovery. *Pharmacol. Rev.* 62, 265–304.

Keov, P., Sexton, P. M., and Christopoulos, A. (2011). Allosteric modulation of G protein-coupled receptors: a pharmacological perspective. *Neuropharmacology* 60, 24–35.

Kiefer, P., Acland, P., Pappin, D., Peters, G., and Dickson, C. (1994). Competition between nuclear localization and secretory signals determines the subcellular fate of a single CUG-initiated form of FGF3. *EMBO J.* 13, 4126–4136.

Kohout, T. A., Nicholas, S. L., Perry, S. J., Reinhart, G., Junger, S., and Struthers, R. S. (2004). Differential desensitization, receptor phosphorylation, beta-arrestin recruitment, and ERK1/2 activation by the two endogenous ligands for the CC chemokine receptor 7. *J. Biol. Chem.* 279, 23214–23222.

Krum, H., and Kemp, W. (2007). Therapeutic potential of blockade of the urotensin II system in systemic hypertension. *Curr. Hypertens. Rep.* 9, 53–58.

Leach, K., Sexton, P. M., and Christopoulos, A. (2007). Allosteric GPCR modulators: taking advantage of permissive receptor pharmacology. *Trends Pharmacol. Sci.* 28, 382–389.

Lee, D. K., Lanca, A. J., Cheng, R., Nguyen, T., Ji, X. D., Gobeil, F. Jr., et al. (2004). Agonist-independent nuclear localization of the Apelin, angiotensin AT1, and bradykinin B2 receptors. *J. Biol. Chem.* 279, 7901–7908.

Lee-Kirsch, M. A., Gaudet, F., Cardoso, M. C., and Lindpaintner, K. (1999). Distinct renin isoforms generated by tissue-specific transcription initiation and alternative splicing. *Circ. Res.* 84, 240–246.

Lescot, E., Sopkova-De Oliveira Santos, J., Colloc'h, N., Rodrigo, J., Milazzo-Segalas, I., Bureau, R., et al. (2008). Three-dimensional model of the human urotensin-II receptor: docking of human urotensin-II and non-peptide antagonists in the binding site and comparison with an antagonist pharmacophore model. *Proteins* 73, 173–184.

Liu, Q., Pong, S. S., Zeng, Z., Zhang, Q., Howard, A. D., Williams, D. L. Jr., et al. (1999). Identification of urotensin II as the endogenous ligand for the orphan G-protein-coupled receptor GPR14. *Biochem. Biophys. Res. Commun.* 266, 174–178.

Maguire, J. J., and Davenport, A. P. (2002). Is urotensin-II the new endothelin? *Br. J. Pharmacol.* 137, 579–588.

Maguire, J. J., Kuc, R. E., and Davenport, A. P. (2000). Orphan-receptor ligand human urotensin II: receptor localization in human tissues and comparison of vasoconstrictor responses with endothelin-1. *Br. J. Pharmacol.* 131, 441–446.

Maguire, J. J., Kuc, R. E., Kleinz, M. J., and Davenport, A. P. (2008). Immunocytochemical localization of the urotensin-II receptor, UT, to rat and human tissues: relevance to function. *Peptides* 29, 735–742.

Marchese, A., Heiber, M., Nguyen, T., Heng, H. H., Saldivia, V. R., Cheng, R., et al. (1995). Cloning and chromosomal mapping of three novel genes, GPR9, GPR10, and GPR14, encoding receptors related to interleukin 8, neuropeptide Y, and somatostatin receptors. *Genomics* 29, 335–344.

Maryanoff, B. E., and Kinney, W. A. (2010). Urotensin-II receptor modulators as potential drugs. *J. Med. Chem.* 53, 2695–2708.

May, L. T., Leach, K., Sexton, P. M., and Christopoulos, A. (2007). Allosteric modulation of G protein-coupled receptors. *Annu. Rev. Pharmacol. Toxicol.* 47, 1–51.

Mori, M., Sugo, T., Abe, M., Shimomura, Y., Kurihara, M., Kitada, C., et al. (1999). Urotensin II is the endogenous ligand of a G-protein-coupled orphan receptor, SENR (GPR14). *Biochem. Biophys. Res. Commun.* 265, 123–129.

Nguyen, T. T., Letourneau, M., Chatenet, D., and Fournier, A. (2012). Presence of urotensin-II receptors at the cell nucleus: specific tissue distribution and hypoxia-induced modulation. *Int. J. Biochem. Cell Biol.* 44, 639–647.

Nothacker, H. P., Wang, Z., McNeill, A. M., Saito, Y., Merten, S., O'Dowd, B., et al. (1999). Identification of the natural ligand of an orphan G-protein-coupled receptor involved in the regulation of vasoconstriction. *Nat. Cell Biol.* 1, 383–385.

Ono, T., Kawaguchi, Y., Kudo, M., Kushikata, T., Hashiba, E., Yoshida, H., et al. (2008). Urotensin II evokes neurotransmitter release from rat cerebrocortical slices. *Neurosci. Lett.* 440, 275–279.

Papadopoulos, P., Bousette, N., and Giaid, A. (2008). Urotensin-II and cardiovascular remodeling. *Peptides* 29, 764–769.

Patel, C. B., Noor, N., and Rockman, H. A. (2010). Functional selectivity in adrenergic and angiotensin signaling systems. *Mol. Pharmacol.* 78, 983–992.

Pearson, D., Shively, J. E., Clark, B. R., Geschwind, I. I., Barkley, M., Nishioka, R. S., et al. (1980). Urotensin II: a somatostatin-like peptide in the caudal neurosecretory system of fishes. *Proc. Natl. Acad. Sci. U.S.A.* 77, 5021–5024.

Petersen, M. C., Munzenmaier, D. H., and Greene, A. S. (2006). Angiotensin II infusion restores stimulated angiogenesis in the skeletal muscle of rats on a high-salt diet. *Am. J. Physiol. Heart Circ. Physiol.* 291, H114–H120.

Prosser, H. C., Forster, M. E., Richards, A. M., and Pemberton, C. J. (2008). Urotensin II and urotensin II-related peptide (URP) in cardiac ischemia-reperfusion injury. *Peptides* 29, 770–777.

Proulx, C. D., Holleran, B. J., Lavigne, P., Escher, E., Guillemette, G., and Leduc, R. (2008). Biological properties and functional determinants of the urotensin II receptor. *Peptides* 29, 691–699.

Re, R. (1999). The nature of intracrine peptide hormone action. *Hypertension* 34, 534–538.

Re, R. N. (2004). A proposal regarding the biology of memory: participation of intracrine peptide networks. *Med. Hypotheses* 63, 887–894.

Roettger, B. F., Ghanekar, D., Rao, R., Toledo, C., Yingling, J., Pinon, D., et al. (1997). Antagonist-stimulated internalization of the G protein-coupled cholecystokinin receptor. *Mol. Pharmacol.* 51, 357–362.

Rondanino, C., Bousser, M. T., Monsigny, M., and Roche, A. C. (2003). Sugar-dependent nuclear import of glycosylated proteins in living cells. *Glycobiology* 13, 509–519.

Roskoski, R. Jr. (2012). ERK1/2 MAP kinases: structure, function, and regulation. *Pharmacol. Res.* 66, 105–143.

Ross, B., McKendy, K., and Giaid, A. (2010). Role of urotensin II in health and disease. *Am. J. Physiol. Regul. Integr. Comp. Physiol.* 298, R1156–R1172.

Shiraishi, Y., Watanabe, T., Suguro, T., Nagashima, M., Kato, R., Hongo, S., et al. (2008). Chronic urotensin II infusion enhances macrophage foam cell formation and atherosclerosis in apolipoprotein E-knockout mice. *J. Hypertens.* 26, 1955–1965.

Silvestre, R. A., Egido, E. M., Hernandez, R., Leprince, J., Chatenet, D., Tollemer, H., et al. (2004). Urotensin-II is present in pancreatic extracts and inhibits insulin release in the perfused rat pancreas. *Eur. J. Endocrinol.* 151, 803–809.

Song, W., Abdel-Razik, A. E., Lu, W., Ao, Z., Johns, D. G., Douglas, S. A., et al. (2006). Urotensin II and renal function in the rat. *Kidney Int.* 69, 1360–1368.

Sorkin, A., and von Zastrow, M. (2009). Endocytosis and signalling: intertwining molecular networks. *Nat. Rev. Mol. Cell Biol.* 10, 609–622.

Spinazzi, R., Albertin, G., Nico, B., Guidolin, D., Di Liddo, R., Rossi, G. P., et al. (2006). Urotensin-II and its receptor (UT-R) are expressed in rat brain endothelial cells, and urotensin-II via UT-R stimulates angiogenesis *in vivo* and *in vitro*. *Int. J. Mol. Med.* 18, 1107–1112.

Stirrat, A., Gallagher, M., Douglas, S. A., Ohlstein, E. H., Berry, C., Kirk, A., et al. (2001). Potent vasodilator responses to human urotensin-II in human pulmonary and abdominal resistance arteries. *Am. J. Physiol. Heart Circ. Physiol.* 280, H925–H928.

Sugo, T., Murakami, Y., Shimomura, Y., Harada, M., Abe, M., Ishibashi, Y., et al. (2003). Identification of urotensin II-related peptide as the urotensin II-immunoreactive molecule in the rat brain. *Biochem. Biophys. Res. Commun.* 310, 860–868.

Tadevosyan, A., Vaniotis, G., Allen, B. G., Hebert, T. E., and Nattel, S. (2012). G protein-coupled receptor signalling in the cardiac nuclear membrane: evidence and possible roles in physiological and pathophysiological function. *J. Physiol.* 590, 1313–1330.

Tal, M., Ammar, D. A., Karpuj, M., Krizhanovsky, V., Naim, M., and Thompson, D. A. (1995). A novel putative neuropeptide receptor expressed in neural tissue, including sensory epithelia. *Biochem. Biophys. Res. Commun.* 209, 752–759.

Terrillon, S., and Bouvier, M. (2004). Receptor activity-independent recruitment of betaarrestin2 reveals specific signalling modes. *EMBO J.* 23, 3950–3961.

Vaniotis, G., Del Duca, D., Trieu, P., Rohlicek, C. V., Hebert, T. E., and Allen, B. G. (2011). Nuclear beta-adrenergic receptors modulate gene expression in adult rat heart. *Cell. Signal.* 23, 89–98.

Vaudry, H., Do Rego, J. C., Le Mevel, J. C., Chatenet, D., Tostivint, H., Fournier, A., et al. (2010). Urotensin, II, from fish to human. *Ann. N.Y. Acad. Sci.* 1200, 53–66.

Watson, A. M., Lambert, G. W., Smith, K. J., and May, C. N. (2003). Urotensin II acts centrally to increase epinephrine and ACTH release and cause potent inotropic and chronotropic actions. *Hypertension* 42, 373–379.

Xu, D., Borges, G. R., Grobe, J. L., Pelham, C. J., Yang, B., and Sigmund, C. D. (2009). Preservation of intracellular renin expression is insufficient to compensate for genetic loss of secreted renin. *Hypertension* 54, 1240–1247.

Yoshimoto, T., Matsushita, M., and Hirata, Y. (2004). Role of urotensin II in peripheral tissue as an autocrine/paracrine growth factor. *Peptides* 25, 1775–1781.

Zhang, Y. G., Li, J., Li, Y. G., and Wei, R. H. (2008). Urotensin II induces phenotypic differentiation, migration, and collagen synthesis of adventitial fibroblasts from rat aorta. *J. Hypertens.* 26, 1119–1126.

6

Taltirelin is a superagonist at the human thyrotropin-releasing hormone receptor

Nanthakumar Thirunarayanan, Bruce M. Raaka and Marvin C. Gershengorn*

Laboratory of Endocrinology and Receptor Biology, National Institute of Diabetes and Digestive and Kidney Diseases, National Institutes of Health, Bethesda, MD, USA

Edited by:
Hubert Vaudry, University of Rouen, France

Reviewed by:
Hubert Vaudry, University of Rouen, France
Ludovic Galas, Institut National de la Santé et de la Recherche Biomédicale, France

****Correspondence:***
Marvin C. Gershengorn, Laboratory of Endocrinology and Receptor Biology, National Institute of Diabetes and Digestive and Kidney Diseases, National Institutes of Health, 50 South Drive, Room 4134, Bethesda, MD 20892, USA.
e-mail: marving@intra.niddk.hih.gov

Taltirelin (TAL) is a thyrotropin-releasing hormone (TRH) analog that is approved for use in humans in Japan. In this study, we characterized TAL binding to and signaling by the human TRH receptor (TRH-R) in a model cell system. We found that TAL exhibited lower binding affinities than TRH and lower signaling potency via the inositol-1,4,5-trisphosphate/calcium pathway than TRH. However, TAL exhibited higher intrinsic efficacy than TRH in stimulating inositol-1,4,5-trisphosphate second messenger generation. This is the first study that elucidates the pharmacology of TAL at TRH-R and shows that TAL is a superagonist at TRH-R. We suggest the superagonism exhibited by TAL may in part explain its higher activity in mediating central nervous system effects in humans compared to TRH.

Keywords: taltirelin, thyrotropin-releasing hormone, human TRH receptor

INTRODUCTION

Based on evidence that thyrotropin-releasing hormone (TRH) modulates a number of central nervous system (CNS) activities including arousal, antidepressant activity, anxiolytic effects, increase in locomotor activity, antagonism of pentobarbital-induced sedation, thermoregulation, and cardiovascular and gastrointestinal autonomic functions (Horita et al., 1986; Horita, 1998; Khomane et al., 2011), many analogs of TRH were synthesized and studied. Taltirelin (TAL) hydrate [(1-methyl-(S)-4,5-dihydroorotyl)-histidyl-prolinamide, TA-0910] is an analog that showed improved CNS activity (Suzuki et al., 1990; Yamamura et al., 1991, 1997) and lower thyrotropin (TSH)-releasing activity (Yamamura et al., 1997) compared to TRH in rodents. Based on these characteristics, TAL was studied as a treatment for neurodegenerative disorders and is the only TRH analog that has been approved for use in humans; it is used in Japan to treat patients with adult spinal muscular atrophy (Ceredist®).

In some mammals, including rodents, there are two subtypes of G protein-coupled (or seven-transmembrane-spanning) receptors for TRH. These are TRH receptor 1 (TRH-R1), which is the primary (or only) receptor in TSH-secreting cells, and TRH-R2, which is expressed throughout the CNS along with TRH-R1 but typically in different areas of the brain (O'Dowd et al., 2000; Sun et al., 2003). In humans, by contrast, only a single type of receptor for TRH, TRH-R, is expressed that is more similar to TRH-R1 than TRH-R2 (Duthie et al., 1993; Matre et al., 1993). It has been reported that TAL binds with lower affinity than TRH to receptors in rat or mouse pituitary and in brain tissue preparations (Kinoshita et al., 1997; Asai et al., 1999, 2005). However, the pharmacology of TAL at TRH-R has not been characterized.

In this study, we characterized TAL binding and signaling by TRH-R in a model cell system and show that TAL is a superagonist at TRH-R.

MATERIALS AND METHODS

MATERIALS

Dulbecco's modified Eagle's medium (DMEM) and fetal bovine serum were purchased from Biosource (Rockville, MD, USA). TRH (pyroGlu-His-ProNH_2) and MeTRH (pGlu-His(1(τ)-methyl)-ProNH_2) were purchased from Sigma (St. Louis, MO, USA). [^{3}H]MeTRH was purchased from PerkinElmer (Waltham, MA, USA). TAL (N-[[(4S)-Hexahydro-1-methyl-2,6-dioxo-4-pyrimidinyl]carbonyl]-L-histidyl-L-prolinamide) was obtained from Tocris (San Diego, CA, USA).

CELL CULTURE AND GENERATION OF CELLS STABLY EXPRESSING TRH-R

HEK-EM 293 (human embryonic kidney) cells stably expressing TRH-R were generated as follows. The human TRH-R cDNA in pcDNA3.1(+) was obtained from the Missouri S&T cDNA Resource Center (Rolla, MO, USA) and was subcloned into the pcDNA3.1(+)/hygromycin vector. HEK-EM 293 cells were transfected with the cDNA of TRH-R using FuGENE 6 transfection reagent (Roche Diagnostics GmbH, Mannheim, Germany) and the cell clones stably expressing TRH-R were selected using hygromycin (250 μg/ml). HEK-EM 293 cells stably expressing TRH-R were grown in DMEM containing 10% fetal bovine serum, 100 U/ml penicillin, 10 μg/ml streptomycin, and 200 μg/ml hygromycin B (Invitrogen, Carlsbad, CA, USA) at 37°C in a humidified 5% CO_2 incubator.

COMPETITION BINDING

Competition binding assays were performed in monolayers of intact HEK cells expressing TRH-Rs. The cells (220,000 cells/well in 24-well plates) were preincubated with various concentrations of unlabeled TAL, TRH, or MeTRH for 15 min before addition of radioligand and then incubated at 37°C for 1 h with 4 nM [^{3}H]MeTRH as described elsewhere (Engel et al., 2006). Non-specific binding was determined in incubations with excess non-radiolabeled MeTRH. IC_{50} is the concentration of unlabeled ligand that reduces specific binding of [^{3}H]MeTRH by 50%. The receptor number per cell was calculated from competition binding curves of various doses of unlabeled MeTRH and 4 nM [^{3}H]MeTRH (**Figure 1**) and found to be 16,000/cell.

MEASUREMENT OF INTRACELLULAR CALCIUM MOBILIZATION

Cells stably expressing TRH-R were seeded in black-walled, clear-bottomed 96-well plates (Corning, NY, USA) at a density of 60,000 cells/well in DMEM with 10% fetal bovine serum and incubated for 24 h at 37°C in 5% CO_2. The following day, the culture media was replaced with 100 μl of Hank's balanced salt solution with 20 mM HEPES, pH 7.5 and the cells were loaded with 100 μl of calcium 4 fluorescent dye (Molecular Devices, Sunnyvale, CA, USA) for 1 h at room temperature before addition of compounds. Transient changes in intracellular [Ca^{++}] induced by TAL, TRH, or MeTRH were measured using the FLIPR^{TETRA} system (Molecular Devices, Sunnyvale, CA, USA). Changes in fluorescence were detected at the emission wavelength ranges from 515 to 575 nm. The agonistic responses of ligands were assessed immediately upon their addition in a concentration range from 0.1 nM to 30 μM. Responses were measured as peak fluorescent intensity minus basal fluorescent intensity at each compound concentration and are presented as % of the maximum response.

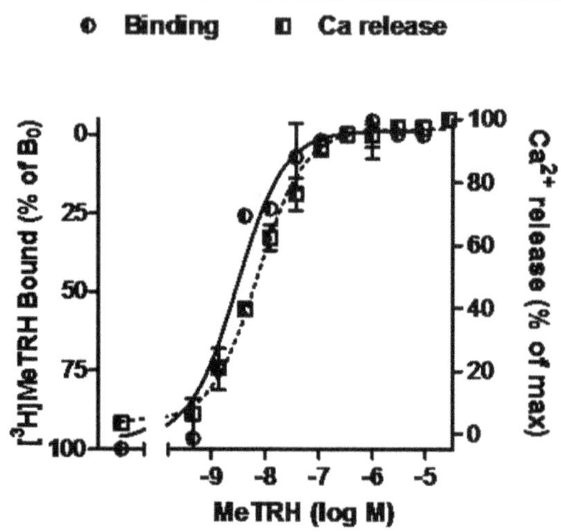

FIGURE 1 | MeTRH binding and signaling via Ca^{2+} in cells expressing TRH-Rs. Competition binding with [^{3}H]MeTRH and changes in cytosolic free Ca^{2+} concentration (Ca^{2+} release) were performed in intact HEK-EM 293 cells stably expressing TRH-Rs as described in Section "Materials and Methods." The competition binding data are presented as the % of [^{3}H]MeTRH bound to cells in the absence of unlabeled ligand (B_0) and represent the results from three experiments conducted with duplicate measurements. Note the left axis is inverted. Intracellular Ca^{2+} release data are shown as a % of the maximal Ca^{2+} increase over basal. The curves represent the non-linear regression analyses of data obtained in one of three experiments with triplicate measurements using a sigmoidal dose–response method.

MEASUREMENT OF IP1 PRODUCTION

Cells were seeded at 220,000/well in white, solid bottom, tissue culture-treated 24-well plates and cultured at 37°C with 5% CO_2 overnight. Serial dilutions of TAL, TRH, or MeTRH, in Hank's balanced salt solution with 20 mM HEPES and 50 mM LiCl, pH 7.4, were added at 200 μl/well on the second day. After 60 min incubation at 37°C in 5% CO_2, inositol monophosphate (IP1) content was measured using the IP-One ELISA kit (Cisbio International, France) according to the manufacturer's protocol. The results were calculated as IP1 nanomoles/well and are presented as % of the maximum response.

DATA ANALYSIS

The dose–response data were analyzed by non-linear regression of curve fit with one-site competition using GraphPad Prism software version 4 (GraphPad, Inc., San Diego, CA, USA) and the significance was determined by *t*-test or ANOVA.

RESULTS

The pharmacology of TAL binding and signaling was studied in HEK-EM 293 cells, which do not endogenously express TRH-Rs, engineered to express 16,000 TRH-Rs/cell (**Table 1**). In competition binding assays using 4 nM [^{3}H]MeTRH and various doses of unlabeled MeTRH, the concentration of MeTRH that half-maximally inhibited [^{3}H]MeTRH binding (IC_{50}) was 3.0 nM (**Figure 1**). The half-maximally effective concentration (EC_{50}) of MeTRH for stimulating an increase in cytosolic Ca^{2+} concentration (Ca^{2+} release) was 7.2 nM, which is not different from the IC_{50} ($p > 0.1$). Thus, MeTRH is an agonist at TRH-R with high potency. We compared the effects of TAL and TRH in competing for [^{3}H]MeTRH binding and on stimulating Ca^{2+} release (**Figure 2**). The IC_{50} values were 910 and 36 nM for TAL and TRH, respectively, and the EC_{50} values were 36 and 5.0 nM for TAL and TRH, respectively. Thus, TRH was a high potency agonist and TAL was a moderate potency agonist at TRH-R. We noted, moreover, that the IC_{50}/EC_{50} ratio was 25 for TAL ($p < 0.02$), 7.2 for TRH ($p < 0.05$), and approximately 0.4 for MeTRH. When comparing two agonists, the agonist with the higher IC_{50}/EC_{50} ratio has a greater intrinsic efficacy (Engel et al., 2006). These findings suggested that TAL may be a more efficacious agonist than TRH and that TRH is more efficacious than MeTRH. We previously showed that TRH exhibited a higher intrinsic efficacy than MeTRH at

Table 1 | Pharmacological parameters for TRH-R.

	IC_{50} for binding (nM)	EC_{50} for Ca signaling (nM)
MeTRH	3.0	7.2
TAL	910	36
TRH	36	5.0

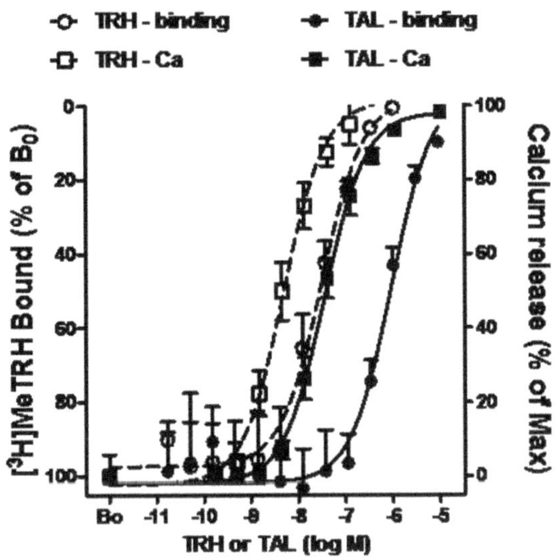

FIGURE 2 | TAL and TRH binding and signaling via Ca^{2+} in cells expressing TRH-Rs. Competition binding with $[^3H]$MeTRH and changes in cytosolic free Ca^{2+} concentration (Ca^{2+} release) were performed in intact HEK-EM 293 cells stably expressing TRH-Rs as described in the legend to Figure 1. The competition binding data are presented as the % of $[^3H]$MeTRH bound to cells in the absence of unlabeled ligand (B_0) and represent the results from three experiments conducted with duplicate measurements. Note the left axis is inverted. Intracellular Ca^{2+} release data are shown as a % of the maximal Ca^{2+} increase over basal. The curves represent the non-linear regression analysis of data obtained in three experiments with duplicate or triplicate measurements using a sigmoidal dose–response method.

mouse TRH-Rs (Engel et al., 2006). As TRH is the natural, full agonist, TAL is termed a superagonist, and MeTRH is a partial agonist.

As Ca^{2+} release is a rapid and transient response to TRH-R activation, it is easier to compare relative intrinsic efficacies by quantifying activation of the inositol-1,4,5-trisphosphate pathway. Inositol-1,4,5-trisphosphate production is the step prior to Ca^{2+} release in signal transduction by TRH-Rs (Gershengorn, 1986) and can be quantified by measuring accumulation of its metabolic product IP1 over time by inhibiting IP1 degradation (**Figure 3A**). The EC_{50} values for IP1 production were found to be 150 nM for TAL and 3.9 nM for TRH. More importantly, TAL was clearly more efficacious than TRH in that TAL stimulated an increase in IP1 production that was 180% of that stimulated by TRH ($p < 0.001$).

Another way of demonstrating relative intrinsic efficacies of agonists is to show that the maximal response of a more efficacious agonist is inhibited by a less efficacious agonist (Engel et al., 2006). **Figure 3B** illustrates the IP1 responses to maximally effective doses of MeTRH, TRH, and TAL. As is evident, TAL (3.5-fold over MeTRH) is more efficacious than TRH (2.1-fold over MeTRH); MeTRH is the least efficacious. As predicted, the least efficacious agonist MeTRH inhibited the response to TRH (full agonist) and to TAL (superagonist).

DISCUSSION

In this study, we characterized the binding and signaling properties of TAL at TRH-R that, to our knowledge, have not been previously reported. The binding properties of TAL at rodent TRH receptors have been studied previously (Asai et al., 1999; Brown, 1999). In agreement with the findings with rodent receptors, we found that TAL binds to TRH-R with lower affinity than TRH. Our most interesting observation, however, is that TAL exhibits higher intrinsic efficacy than TRH; that is, TAL can stimulate the same level of signaling as TRH but at lower levels of receptor occupancy and could induce higher levels of signaling than TRH at full occupancy (**Figure 3**). Since TRH is the natural, full agonist for TRH-R, TAL is termed a superagonist. We previously reported that other TRH analogs displayed higher intrinsic efficacies than TRH at rodent TRH receptors (Engel et al., 2006). In the same study, we showed that MeTRH, the only TRH analog with higher affinity and potency than TRH, was a partial agonist that displayed lower intrinsic efficacy than TRH and that when high levels of TRH and MeTRH were added simultaneously the level of signaling was lowered to that of MeTRH. This is the predicted effect of adding a

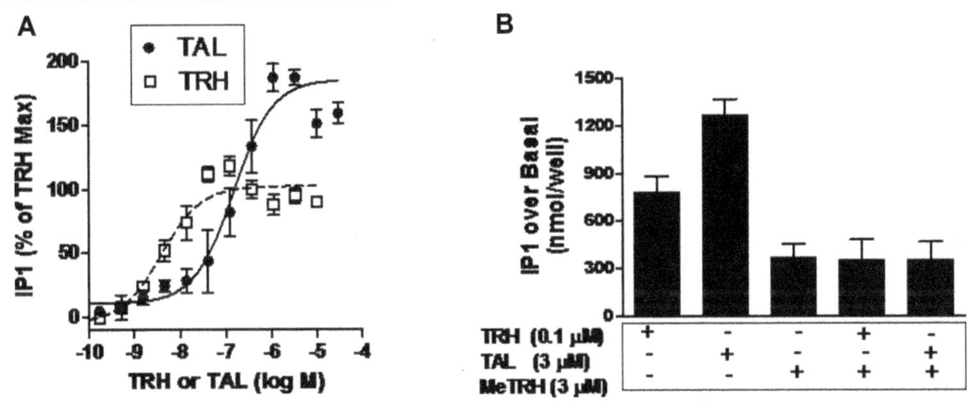

FIGURE 3 | TAL is a superagonist at TRH-R. (A) IP1 production was determined in HEK 293 cells expressing TRH-R in the presence of increasing doses of TAL or TRH as described in Section "Materials and Methods." The data represent the mean of duplicate points from five experiments. **(B)** MeTRH inhibits IP1 formation stimulated by TAL and TRH. IP1 production was determined in the presence of TRH (0.1 μM), TAL (3 μM), MeTRH (3 μM), TRH + MeTRH, or TAL + MeTRH. The data are expressed as mean ± SEM performed in duplicate of two experiments.

partial agonist along with a full agonist. We used a similar experimental design herein to confirm that TAL is a superagonist at TRH-R; MeTRH antagonized IP1 production stimulated by both TRH and TAL (**Figure 3B**).

Previous reports in rodents showed that TAL displayed more activity in stimulating CNS effects than TRH (Suzuki et al., 1990; Brown, 1999). TAL may have similar CNS effects in humans (Gary et al., 2003; Khomane et al., 2011). The differences in the activities of TAL and TRH in the CNS have been attributed to the higher stability in blood and increased penetration of the blood–brain barrier of TAL compared to TRH. Although this is likely true, our new findings of the signaling efficacy of TAL at TRH-R suggest that the higher intrinsic efficacy of TAL may be contributing to its CNS activity in humans also.

In summary, we have described characterization of the pharmacology of TAL at TRH-R. Most importantly, we showed that TAL is a superagonist when signaling at TRH-R via the $G_{q/11}$ protein-phospholipase C-phosphatidylinositol-4,5-bisphosphate-inositol-1,4,5-trisphosphate-calcium pathway. We suggest the superagonism exhibited by TAL may, in addition to its relative metabolic stability and ability to cross the blood–brain barrier, explain its higher activity in mediating CNS effects in humans compared to TRH.

ACKNOWLEDGMENTS

This work was supported by the Intramural Research Program of the National Institutes of Diabetes and Digestive and Kidney Diseases, US National Institutes of Health (1 Z01 DK011006).

REFERENCES

Asai, H., Asahi, T., Yamamura, M., Yamauchi-Kohno, R., and Saito, A. (2005). Lack of behavioral tolerance by repeated treatment with taltirelin hydrate, a thyrotropin-releasing hormone analog, in rats. *Pharmacol. Biochem. Behav.* 82, 646–651.

Asai, H., Kinoshita, K., Yamamura, M., and Matsuoka, Y. (1999). Diversity of thyrotropin-releasing hormone receptors in the pituitary and discrete brain regions of rats. *Jpn. J. Pharmacol.* 79, 313–317.

Brown, W. (1999). Taltirelin. Tanabe Seiyaku. *IDrugs* 2, 1059–1068.

Duthie, S. M., Taylor, P. L., and Eidne, K. A. (1993). Characterization of the mouse thyrotrophin-releasing hormone receptor gene: an exon corresponds to a deletion in the rat cDNA. *J. Mol. Endocrinol.* 11, 141–149.

Engel, S., Neumann, S., Kaur, N., Monga, V., Jain, R., Northup, J., et al. (2006). Low affinity analogs of thyrotropin-releasing hormone are super-agonists. *J. Biol. Chem.* 281, 13103–13109.

Gary, K. A., Sevarino, K. A., Yarbrough, G. G., Prange, A. J. Jr., and Winokur, A. (2003). The thyrotropin-releasing hormone (TRH) hypothesis of homeostatic regulation: implications for TRH-based therapeutics. *J. Pharmacol. Exp. Ther.* 305, 410–416.

Gershengorn, M. C. (1986). Mechanism of thyrotropin releasing hormone stimulation of pituitary hormone secretion. *Annu. Rev. Physiol.* 48, 515–526.

Horita, A. (1998). An update on the CNS actions of TRH and its analogs. *Life Sci.* 62, 1443–1448.

Horita, A., Carino, M. A., and Lai, H. (1986). Pharmacology of thyrotropin-releasing hormone. *Annu. Rev. Pharmacol. Toxicol.* 26, 311–332.

Khomane, K. S., Meena, C. L., Jain, R., and Bansal, A. K. (2011). Novel thyrotropin-releasing hormone analogs: a patent review. *Expert Opin. Ther. Pat.* 21, 1673–1691.

Kinoshita, K., Yamamura, M., and Sugihara, J. (1997). Distribution of thyrotropin-releasing hormone (TRH) receptors in the brain of the ataxic mutant mouse, rolling mouse Nagoya. *Biol. Pharm. Bull.* 20, 86–87.

Matre, V., Karlsen, H. E., Wright, M. S., Lundell, I., Fjeldheim, Å. K., Gabrielsen, O. S., et al. (1993). Molecular cloning of a functional human thyrotropin-releasing hormone receptor. *Biochem. Biophys. Res. Commun.* 195, 179–185.

O'Dowd, B. F., Lee, D. K., Huang, W., Nguyen, T., Cheng, R., Liu, Y., et al. (2000). TRH-R2 exhibits similar binding but distinct regulation and anatomic distribution compared to TRH-R1. *Mol. Endocrinol.* 14, 183–193.

Sun, Y., Lu, X., and Gershengorn, M. C. (2003). Thyrotropin-releasing hormone receptors – similarities and differences. *J. Mol. Endocrinol.* 30, 87–97.

Suzuki, M., Sugano, H., Matsumoto, K., Yamamura, M., and Ishida, R. (1990). Synthesis and central nervous system actions of thyrotropin-releasing hormone analogues containing a dihydroorotic acid moiety. *J. Med. Chem.* 33, 2130–2137.

Yamamura, M., Kinoshita, K., Nakagawa, H., and Ishida, R. (1991). Pharmacological study of TA-0910, a new thyrotropin-releasing hormone (TRH) analog (III): inhibition of pentobarbital anesthesia. *Jpn. J. Pharmacol.* 55, 69–80.

Yamamura, M., Suzuki, M., and Matsumoto, K. (1997). Synthesis and pharmacological action of TRH analog peptide (taltirelin). *Nihon Yakurigaku Zasshi* 110(Suppl. 1), P33–P38.

7

Galanin receptors and ligands

Kristin E. B. Webling[1]*, Johan Runesson[1], Tamas Bartfai[2] and Ülo Langel[1,3]

[1] Department of Neurochemistry, Arrhenius Laboratories for Natural Science, Stockholm University, Stockholm, Sweden
[2] Molecular and Integrative Neurosciences Department, The Scripps Research Institute, La Jolla, CA, USA
[3] Institute of Technology, University of Tartu, Tartu, Estonia

Edited by:
Jae Young Seong, Korea University, Korea

Reviewed by:
Jong-Ik Hwang, Korea University, Korea
Sebastien G. Bouret, University of Southern California, USA

***Correspondence:**
Kristin E. B. Webling, Department of Neurochemistry, Arrhenius Laboratories for Natural Science, Stockholm University, Svante Arrheniusv. 21A, 10691 Stockholm, Sweden.
e-mail: kristin.webling@neurochem.su.se

The neuropeptide galanin was first discovered 30 years ago. Today, the galanin family consists of galanin, galanin-like peptide (GALP), galanin-message associated peptide (GMAP), and alarin and this family has been shown to be involved in a wide variety of biological and pathological functions. The effect is mediated through three GPCR subtypes, GalR1-3. The limited number of specific ligands to the galanin receptor subtypes has hindered the understanding of the individual effects of each receptor subtype. This review aims to summarize the current data of the importance of the galanin receptor subtypes and receptor subtype specific agonists and antagonists and their involvement in different biological and pathological functions.

Keywords: galanin, galanin-like peptide, GMAP, alarin, epilepsy

THE GALANIN FAMILY

Since the discovery of galanin 30 years ago, several bioactive peptides have been reported to be part of the galanin family. The discovery of galanin was followed by the characterization of a second peptide originating from the same prepropeptide as galanin, the galanin message associated peptide (GMAP). Furthermore, a third peptide, GALP, was identified with capacity to bind to the galanin receptor subtypes, GalR1-3, followed by the characterization of a splice variant of GALP named alarin.

GALANIN

Galanin was discovered among several other bioactive peptides with C-terminal α-amide motif, using a new method by Professor Viktor Mutt and colleagues at Karolinska Institute, Stockholm (Tatemoto et al., 1983; Hökfelt, 2005; Lang et al., 2007). The 29 amino acid long peptide (30 amino acids in humans) was named galanin after its N-terminal glycine and its C-terminal alanine. The N-terminal end of galanin is crucial for its biological activity and the first 15 amino acids are conserved in all species (the tuna fish being the exception; Kakuyama et al., 1997). Interestingly, the C-terminal region (residues 17–29) varies among species and it lacks receptor affinity (**Table 2**), which is also true for N-terminal fragments shorter than galanin (1–11) (Land et al., 1991b). The C-terminus is believed to primarily serve as a protector against proteolytic attacks (Land et al., 1991a; Bedecs et al., 1995). In a membrane-mimicking environment, galanin adopts a horseshoe-like shape, where the N-terminus is organized in an α-helical conformation, followed by a β-bend around the proline in position 13 and a more uncertain configuration of the C-terminal region (Wennerberg et al., 1990; Morris et al., 1995, Öhman et al., 1998).

Galanin has been ascribed a large range of different functions. To accomplish these, the galanin gene has a highly plastic expression pattern, which has been portrayed numerous times in the literature. Galanin was early shown to be induced by estrogens (Vrontakis et al., 1987, 1989; Kaplan et al., 1988), and later, three copies of estrogen responsive element, ERE, were identified in the promoter region of the human galanin gene (Kofler et al., 1995). Thereafter, the galanin expression has also been shown to be up-regulated by the leukemia inhibitory factor (LIF; Corness et al., 1996; Sun and Zigmond, 1996), and down-regulated by the nerve growth factor (NGF; Verge et al., 1995).

Galanin is widely expressed in the central and peripheral nervous system as well as in the endocrine system and co-exists with a number of classical neurotransmitters, including acetyl choline, serotonin, glutamate, GABA, noradrenalin, and dopamine (Melander et al., 1986; Hökfelt et al., 1987; Xu et al., 1998; Liu et al., 2003). Galanin also co-exists with other neuropeptides like enkephalin, NPY, substance P, vasopressin, calcitonin gene-regulated peptide, and gonadotropin-releasing hormone (Rökaeus and Carlquist, 1988; Merchenthaler et al., 1990; Zhang et al., 1993a,b, 1995).

An extensive up-regulation of galanin was seen during development of sensory and motor systems (Gabriel et al., 1989; Xu et al., 1996) and after nerve injury, both in PNS and CNS (Hökfelt et al., 1987) and also, an extensive up-regulation in the basal forebrain of patients with Alzheimer's disease (AD; Chan-Palay, 1988a,b). Epileptic seizures have been shown to rapidly deplete galanin (Mazarati et al., 1998).

Galanin has also been shown to be expressed in keratinocytes, eccrine sweat glands and around blood vessels (Kofler et al., 2004). Furthermore, galanin has been proposed to be expressed in macrophages of the dermis (reviewed in Bauer et al., 2010).

GALANIN MESSAGE ASSOCIATED PEPTIDE

There are very few studies regarding the localization, function, and pharmacological potential of GMAP. It was early shown that the sequence of GMAP displays a much greater divergence between species than galanin (Lundkvist et al., 1995). Immunohistochemistry has shown that GMAP distribution generally parallels that of galanin (Hökfelt et al., 1992) although heterologous distribution was observed in certain areas. Xu et al. (1995a,b) showed that GMAP has a pharmacological action in spinal nociceptive transmission in rat spinal cord (Andell-Jonsson et al., 1997; Hao et al., 1999). GMAP has also been assigned anti-microbial activities and hypothesized to be part of the innate immune system, since it suppresses *Candida albicans* growth and the budded-to-hyphal-form transition of *C. albicans* (Rauch et al., 2007) (**Table 1**). Recently, in an extended study, it was shown that GMAP could significantly reduce growth in six out of seven *Candida* strains (Holub et al., 2011).

GALANIN-LIKE PEPTIDE

Ohtaki et al. (1999) characterized a third peptide, isolated from porcine hypothalamus, that was recognized to induce GTP-binding to a membrane preparation of GalR2-transfected cells. They named this new peptide galanin-like peptide, or GALP. Porcine GALP was shown to act as an agonist in a GTPγS binding

Table 1 | A short summary of the involvement of the galanin family in different physiological and pathological functions.

Agonist	Antagonist
GALANIN RECEPTOR 1	
Reduces acetylcholine release in cardiac neurons (Potter and Smith-White, 2005)	Anxiolytic and antidepressant (Kuteeva et al., 2008)
Antinocicepive effects for neuropathic pain (Liu et al., 2001)	Improving memory and learning (Wrenn et al., 2004; Bailey et al., 2007)
Treatment for diseases of altered extrinsic afferent signaling around that gastrointestinal tract (Page et al., 2007)	
Anticonvulsant, reduces initiation of seizures (Mazarati et al., 2004b; Bulaj et al., 2008)	
GALANIN RECEPTOR 2	
Neuroprotective effects against Alzheimer's disease (Pirondi et al., 2010)	
Anxiolytic and antidepressant (Kuteeva et al., 2008)	
Anticonvulsant by reduction of severity of seizures (Mazarati et al., 2004a; Robertson et al., 2010)	
GALANIN RECEPTOR 3	
Inhibit oxytocin secretion (Radács et al., 2010)	Anxiolytic and antidepressant (Swanson et al., 2005; Kuteeva et al., 2008; Ash et al., 2011)
	Reduced alcohol consumption (Ash et al., 2011)
	Reduces severity of acute pancreatitis (Barreto et al., 2011)
EXOGENOUS GALANIN	
Increases heart rate, induces tachycardia and a weak vasodepressor response (Narváez et al., 2000)	
Impaired performance in memory tests (Wrenn et al., 2004; Bailey et al., 2007)	
Increases alcohol intake (Schneider et al., 2007)	
Inhibit the secretion of vasopressin and oxycotin (Ciosek and Cisowska, 2003; Izdebska and Ciosek, 2010; Radács et al., 2010)	
Anticonvulsant effects (Mazarati et al., 1992, 1998, 2000, 2004b; Chepurnov et al., 1998; Lu et al., 2010; Robertson et al., 2010,)	
Anti-nociceptive (Xu et al., 2012)	
Neuroprotective effects against Alzheimer's disease (Pirondi et al., 2010) Anxiolytic- and antidepressant (Kuteeva et al., 2008)	
EXOGENOUS GALP	
In rats: an acute increase (30–60 min) of food intake, followed by reduction in food intake (Lawrence, 2009), increased sexual behavior in male rats (Fraley et al., 2004)	
In mice: decreased food intake (Lawrence, 2009), an acute decrease in body temperature followed by an increase in body temperature (Man and Lawrence, 2008a)	
Inhibition of male sexual behavior in mice (Kauffman et al., 2005)	
EXOGENOUS ALARIN	
In male mice: Increase of acute food intake, acute increase of body weight, increased LH levels, decrease of neurogenic inflammation, no change in body temperature (Fraley et al., 2012)	
Anti-edema and vasoconstrictive effects (Santic et al., 2007)	
Increases LH levels in mice and rats (Boughton et al., 2010; van Der Kolk et al., 2010; Fraley et al., 2012)	
EXOGENOUS GMAP	
Anti-microbial activities (Rauch et al., 2007; Holub et al., 2011)	
Facilitation of the flexor reflex, decrease of spinal cord blood flow (Xu et al., 1995a)	

Table 2 | Affinities of galanin, GALP, GMAP, and alarin, as well as fragments of galanin and GALP, for the three galanin receptor subtypes, determined as K_i.

Ligand	K_i (nM)			Reference
	GalR1	GalR2	GalR3	
Rat galanin(1–29)	1.0	1.5	1.5	Wang et al. (1997b)
	0.3 (h)	1.6 (h)	12 (h)	Borowsky et al. (1998)
	0.9 (h)	1.2 (h)	7.4 (h)	Lu et al. (2005b)
Human galanin(1–30)	0.4 (h)	2.3 (h)	69 (h)	Borowsky et al. (1998)
Porcine galanin(1–29)	0.23 (h)	0.95 (h)	9.8 (h)	Borowsky et al. (1998)
Galanin(1–16)	4.8	5.7	50	Wang et al. (1997b)
Galanin(2–29)	85	1.9	12	Wang et al. (1997b)
Galanin(3–29)	>1000	>1000	>1000	Wang et al. (1997b)
Galanin(2–11)	>5000 (h)	88	271	Lu et al. (2005a)
	879[a] (h)	1.8[a]	–	Liu et al. (2001)
Porcine GALP	4.3	0.24	–	Ohtaki et al. (1999)
Human GALP	77[a] (h)	28[a] (h)	10[a] (h)	Lang et al. (2005)
Human GALP(1–32)	129[a] (h)	69[a] (h)	–	Lang et al. (2005)
Human GALP(3–32)	33[a] (h)	15[a] (h)	–	Lang et al. (2005)
Rat GALP	45[a]	18.7[a]	1530[a] (h)	Boughton et al. (2010)
Alarin	>1000	>1000	>1000000	Boughton et al. (2010)
GMAP(1–41)	–	>840	–	Wang et al. (1997a)
	–	–	>1000	Wang et al. (1997b)
GMAP(44–59)	–	>1000	>1000	Wang et al. (1997b)

Displacement is performed on the rat galanin receptor unless indicated otherwise. (h) human; [a]presented as IC_{50} values; – not determined.

assay and to have a preferential binding (20 times) toward GalR2 (Ohtaki et al., 1999). A later study using human GALP showed that GALP interacts with GalR3 with three times preferential selectivity as compared to GalR2 (Lang et al., 2005) (**Table 2**).

The amino acid sequence of GALP (9–21) is identical to that of galanin (1–13).

Galanin-like peptide distribution in the CNS appears to be rather restricted, disparate to the much broader expression pattern seen for galanin. Cells identified to produce GALP mRNA and protein have only been found in the hypothalamic arcuate nucleus (ARC), the median eminence and infundibular stalk, and the posterior pituitary when studied in the rat, mouse, and macaque (Juréus et al., 2000, 2001; Kerr et al., 2000; Larm and Gundlach, 2000; Takatsu et al., 2001; Cunningham et al., 2002; Fujiwara et al., 2002). GALP-immunoreactive (IR) fibers were shown to project to several regions of the forebrain (Takatsu et al., 2001).

Galanin-like peptide has also been shown to be expressed by specialized glia-like cells known as pituicytes in the neuronal lobe of dehydrated and salt loaded rats, where the expression is strongly regulated by osmotic stimuli (Shen et al., 2001; Fujiwara et al., 2002; Saito et al., 2003; Shen and Gundlach, 2004). Furthermore, studies show that the GALP gene expression, especially in the pituicytes, is induced by both acute and chronic inflammatory stimuli (Saito et al., 2003, 2005). Central administration of GALP increases IL-1α and IL-1β and it has been suggested that IL-1 mediates both the anorectic and febrile actions of GALP (Man and Lawrence, 2008b).

Intracerebroventricular (i.c.v.) injection of GALP profoundly stimulates male sex behaviors in rat (Fraley et al., 2004), seemingly independent of the testosterone milieu (Stoyanovitch et al., 2005) (**Table 1**). Interestingly, the opposite is seen in mice were GALP instead inhibits male sex behavior (Kauffman et al., 2005). Recently, Taylor et al. (2009) presented evidence supporting the hypothesis that this effect of GALP depends upon hypothalamic dopamine input to the medial preoptic area (mPOA).

Several studies have proposed that GALP does not solely interact with the three known galanin receptor subtypes (Man and Lawrence, 2008a). Krasnow et al. (2004) reported that GALP injection affect food intake and body weight in a similar manner in both GalR1-KO and GalR2-KO mice compared to wild type littermates. Furthermore, to somewhat exclude the possibility that this effect was mediated through GalR3, the authors showed that the GALP fragment, GALP (1–21), failed to mimic the effect of full length GALP (Krasnow et al., 2004).

ALARIN

The newest member of the galanin peptide family, alarin, a 25 amino acid long peptide named after its N-terminal alanine and its C-terminal serine originating as a splice variant of the GALP mRNA (Santic et al., 2006). The alarin peptide has been isolated from murine brain, thymus, skin (Santic et al., 2007), human neuroblastic tumors, and human skin (Santic et al., 2006, 2007) and has no detectable affinity toward either of the three galanin receptor subtypes (Boughton et al., 2010) (**Table 2**). Recently, two publications characterized in more detail the alarin-LI in the murine brain (van Der Kolk et al., 2010; Eberhard et al., 2012). Alarin-LI has a much broader expression pattern than GALP and was found in such diverse areas as the accessory olfactory bulb, different nucleus in the hypothalamus, within the locus coeruleus (LC) and locus subcoeruleus of the midbrain.

When first discovered, alarin was ascribed vasoconstrictive and anti-edema activities (Santic et al., 2007) (**Table 1**). Contradictory to the effect of GALP, alarin has neither an effect on body temperature nor an effect on male sex behaviors in rodents (van Der Kolk et al., 2010; Fraley et al., 2012). Recently, it was shown that alarin stimulates acute food intake and some studies have reported a significant increase in body weight after 24 h, although other studies were unable to confirm this (Boughton et al., 2010; van Der Kolk et al., 2010; Fraley et al., 2012). Central injection of alarin elicit a gonadotrophin-releasing hormone (GnRH)-mediated increase in leutizing hormone (LH)-levels in both rats and mice (Boughton et al., 2010; van Der Kolk et al., 2010; Fraley et al., 2012).

GALANIN RECEPTOR SUBTYPES

All three galanin receptor subtypes are members of the GPCR superfamily but the subtypes have substantial differences in sites of expression as well as their functional coupling and subsequent signaling activities. These differences between the receptor subtypes contributes to the diversity of possible physiological effects and the plausible pharmacological relevance of targeting the galanin family (**Table 1**).

GALANIN RECEPTOR TYPE 1

The first known galanin receptor, galanin receptor type 1 (GalR1), was isolated from the Bowes human melanoma cell line (Habert-Ortoli et al., 1994) and subsequently rat (Burgevin et al., 1995; Parker et al., 1995) and mouse (Jacoby et al., 1997; Wang et al., 1997c) receptor was cloned.

The human GalR1 gene contains three exons and the hGalR1 gene translates into a 349 amino acid long protein (Jacoby et al., 1997). The homology between species is rather high, as 93% of the residues in rat GalR1 are identical to those of human GalR1 (Jacoby et al., 1997). The expression of GalR1, but neither GalR2 nor GalR3, is regulated by cyclic adenosine monophosphate (cAMP) through the transcription factor CREB (cAMP regulatory element binding protein; Zachariou et al., 2001; Hawes et al., 2005). The GalR1 expression does not fluctuate during development (Branchek et al., 2000; Burazin et al., 2000).

GalR1 mRNA was initially identified by northern blot to be found in the fetal brain and small intestinal tissues (Habert-Ortoli et al., 1994). It has, thereafter, been identified by reverse transcript polymerase chain reaction (RT-PCR) in the gastrointestinal tract (Lorimer and Benya, 1996). However, a later study identified the GalR1 expression to be exclusively in the central and peripheral nervous system (Waters and Krause, 2000), where it was detected in hippocampus, hypothalamus, amygdala, thalamus, cortex, brainstem (medulla oblongata), spinal cord, and dorsal root ganglia (DRG; Gustafson et al., 1996; Waters and Krause, 2000), even if broader central and peripheral tissue distribution has also been reported (Sullivan et al., 1997).

Activation of GalR1 results in a pertussis toxin (PTX) sensitive inhibition of adenylate cyclase (AC) through interaction with $G\alpha_i/\alpha_o$ types of G-proteins (Habert-Ortoli et al., 1994; Parker et al., 1995; Wang et al., 1997c) which leads to opening of GIRK channels. Activation of GalR1 can also stimulate a mitogen associated protein kinase (MAPK) activity, through a PKC-independent mechanism, consistent with that the mediator is the $\beta\gamma$-subunit of $G\alpha_i$ (Wang et al., 1998).

GALANIN RECEPTOR TYPE 2

The second galanin receptor type (GalR2) was identified in rat hypothalamus, spinal cord, and DRG (Fathi et al., 1997; Howard et al., 1997; Smith et al., 1997; Ahmad and Dray, 2004) and subsequently in mouse spleen (Pang et al., 1998) as well as from various human tissues (Bloomquist et al., 1998; Borowsky et al., 1998). The human GalR2 has rather high sequence identity to rat GalR2 (92%), although there is one notable difference; the 15 amino acid extension of the C-terminal end in human GalR2 (Kolakowskim et al., 1998; Waters and Krause, 2000).

GalR2 is able to activate the stimulatory pathway of $G\alpha_{q/11}$ class of G-proteins, i.e., PTX-insensitive. This triggers PLC activity and intracellular phosphoinositol turnover, mediating the release of Ca^{2+} into the cytoplasm from intracellular stores and opening Ca^{2+}-dependent channels (Smith et al., 1997; Kolakowskim et al., 1998; Wang et al., 1998). GalR2 is also able to activate MAPK through a PKC and $G\alpha_o$ class of G-proteins dependent mechanism (Wang et al., 1998). This may in turn lead to the downstream PI3K-dependent phosphorylation of Protein Kinase B (PKB) leading to suppression of caspase-3 and caspase-9 activity (Ding et al., 2006; Elliott-Hunt et al., 2007). GalR2 activation may also inhibit forskolin stimulated cAMP production in a PTX-sensitive manner, suggesting the activation of $G\alpha_i/\alpha_o$ types of G-proteins (Fathi et al., 1997; Wang et al., 1997a). Consequently, both GalR1 and GalR2 activation can inhibit CREB (Badie-Mahdavi et al., 2005).

GalR2 is expressed in a wider pattern, compared to GalR1, as it is found in several peripheral tissues including the pituitary gland, gastrointestinal tract, skeletal muscle, heart, kidney, uterus, ovary, and testis as well as in regions in the CNS (Smith et al., 1997; Bloomquist et al., 1998; Waters and Krause, 2000). In the brain, the highest levels of GalR2 are detected in hypothalamus, dentate gyrus, amygdala, piriform cortex, and mammillary nuclei (Mitchell et al., 1999; O'Donnell et al., 1999; Waters and Krause, 2000).

Interestingly, GalR2 expression levels vary during the development of the rat brain with a broader distribution with a peak in expression before postnatal day 7, particularly in cortex and thalamus, and much reduced levels after postnatal day 14 (Burazin et al., 2000).

GALANIN RECEPTOR TYPE 3

Galanin receptor type 3 (GalR3) was first isolated from rat hypothalamic cDNA libraries (Wang et al., 1997b) and later from human cDNA (Kolakowskim et al., 1998; Smith et al., 1998). The 368 amino acid long hGalR3 shares 36% amino acids identity with hGalR1 and 58% with hGalR2 and approximately 90% with rGalR3 (Kolakowskim et al., 1998).

The distribution pattern of GalR3 is somewhat unclear but it is assumed that this receptor has a more restricted expression pattern in relation to the other two receptors. Transcript levels is most prominent in the hypothalamus (Wang et al., 1997b; Smith et al., 1998; Mennicken et al., 2002) although, some studies report a wider distribution of GalR3 throughout central and peripheral tissues (Kolakowskim et al., 1998; Waters and Krause, 2000).

Signaling properties of GalR3 are still ill-defined. Activation of GalR3 expressed in *Xenopus* oocytes or *Xenopus* melanophores leads to the activation of $G\alpha_i/\alpha_o$ type of G-proteins inhibiting AC which results in the opening of GIRK channels (Kolakowskim et al., 1998; Smith et al., 1998).

PEPTIDE LIGANDS FOR THE GALANIN RECEPTORS

Endogenous galanin has high affinity for all three galanin receptors (Wang et al., 1997b). The N-terminal part of galanin is crucial for receptor interaction and the galanin fragment galanin (1–16) retains the high affinity of its parental peptide. When galanin (1–16) underwent an L-alanine scan and subsequent testing on rat hypothalamus membranes, Gly^1, Trp^2, Asn^5, Tyr^9, and Gly^{12} were identified as pharmacophores (Land et al., 1991b). A later study, which tested an identical set of peptides on separated GalR1 and GalR2 membranes, identified Trp^2, Tyr^9, and Leu^{10} as pharmacophores on both receptor subtypes (Carpenter et al., 1999).

Several N-terminal truncated galanin fragments have been shown to have a preference for GalR2 (Wang et al., 1997b; Liu et al., 2001), in concurrence with the fact that Gly^1 is of great importance for ligand binding to GalR1. Further truncation, with as little as two amino acids, leads to a complete loss of receptor affinity to all receptor subtypes (Wang et al., 1997a).

Liu et al. (2001) published the galanin fragment galanin (2–11) as a GalR2 selective agonist, although they did not test it on GalR3 (**Table 3**). Later publication has unfortunately shown that it has similar affinity toward GalR3 (Lu et al., 2005a), without testing receptor signaling, even so, it has been used extensively as a non-GalR1 agonist. Lundström and colleagues showed that Trp^2, Asn^5, Gly^8, Tyr^9, and Leu^{10} were identified as crucial for interactions with GalR2 by performing Ala-scan on the peptide (Lundström et al., 2005a).

The interaction between the galanin receptor subtypes and GALP has received less attention. GALP, isolated from porcine tissues, was original published as a GalR2 preferring ligand, with a 20 times difference in affinity between GalR1 and GalR2 (Ohtaki et al., 1999). Later it was shown, using human GALP, that GALP also interacts with GalR3. In this study GALP was ascribed a GalR3 preferential selectivity (3 times differences; Lang et al., 2005). Recently, Boughton et al. (2010) showed a more than 10 times preferential binding toward GalR3 for the rat GALP (**Table 2**).

Several chimeric ligands have been synthesized, conjugating galanin (1–13) to other bioactive molecules, yielding M15 (also called galantide; Bartfai et al., 1991), M32 (Wiesenfeld-Hallin et al., 1992b), M35 (Wiesenfeld-Hallin et al., 1992b, Ögren et al., 1992, Kask et al., 1995), C7 (Langel et al., 1992), and M40 (Langel et al., 1992; Bartfai et al., 1993). Although, they all maintain antagonistic properties *in vivo* at doses between 0.1 and 10 nmol when delivered i.c.v. or intrathecally (i.t.; Parker et al., 1995; Lu et al., 2005b), they all have a partial agonistic nature *in vivo* at doses higher than 10 nmol when delivered i.c.v. or i.t. (Kask et al., 1995; Lu et al., 2005b).

The first introduced chimeric peptide which acts as an antagonist of the galanin receptor family was M15 (Bartfai et al., 1991).

Table 3 | Published ligands and their affinities for the galanin receptor subtypes.

Peptide	K_i (nM)			K_i (GalR1)/ K_i (GalR2)	K_i (GalR3)/ K_i (GalR2)	Reference
	GalR1	GalR2	GalR3			
M1151	98.6	28.9	874	3.4	30	Saar et al. (2011)
M1152	2370	36.4	656	65	18	Saar et al. (2011)
M1153	1890	4.98	230	380	46	Saar et al. (2011)
M1145	587	6.55	497	90	76	Runesson et al. (2009)
M15	0.65	1.0	1.0	0.65	1	Smith et al. (1998)
M35	0.11 (h)	2.0 (h)	–	0.055	–	Borowsky et al. (1998)
	0.325	3.24	2.09	0.1	0.64	Smith et al. (1998)
	4.8	8.2	4.7	0.58	0.57	Lu et al. (2005b)
M40	2.4 (h)	4.1 (h)	–	0.58	–	Borowsky et al. (1998)
	6.76	3.55	79.4	1.9	22.3	Smith et al. (1998)
	1.8	5.1	63	0.35	12.3	Lu et al. (2005b)
M617	0.23 (h)	5.7 (h)	–	0.04	–	Lundström et al. (2005b)
	–	–	49 (h)	–	–	Sollenberg Eriksson et al. (2010)
M871	420 (h)	13 (h)	–	32.3	–	Sollenberg Eriksson et al. (2006)
	–	–	>10000 (h)	–	–	Sollenberg Eriksson et al. (2010)
Gal-B2	3.5 (h)	51.5 (h)	–	0.019	–	Bulaj et al. (2008)
[N-Me,des-Sar]Gal-B2	364 (h)	20 (h)	-	18.2	–	Robertson et al. (2010)
Gal2–11	>5000 (h)	88	271	56.8	3.08	Lu et al. (2005a)

The sequences and structures of the ligands are listed in ***Table 4****.*

Displacement was performed on the rat galanin receptor unless indicated otherwise. (h) human; – not determined.

Table 4 | The sequences for the galanin family peptides along with the discussed analogs.

Name	Sequence	
GALANINFAMILY		
Rat galanin(1–29)	GWTLNSAGYLLGPHAIDNHRSFSDKHGLT-amide	
Human galanin(1–30)	GWTLNSAGYLLGPHAVGNHRSFSDKNGLTS	
Porcine galanin(1–29)	GWTLNSAGYLLGPHAIDNHRSFHDKYGLA-amide	
Galanin(1–16)	GWTLNSAGYLLGPHAI-amide (rat/porcine) GWTLNSAGYLLGPHAV-amide (human)	
Rat Galanin(2–29)	WTLNSAGYLLGPHAIDNHRSFSDKHGLT-amide	
Rat Galanin(3–29)	TLNSAGYLLGPHAIDNHRSFSDKHGLT-amide	
Galanin(2–11)	WTNLSAGYLL-amide	
Porcine GALP	APVHRGRGGWTLNSAGYLLGPVLHPPSRAEGGGKGKTALGILDWKAIDGLPYPQSQLAS	
Human GALP	APAHRGRGGWTLNSAGYLLGPVLHLPQMGDQDGKRETALEILDLWKAIDGLPYSHPPQPS	
Human GALP(1–32)	APAHRGRGGWTLNSAGYLLGPVLHLPQMGDQD	
Human GALP(3–32)	AHRGRGGWTLNSAGYLLGPVLHLPQMGDQD	
Rat GALP	APAHRGRGGWTLNSAGYLLGPVLHPPSRAEGGGKGKTALGILDLWKAIDGLPYPQSQLAS	
Alarin	APAHRSSTFPKWVTKTERGRQPLRS (human) APAHRSSPFPPRPTRAGRETQLLRS (mouse)	
GMAP(1–41)	ELPLEVEEGRLGSVAVPLPESNIVRTIMEFLSFLHLKEAGA (rat)	
GMAP(44–59)	SLGIPLATSSEDLEQS (rat)	
PEPTIDE LIGANDS		
M1151	GWTLNSAGYLLGPK(ε-NH-C(O)Glu)-amide	
M1152	WTLNSAGYLLGPK(ε-NH-C(O)Glu)-amide	
M1153	RGRGNWTLNSAGYLLGPK(ε-NH-C(O)Glu)-amide	
M1145	RGRGNWTLNSAGYLLGPVLPPPALALA-amide	
M15	GWTLNSAGYLLGPQQFFGLM-amide	
M35	GWTLNSAGYLLGPPPGFSPFR-amide	
M40	GWTLNSAGYLLGPPPALALA-amide	
M617	GWTLNSAGYLLGPQPGFSPFR-amide	
M871	WTLNSAGYLLGPEHPPPALALA-amide	
Gal-B2	(Sar)WTLNSAGYLLGPKKK(palmitoyl)K-amide	
[N-Me,des-Sar]Gal-B2	(N-Me)WTLNSAGYLLGPKKK(palmitoyl)K-amide	
NON-PEPTIDE LIGANDS		
Galnon	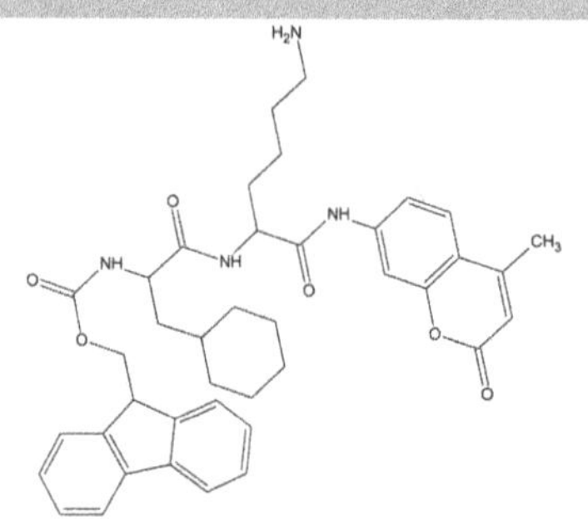	GalR1–3 agonist
Galmic	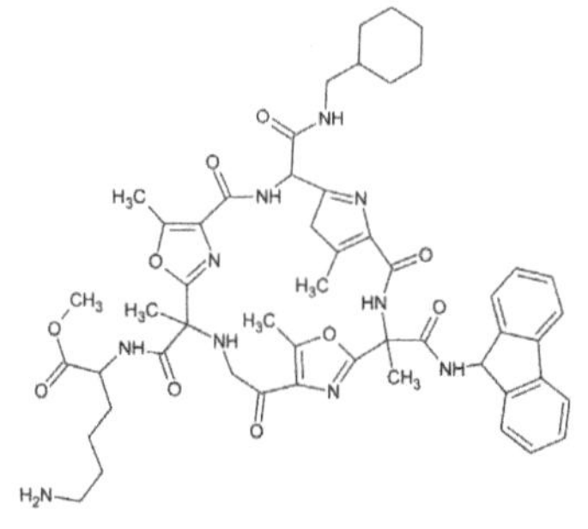	GalR1 agonist

(Continued)

Table 4 | Continued

Name	Sequence	
Sch 202596	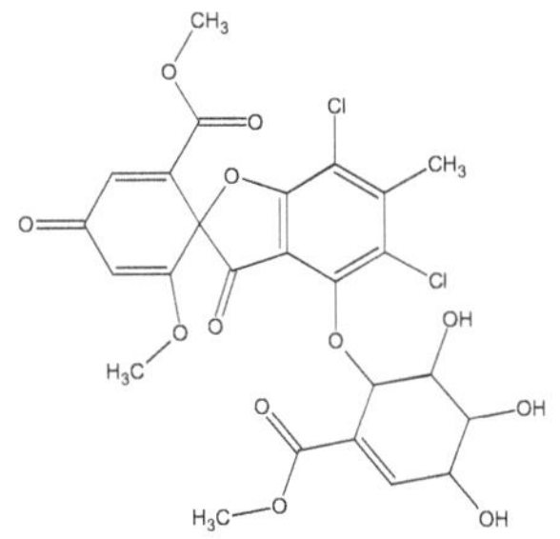	GalR1 antagonist
Dithiepine-1,1,4,4,-tetroxide	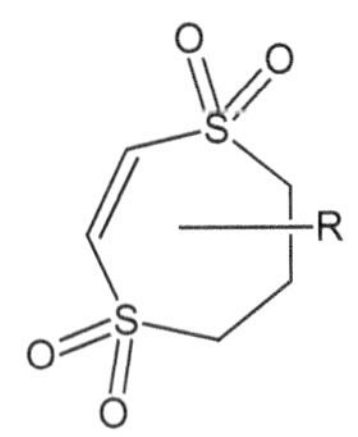	
SNAP 37889	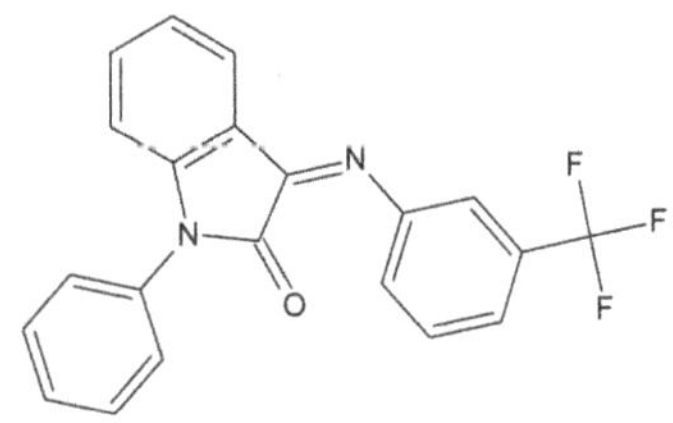	GalR3 antagonist
SNAP 398299	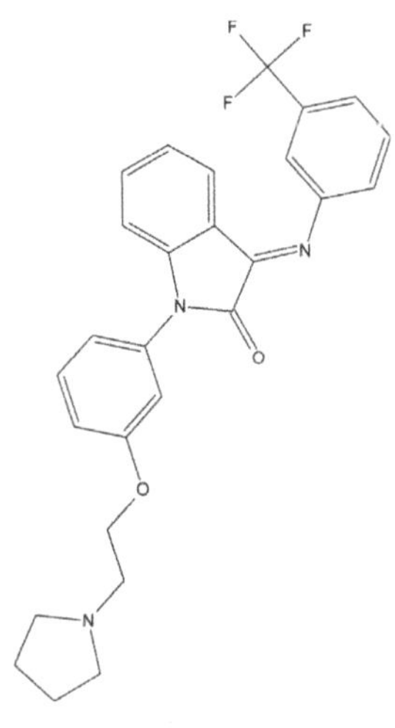	GalR3 antagonist

(Continued)

Here, the galanin (1–13) fragment, was coupled to a C-terminal fragment in substance P (residue 5–11), reported to have agonistic effect on the substance P receptor. M15 showed an about 10-fold higher affinity than the endogenous galanin to unspecified subtypes of the galanin receptor family in membrane preparations of rat tissues. Later, M35 was synthesized (Ögren et al., 1992) with an improved *in vivo* stability (Wiesenfeld-Hallin et al., 1992b). M15, M32, M35, and M40 have similar affinity as galanin and have been valuable tools in galanin research but are limited by their relative non-specificity toward the different galanin receptors (Ögren et al., 1992) and by their weak interactions with other receptors than the galanin receptors (Wiesenfeld-Hallin et al., 1992a).

M617 resembles the M35 peptide, with the substitution of proline at position 14 to a glutamine, which results in a 25-fold selectivity for GalR1 over GalR2 *in vitro* (**Table 3**). M617

Table 4 | Continued

Name	Sequence	
GalR3ant	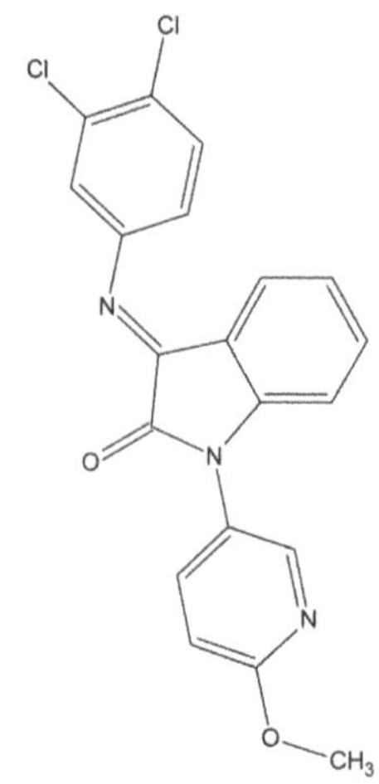	GalR3 antagonist

Sar, sarcosine.

has thereafter been shown to produce anti-nociceptive effects (Jimenez-Andrade et al., 2006) and to delay the development of seizure in an animal model (Mazarati et al., 2006). The M871 peptide is N-terminally truncated and has two additional amino acid residues compared to the M40 peptide and function as a partial agonist, selective for GalR2 (Sollenberg Eriksson et al., 2006, 2010). M871 has been used in several *in vivo* studies (Jimenez-Andrade et al., 2006; Alier et al., 2007; Kuteeva et al., 2008). Several GalR2 selective agonists have been reported over the years (Pooga et al., 1998; Runesson et al., 2009; Saar et al., 2011). Small changes in the N-terminus of galanin have been associated with lost binding affinity. However, recently analogues with modifications at both N-terminus and C-terminus have been presented, namely M1145 (Runesson et al., 2009) and M1153 (Saar et al., 2011). M1145 was reported as the first specific GalR2 agonist with a 90-fold binding preference for GalR2 over GalR1 and 76-fold preference over GalR3 (Runesson et al., 2009). The importance of the development of M1145 and M871 and other subtype selective agonists and antagonists can almost not be overestimated and is the key to a successful delineation of galaninergic system and to identify its potential as a therapeutic target.

Recently, several galanin analogs, all modified by introducing several cationic amino acid residues and a palmitoyl moiety was shown to exhibit improved bioavailability after systemic administration (Bulaj et al., 2008; White et al., 2009). One of these, the Gal-B2, with a slight selectivity toward GalR1 (**Table 3**), was shown to have anticonvulsant effect in several tested animal models (White et al., 2009). In a later study, Bulaj and colleagues modified Gal-B2 to obtain a ligand with an 18 times preferential binding toward GalR2, which displayed similar anticonvulsant activity as the parental peptide (Robertson et al., 2010). Future characterization will probably identify other potential application of Gal-B2 and other systemically active galanin analogs.

NON-PEPTIDE LIGANDS

The non-peptide ligand galnon was identified after screening a combinatorial peptidomimetic library (**Table 5**). It acts as an agonist in functional studies both *in vitro* and *in vivo* (Saar et al., 2002; Bartfai et al., 2004). It has been evaluated in models of anxiety and depression (Rajarao et al., 2007), feeding (Abramov et al., 2004), and pain (Wu et al., 2003). Galmic (**Table 5**) is a non-peptide agonist with higher affinity for GalR1 compared to GalR2, which under conditions of intrahippocampal administration was 6-fold more potent than galnon in inhibiting self-sustaining status epilepticus (SE), an *in vivo* model for epilepsy (Bartfai et al., 2004; Ceide et al., 2004). Nevertheless, both galnon and galmic potentials are limited by the fact that they have multiple sites of interactions, i.e., D2 dopamine receptors, grehlin and melanocortin receptors, which produce unwanted physiological effects (Florén et al., 2005; Lu et al., 2005b).

The metabolite Sch 202596 (**Table 5**), originated from an *Aspergillus* sp. culture found in an abandoned uranium mine in Tuolemene County California, was found to have a modest affinity to GalR1 *in vitro* (Chu et al., 1997). Sch 202596 was characterized as a molecule with a spirocoumaranone skeleton and has only partly been synthesized so far (Katoh et al., 2002). Several 1,4-dithiins and dithiipine-1,1,4,4-tetroxides with binding affinity to GalR1 were identified at the R. W. Johnson Pharmaceutical Institute (Scott et al., 2000). The compound 2,3-dihydro-2-(4-methylphenyl)-1,4-dithiepine-1,1,4,4-tetroxide (**Table 5**) was shown to be a submicromolar antagonist. It has an IC_{50} of 190 nM for GalR1 and above the highest tested concentration (30 μM) for GalR2. However, its reactive nature and its low solubility makes it unattractive from a therapeutic point of view. Nevertheless, it has been used and evaluated in several studies (Mahoney et al., 2003; Kozoriz et al., 2006).

A series of 3-imonio-2-indolones were identified as specific GalR3 antagonists, with K_i-values for GalR3 as low as 17 nM

Table 5 | Affinities of non-peptidergic galanin receptor ligands for the three galanin receptor subtypes, determined as K_i on human receptor subtypes.

Ligand	K_i (nM)			Reference
	GalR1	**GalR2**	**GalR3**	
Galnon	11700	34100	–	Saar et al. (2002)
Galmic	34200	>100000	–	Saar et al. (2002)
Sch 202596	1700	–	–	Chu et al. (1997)
Dithiepine-1,1,4,4-tetroxide	190[a]	>30000[a]	–	Scott et al. (2000)
SNAP 37889	>10000	>10000	17.4	Swanson et al. (2005)
SNAP 398299	>1000	>1000	5.3	Swanson et al. (2005)
GalR3ant	>10000	>10000	15	Barr et al. (2006)

The structures of the ligands are listed in ***Table 4****.*
Displacement is performed on the rat galanin receptor unless indicated otherwise.
[a]presented as IC_{50} values; – not determined.

and above the tested 10 μM for the other receptors studied (Konkel et al., 2006a). One of these was referred as SNAP37889 (Swanson et al., 2005) (**Table 5**). One drawback of the above mentioned indolones is the low aqueous solubility (less than 1 μg/ml) which motivated further studies, leading to the identification of a compound with an increased water solubility and selectivity, 1,3-dihydro-1-[3-(2-pyrrolidinylethoxy)phenyl]-3-[[3-(trifluoromethyl)phenyl]imino]-2*H*-indol-2-one, referred as SNAP398299 (Swanson et al., 2005; Konkel et al., 2006b) (**Table 5**). Another of the synthesized indolones (**Table 5**) was evaluated *in vivo* by Barr et al. (2006), which together with the other articles and several patent applications (Konkel et al., 2004) indicates that specific GalR3 ligands are in development.

A series of 2,4,6-triaminopyrimidines were recently introduced by The Scripps Research Institute (Sagi et al., 2011). They present both GalR1 and GalR2 selective compounds with K_i-values starting from 330 nM. Further development of these compounds is likely ongoing and published in due course. Studies from the same institute led to characterization of the first identified allosteric modulator, named CYM2503, for the galanin receptor family, i.e., GalR2 (Lu et al., 2010). CYM2503 failed to displace galanin in binding studies and showed no detectable signaling by itself, but potentiated the effect of galanin when administered simultaneously (Lu et al., 2010).

GALANIN LIGANDS AS POSSIBLE THERAPEUTICS FOR EPILEPSY

Among the early reported biological effects of galanin were the decreased excitability of myenteric neurons (Tamura et al., 1988) and cardiac ganglia (Konopka et al., 1989). These findings, together with reports that the hippocampus, which is a key structure for the initiation and maintenance of seizures, have a considerable amount of galaninergic innervation (Lu et al., 2005b) draw attention to galanin as a possible anticonvulsant (Mitsukawa et al., 2008).

Mazarati et al. (1992) reported that galanin had an anticonvulsant effect in a picrotoxin-kindled seizure model. Since then, galanin has been shown to up-regulated in several models of SE (in adult rats), i.e., in kainic acid-induced SE (Wilson et al., 2005) and after perforant path stimulation-induced SE (Mazarati et al., 1998). Galanin administrated i.c.v. had anticonvulsant activity in rodents exposed to either PTZ or Li-pilocarpine (Chepurnov et al., 1998; Mazarati et al., 1998, 2000). Similar results were obtained when SE was induced by perforant path stimulation (Mazarati et al., 1998, 2004a).

The galanin receptor subtypes present in the hippocampus have been investigated and both GalR1 and GalR2 are present in relatively high levels (Lu et al., 2005b) with GalR1 mRNA in CA-fields and GalR2-mRNA in the dentate gyrus (Burazin et al., 2000). The involvement of GalR3 in hippocampus is still not well characterized.

GalR1-KO mice displayed a more severe seizure phenotype when SE is induced by either perforant path stimulation or Li-pilocarpine exposure but not when induced by KA exposure compared to WT (Mazarati et al., 2004b). Li-pilocarpine exposure resulted in cell death in CA1, an effect that was elevated in GalR1-KO mice (Mazarati et al., 2004b). Inbred mice with a lower expression of GalR1 has a larger cell loss than wildtype littermates in several hippocampal regions when exposed to KA (Kong et al., 2008; Schauwecker, 2010) without any alteration in seizure parameters. Some studies has also reported that GalR1-KO mice exhibit spontaneous epilepsy (Jacoby et al., 2002; Fetissov et al., 2003; McColl et al., 2006) although other studies could not replicate this phenotype (Mazarati et al., 2004b).

GalR2-KO mice display no difference in seizure susceptibility in two model of SE compared to WT (Gottsch et al., 2005). In contrast to the knockout mice, application of a putative GalR2 specific ligand shorten the SSSE duration and decreased the seizure density and seizure episodes in the perforant path stimulation model, but not the duration of single seizure episodes (Mazarati et al., 2004a). Similar effects were reported after addition peptide nucleic antisense (PNA) oligonucleotide that mediated transient downregulation of GalR2. PNA-treatment resulted in an increase in the severity of SSSE after perforant path stimulation (Mazarati et al., 2004a). Increased damage to hilar interneurons was also seen after PNA-application (Mazarati et al., 2004a).

Acute administration of two systemically active non-selective subtype galanin receptor agonists, galnon, and galmic, has been shown to prevent self-sustained seizure activity (Saar et al.,

2002; Bartfai et al., 2004) and penthylenetetrazole (PTZ)-induced seizures (Saar et al., 2002). Galnon has shown to interact with several other receptors (Florén et al., 2005), although the anticonvulsant effect seems to be mediated via GalR1, as pretreatment with a GalR1-specific PNA attenuates its anticonvulsant properties (Saar et al., 2002).

In concordance with this, application of non-selective subtype galanin receptor antagonists has been shown to worsen the severity of SE in several models, i.e., kainic acid-induced seizures (Reiss et al., 2009), hippocampal kindling model (Kokaia et al., 2001), self-sustained SE (SSSE), and PTZ-induced convulsions (Chepurnov et al., 1998; Mazarati et al., 1998, 2000; Saar et al., 2002). A recent study showed that M15, a non-selective subtype galanin receptor antagonist significantly induced cell death in several hippocampal areas although no differences in the latency of onset or duration of severe seizures were seen (Schauwecker, 2010).

Galanin-KO mice have a lower threshold for developing SE after perforant path stimulation or KA exposure compared to WT (Mazarati et al., 2000). Furthermore, Gal-KO mice displayed a neuronal injury in the CA3-region that was not present in WT littermates (Mazarati et al., 2000). In concordance with this, Galanin-OE mice have a higher threshold for SE induced by either perforant path stimulation or PTZ and KA exposure compared to WT (Mazarati et al., 2000). Gal-OE mice have been shown to be less affected during hippocampal kindling, a model for human complex partial epilepsy (Kokaia et al., 2001).

Utilizing a recombinant adeno-associated viral (AAV) system that overexpresses galanin resulted in a dramatic reduction in KA-induced seizure episodes and the total time spent in seizures although no reduction of cell damage was seen (Lin et al., 2003). The same vector delayed the initiation of convulsions at generalized seizure stages and shortened the duration of electrographic after discharges in rats undergoing hippocampal kindling (Kanter-Schlifke et al., 2007). A similar AAV system that overexpresses galanin together with the fibronectin secretory signal sequence succeeded to the attenuation of KA-induced seizures and the neuronal death after KA exposure (Haberman et al., 2003).

A recent study showed that a GalR2 allosteric modulator increased the latency to the first electrographic seizure, decrease the total time in seizure and decreased the mortality in the Li-pilocarpine SE-model (Lu et al., 2010).

Furthermore, acute administration of the systemically active subtype galanin receptor agonist, Gal-B2, with a moderate GalR1 preferential binding, prevents seizures in the 6 Hz mouse model of pharmacoresistant epilepsy (Bulaj et al., 2008). It was later shown to be active also in other seizure and epilepsy models (White et al., 2009). An analog with a moderate GalR2 preferential binding [N-me, des-Sar]Gal-B2, also prevent seizure in the 6 Hz mouse model (Robertson et al., 2010). The authors conclude that these GalR1- and GalR2 preferential analogs (with 15 and 18 times selectivity, respectively) exhibit similar levels of anticonvulsant activity in the 6 Hz mouse model.

In summary, the wide involvement of galanin family peptides in physiological and pathological conditions has drawn attention to this neuropeptide family. Among the earliest areas of interests was the usage of galanin as a possible anticonvulsant.

Due to the three different galanin receptors specific expression in the CNS, several attempts have been made trying to characterize the contribution of each receptor and delineate their effects. Unfortunately, more selective or specific ligands are still needed.

Recent publications of stable peptide ligands have made new administration routes available as well as attract attention from the pharmaceutical industry.

REFERENCES

Abramov, U., Florén, A., Echevarria, D. J., Brewer, A., Manuzon, H., Robinson, J. K., et al. (2004). Regulation of feeding by galnon. *Neuropeptides* 38, 55–61.

Ahmad, S., and Dray, A. (2004). Novel G protein-coupled receptors as pain targets. *Curr. Opin. Investig. Drugs* 5, 67–70.

Alier, K. A., Chen, Y., Sollenberg Eriksson, U., Langel, Ü., and Smith, P. A. (2007). Selective stimulation of GalR1 and GalR2 in rat substantia gelatinosa reveals a cellular basis for the anti- and pronociceptive actions of galanin. *Pain* 137, 138–146.

Andell-Jonsson, S., Xu, I. S., Bartfai, T., Xu, X. J., and Wiesenfeld-Hallin, Z. (1997). The effect of naturally occurring fragments of galanin message-associated peptide on spinal cord excitability in rats. *Neurosci. Lett.* 235, 154–156.

Ash, B. L., Zanatta, S. D., Williams, S. J., and Djouma, E. (2011). The galanin-3 receptor antagonist, SNAP 37889, reduces operant responding for ethanol in alcohol-preferring rats. *Regul. Pept.* 166, 59–67.

Badie-Mahdavi, H., Lu, X., Behrens, M. M., and Bartfai, T. (2005). Role of galanin receptor 1 and galanin receptor 2 activation in synaptic plasticity associated with 3′,5′-cyclic AMP response element-binding protein phosphorylation in the dentate gyrus: studies with a galanin receptor 2 agonist and galanin receptor 1 knockout mice. *Neuroscience* 133, 591–604.

Bailey, K. R., Pavlova, M. N., Hohmann, J. G., and Crawley, J. N. (2007). Galanin receptor subtype 2 (GalR2) null mutant mice displays an anxiogenic-like phenotype specific to the elevated plus-maze. *Pharmacol. Biochem. Behav.* 86, 8–20.

Barr, A. M., Kinney, J. W., Hill, M. N., Lu, X., Biros, S., Rebek, J. Jr., et al. (2006). A novel, systemically active, selective galanin receptor type-3 ligand exhibits antidepressant-like activity in preclinical tests. *Neurosci. Lett.* 405, 111–115.

Barreto, S. G., Bazargan, M., Zotti, M., Hussey, D. J., Sukocheva, O. A., Peiris, H., et al. (2011). Galanin receptor 3 – a potential target for acute pancreatitis therapy. *Neurogastroenterol. Motil.* 23, e141–e151.

Bartfai, T., Bedecs, K., Land, T., Langel, Ü., Bertorelli, R., Girotti, P., et al. (1991). M-15: high-affinity chimeric peptide that blocks the neuronal actions of galanin in the hippocampus, locus coeruleus, and spinal cord. *Proc. Natl. Acad. Sci. U.S.A.* 88, 10961–10965.

Bartfai, T., Langel, Ü., Bedecs, K., Andell, S., Land, T., Gregersen, S., et al. (1993). Galanin-receptor ligand M40 peptide distinguishes between putative galanin-receptor subtypes. *Proc. Natl. Acad. Sci. U.S.A.* 90, 11287–11291.

Bartfai, T., Lu, X., Badie-Mahdavi, H., Barr, A. M., Mazarati, A., Hua, X. Y., et al. (2004). Galmic, a nonpeptide galanin receptor agonist, affects behaviors in seizure, pain, and forced-swim tests. *Proc. Natl. Acad. Sci. U.S.A.* 101, 10470–10475.

Bauer, J. W., Lang, R., Jakab, M., and Kofler, B. (2010). "Galanin family of peptides in skin function"in *Experientia Supplementum*, ed. T. Hökfelt (Basel: Springer), 51–59.

Bedecs, K., Langel, Ü., and Bartfai, T. (1995). Metabolism of galanin and galanin (1–16) in isolated cerebrospinal fluid and spinal cord membranes from rat. *Neuropeptides* 29, 137–143.

Bloomquist, B. T., Beauchamp, M. R., Zhelnin, L., Brown, S. E., Gore-Willse, A. R., Gregor, P., et al. (1998). Cloning and expression of the human galanin receptor GalR2. *Biochem. Biophys. Res. Commun.* 243, 474–479.

Borowsky, B., Walker, M. W., Huang, L. Y., Jones, K. A., Smith, K. E., Bard, J., et al. (1998). Cloning and characterization of the human galanin GALR2 receptor. *Peptides* 19, 1771–1781.

Boughton, C. K., Patterson, M., Bewick, G. A., Tadross, J. A., Gardiner, J. V., Beale, K. E., et al. (2010). Alarin stimulates food intake and gonadotrophin release in male rats. *Br. J. Pharmacol.* 161, 601–613.

Branchek, T. A., Smith, K. E., Gerald, C., and Walker, M. W. (2000). Galanin receptor subtypes. *Trends Pharmacol. Sci.* 21, 109–117.

Bulaj, G., Green, B. R., Lee, H. K., Robertson, C. R., White, K., Zhang, L., et al. (2008). Design, synthesis, and characterization of high-affinity, systemically-active galanin analogues with potent anticonvulsant activities. *J. Med. Chem.* 51, 8038–8047.

Burazin, T. C., Larm, J. A., Ryan, M. C., and Gundlach, A. L. (2000). Galanin-R1 and -R2 receptor mRNA expression during the development of rat brain suggests differential subtype involvement in synaptic transmission and plasticity. *Eur. J. Neurosci.* 12, 2901–2917.

Burgevin, M. C., Loquet, I., Quarteronet, D., and Habert-Ortoli, E. (1995). Cloning, pharmacological characterization, and anatomical distribution of a rat cDNA encoding for a galanin receptor. *J. Mol. Neurosci.* 6, 33–41.

Carpenter, K. A., Schmidt, R., Yue, S. Y., Hodzic, L., Pou, C., Payza, K., et al. (1999). The glycine residue in cyclic lactam analogues of galanin(1-16)-NH2 is important for stabilizing an N-terminal helix. *Biochemistry* 38, 15295–15304.

Ceide, S. C., Trembleau, L., Haberhauer, G., Somogyi, L., Lu, X., Bartfai, T., et al. (2004). Synthesis of galmic: a nonpeptide galanin receptor agonist. *Proc. Natl. Acad. Sci. U.S.A.* 101, 16727–16732.

Chan-Palay, V. (1988a). Galanin hyperinnervates surviving neurons of the human basal nucleus of Meynert in dementias of Alzheimer's and Parkinson's disease: a hypothesis for the role of galanin in accentuating cholinergic dysfunction in dementia. *J. Comp. Neurol.* 273, 543–557.

Chan-Palay, V. (1988b). Neurons with galanin innervate cholinergic cells in the human basal forebrain and galanin and acetylcholine coexist. *Brain Res. Bull.* 21, 465–472.

Chepurnov, S. A., Chepurnova, N. E., and Berdiev, R. K. (1998). Galanin controls excitability of the brain. *Ann. N. Y. Acad. Sci.* 865, 547–550.

Chu, M., Mierzwa, R., Truumees, I., King, A., Sapidou, E., Barrabee, E., et al. (1997). A new fungal metabolite, Sch 202596, with inhibitory activity in the galanin receptor GALR1 assay. *Tetrahedron Lett.* 38, 6111–6114.

Ciosek, J., and Cisowska, A. (2003). Centrally administrered galanin modifies vasopressin and oxytocin release from the hypothalamoneurohypophysial system of euhydrated and dehydrated rats. *J. Physiol. Pharmacol.* 54, 625–641.

Corness, J., Shi, T. J., Xu, Z. Q., Brulet, P., and Hökfelt, T. (1996). Influence of leukemia inhibitory factor on galanin/GMAP and neuropeptide Y expression in mouse primary sensory neurons after axotomy. *Exp. Brain Res.* 112, 79–88.

Cunningham, M. J., Scarlett, J. M., and Steiner, R. A. (2002). Cloning and distribution of galanin-like peptide mRNA in the hypothalamus and pituitary of the macaque. *Endocrinology* 143, 755–763.

Ding, X., MacTavish, D., Kar, S., and Jhamandas, J. H. (2006). Galanin attenuates beta-amyloid (Abeta) toxicity in rat cholinergic basal forebrain neurons. *Neurobiol. Dis.* 21, 413–420.

Eberhard, N., Mayer, C., Santic, R., Navio, R. P., Wagner, A., Bauer, H. C., et al. (2012). Distribution of alarin immunoreactivity in the mouse brain. *J. Mol. Neurosci.* 46, 18–32.

Elliott-Hunt, C. R., Pope, R. J., Vanderplank, P., and Wynick, D. (2007). Activation of the galanin receptor 2 (GalR2) protects the hippocampus from neuronal damage. *J. Neurochem.* 100, 780–789.

Fathi, Z., Cunningham, A. M., Iben, L. G., Battaglino, P. B., Ward, S. A., Nichol, K. A., et al. (1997). Cloning, pharmacological characterization and distribution of a novel galanin receptor. *Mol. Brain Res.* 51, 49–59.

Fetissov, S. O., Jacoby, A. S., Brumovsky, P. R., Shine, J., Iismaa, T. P., and Hökfelt, T. (2003). Altered hippocampal expression of neuropeptides in seizure-prone GALR1 knockout mice. *Epilepsia* 44, 1022–1033.

Florén, A., Sollenberg, U., Lundström, L., Zorko, M., Stojan, J., Budihna, M., et al. (2005). Multiple interaction sites of galnon trigger its biological effects. *Neuropeptides* 39, 547–558.

Fraley, G. S., Leathley, E., Lundy, N., Cheng, E., King, I., and Kofler, B. (2012). Effects of alarin on food intake, body weight and luteinizing hormone secretion in male mice. *Neuropeptides* 46, 99–104.

Fraley, G. S., Scarlett, J. M., Shimada, I., Teklemichael, D. N., Acohido, B. V., Clifton, D. K., et al. (2004). Effects of diabetes and insulin on the expression of galanin-like peptide in the hypothalamus of the rat. *Diabetes* 53, 1237–1242.

Fujiwara, K., Adachi, S., Usui, K., Maruyama, M., Matsumoto, H., Ohtaki, T., et al. (2002). Immunocytochemical localization of a galanin-like peptide (GALP) in pituicytes of the rat posterior pituitary gland. *Neurosci. Lett.* 317, 65–68.

Gabriel, S. M., Kaplan, L. M., Martin, J. B., and Koenig, J. I. (1989). Tissue-specific sex differences in galanin-like immunoreactivity and galanin mRNA during development in the rat. *Peptides* 10, 369–374.

Gottsch, M. L., Zeng, H., Hohmann, J. G., Weinshenker, D., Clifton, D. K., and Steiner, R. A. (2005). Phenotypic analysis of mice deficient in the type 2 galanin receptor (GALR2). *Mol. Cell. Biol.* 25, 4804–4811.

Gustafson, E. L., Smith, K. E., Durkin, M. M., Gerald, C., and Branchek, T. A. (1996). Distribution of a rat galanin receptor mRNA in rat brain. *Neuroreport* 7, 953–957.

Haberman, R. P., Samulski, R. J., and McCown, T. J. (2003). Attenuation of seizures and neuronal death by adeno-associated virus vector galanin expression and secretion. *Nat. Med.* 9, 1076–1080.

Habert-Ortoli, E., Amiranoff, B., Loquet, I., Laburthe, M., and Mayaux, J. F. (1994). Molecular cloning of a functional human galanin receptor. *Proc. Natl. Acad. Sci. U.S.A.* 91, 9780–9783.

Hao, J. X., Shi, T. J., Xu, I. S., Kaupilla, T., Xu, X. J., Hökfelt, T., et al. (1999). Intrathecal galanin alleviates allodynia-like behaviour in rats after partial peripheral nerve injury. *Eur. J. Neurosci.* 11, 427–432.

Hawes, J. J., Brunzell, D. H., Wynick, D., Zachariou, V., and Picciotto, M. R. (2005). GalR1, but not GalR2 or GalR3, levels are regulated by galanin signaling in the locus coeruleus through a cyclic AMP-dependent mechanism. *J. Neurochem.* 93, 1168–1176.

Hökfelt, T. (2005). Galanin and its receptors: introduction to the Third International Symposium San Diego, CA, USA, 21–22 October 2004. *Neuropeptides* 39, 125–142.

Hökfelt, T., Aman, K., Arvidsson, U., Bedecs, K., Ceccatelli, S., Hulting, A. L., et al. (1992). Galanin message-associated peptide (GMAP)- and galanin-like immunoreactivities: overlapping and differential distributions in the rat. *Neurosci. Lett.* 142, 139–142.

Hökfelt, T., Wiesenfeld-Hallin, Z., Villar, M., and Melander, T. (1987). Increase of galanin-like immunoreactivity in rat dorsal root ganglion cells after peripheral axotomy. *Neurosci. Lett.* 83, 217–220.

Holub, B. S., Rauch, I., Radner, S., Sperl, W., Hell, M., and Kofler, B. (2011). Effects of galanin message-associated peptide and neuropeptide Y against various non-albicans Candida strains. *Int. J. Antimicrob. Agents* 38, 76–80.

Howard, A. D., Tan, C., Shiao, L. L., Palyha, O. C., McKee, K. K., Weinberg, D. H., et al. (1997). Molecular cloning and characterization of a new receptor for galanin. *FEBS Lett.* 405, 285–290.

Izdebska, K., and Ciosek, J. (2010). Galanin influences on vasporessin and oxytocin release: in vitro studies. *Neuropeptides* 44, 341–348.

Jacoby, A. S., Hort, Y. J., Constantinescu, G., Shine, J., and Iismaa, T. P. (2002). Critical role or GALR1 galanin receptor in galanin regulation of neuroendocrine function and seizure activity. *Brain Res. Mol. Brain Res.* 107, 195–200.

Jacoby, A. S., Webb, G. C., Liu, M. L., Kofler, B., Hort, Y. J., Fathi, Z., et al. (1997). Structural organization of the mouse and human GALR1 galanin receptor genes (Galnr and GALNR) and chromosomal localization of the mouse gene. *Genomics* 45, 496–508.

Jimenez-Andrade, J. M., Lundström, L., Sollenberg Eriksson, U., Langel, Ü., Castañeda-Hernandez, G., and Carlton, S. M. (2006). Activation of peripheral galanin receptors: differential effects on nociception. *Pharmacol. Biochem. Behav.* 85, 273–280.

Juréus, A., Cunningham, M. J., Li, D., Johnson, L. L., Krasnow, S. M., Teklemichael, D. N., et al. (2001). Distribution and regulation of galanin-like peptide (GALP) in the hypothalamus of the mouse. *Endocrinology* 142, 5140–5144.

Juréus, A., Cunningham, M. J., McClain, M. E., Clifton, D. K., and Steiner, R. A. (2000). Galanin-like peptide (GALP) is a target for regulation by leptin in the hypothalamus of the rat. *Endocrinology* 141, 2703–2706.

Kakuyama, H., Kuwahara, A., Mochizuki, T., Hoshino, M., and Yanaihara, N. (1997). Role of N-terminal active sites of galanin in neurally evoked circular muscle contractions in the guinea-pig ileum. *Eur. J. Pharmacol.* 329, 85–91.

Kanter-Schlifke, I., Toft Sørensen, A., Ledri, M., Kuteeva, E., Hökfelt, T., and Kokaia, M. (2007). Galanin gene transfer curtails generalized seizures in kindled rats without altering hippocampal synaptic plasticity. *Neuroscience* 150, 984–992.

Kaplan, L. M., Gabriel, S. M., Koenig, J. I., Sunday, M. E., Spindel, E. R., Martin, J. B., et al. (1988). Galanin is an estrogen-inducible, secretory product of the rat anterior pituitary. *Proc. Natl. Acad. Sci. U.S.A.* 85, 7408–7412.

Kask, K., Berthold, M., Bourne, J., Andell, S., Langel, Ü., and Bartfai, T. (1995). Binding and agonist/antagonist actions of M35, galanin(1-13)-bradykinin(2-9)amide chimeric peptide, in Rin m 5F insulinoma cells. *Regul. Pept.* 59, 341–348.

Katoh, T., Ohmori, O., Iwasaki, K., and Inoue, M. (2002). Synthetic studies on Sch 202596, an antagonist of the galanin receptor GalR1: an efficient synthesis of (±)-geodin, the spirocoumaranone part of Sch 202596. *Tetrahedron* 58, 1289–1299.

Kauffman, A. S., Buenzle, J., Fraley, G. S., and Rissman, E. F. (2005). Effects of galanin-like peptide (GALP) on locomotion, reproduction, and body weight in female and male mice. *Horm. Behav.* 48, 141–151.

Kerr, N. C., Holmes, F. E., and Wynick, D. (2000). Galanin-like peptide (GALP) is expressed in rat hypothalamus and pituitary, but not in DRG. *Neuroreport* 11, 3909–3913.

Kofler, B., Berger, A., Santic, R., Moritz, K., Almer, D., Tuechler, C., et al. (2004). Expression of neuropeptide galanin and galanin receptors in human skin. *J. Invest. Dermatol.* 122, 1050–1053.

Kofler, B., Evans, H. F., Liu, M. L., Falls, V., Iismaa, T. P., Shine, J., et al. (1995). Characterization of the 5′-flanking region of the human preprogalanin gene. *DNA Cell Biol.* 14, 321–329.

Kokaia, M., Holmberg, K., Nanobashvili, A., Xu, Z. Q., Kokaia, Z., Lendahl, U., et al. (2001). Suppressed kindling epileptogenesis in mice with ectopic overexpression of galanin. *Proc. Natl. Acad. Sci. U.S.A.* 98, 14006–14011.

Kolakowskim, L. F. Jr., O'Neill, G. P., Howardm, A. D., Broussard, S. R., Sullivan, K. A., Feighner, S. D., et al. (1998). Molecular characterization and expression of cloned human galanin receptors GALR2 and GALR3. *J. Neurochem.* 71, 2239–2251.

Kong, S., Lorenzana, A., Deng, Q., McNeill, T. H., and Schauwecker, P. E. (2008). Variation in Galr1 expression determines susceptibility to excitotoxin-induced cell death in mice. *Genes Brain Behav.* 7, 587–598.

Konkel, M., Wetzel, J. M., and Talisman, I. J. (2004). 3-Imino-2-indolones for the treatment of depression and/or anxiety. *United States Patent.* US7,166,635 B2 (accessed January 23, 2007).

Konkel, M. J., Lagu, B., Boteju, L. W., Jimenez, H., Noble, S., Walker, M. W., et al. (2006a). 3-arylimino-2-indolones are potent and selective galanin GAL3 receptor antagonists. *J. Med. Chem.* 49, 3757–3758.

Konkel, M. J., Packiarajan, M., Chen, H., Topiwala, U. P., Jimenez, H., Talisman, I. J., et al. (2006b). Amino substituted analogs of 1-phenyl-3-phenylimino-2-indolones with potent galanin Gal3 receptor binding affinity and improved solubility. *Bioorg. Med. Chem. Lett.* 16, 3950–3954.

Konopka, L. M., McKeon, T. W., and Parsons, R. L. (1989). Galanin-induced hyperpolarization and decreased membrane excitability of neurones in mudpuppy cardiac ganglia. *J. Physiol.* 410, 107–122.

Kozoriz, M. G., Kuzmiski, J. B., Hirasawa, M., and Pittman, Q. J. (2006). Galanin modulates neuronal and synaptic properties in the rat supraoptic nucleus in a use and state dependent manner. *J. Neurophysiol.* 96, 154–164.

Krasnow, S. M., Hohmann, J. G., Gragerov, A., Clifton, D. K., and Steiner, R. A. (2004). Analysis of the contribution of galanin receptors 1 and 2 to the central actions of galanin-like peptide. *Neuroendocrinology* 79, 268–277.

Kuteeva, E., Wardi, T., Lundström, L., Sollenberg, U., Langel, Ü., Hökfelt, T., et al. (2008). Differential role of galanin receptors in the regulation of depression-like behavior and monoamine/stress-related genes at the cell body level. *Neuropsychopharmacology* 33, 2573–2585.

Land, T., Langel, Ü., and Bartfai, T. (1991a). Hypothalamic degradation of galanin(1-29) and galanin(1-16): identification and characterization of the peptidolytic products. *Brain Res.* 558, 245–250.

Land, T., Langel, Ü., Low, M., Berthold, M., Undén, A., and Bartfai, T. (1991b). Linear and cyclic N-terminal galanin fragments and analogs as ligands at the hypothalamic galanin receptor. *Int. J. Pept. Prot. Res.* 38, 267–272.

Lang, R., Berger, A., Santic, R., Geisberger, R., Hermann, A., Herzog, H., et al. (2005). Pharmacological and functional characterization of galanin-like peptide fragments as potent galanin receptor agonists. *Neuropeptides* 39, 179–184.

Lang, R., Gundlach, A. L., and Kofler, B. (2007). The galanin peptide family: Receptor pharmacology, pleiotropic biological actions, and implications in health and disease. *Pharmacol. Ther.* 115, 177–207.

Langel, Ü., Land, T., and Bartfai, T. (1992). Design of chimeric peptide ligands to galanin receptors and substance P receptors. *Int. J. Pept. Protein Res.* 39, 516–522.

Larm, J. A., and Gundlach, A. L. (2000). Galanin-like peptide (GALP) mRNA expression is restricted to arcuate nucleus of hypothalamus in adult male rat brain. *Neuroendocrinology* 72, 67–71.

Lawrence, C. B. (2009). Galanin-like peptide modulates energy balance by affecting inflammatory mediators. *Physiol. Behav.* 97, 515–519.

Lin, E.-J. D., Richichi, C., Young, D., Baer, K., Vezzani, D., and During, M. J. (2003). Recombinant AAV-mediated expression of galanin in rat hippocampus suppresses seizure development. *Eur. J. Neurosci.* 18, 2087–2092.

Liu, E. J., Richichi, C., Young, D., Baer, K., Vezzani, A., and During, M. J. (2003). Recombinant AAV-mediated expression of galanin in rat hippocampus suppresses seizure development. *Eur. J. Neurosci.* 18, 2087–2092.

Liu, H. X., Brumovsky, P., Schmidt, R., Brown, W., Payza, K., Hodzic, L., et al. (2001). Receptor subtype-specific pronociceptive and analgesic actions of galanin in the spinal cord: selective actions via GalR1 and GalR2 receptors. *Proc. Natl. Acad. Sci. U.S.A.* 98, 9960–9964.

Lorimer, D. D., and Benya, R. V. (1996). Cloning and quantification of galanin-1 receptor expression by mucosal cells lining the human gastrointestinal tract. *Biochem. Biophys. Res. Commun.* 222, 379–385.

Lu, X., Lundström, L., and Bartfai, T. (2005a). Galanin (2-11) binds to GalR3 in transfected cell lines: limitations for pharmacological definition of receptor subtypes. *Neuropeptides* 39, 165–167.

Lu, X., Lundström, L., Langel, Ü., and Bartfai, T. (2005b). Galanin receptor ligands. *Neuropeptides* 39, 143–146.

Lu, X., Roberts, E., Xia, F., Sanchez-Alavez, M., Liu, T., Baldwin, R., et al. (2010). GalR2-positive allosteric modulator exhibits anticonvulsant effects in animal models. *Proc. Natl. Acad. Sci. U.S.A.* 107, 15229–15234.

Lundkvist, J., Land, T., Kahl, U., Bedecs, K., and Bartfai, T. (1995). cDNA sequence, ligand biding, and regulation of galanin/GMAP in mouse brain. *Neurosci. Lett.* 200, 121–124.

Lundström, L., Lu, X., Langel, Ü., and Bartfai, T. (2005a). Important pharmacophores for binding to galanin receptor 2. *Neuropeptides* 39, 169–171.

Lundström, L., Sollenberg, U., Brewer, A., Kouya, P. F., Zheng, K., Xu, X. J., et al. (2005b). A Galanin Receptor Subtype 1 Specific Agonist. *Int. J. Pept. Res. Ther.* 11, 17–27.

Mahoney, S. A., Hosking, R., Farrant, S., Holmes, F. E., Jacoby, A. S., Shine, J., et al. (2003). The second galanin receptor GalR2 plays a key role in neurite outgrowth from adult sensory neurons. *J. Neurosci.* 23, 416–421.

Man, P. S., and Lawrence, C. B. (2008a). The effects of galanin-like peptide on energy balance, body temperature and brain activity in the mouse and rat are independent of the GALR2/3 receptor. *J. Neuroendocrinol.* 20, 128–137.

Man, P. S., and Lawrence, C. B. (2008b). Interleukin-1 mediates the anorexic and febrile actions of galanin-like Peptide. *Endocrinology* 149, 5791–5580.

Mazarati, A., Lu, X., Kilk, K., Langel, Ü., Wasterlain, C., and Bartfai, T. (2004a). Galanin type 2 receptors regulate neuronal survival, susceptibility to seizures and seizure-induces neurogenesisin the dentate gyrus. *Eur. J. Neurosci.* 19, 3235–3244.

Mazarati, A., Lu, X., Shinmei, S., Badie-Mahdavi, H., and Bartfai, T. (2004b). Patterns of seizures, hippocampal injury and neurogenesis in the three models of status epilepticus in galanin receptor type 1 (GalR1) knockout mice. *Neuroscience* 128, 431–441.

Mazarati, A., Lundström, L., Sollenberg, U., Shin, D., Langel, Ü., and Sankar, R. (2006). Regulation of kindling epileptogenesis by hippocampal galanin type 1 and type 2 receptors: The effects of subtype-selective agonists and the role of G-protein-mediated signaling. *J. Pharm. Exp. Ther.* 318, 700–708.

Mazarati, A. M., Liu, H., Soomets, U., Sankar, R., Shin, D., Katsumori, H., et al. (1998). Galanin modulation of seizures and seizure modulation of hippocampal galanin in animal models of status epilepticus. *J. Neurosci.* 814, 179–185.

Mazarati, A. M., Halászi, E., and Telegdy, G. (1992). Anticonvulsive effects of galanin administered into the central nervous system upon picrotoxin-kindeled seizure syndrome in rats. *Brain Res.* 589, 164–166.

Mazarati, A. M., Hohmann, J. G., Bacon, A., Liu, H., Sankar, R., Steiner, R. A., et al. (2000). Modulation of hippocampal excitability and seizures by galanin. *J. Neurosci.* 20, 6276–6281.

McColl, C. D., Jacoby, A. S., Shine, J., Iismaa, T. P., and Bekkers, J. M. (2006). Galanin receptor-1 knockout mice exhibit spontaneous epilepsy, abnormal EEGs and altered inhibition in the hippocampus. *Neuropharmacology* 50, 209–218.

Melander, T., Hökfelt, T., Rökaeus, Å., Cuello, A. C., Oertel, W. H., Verhofstad, A., et al. (1986). Coexistence of galanin-like immunoreactivity with catecholamines, 5-hydroxytryptamine, GABA and neuropeptides in the rat CNS. *J. Neurosci.* 6, 3640–3654.

Mennicken, F., Hoffert, C., Pelletier, M., Ahmad, S., and O'Donnell, D. (2002). Restricted distribution of galanin receptor 3 (GalR3) mRNA in the adult rat central nervous system. *J. Chem. Neuroanat.* 24, 257–268.

Merchenthaler, I., Lopez, F. J., and Negro-Vilar, A. (1990). Colocalization of galanin and luteinizing hormone-releasing hormone in a subset of preoptic hypothalamic-neurons: anatomical and functional correlates. *Proc. Natl. Acad. Sci. U.S.A.* 87, 6326–6330.

Mitchell, V., Bouret, S., Howard, A. D., and Beauvillain, J. C. (1999). Expression of the galanin receptor subtype Gal-R2 mRNA in the rat hypothalamus. *J. Chem. Neuroanat.* 16, 265–277.

Mitsukawa, K., Lu, X., and Bartfai, T. (2008). Galanin, galanin receptors and drug targets. *Cell. Mol. Life. Sci.* 65, 1796–1805.

Morris, M. B., Ralston, G. B., Biden, T. J., Browne, C. L., King, G. F., and Iismaa, T. P. (1995). Structural and biochemical studies of human galanin: NMR evidence for nascent helical structures in aqueous solution. *Biochemistry* 34, 4538–4545.

Narváez, J. A., Diaz-Cabiale, Z., Hedlund, P. B., Aguirre, J. A., Coveñas, R., González-Barón, S., et al. (2000). The galanin receptor antagonist M40 blocks the central cardiovascular actions of the galanin N-terminal fragment (1-15). *Eur. J. Pharmacol.* 399, 197–203.

O'Donnell, D., Ahmad, S., Wahlestedt, C., and Walker, P. (1999). Expression of the novel galanin receptor subtype GALR2 in the adult rat CNS: distinct distribution from GALR1. *J. Comp. Neurol.* 409, 469–481.

Ögren, S. O., Hökfelt, T., Kask, K., Langel, Ü., and Bartfai, T. (1992). Evidence for a role of the neuropeptide galanin in spatial learning. *Neuroscience* 51, 1–5.

Öhman, A., Lycksell, P. O., Juréus, A., Langel, Ü., Bartfai, T., and Gräslund, A. (1998). NMR study of the conformation and localization of porcine galanin in SDS micelles. Comparison with an inactive analog and a galanin receptor antagonist. *Biochemistry* 37, 9169–9178.

Ohtaki, T., Kumano, S., Ishibashi, Y., Ogi, K., Matsui, H., Harada, M., et al. (1999). Isolation and cDNA cloning of a novel galanin-like peptide (GALP) from porcine hypothalamus. *J. Biol. Chem.* 274, 37041–37045.

Page, A. J., Slattery, J. A., Brieerley, S. M., Jacoby, A. S., and Blackshaw, L. A. (2007). Invovlement of galanin receptors 1 and 2 in the modulation of mouse vagal afferent mechanosensitivity. *J. Physiol.* 583, 675–684.

Pang, L., Hashemi, T., Lee, H. J., Maguire, M., Graziano, M. P., Bayne, M., et al. (1998). The mouse GalR2 galanin receptor: genomic organization, cDNA cloning, and functional characterization. *J. Neurochem.* 71, 2252–2259.

Parker, E. M., Izzarelli, D. G., Nowak, H. P., Mahle, C. D., Iben, L. G., Wang, J., et al. (1995). Cloning and characterization of the rat GALR1 galanin receptor from Rin14B insulinoma cells. *Mol. Brain Res.* 34, 179–189.

Pirondi, S., Giuliani, A., Del Vecchio, G., Hökfelt, T., and Calzà, L. (2010). The galanin receptor 2/3 agonist Gal2-11 protects the SN56 cells against (β-amyloid25-35 toxicity. *J. Neurosci. Res.* 88, 1064–1073.

Pooga, M., Juréus, A., Razaei, K., Hasanvan, H., Saar, K., Kask, K., et al. (1998). Novel galanin receptor ligands. *J. Pept. Res.* 51, 65–74.

Potter, E. K., and Smith-White, M. A. (2005). Galanin modulates cholinergic neurotransmission in the heart. *Neuropeptides* 39, 345–348.

Radács, M., Molnár, A. H., László, F. A., Varga, C., László, F., and Gálfi, M. (2010). Inhibitory Effect of galanin on adrenaline- and noradrenaline-induced increased oxytocin secretion in rat neurohypophyseal cell cultures. *J. Mol. Neurosci.* 42, 59–66.

Rajarao, S. J., Platt, B., Sukoff, S. J., Lin, Q., Bender, C. N., Nieuwenhuijsen, B. W., et al. (2007). Anxiolytic-like activity of the non-selective galanin receptor agonist, galnon. *Neuropeptides* 41, 307–320.

Rauch, I., Lundström, L., Hell, M., Sperl, W., and Kofler, B. (2007). Galanin message-associated peptide suppresses growth and the budded-to-hyphal-form transition of *Candida albicans. Antimicrob. Agents Chemother.* 51, 4167–4170.

Reiss, J. I., Dishman, R. K., Boyd, H. E., Robinson, J. K., and Holmes, P. V. (2009). Chronic activity wheel running reduces the severity of kainic acid-induced seizures in the rat: possible role of galanin. *Brain Res.* 1266, 54–63.

Robertson, C. R., Scholl, E. A., Pruess, T. H., Green, B. R., White, H. S., and Bulaj, G. (2010). Engineering galanin analogues that discriminate between GalR1 and GalR2 receptor subtypes and exhibit anticonvulsant activity following systemic delivery. *J. Med. Chem.* 53, 1871–1875.

Rökaeus, Å., and Carlquist, M. (1988). Nucleotide sequence analysis of cDNAs encoding a bovine galanin precursor protein in the adrenal medulla and chemical isolation of bovine gut galanin. *FEBS Lett.* 234, 400–406.

Runesson, J., Saar, I., Lundström, L., Järv, J., and Langel, Ü. (2009). A novel GalR2-specific peptide agonist. *Neuropeptides* 43,187–192.

Saar, I., Runesson, J., McNamara, I., Järv, J., Robinson, J. K., and Langel, Ü. (2011). Novel galanin receptor subtype specific ligands in feeding regulation. *Neurochem. Int.* 58, 714-720

Saar, K., Mazarati, A. M., Mahlapuu, R., Hallnemo, G., Soomets, U., Kilk, K., et al. (2002). Anticonvulsant activity of a nonpeptide galanin receptor agonist. *Proc. Natl. Acad. Sci. U.S.A.* 99, 7136–7141.

Sagi, V. N., Liu, T., Lu, X., Bartfai, T., and Roberts, E. (2011). Synthesis and biological evaluation of novel pyrimidine derivatives as sub-micromolar affinity ligands of GalR2. *Bioorg. Med. Chem. Lett.* 21, 7210–7215.

Saito, J., Ozaki, Y., Kawasaki, M., Ohnishi, H., Okimoto, N., Nakamura, T., et al. (2005). Induction of galanin-like peptide gene expression in the arcuate nucleus of the rat after acute but not chronic inflammatory stress. *Mol. Brain Res.* 133, 233–241.

Saito, J., Ozaki, Y., Ohnishi, H., Nakamura, T., and Ueta, Y. (2003). Induction of galanin-like peptide gene expression in the rat posterior pituitary gland during endotoxin shock and adjuvant arthritis. *Mol. Brain Res.* 113, 124–132.

Santic, R., Fenninger, K., Graf, K., Schneider, R., Hauser-Kronberger, C., Schilling, F. H., et al. (2006). Gangliocytes in neuroblastic tumors express alarin, a novel peptide derived by differential splicing of the galanin-like peptide gene. *J. Mol. Neurosci.* 29, 145–152.

Santic, R., Schmidhuber, S. M., Lang, R., Rauch, I., Voglas, E., Eberhard, N., et al. (2007). Alarin is a vasoactive peptide. *Proc. Natl. Acad. Sci. U.S.A.* 104, 10217–10222.

Schauwecker, P. E. (2010). Galanin receptor 1 deletion exacerbates hippocampal neuronal loss after systemic kainate administration in mice. *PLoS ONE* 15:e15657. doi:10.1371/journal.pone.0015657

Schneider, E. R., Rada, P., Darby, R., Leibowitz, S. F., and Hoebel, B. G. (2007). Orexigenic peptides and alcohol intake: differential effects of orexin, galanin, and ghrelin. *Alcohol. Clin. Exp. Res.* 31, 1858–1865.

Scott, M. K., Ross, T. M., Lee, D. H., Wang, H. Y., Shank, R. P., Wild, K. D., et al. (2000). 2,3-Dihydro-dithiin and -dithiepine-1,1,4,4-tetroxides: small molecule non-peptide antagonists of the human galanin hGAL-1 receptor. *Bioorg. Med. Chem.* 8, 1383–1391.

Shen, J., and Gundlach, A. L. (2004). Galanin-like peptide mRNA alterations in arcuate nucleus and neural lobe of streptozotocin-diabetic and obese zucker rats. Further evidence for leptin-dependent and independent regulation. *Neuroendocrinology* 79, 327–337.

Shen, J., Larm, J. A., and Gundlach, A. L. (2001). Galanin-like peptide mRNA in neural lobe of rat pituitary. Increased expression after osmotic stimulation suggests a role for galanin-like peptide in neuron-glial interactions and/or neurosecretion. *Neuroendocrinology* 73, 2–11.

Smith, K. E., Forray, C., Walker, M. W., Jones, K. A., Tamm, J. A., Bard, J., et al. (1997). Expression cloning of a rat hypothalamic galanin receptor coupled to phosphoinositide turnover. *J. Biol. Chem.* 272, 24612–24616.

Smith, K. E., Walker, M. W., Artymyshyn, R., Bard, J., Borowsky, B., Tamm, J. A., et al. (1998). Cloned human and rat galanin GALR3 receptors. Pharmacology and activation of G-protein inwardly rectifying K+ channels. *J. Biol. Chem.* 273, 23321–23326.

Sollenberg Eriksson, U., Lundström, L., Bartfai, T., and Langel, Ü. (2006). M871 – a novel peptide antagonist selectively recognizingthe galanin receptor type 2. *Int. J. Pept. Res. Ther.* 12, 115–119.

Sollenberg Eriksson, U., Runesson, J., Sillard, R., and Langel, Ü. (2010). Binding of chimeric peptides M617 and M871 to galanin receptor type 3 reveals characteristics of galanin receptor-ligand interaction. *Int. J. Pept. Res. Ther.* 16, 17–22.

Stoyanovitch, A. G., Johnson, M. A., Clifton, D. K., Steiner, R. A., and Fraley, G. S. (2005). Galanin-like peptide rescues reproductive function in the diabetic rat. *Diabetes* 54, 2471–2476.

Sullivan, K. A., Shiao, L. L., and Cascieri, M. A. (1997). Pharmacological characterization and tissue distribution of the human and rat GALR1 receptors. *Biochem. Biophys. Res. Commun.* 233, 823–828.

Sun, Y., and Zigmond, R. E. (1996). Involvement of leukemia inhibitory factor in the increases in galanin and vasoactive intestinal peptide mRNA and the decreases in neuropeptide Y and tyrosine hydroxylase mRNA in sympathetic neurons after axotomy. *J. Neurochem.* 67, 1751–1760.

Swanson, C. J., Blackburn, T. P., Zhang, X., Zheng, K., Xu, Z. Q., Hökfelt, T., et al. (2005). Anxiolytic- and antidepressant-like profiles of the galanin-3 receptor (Gal3) antagonists SNAP 37889 and SNAP 398299. *Proc. Natl. Acad. Sci. U.S.A.* 102, 17489–17494.

Takatsu, Y., Matsumoto, H., Ohtaki, T., Kumano, S., Kitada, C., Onda, H., et al. (2001). Distribution of galanin-like peptide in the rat brain. *Endocrinology* 142, 1626–1634.

Tamura, K., Palmer, J. M., Winkelmann, C. K., and Wood, J. D. (1988). Mechanism of action of galanin on myenteric neurons. *J. Neurophysiol.* 60, 966–979.

Tatemoto, K., Rökaeus, Å., Jornvall, H., McDonald, T. J., and Mutt, V. (1983). Galanin – a novel biologically active peptide from porcine intestine. *FEBS Lett.* 164, 124–128.

Taylor, A., Madison, F. N., and Fraley, G. S. (2009). Galanin-like peptide stimulates feeding and sexual behavior via dopaminergic fibers within the medial preoptic area of adult male rats. *J. Chem. Neuroanat.* 37, 105–111.

van Der Kolk, N., Madison, F. N., Mohr, M., Eberhard, N., Kofler, B., and Fraley, G. S. (2010). Alarin stimulates food intake in male rats and LH secretion in castrated male rats. *Neuropeptides* 44, 333–340.

Verge, V. M., Richardson, P. M., Wiesenfeld-Hallin, Z., and Hökfelt, T. (1995). Differential influence of nerve growth factor on neuropeptide expression in vivo: a novel role in peptide suppression in adult sensory neurons. *J. Neurosci.* 15, 2081–2096.

Vrontakis, M. E., Peden, L. M., Duckworth, M. L., and Friesen, H. G. (1987). Isolation and characterization of a complementary DNA (galanin) clone from estrogen-induced pituitary tumor messenger RNA. *J. Biol. Chem.* 262, 16755–16758.

Vrontakis, M. E., Yamamoto, T., Schroedter, I. C., Nagy, J. I., and Friesen, H. G. (1989). Estrogen induction of galanin synthesis in the rat anterior pituitary gland demonstrated by in situ hybridization and immunohistochemistry. *Neurosci. Lett.* 100, 59–64.

Wang, S., Hashemi, T., Fried, S., Clemmons, A. L., and Hawes, B. E. (1998). Differential intracellular signaling of the GalR1 and GalR2 galanin receptor subtypes. *Biochemistry* 37, 6711–6717.

Wang, S., Hashemi, T., He, C., Strader, C., and Bayne, M. (1997a). Molecular cloning and pharmacological characterization of a new galanin receptor subtype. *Mol. Pharmacol.* 52, 337–343.

Wang, S., He, C., Hashemi, T., and Bayne, M. (1997b). Cloning and expressional characterization of a novel galanin receptor. Identification of different pharmacophores within galanin for the three galanin receptor subtypes. *J. Biol. Chem.* 272, 31949–31952.

Wang, S., He, C., Maguire, M. T., Clemmons, A. L., Burrier, R. E., Guzzi, M. F., et al. (1997c). Genomic organization and functional characterization of the mouse GalR1 galanin receptor. *FEBS Lett.* 411, 225–230.

Waters, S. M., and Krause, J. E. (2000). Distribution of galanin-1, -2 and -3 receptor messenger RNAs in central and peripheral rat tissues. *Neuroscience* 95, 265–271.

Wennerberg, A. B., Cooke, R. M., Carlquist, M., Rigler, R., and Campbell, I. D. (1990). A 1H NMR study of the solution conformation of the neuropeptide galanin. *Biochem. Biophys. Res. Commun.* 166, 1102–1109.

White, H. S., Scholl, E. A., Klein, B. D., Flynn, S. P., Pruess, T. H., Green, B. R., et al. (2009). Developing novel antiepileptic drugs: characterization of NAX 5055, a systemically-active galanin analog, in epilepsy models. *Neurotherapeutics* 6, 372–380.

Wiesenfeld-Hallin, Z., Bartfai, T., and Hökfelt, T. (1992a). Galanin in sensory neurons in the spinal cord. *Front. Neuroendocrinol.* 13, 319–343.

Wiesenfeld-Hallin, Z., Xu, X. J., Langel, Ü., Bedecs, K., Hökfelt, T., and Bartfai, T. (1992b). Galanin-mediated control of pain: enhanced role after nerve injury. *Proc. Natl. Acad. Sci. U.S.A.* 89, 3334–3337.

Wilson, D. N., Chung, H., Elliott, R. C., Bremer, E., George, D., and Koh, S. (2005). Microarray analysis of postical transcriptional regulation of neuropeptides. *J. Mol. Neurosci.* 25, 285–298.

Wrenn, C. C., Kinney, J. W., Marriott, L. K., Holmes, A., Harris, A. P., Saavedra, M. C., et al. (2004). Learning and memory performance in mice lacking the Gal-R1 subtype of galanin receptor. *Eur. J. Neurosci.* 19, 1384–1396.

Wu, W. P., Hao, J. X., Lundström, L., Wiesenfeld-Hallin, Z., Langel, Ü., Bartfai, T., et al. (2003). Systemic galnon, a low-molecular weight galanin receptor agonist, reduces heat hyperalgesia in rats with nerve injury. *Eur. J. Pharmacol.* 482, 133–137.

Xu, X., Yang, X., Zhang, P., Chen, X., Liu, H., and Li, Z. (2012). Effects of exogenous galanin on neuropathic pain state and change of galanin and its receptors in DRG and SDH after sciatic nerve-pinch injury in rat. *PLoS ONE* 7:e37621. doi:10.1371/journal.pone.0037621

Xu, X. J., Andell, S., Hao, J. X., Wiesenfeld-Hallin, Z., and Bartfai, T. (1995a). The effects of intrathecal galanin message-associated peptide (GMAP) on the flexor reflex in rats. *Regul. Pept.* 58, 19–24.

Xu, X. J., Andell, S., Zhang, X., Wiesenfeld-Hallin, Z., Langel, Ü., Bedecs, K., et al. (1995b). Peripheral axotomy increases the expression of galanin message-associated peptide (GMAP) in dorsal root ganglion cells and alters the effects of intrathecal GMAP on the flexor reflex in the rat. *Neuropeptides* 28, 299–307.

Xu, Z. Q., Shi, T. J., and Hökfelt, T. (1996). Expression of galanin and a galanin receptor in several sensory systems and bone anlage of rat embryos. *Proc. Natl. Acad. Sci. U.S.A.* 93, 14901–14905.

Xu, Z. Q., Shi, T. J., and Hökfelt, T. (1998). Galanin/GMAP- and NPY-like immunoreactivities in locus coeruleus and noradrenergic nerve terminals in the hippocampal formation and cortex with notes on the galanin-R1 and -R2 receptors. *J. Comp. Neurol.* 392, 227–251.

Zachariou, V., Georgescu, D., Kansal, L., Merriam, P., and Picciotto, M. R. (2001). Galanin receptor 1 gene expression is regulated by cyclic AMP through a CREB-dependent mechanism. *J. Neurochem.* 76, 191–200.

Zhang, X., Nicholas, A. P., and Hökfelt, T. (1993a). Ultrastructural studies on peptides in the dorsal horn of the spinal cord-I. Co-existence of galanin with other peptides in primary afferents in normal rats. *Neuroscience* 57, 365–384.

Zhang, X., Verge, V. M., Wiesenfeld-Hallin, Z., Piehl, F., and Hökfelt, T. (1993b). Expression of neuropeptides and neuropeptide mRNAs in spinal cord after axotomy in the rat, with special reference to motoneurons and galanin. *Exp. Brain Res.* 93, 450–461.

Zhang, X., Nicholas, A. P., and Hökfelt, T. (1995). Ultrastructural studies on peptides in the dorsal horn of the rat spinal cord-II. Co-existence of galanin with other peptides in local neurons. *Neuroscience* 64, 875–891.

8

Mechanisms underlying the tissue-specific and regulated activity of the *Gnrhr* promoter in mammals

Anne-Laure Schang, Bruno Quérat, Violaine Simon, Ghislaine Garrel, Christian Bleux, Raymond Counis, Joëlle Cohen-Tannoudji and Jean-Noël Laverrière*

Physiologie de l'Axe Gonadotrope, Biologie Fonctionnelle et Adaptative, EAC CNRS 4413, Sorbonne Paris Cité, Université Paris Diderot-Paris 7, Paris, France

Edited by:
Hubert Vaudry, University of Rouen, France

Reviewed by:
Jae Young Seong, Korea University, South Korea
Ursula B. Kaiser, Brigham and Women's Hospital, USA

***Correspondence:**
Jean-Noël Laverrière, Physiologie de l'Axe Gonadotrope, Biologie Fonctionnelle et Adaptative, EAC CNRS 4413, Sorbonne Paris Cité, Université Paris Diderot-Paris 7, Bâtiment Buffon, case courrier 7007, 4 rue MA Lagroua Weill-Hallé, 75205 Paris Cedex 13, France.
e-mail: jean-noel.laverriere@univ-paris-diderot.fr

The GnRH receptor (GnRHR) plays a central role in the development and maintenance of reproductive function in mammals. Following stimulation by GnRH originating from the hypothalamus, GnRHR triggers multiple signaling events that ultimately stimulate the synthesis and the periodic release of the gonadotropins, luteinizing-stimulating hormone (LH) and follicle-stimulating hormones (FSH) which, in turn, regulate gonadal functions including steroidogenesis and gametogenesis. The concentration of GnRHR at the cell surface is essential for the amplitude and the specificity of gonadotrope responsiveness. The number of GnRHR is submitted to strong regulatory control during pituitary development, estrous cycle, pregnancy, lactation, or after gonadectomy. These modulations take place, at least in part, at the transcriptional level. To analyze this facet of the reproductive function, the 5′ regulatory sequences of the gene encoding the GnRHR have been isolated and characterized through *in vitro* and *in vivo* approaches. This review summarizes results obtained with the mouse, rat, human, and ovine promoters either by transient transfection assays or by means of transgenic mice.

Keywords: GnRH receptor, promoter regions, transcription, gonadotrope cell lines, steroidogenic factor 1, homeodomain proteins, transgenic mice

INTRODUCTION

Two GnRH systems (GnRH decapeptides and specific receptors) originally existed in the common mammalian ancestor but a large number of extant species have lost either the second type GnRH or its receptor (Stewart et al., 2009). Humans possess GnRH-II but lack a functional type-II receptor whereas mouse and rats lack both of them. In this paper, we will be dealing with the only GnRH system that has been proved to be involved in the reproductive hormonal cascade and that was retained in either humans or the two rodent models. The pituitary GnRH receptor (GnRHR) plays a central role in mammalian reproductive function since it establishes a unique molecular link between its ligand, the decapeptide GnRH originating from the hypothalamus, and the gonadotrope cells in the anterior pituitary. The hypothalamic GnRH is released into the portal hypophyseal vasculature in a periodic manner through a pulse generator that, likely by means of both gap junctions and voltage-gated calcium channels, coordinates the activity of individual neurons diffusely distributed in the hypothalamus (Vazquez-Martinez et al., 2001). Within the anterior pituitary, GnRH binds to specific high-affinity receptors present at the surface of the gonadotrope cells and induces increase in the synthesis and pulsatile release of the gonadotropins, luteinizing and follicle-stimulating hormones (LH and FSH). The pituitary hormones, which are composed of a common α- and distinct β-subunits, then enter the systemic circulation and, *via* specific receptors, modulate gonadal functions including gametogenesis, steroidogenesis, and ovulation. The amplitude and frequency of GnRH pulses relayed by the GnRHR appear critical in the development of the reproductive function, in the onset of puberty and throughout the menstrual or estrous cycle.

INTRACELLULAR SIGNALING AND GnRHR-MEDIATED EFFECTS

The activation of GnRHR may trigger several intracellular signaling pathways in gonadotrope cells depending on the cellular context. Two mouse gonadotrope tumor-derived cell lines expressing the GnRHR, αT3-1 and LβT2 cell lines, have been used as homogenous cell models to study gonadotrope function (Windle, et al., 1990; Alarid et al., 1996; Thomas et al., 1996; Turgeon et al., 1996). In both cell lines, GnRH activates the protein kinase C (PKC)-dependent signaling pathway through coupling to G proteins of the Gq/G11 family (see review in Anderson, 1996). In primary culture of rat pituitary cells under sustained GnRH stimulation, a cAMP/PKA pathway is preferentially recruited (Garrel et al., 2010). In the gonadotrope-derived LβT2 cell line, sustained stimulation of GnRHR activates the cAMP signaling pathway through PKC δ and ε (Larivière et al., 2007). Also, in these cells, GnRHR signaling has been shown to further involve the three mitogen-activator protein kinases (MAPK) subfamilies (Liu et al., 2002). In non-gonadotrope cells like insect or rat lactosomatotrope cells stably transfected with GnRHR, the signaling mechanisms may involve the PKA pathway *via* Gs or Gi (Stanislaus et al., 1996; Delahaye et al., 1997; see review in Kraus et al., 2001). GnRHR activation generates several intracellular processes in the gonadotropes leading to enhanced transcription of the common α and specific LH and FSHβ subunit genes and secretion of these gonadotropins. Among these processes have been described activation of the neuronal nitric oxide synthase, induction of *cfos* expression, increase in the early growth response protein 1, increase in mRNA for annexin 5 and activation of translation and phosphorylation of the pituitary adenylate cyclase activating polypeptide (PACAP) type 1 receptor (see review in Garrel et al., 1995, 1997, 1998; Lozach et al., 1998; Brown and McNeilly, 1999; Sosnowski et al., 2000; Bachir et al., 2001, 2003; Duan et al., 2002; Kawaminami et al., 2002; Liu et al., 2002; Larivière et al., 2008). A global profile of genes regulated by GnRH in the LβT2 gonadotrope cell line was established through microarray analysis showing that more than 200 genes are either up- or down-regulated after GnRH agonist treatment (Kakar et al., 2003). The amplitude of these events is strictly dependent on the number of GnRHR molecules at the surface of the pituitary gonadotropes that is itself dependent, at least in part, on the transcriptional level of GnRHR gene (*Gnrhr*).

GENE STRUCTURE AND PATHOLOGIES ASSOCIATED WITH MUTATIONS AFFECTING THE HUMAN GENE

The cloning of its encoding cDNA, firstly in the mouse and subsequently in other mammalian species, revealed that GnRHR is 325–328 amino acid long (327 in mouse and rat, 328 in human) and confirmed that this receptor belongs to the serpentine family of transmembrane G protein-coupled receptors (review in Norwitz et al., 1999a and references therein). The cDNA probes have subsequently been used to characterize the gene and its chromosomal localization in various mammalian species. *Gnrhr* is composed of three exons and two introns and is approximately 15–31 kb in size depending on the species (**Figure 1**). It is localized to chromosome 4q21.2 in human, chromosome 4, 5, 6, or 8 in bovine, murine, ovine, and porcine species, respectively (Fan et al., 1994; Kaiser et al., 1994; Morrison et al., 1994; Kakar and Neill, 1995; Kottler et al., 1995; Leung et al., 1995; Montgomery et al., 1995; Connor et al., 1999; Jiang et al., 2001). Cloning of the human *GNRHR* cDNA has led to the identification of mutations in the coding sequence that are associated with variable clinical features ranging from partial to complete hypogonadotropic hypogonadism (Achermann et al., 2001; de Roux and Milgrom, 2001). Two separate groups initially reported loss-of-function mutations in the *GNRHR* gene in patients with isolated hypogonadotropic hypogonadism (de Roux et al., 1997; Layman et al., 1998). A natural knockout of the human *GNRHR* resulting from aberrant splicing that eliminates exon 2 and creates a frame shift in the coding sequence was reported (Silveira et al., 2002). The woman affected by this homozygous mutation presented with primary amenorrhea, absence of gonadotropin pulsatility and did not respond to exogenous pulsatile or acute GnRH administration. To date, at least 20 additional mutations in *GNRHR* have been identified in patients with sporadic and familial isolated hypogonadotropic hypogonadism (Chevrier et al., 2011; Noel and Kaiser, 2011). These data again lay emphasis on the predominant role of *GNRHR* in the development of reproductive function in humans.

TISSUE- AND CELL-SPECIFIC EXPRESSION OF THE GnRHR

The isolation of the cDNA also provided the basic tools for initiating studies on the regulation of *Gnrhr* expression by *in situ* hybridization, northern blotting, and semi quantitative RT-PCR. The presence of transcripts for the GnRHRs have notably been observed in brain regions previously shown to bind radiolabeled GnRH, thus confirming that *Gnrhr* is expressed in non-pituitary tissues, notably in the hippocampus and hypothalamus (see review in Jennes et al., 1997). *Gnrhr* is also expressed in granulosa cells of atretic follicles in the ovary, in Leydig cells in the testis, in prostate, breast, and placenta (Stojilkovic et al., 1994). In the pituitary, the expression of *Gnrhr* is restricted to the gonadotrope cells despite the common origin of the six different secreting cell types that composed the anterior pituitary (Scully and Rosenfeld, 2002).

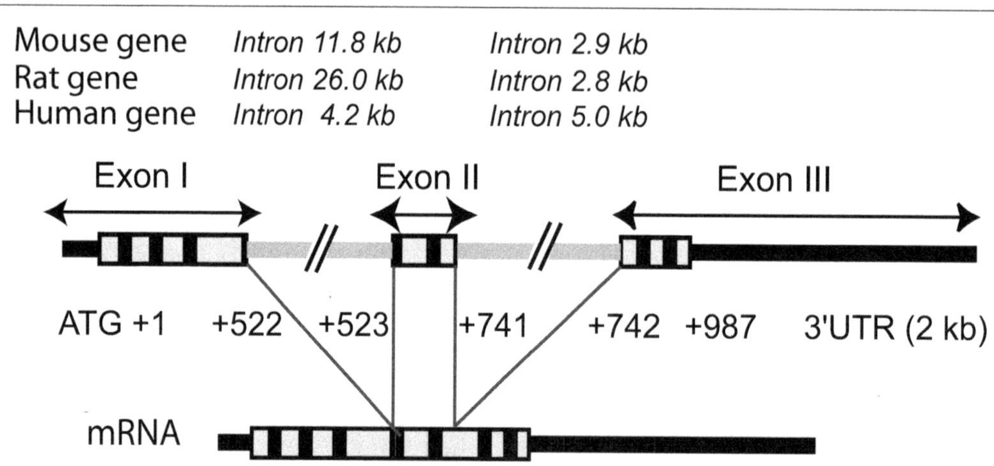

FIGURE 1 | Structure of the GnRH receptor gene. The GnRH receptor gene is 15–31 kb in size depending on the species. This is primarily due to differences in intron sizes which are indicated at the top of the figure for mouse, rat, and human species. The coding sequence is boxed with the trans-membrane domains specified in black. The 5′ and 3′ untranslated regions (UTR) are designated by thick black lines whereas the two introns are specified by thick gray lines. The mature mRNA resulting from usual intron splicing is illustrated below the gene. Sizes of translated sequences included in the human mature transcript are indicated (987 bp corresponding to 328 codons excluding the stop codon). Rat and mouse translated sequences are 327 amino acids long, the exon II being three bases shorter (+523/+738).

These diverse and discrete sites of expression raise the question of the mechanisms that determine the tissue-specific expression of *Gnrhr*. In addition, *Gnrhr* is regulated by extracellular signals, the first of them being GnRH itself. Endocrine factors such as estradiol (E_2), progesterone, or testosterone also regulate the levels of *Gnrhr* mRNA (Stojilkovic et al., 1994). Altogether, these data led several groups to investigate the mechanisms that underlie the tissue-specific expression and regulation of *Gnrhr* (see review in Hapgood et al., 2005).

To this aim, the 5′ regulatory sequences of the rat, mouse, and human receptor genes have been isolated and characterized essentially by transient transfection assays and gel-shift analyses. A limited number of studies have also been conducted *in vivo* through the elaboration of transgenic mouse lines harboring a reporter gene under the control of the mouse, rat, or ovine promoter. This review focuses on the present state of knowledge related to the cell-specific and regulated activity of the promoter of the *Gnrhr in vitro* and *in vivo*.

IN VITRO ANALYSIS OF THE MOUSE, RAT, AND HUMAN PROMOTERS

The tissue-specific and regulated activity of the rodent promoters have been evaluated using three main cellular models; the αT3-1 and LβT2 mouse gonadotrope-derived cell lines that are commonly used for studying the expression of marker genes of the gonadotrope lineage (Windle, et al., 1990; Alarid et al., 1996; Thomas et al., 1996; Turgeon et al., 1996) and a rat cell line of lactosomatotrope origin, the GGH(3) cells which were obtained by stable transfection with GnRHR of the tumor-derived GH3 cell line (Janovick et al., 1994; Kaiser et al., 1994; Stanislaus et al., 1994). αT3-1 cells express early marker genes of the developing gonadotrope in mouse, the gene encoding the common α-subunit of the three pituitary glycoprotein hormones (*Cga*) detected at embryonic day 11.5 (E11.5), *Gnrhr* detected at E13.5 and steroidogenic factor 1 (*Sf1*, formally nuclear receptor subfamily 5, member 1, NR5A1) detected at E14.5. The LβT2 cell line further expresses later marker genes, namely those encoding the β-subunits of LH (*Lhb*), from E16.5 onward, and FSH (*Fshb*), from E17.5. These data together with the way by which these cell lines were generated – by targeted oncogenesis using the promoter of *Cga* and *Lhb*, respectively – strongly suggest that the αT3-1 cell line may be representative of the gonadotrope lineage at early developmental stages, between E14 and E16.5. In contrast, the LβT2 cell line would be derived from cells at later stage, beyond E17.5 (Ingraham et al., 1994; Japón et al., 1994; Granger et al., 2004). It has to be emphasized that GGH3 cells express different tissue-specific transcription factors such as pituitary-specific transcription factor 1 (PIT1 formally POU domain class 1 transcription factor 1, POU1F1) that directs the expression of *Prl*, *Gh*, and *Tshb* (Bodner et al., 1988; Ingraham et al., 1988; Li et al., 1990; Ngô et al., 1995). Also, gonadotrope and lactosomatotrope cells likely express ubiquitous transcription factors at different levels. Moreover, as already mentioned above, the GnRHR seems to be coupled to slightly different signal transduction pathways in these cell lines. Consequently, the results obtained with these cellular models may reflect these major differences.

ELEMENTS INVOLVED IN THE GONADOTROPE-SPECIFIC ACTIVITY OF THE MOUSE AND RAT *Gnrhr*

The mouse promoter (Figure 2A)

SF1, AP1, and GRAS elements. The 1.2 kb promoter of the mouse *Gnrhr* was the first to be isolated and characterized in 1994 by Albarracin et al. (1994) Shortly after, a 1.9 kb mouse promoter was further isolated and functionally characterized (Clay et al., 1995). Both studies allowed identification of multiple transcription start sites within the first 100 bp immediately upstream from the ATG codon, the major one being located 62 nucleotides from the translation start codon. This transcription start site was referred to as position +1 in papers dealing with the mouse promoter. However, owing to the presence of multiple transcription start sites in GnRHR promoters and in order to facilitate the comparison between promoters of different species, we chose to use the translation start site as the position +1 in this review. Consequently, numbering in this review differs by +63 nucleotides from that currently used for the mouse promoter. This core promoter domain does not exhibit any typical CAAT or TATA boxes close to the transcription start sites. Both studies also demonstrated that the highest levels of promoter activity after transient transfection were obtained in mouse αT3-1 gonadotrope-derived cells. In rat lactosomatotrope cell line (GH3) or human JEG-3 placental cells, the activity of the mouse promoter was considerably weaker and represented only 17 and 5% of that observed in αT3-1 cells, respectively. Progressively, it appeared that all the positive regulatory elements involved in the tissue-specific activity of the mouse promoter in gonadotrope cells were confined into the 500 bp proximal region (Duval et al., 1997a,b). Three distinct motifs making up a tripartite basal enhancer are essentially required: a SF1 (NR5A1) response element (−243 5′-TGGCCTTCA-3′ −235), a canonical activating protein 1 (AP1) motif (−336 5′-TGACTCA-3′ −330), and a novel element termed GnRHR activating sequence (GRAS; −391 5′-CTAGTCACAACA-3′ −380; **Figure 2**). Mutation of all three elements fully abrogates promoter activity. The identity of SF1 was further corroborated by gel-shift and antibody super-shift assays. Using similar approaches, the AP1 complex has been found to involve factors likely belonging to the FOS and JUN families. The nature of the factors that bind the GRAS element were also deciphered. They consist of SMAD3 (mothers against decapentaplegic homolog 3) which interacts with SMAD4 and bind to the 5′ end of the GRAS motif, AP1 that binds within the middle of the motif, and FOXL2, a member of the forkhead family, that interacts with the 3′ end of the GRAS motif. GRAS is thus a composite regulatory element whose functional activity is dependent on a multi-protein complex (Ellsworth et al., 2003a).

Homeobox transcription factors. Several homeobox factors further participate in the combinatorial code that directs gonadotrope-specific expression of the mouse *Gnrhr* promoter. The paired-like homeodomain transcription factor 1 (PITX1) belongs to the expanding family of bicoid-related vertebrate homeobox genes. It appears very early, being involved in the specification of the adenohypophyseal placode and its expression in the anterior pituitary persists afterward until adulthood (Drouin et al., 1998; Schlosser, 2006). PITX1 regulates different marker genes in

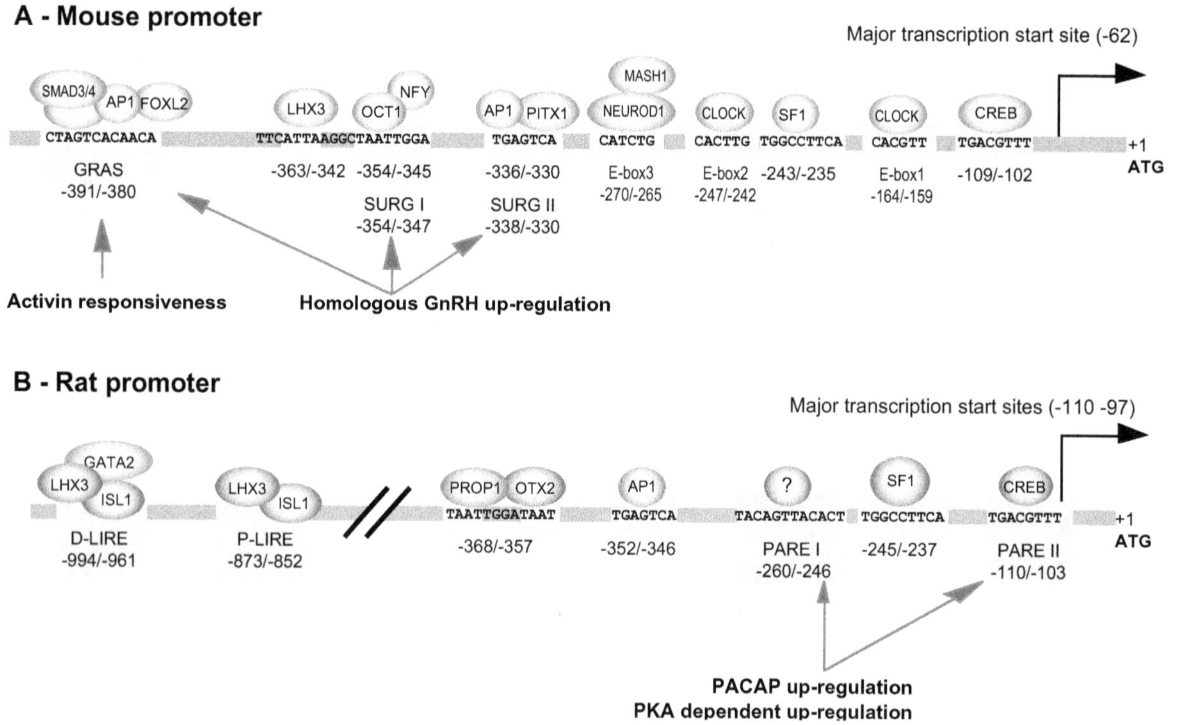

FIGURE 2 | Response elements identified within the mouse and rat promoters. The schema summarizes the functional elements characterized on mouse **(A)** and rat **(B)** promoters. These elements are involved in tissue-specific expression in gonadotrope cell lines, some of them being also involved in activin-, GnRH-, and PACAP-dependent regulation. Note that response elements directing gonadotrope-specific expression of the rat promoter are located within 1000 bp 5′ upstream of the ATG codon whereas those of the mouse promoter are confined within the most proximal 400 bp. The numbering is relative to the translation start codon, the adenine being considered at position +1. This numbering may therefore be different from that used in the original publications.

the adult pituitary notably *Cga*, *Lhb*, *Fshb*, *Tshb*, *Gh*, *Prl*, *Pomc*, and *Gnrhr* (Drouin et al., 1998). PITX1 activates the *Gnrhr* promoter by interacting with c-JUN in the AP1 complex and by binding to several low affinity response elements scattered within the −370/−326 region of the mouse promoter that includes the AP1 response element (Jeong et al., 2004). Octamer-binding transcription factor 1 (OCT1, formally POU2F1) belongs to the other members of homeodomain transcription factors that regulate the *Gnrhr* promoter activity. This was demonstrated by several convergent approaches including targeted mutagenesis coupled with gel-shift assays and transient transfection in gonadotrope cell lines, chromatin immunoprecipitation (ChIP) assay, and short interfering RNA strategy (Kam et al., 2005). Together with the discovery of the OCT1 response element that contains a core TAAT motif at position −352/−349, a functional binding site for nuclear factor Y (NFY) was identified in the course of this study. It partially overlaps the OCT1 response element. Both transcription factors contribute to the tissue-specific activity of the mouse *Gnrhr* promoter. Several other TAAT motifs are present in the sequence of the mouse promoter. One of them, located at position −164/−159, mediates OCT1 trans-acting stimulation of *Gnrhr* promoter in addition to the distal OCT1 interacting motif (Lents et al., 2009). Additional homeodomain factors are involved in promoter activity. LHX3 that belongs to the LIM homeodomain (LIM-HD) proteins is expressed in the early stages of pituitary ontogenesis at E9.5 and its expression persists in the adulthood (Ericson et al., 1998). Similarly to PITX1, LHX3 is involved in the expression of several pituitary marker genes. An ATTA motif located at −360/−357 was found to mediate the mouse *Gnrhr* promoter responsiveness to LHX3. Also, the presence of LHX3 on the mouse promoter was demonstrated *in vivo* by ChIP assay (McGillivray et al., 2005). A complementary study showed that responsiveness to LHX3 was further dependent on a second TAAT motif located only 4 bp downstream (Cherrington et al., 2006). The integrity as well as the specific helical orientation of the two motifs are required for full LHX3 activity.

E-box transcription factors. Seven non-canonical E-boxes have been identified along the *Gnrhr* promoter sequence suggesting that basic/helix-loop-helix (b/HLH) transcription factors might be involved in tissue-specific promoter activity. b/HLH transcription factors (124 in numbers in mouse) have been classified into six groups based on their evolutionary relationship, protein structure characteristics, and sequence binding affinities (Li et al., 2006). Four of them, belonging to class A, B, and C, are suspected to modulate the activity of the mouse *Gnrhr* promoter. Indeed, mutation of each E-box in the mouse promoter resulted in full or severe decrease in promoter activity as measured by transient transfection assays using the αT3-1 gonadotrope cell line (Resuehr et al., 2007). One at least out of the three most proximal E-boxes (E-box 1, 2, and 3), binds the CLOCK (circadian locomotor output cycles kaput) transcription factor as demonstrated by ChIP assay. This strongly suggested that the mouse promoter is under the control of CLOCK/BMAL1 (brain and muscle arnt-like protein 1) heterodimer. In addition, transcripts encoding *Drosophila* homolog of period 1 (PER1), PER2, cryptochrome 1 (CRY1), and CRY2 were detected, signifying that dynamic inhibition by CRY/PER of CLOCK/BMAL1-directed gene transcription may take place in this gonadotrope cell line. Although the actors of the molecular loop essential for rhythmic timekeeping are all present, circadian rhythms of *Gnrhr* expression were not observed in cultured gonadotrope αT3-1 cells. Subsequent study considering E-box transcription factors has demonstrated the involvement of two other b/HLH transcription factors, neurogenic differentiation 1 (NEUROD1) and mammalian achaete-scute homolog 1 (MASH1), that both interact with E-box 3, suggesting that the CLOCK/BMAL1 heterodimer bind to either E-box 1 or 2 but not to E-box 3 (Cherrington et al., 2008). Interestingly, the αT3-1 gonadotrope cell line preferentially expresses NEUROD1 whereas LβT2 cells preferentially express MASH1. Consequently, *Gnrhr* E-box 3 binds NEUROD1 from αT3-1 cells, but binds MASH1 from LβT2 cells. This difference may be related to the differentiation state of these cell lines as mentioned above.

The rat promoter (Figure 2B)

SF1, CRE, SAP, and AP1 elements in the proximal active domain. The 5′ flanking sequence of the rat promoter has been successively isolated by Reinhart et al. (1997) and by Pincas et al. (1998) in our laboratory. Comparative analyses reveal 82–84% sequence identity with the corresponding 1.9 and 1.2 kb mouse promoter region. Sequence homology is well illustrated by dot matrix pairwise alignment of rat versus mouse sequence (**Figure 3A**). The analysis further reveals full lack of homology beyond 2.1 kb, suggesting that master regulatory domains in rodents are constrained within 2 kb upstream of the ATG codon. Furthermore, the transcriptional start sites appear similarly clustered within the 110 bp proximal region. A first set of major sites is located between −110 and −103, depending on the authors and a second set of both major and minor sites is located around position −30. The rat promoter was proved to be strongly active in αT3-1 and LβT2 gonadotrope-derived cells as well as in GT1-7 hypothalamic-derived cell line. Within the proximal domain, two elements that are identical to the AP1 (−352/−346) and SF1 (−245/−237) response elements of the mouse promoter are required to mediate gonadotrope-specific activity (Pincas et al., 2001a). However, despite these remarkable similarities, the rat promoter displays functional characteristics that distinguish it from the mouse promoter. Two additional response elements are required in the proximal active domain for full cell-specific activity (Granger et al., 2006) a CRE (cAMP response element) element (−110 TGACGTTT −103) that binds CRE binding protein (CREB) with a lower affinity than the consensus TGACGTCA sequence (Pincas et al., 2001b) and an element located at −252/−245 that binds a yet unidentified factor referred to as SAP for SF1 adjacent protein. Despite its immediate proximity with the SF1 response element, the SAP element acts independently of SF1. Furthermore, a GRAS-like element is present in the rat promoter but was proved inactive despite the close sequence identity with its mouse counterpart (Pincas et al., 2001a; Cherrington et al., 2005).

Homeodomain factor response elements in the distal and proximal regulatory domains. The distribution of response elements along the promoter constitutes the most important difference between the rat and mouse species. In contrast with the mouse promoter where all known response elements are clustered within the 500 bp proximal region, an additional regulatory region containing a bipartite enhancer that we named *Gnrhr*-specific enhancer (GnSE) lies on a more distal part of the rat promoter (−1135/−753). Two major response elements located at positions −994/−960 and −871/−862 are responsible for GnSE action (Pincas et al., 2001a; Granger et al., 2006). Interestingly, GnSE activity is dependent on both cellular and promoter contexts. Maximal activity required the presence of the SF1 response element that lies on the proximal promoter domain, 600 bp downstream. Thus, the GnSE belongs to a class of promoter-specific enhancers, capable of acting at a distance as classical enhancers do, but requiring a specific context, in our case, a SF1 element containing promoter. Regarding the proximal GnSE element (−871/−862), it was found to bind the pair of LIM-HD proteins LHX3 and ISL1 (Granger et al., 2006). This was demonstrated by several convergent approaches, notably using overexpression of the LIM HD proteins and a LHX3 dominant negative in co-transfection assays, gel-shift and super-shift assays, and DNA affinity chromatography. This element displays high sequence identity in the antisense orientation with the −363/−342 region of the mouse promoter that was itself shown to interact with LHX3 (McGillivray et al., 2005; Cherrington et al., 2006). Using antibodies against LHX3 and ISL1 in ChIP assays, we were able to show that the mouse sequence did recruit ISL1 in addition to LHX3 (Schang et al., 2012b) as already demonstrated by McGillivray et al. (2005). Nevertheless, deletion of the LIM-HD response element in the rat promoter does not fully abolish the trans-acting effect of the ISL1/LHX3 pair. This led us to identify the upstream element of the GnSE as a second LIM-HD response element. It displays similar properties and specificity as the first characterized one (Schang et al., 2012b). These elements were then referred to as proximal and distal LIM-HD response elements, P-LIRE and D-LIRE, respectively. Finally, recent work from our laboratory has permitted to the identification of a prophet of PIT1 (PROP1)/orthodenticle drosophila homolog 2 (OTX2) response element in the proximal regulatory domain of the rat promoter, located at −368/−357. Interestingly, OTX2 (or OTX1) stimulates promoter activity in synergy with PROP1 by interacting with this element in gonadotrope-derived cell lines. In contrast, in non-gonadotrope cells, notably in the neutral Chinese hamster ovary (CHO) cell line, OTX2 acts synergistically with CREB through another OTX2 response element involving a ATTA core motif located at position −163/−160, close to the CRE element (Schang et al., 2012a).

Negative regulatory elements in the proximal part of the mouse promoter

As underlined above, the GH3 lactosomatotrope-derived cell line expresses the mouse promoter at a low but detectable level. The

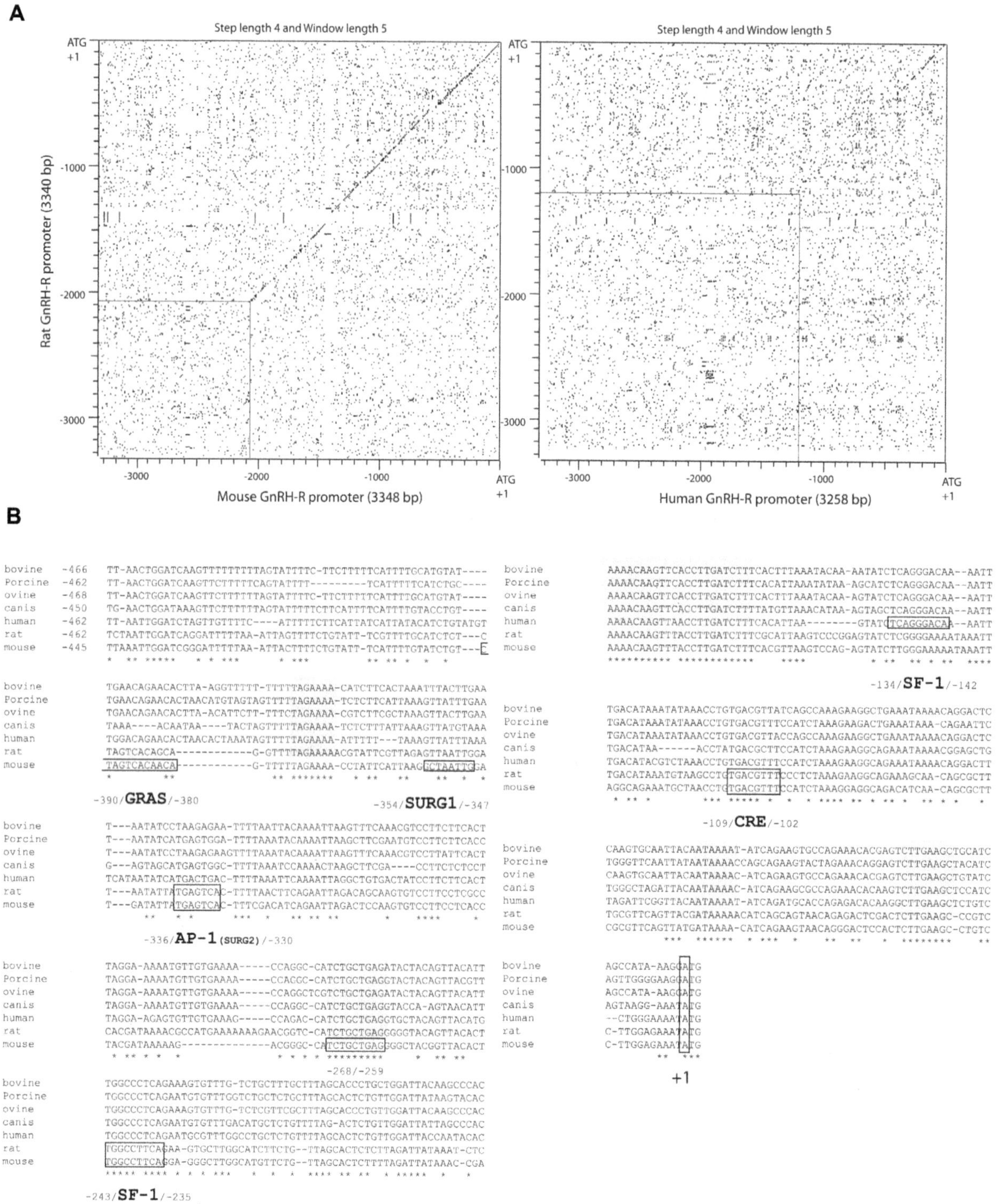

FIGURE 3 | Sequence comparison of *Gnrhr* promoters in different mammalian species. (A) Dot matrix representation of pairwise alignment of rat versus mouse (left panel) or human (right panel) sequences. A strong sequence conservation between mouse and rat 5′ upstream flanking regions extends over 2 kb whereas that between rat (or mouse) and human sequences is limited to a proximal 0.5 kb region upstream of the ATG codon. Relaxed sequence identity between rat and human sequences is further observed between 0.5 and 1.2 kb upstream of the ATG codon. **(B)** Multiple sequence alignment of mammalian *Gnrhr* proximal promoters. Blocks of full identity are highlighted in gray. Some motifs of interest are boxed in the sequences of the species where they have been characterized (e.g., SURG1 in the mouse, AP1 in rat and mouse). Note that the SF1 response element characterized in the rat and mouse promoter sequences (−243/−235) is particularly well conserved among species contrasting with the human SF1 response element (−134/−142). The latter appears to be shared by bovine, porcine, ovine and canis species but not by rat and mouse.

stably transfected GGH(3) cell, first designed in order to evaluate GnRH action, was thereafter used to identify the elements that allow constitutive expression in this non-gonadotrope, SF1-lacking cell line (Maya-Nunez and Conn, 1999). A CRE element (−109 5′-TGACGTTT-3′ −102) contributed to basal promoter activity, suggesting that constitutive activation of the PKA-dependent signaling pathway may also participate in cell-specific activity in pituitary gonadotropes as well as in other GnRHR expressing tissues. Importantly, several negative regulatory regions were identified (−213/−207; −268/−259; −354/−342) that may serve to repress the activity of the *Gnrhr* in non-gonadotrope pituitary cells. Among them the −268/−259 (5′-TCTGCTGA-3′) region is strictly conserved among bovine, porcine, ovine, canis, human, rat, and mouse sequences (**Figure 3B**). However, the inhibitory effects of these sequences are modest and cannot account for the whole lack of *Gnrhr* expression in non gonadotrope pituitary cells. Furthermore, they partially overlap regulatory regions characterized as positive in a gonadotrope cell context.

RESPONSE ELEMENTS INVOLVED IN TISSUE-SPECIFIC MOUSE AND RAT PROMOTER ACTIVITY ARE ALSO INVOLVED IN REGULATION BY EXTRA-CELLULAR SIGNALS

It is often noticed that tissue-specific transcription factors participate either directly or as co-regulators in the modulation of promoter activity by extra-cellular signals. This is also true for the rodent *Gnrhr* since, as we shall see in more detail below, SF1 is involved in PACAP- and PKA-regulated activity, AP1 in the homologous up-regulation by GnRH, and GRAS in the up-regulation by activin.

GnRH homologous up-regulation in gonadotrope-derived cells (Figure 4)

Two independent studies using transient transfection in αT3-1 cells demonstrated a time- and dose-dependent increase in the activity of the mouse *Gnrhr* promoter under GnRH treatment (Norwitz et al., 1999b; White et al., 1999). By using 3′ and 5′ deletion analyses combined with functional transfection studies, White et al. (1999) showed that a 54 bp fragment extending from −370 to −326 and thus including the AP1 element was sufficient to mediate GnRH response when placed upstream of a minimal heterologous promoter. Further analysis by Norwitz et al. (1999a) using linker scanning mutagenesis led to identifying two sequences of 8 bp, SURG-1 (sequence underlying responsiveness to GnRH-1; −354/−347) and SURG-2 (−338/−331) that are necessary for full GnRH responsiveness (**Figure 3B**). The SURG-2 element corresponds to the AP1 element and is absolutely required since mutations within this sequence totally abolished GnRH-induced stimulation of promoter activity whereas mutations within the SURG-1 element (5′-GCTAATTG-3′) only attenuated the response. Based on targeted mutagenesis of each of the GRAS, AP1, and SF1 elements that compose the tripartite basal enhancer, the study by White et al. (1999) has led to a rather similar conclusion regarding the AP1 element involvement. Both studies, using antibodies directed against conserved protein domains of either the JUN or FOS families in electrophoretic mobility shift assays strongly suggest that an AP1/DNA complex mediates GnRH homologous up-regulation. The MAPK kinase (MEK1/2) inhibitor PD98059 abrogates both GnRH-induced stimulation of promoter activity and GnRH-induced phosphorylation of extra-cellular signal-regulated kinases (ERK) 1 and 2 (White et al., 1999) and of c-Jun N-terminal kinase (JNK; Ellsworth et al., 2003b). GnRH induction of mouse *Gnrhr* promoter activity may thus require functional activation of a PKC-dependent pathway that involves the ERK- or JNK-signaling cascade or both and ultimately converges to AP1. However, accurate analysis of the intracellular events induced by GnRH treatment of αT3-1 cells strongly suggested that the JNK-signaling cascade is predominantly involved (Ellsworth et al., 2003b). Accordingly, in pituitary-targeted ERK1/2 double-knockout mice, *Gnrhr* expression was not altered as compared with wild-type animals (Bliss et al., 2009), suggesting that ERK signaling is not primarily involved in gonadotrope specific expression of the *Gnrhr*. Moreover, the activation of the JNK-signaling cascade induced post-translational modifications of FOSB and JUND that led to increased binding of both factors on the SURG-2, the AP1 response element of the *Gnrhr* promoter (Ellsworth et al., 2003b). More recently, the factors that interact with SURG-1 have been identified as OCT1 and NFY. They are not only involved in the tissue-specific expression as mentioned above but also in GnRH homologous up-regulation. ChIP assays demonstrated that both factors are recruited on the mouse promoter in a time-dependent manner after GnRH treatment (Kam et al., 2005). It is important to point out that, in the context of the 600 bp mouse promoter, the adenylate cyclase activator forskolin inhibits GnRH-induced stimulation, suggesting a cross-talk between these two pathways (White et al., 1999). However, in the context of the chimera promoter made up with the mouse −370/−326 bp promoter fragment linked to the minimal GH heterologous promoter, forskolin is inefficient even if the GnRH response is maintained. This may indicate that the cross-talk takes place at the promoter level and requires response element(s) that are present within the 600 bp mouse promoter fragment and absent from the −370/−326 bp promoter fragment, notably the CRE element located at −109/−102 bp.

GnRH homologous up-regulation in non-gonadotrope cells (Figure 4)

The GnRHR is known to be expressed in several extra-pituitary tissues, notably in some areas of the brain, as well as in gonads and placenta. In this regard, it is important to consider the modalities of expression and regulation of the *Gnrhr* in cells distinct from gonadotropes. The availability of the stably transfected GGH3 cell line has permitted evaluating GnRH action on the transfected mouse promoter in a non-gonadotrope context. Consistent with the data obtained with αT3-1 cells, the activity of the mouse promoter was significantly increased in GGH3 cells following GnRH treatment (Lin and Conn, 1998). Subsequent analysis suggested that GnRH action is likely mediated by both PKA- and PKC-dependent signaling pathways (Lin and Conn, 1998, 1999; Maya-Nunez and Conn, 1999, 2001). Accordingly, GnRH stimulation was partly prevented by the adenylate cyclase inhibitor SQ22536 while treatment with the PKC inhibitor GF109203X led to nearly complete blockade. These data are in accordance with other results obtained using cholera toxin or cAMP analogs as well as following treatment with phorbol ester (Lin and Conn,

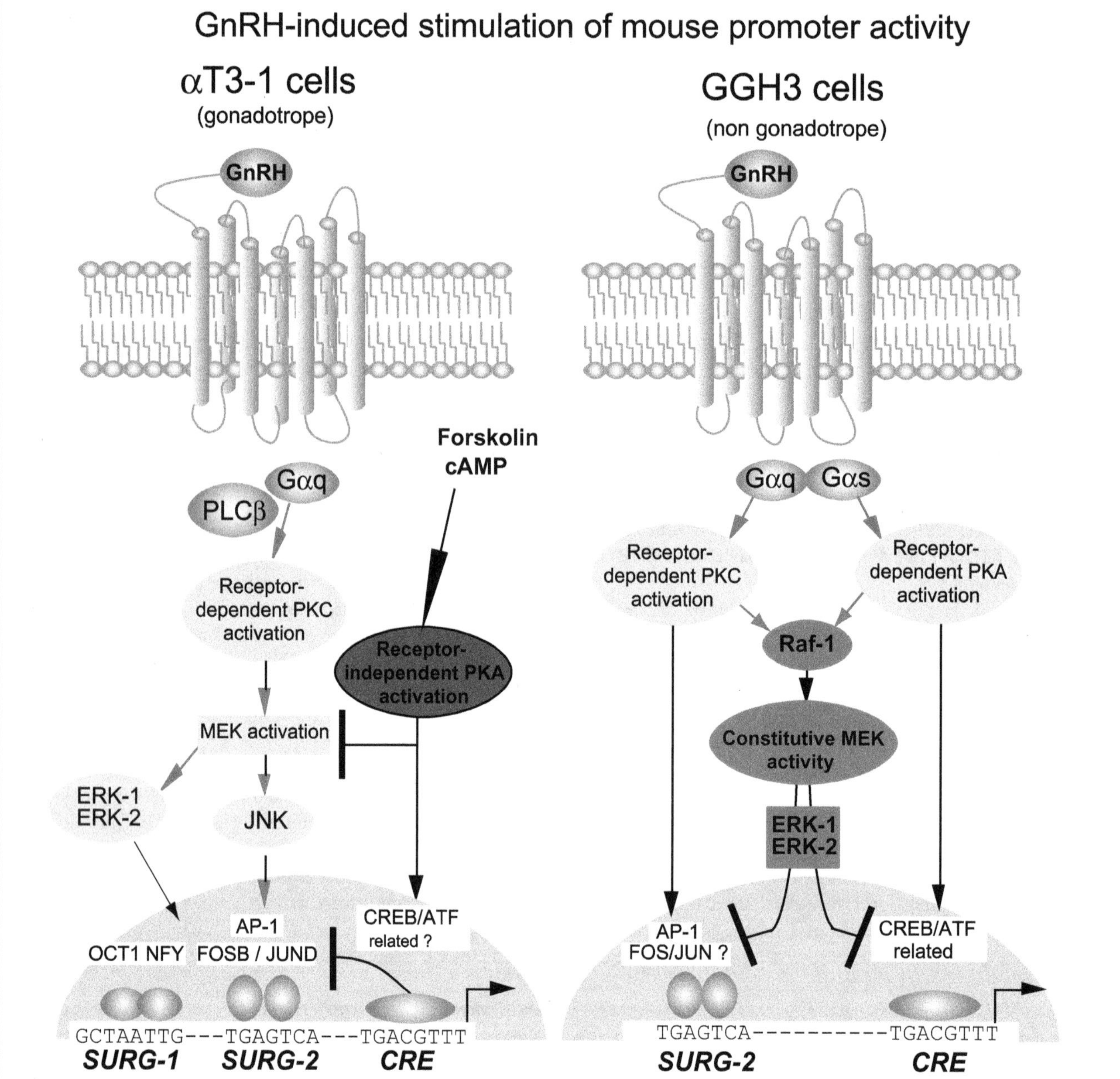

FIGURE 4 | Signaling pathways in the homologous up-regulation of the mouse GnRHR promoter by GnRH in gonadotrope and non-gonadotrope cells. In αT3-1 cells, GnRH-induced activation of the PKC-dependent pathway stimulates promoter activity through the MAP kinase signaling pathway, involving ERK1 and ERK2. Receptor-independent activation of the PKA-dependent pathway inhibits GnRH-stimulated promoter activity. In GGH3 cells, GnRH induces the simultaneous activation of the PKC and PKA-dependent pathways for stimulating promoter activity. Constitutive activation of the MAP kinase signaling pathway, involving ERK1 and ERK2, inhibits basal and GnRH-stimulated promoter activity. The three elements, SURG-1, SURG-2, and CRE therefore participate in GnRH up-regulation in both αT3-1 and GGH3 cells. In αT3-1 cells, the positive involvement of SURG-1 and SURG-2 have been demonstrated whereas that of the CRE element is only suspected to be inhibitory. In GGH3 cells, the CRE element is required for promoter stimulation and appears as the ultimate target of the PKA-dependent pathway. AP1, also referred to as SURG-2 is only potentially involved essentially because GnRH also activates the PKC-dependent signaling pathway in these cells.

1998, 1999). It is important to specify that all these treatments resulted in the stimulation of the MAPK pathway in GGH3 cells (Han and Conn, 1999). However, agents that inhibit the activation of the MAPK pathway such as the drug PD98059 or ERK1 and ERK2 mutants together increased both tissue-specific and GnRH-stimulated promoter activity. Conversely, transfection of vectors expressing agents that mimic the activation of the MAPK pathway such as Raf1 or wild-type ERK1 and ERK2 inhibited tissue-specific and GnRH-stimulated promoter activity. Altogether, these data indicate that activation of the MAPK pathway is inhibitory in the lactosomatotrope GGH3 cell line whereas it is stimulatory in gonadotropes. Furthermore, GnRH action in

GGH3 cells resulted in two opposite effects on the activity of the mouse *Gnrhr* promoter: a negative effect through the activation of the MAPK pathway and a positive one through the activation of PKA- and PKC-dependent pathways. The CRE element (−109/−102) that is involved in tissue-specific activity seems to be also involved in the GnRH and PKA-dependent regulation. The stimulatory effect of GnRH was indeed partially abolished and that of cAMP analog fully abrogated by targeted mutations of the CRE element. It is then rather probable that GnRH action also occurs through the SURG2 element in GGH3 cells.

Activin up-regulation

Activin, a member of the transforming growth factor-β superfamily, has first been shown to enhance the GnRH-induced FSH and LH release and to enhance the rate of GnRHR synthesis in rat pituitary cells (Braden and Conn, 1992; Weiss et al., 1993). This led to question its potential action at the transcriptional level. Exogenous activin B treatment of αT3-1 cells was shown to increase *Gnrhr* promoter activity as demonstrated by nuclear run-off assays or after transient transfection of the 1.2 kb mouse promoter linked to the luciferase reporter gene (Fernandez-Vazquez et al., 1996). However, since αT3-1 cells and pituitary gonadotropes both produce activin B, responsiveness to activin has then been mainly monitored by follistatin-induced inhibition of activin action in subsequent analyses (Duval et al., 1999). Using transient transfection in αT3-1 cells, follistatin inhibition of promoter activity was demonstrated to be mediated through the GRAS element. Indeed, mutation of this motif abrogated follistatin inhibition whereas alteration of the SF1 or AP1 elements was minimally efficient. Consistent with these results, three copies of the GRAS element were sufficient to confer activin responsiveness to a minimal heterologous promoter. The GRAS motif also exhibits sequence similarities with the element (GTCTAGAC) that binds the receptor-activated SMAD2/SMAD3 and the common SMAD4 (Stopa et al., 2000), involved in activin signaling (Walton et al., 2012). The autocrine/paracrine action of activin also explains why the GRAS motif has been classified as a paracrine/autocrine cell-specific response element. Comparison with the rat promoter sequence that does not exhibit activin responsiveness led to the characterization of a second region involved in activin-mediated up-regulation of the mouse promoter, a region referred to as "downstream activin regulatory element" or DARE (Cherrington et al., 2005). This 18 bp-long region lies between −366 and −349 and overlaps LHX3, OCT1, and NFY response elements. However, none of these factors seems to be involved in activin responsiveness. The integrity of the two TAAT motifs identified in this sequence was mandatory for functional DARE. Furthermore, appropriate helical orientation of this region relatively to the GRAS element located 20 bp downstream is required suggesting that factors that bind to DARE interact with GRAS binding factors (SMAD, AP1, FOXL2; Cherrington et al., 2006).

Norwitz et al. (2002a,b) have investigated the potential synergy between GnRH and activin treatment on the mouse promoter activity. They found that activin was able to increase the stimulatory effect of GnRH by approximately twofold. Interestingly, deletion of the promoter region that contains the GRAS element as well as mutation that alters the 5′ part of the GRAS element abrogated the effect of activin on GnRH stimulation. They also showed that overexpression of SMAD4 together with SMAD2 or SMAD3 increased both tissue-specific promoter activity and GnRH homologous up-regulation. However, it remains to be established if mutation of the presumed Smad binding element (SBE box −393/−386) in the GRAS element may prevent the stimulatory effect induced by SMAD overexpression. Competition and super-shift experiments further indicated that a second factor, belonging to the AP1 family, may bind the 3′ part of the GRAS element, suggesting that JUN/FOS related factors and SMAD protein functionally interact.

PACAP up-regulation

Specific type 1 receptors for PACAP are present in gonadotrope cells of the anterior pituitary gland as well as in mouse gonadotrope derived αT3-1 cells. By transient transfection in αT3-1 cells, Pincas et al. (2001b) provided evidence that PACAP stimulates rat *Gnrhr* promoter activity. The EC50 of this stimulation was compatible with PACAP activation of the cyclic AMP-dependent signaling pathway and, consistently, co-transfection of an expression vector expressing the PKA inhibitor caused reduction in PACAP – as well as cholera toxin –stimulated promoter activity. Deletion and mutational analyses indicated that PACAP activation necessitated a bipartite response element that consists of a first region (−272/−237) termed PACAP response element (PARE) I that includes the SF1-binding site and a second region (−136/−101) referred to as PARE II that contains the CRE (TGACGTTT). Gel-shift experiments revealed that SF1 and SAP together bind to PARE I while a protein immunologically related to the CREB interacted with PARE II. Altogether, these findings indicated that PACAP regulates the rat *Gnrhr* at the transcriptional level in αT3-1 cells. Interestingly, the mouse promoter was similarly proved to be regulated by PACAP (Sadie et al., 2003). However, the response elements were not identified, nor were those involved in the PKA-induced stimulation of the mouse promoter. Notably, the ability of the CRE located at −109/−102 (i.e., equivalent to the rat promoter one) to mediate the PKA-dependent stimulation of the mouse promoter was not assessed. Nevertheless, two other response elements were shown to modulate PKA responsiveness (Sadie et al., 2003), the SF1 response element and a newly identified response element located at −15/−7, close to the translation initiation site (ATG). Both elements were able to bind NUR77 (NR4A1) and SF1 and exerted opposite effects. Mutation of the element close to the ATG codon together with overexpression of SF1 dramatically amplified PKA-induced stimulation. In contrast, overexpression of NUR77 repressed PKA-dependent regulation, most probably through the −15/−7 element. PACAP has been shown to stimulate follistatin (*Fst*) gene expression which restrains activin signaling and thus represses *Fshb* and *Gnrhr* expression as well as other activin-responsive genes. Therefore, in mouse gonadotrope cells, the PACAP direct stimulatory effect on *Gnrhr* promoter may be weakened by the indirect inhibitory action of PACAP on activin-stimulated promoter activity. The rat promoter is not submitted to this down-regulation because both the GRAS element and the DARE region are inactive. Whether PACAP regulation also occurs *in vivo* and is a common trait in mammals remains to be elucidated however.

FUNCTIONAL CHARACTERISTICS OF THE HUMAN *Gnrhr* PROMOTER *IN VITRO*

The human *Gnrhr* promoter has been independently isolated by two groups (Fan et al., 1995; Kakar, 1997). It displays several features that distinguish it from rodent promoters (Cheng and Leung, 2005). Firstly, a significant sequence identity with the above-described promoters does not extend beyond approximately −1200 bp from the ATG codon (**Figure 3A**). Secondly, in contrast to the rodent promoters, the transcription start sites are located far upstream of the ATG codon and disperse within two domains localized between −578 and −826 and between −1347 and −1751, indicating the existence of two core promoter regions (Fan et al., 1995; Kakar, 1997). A further difference with mouse and rat promoters is the presence of several TATA boxes well scattered among the transcription start sites, suggesting that transcription initiation occurs through different mechanisms in rodent and human.

Given that GnRHR is expressed in several tissues in addition to the pituitary gland, functional studies with the human promoter have been performed in non-pituitary cell lines, notably cells derived from placenta, endometrium, trophoblast, and ovary. This strategy has also been motivated by the absence of pituitary cell line of human origin. These studies led to the discovery of several positive and negative regulatory regions, the efficacy of which being strongly dependent on the considered cell line. They essentially confirmed the existence of distinct promoters within the 2 kb human 5′ flanking sequence.

The proximal core promoter is predominantly active in gonadotrope-derived cells (Figure 5A)

Following transfection in αT3-1 cells, it appeared that crucial elements are located in the close vicinity of the translation start codon because the −173/+1 deletion abolished promoter activity (Ngan et al., 1999; Kang et al., 2000). Targeted mutagenesis of a SF1 response element located at −142/−134 (5′-CAGGGACAA-3′) altered overall promoter strength suggesting that it is likely contributing to the gonadotrope-specific activity. The involvement of SF1 has been further evidenced by electrophoretic mobility shift and super-shift assays as well as by overexpression of SF1 (Ngan et al., 1999). However, silencer elements present in the middle part of the human promoter (−1018/−707) weaken promoter strength. Indeed, 5′ deletion to −707 increased tissue-specific activity in αT3-1 cells, the deleted promoter (−707/+1) being approximately threefold more active than the entire promoter (−2200/+1; Cheng and Leung, 2001). These data are in agreement with the existence of a proximal core promoter region (−816/−577) previously documented (Fan et al., 1995) and with the presence of a positive regulatory region (−771/−557) identified by 3′ deletion analysis (Kang et al., 2000). This also suggests that positive regulatory regions either overlap the core promoter region or are situated downstream from the transcription start sites as is the SF1 element cited above. Subsequent analysis by scanning mutations in αT3-1 cells has allowed precise delimitation of this proximal promoter that extends from −607 to −568. It contains two pyrimidine-rich initiator elements (−602/−597 and −589/−584) that bind similar proteins notably TFIID (Hoo et al., 2003). The distal promoter of the human gene is constitutively active in both gonadotrope and non-pituitary cell lines (**Figure 5B**).

The existence of a distal promoter active in non-pituitary cell lines has been strongly suggested in the early study by Kakar (1997). In this work, it is indeed shown that the −2300/−1020 human flanking sequence is highly active in human endometrial (HEC-1A) and breast tumor cell (MCF-7) lines. This upstream promoter was further characterized in either gonadotrope or non-pituitary cells by Ngan et al. (2000) and Cheng et al. (2001a), respectively. It appears to be less active in αT3-1 pituitary than in JEG-3 placental cells (Cheng et al., 2001a) and thus contrasts with the core proximal promoter that displays opposite characteristics. Also, the distal promoter seems to be more ubiquitous than the proximal promoter since it was active in gonadotrope, ovarian, endometrial, mammary, placental, and kidney cells. The in-depth analysis of the distal promoter in gonadotrope-derived αT3-1 cells (Ngan et al., 2000) and placental JEG-3 cells (Cheng et al., 2001a) reveals cell-specific differences.

In gonadotrope-derived cells, the active elements of the upstream promoter are located within a −1705/−1674 region and are not functional in the reverse orientation. They consist of a pyrimidine-rich initiator (−1685/−1676) and additional upstream motifs (−1705/−1687) that include a CCAAT box. Multiple proteins ranging from 40 to 54 K are capable of binding this upstream promoter. Interestingly, a downstream silencer element (−1674/−1577) prevents upstream promoter activity, at least in gonadotrope cells. This silencer is efficient only when positioned downstream of the promoter in either reverse or forward orientation. Two sequence-specific repressor motifs of 28 and 8 bp (−1670/−1643 and −1630/−1623) are essential for silencer activity as evidenced by linker-scanning mutagenesis and gel mobility shift assays (Ngan et al., 2001).

In JEG-3 and IEVT placental cell lines, a similar organization seems to occur, combining positive regulatory sequence and downstream silencer, however with different localization and distinct response elements (Cheng et al., 2001a). The placental cell-specific upstream promoter is located within a −1737/−1346 region and thus overlaps the gonadotrope cell-specific promoter. In JEG-3 cells, four motifs related to OCT1 (−1718/−1710), CRE (−1649/−1641), GATA (−1602/−1597), and AP1 (−1518/−1511) response elements are contributing to promoter activity. The characterization of these motifs has been further assessed by gel mobility shift and antibody super-shift assays. The downstream silencer is located between −1017 and −771 and abrogates upstream promoter activity in a manner similar to what is observed with the gonadotrope promoter. The silencer was further characterized in the context of the −1300/−1018 promoter described below. Under these conditions, it appeared that most of the silencing activity of this negative regulatory element resides in an octamer responsive sequence activated by OCT1 (Cheng et al., 2002b).

Distal promoter usages in granulosa and neuronal cell lines

A third distal promoter was characterized in human ovarian granulosa-luteal cells. It extends from −1300 to −1018 and exhibited the highest promoter activity in SVOG-4o and SVOG-4m immortalized granulosa-luteal cells (Cheng et al., 2002a).

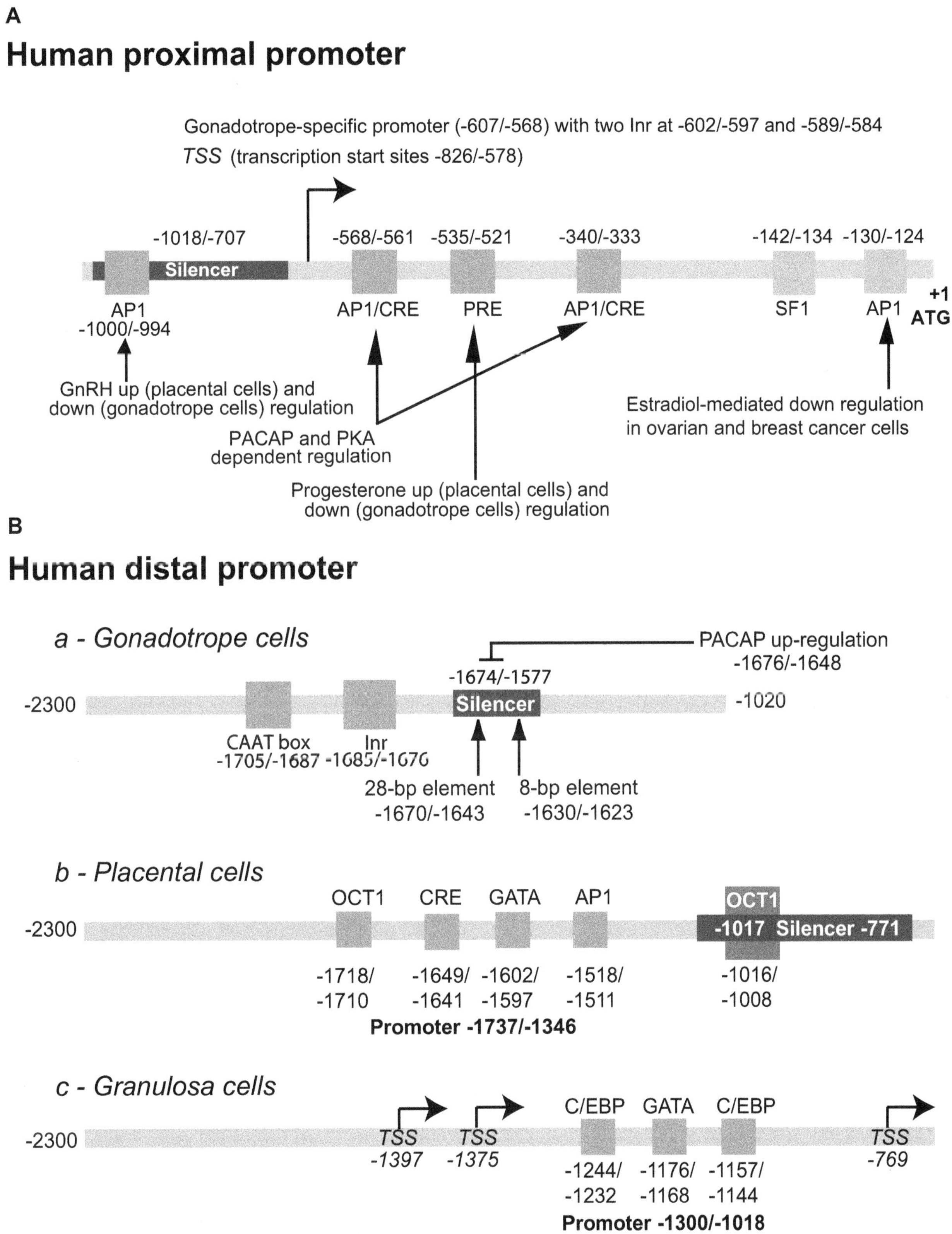

FIGURE 5 | Structure of the human GnRHR promoter. The elements identified in the proximal **(A)** and distal **(B)** promoter of the human gene and involved either in the tissue-specific or regulated activity are indicated. To facilitate comparison with the rodent promoters, the first nucleotide of the ATG codon was considered as position +1. The numbering may therefore be different from that used in the original publications.

However, it was also active in placental, ovarian, and gonadotrope cells. Two CCAAT enhancer binding protein (C/EBP) located at −1244/−1232 and −1157/−1144 and one GATA response element located at −1176/−1168 were required for full promoter activity because simultaneous mutations of these three elements led to more than 75% decrease in promoter activity in granulosa cells. Interestingly, the same mutations induced minimal or no significant decrease in promoter activity in ovarian, placental, and gonadotrope cells suggesting that different response elements and different transcription factors are involved in these cell contexts.

Human GnRHR was further expressed in the human cerebellar medulloblastoma cell line TE-671. In these neuronal cells, promoter activity was dependent on an upstream region located between −2197 and −1018. Important *cis*-acting regulatory elements were identified at −1300/−1018 and −2197/−1900, as deletion of either region induced a dramatic decrease in promoter activity (Yeung et al., 2005).

REGULATION OF HUMAN PROMOTER ACTIVITY BY EXTRACELLULAR SIGNALS (FIGURE 5)

Homologous up- and down-regulation by GnRH and the PKC-dependent pathway

Surprisingly, when compared to rodents, a 6–24 h-long treatment with 0.1 μM GnRH reduced activity of the 2.3 kb human *GnRHR* promoter by 31–71% in αT3-1 cells. This inhibitory effect was mimicked by phorbol ester and prevented by GnRH antagonists or specific PKC inhibitors (Cheng et al., 2000) strongly suggesting that GnRH action is mediated through receptor-dependent activation of the PKC pathway. Subsequent 5′ deletion analyses combined with site-directed mutagenesis revealed that an AP1 related element located at −1000/−994 (TTAGACA) is responsible for the homologous down-regulation of promoter activity by forming an AP1 complex involving the c-JUN and c-FOS protooncogenes. This AP1 element is unrelated to the AP1/CRE element involved in tissue-specific expression. It is worth stressing that similar GnRH treatment applied to placental JEG-3 or IEVT cell lines led to significant increases in promoter activity, contrasting again with data obtained in gonadotrope-derived cells (Cheng et al., 2000). The mechanisms underlying these positive and negative regulations remain to be elucidated, notably whether differential promoter usage (upstream versus proximal) may be related to such difference in GnRH regulation.

Up-regulation by PACAP and PKA-dependent pathway

The regulation of the human promoter by PACAP and the PKA-dependent activation pathway has been investigated in two different studies and led to the identification of distinct regulatory domains located within either the upstream or the proximal promoter, respectively (Cheng and Leung, 2001; Ngan et al., 2001). The former study (Ngan et al., 2001) indicated that both the gonadotrope cell-specific upstream promoter as well as the downstream silencer are involved in PACAP and PKA-dependent regulation. In support, PACAP treatment enhanced the formation of a complex with the 28 bp sequence-specific repressor motif (see above). Whether this may contribute to suppress silencer function and in turn to activate promoter remains to be demonstrated. The mechanisms underlying this positive regulation are not yet clearly identified. The latter study by Cheng and Leung (2001) led to the conclusion that PACAP and CREs reside within a 412 bp fragment (−577/−167) of the proximal promoter. Indeed, mutation of the (−568/−561 and −340/−333) AP1/CRE related motifs nearly abrogated the stimulation.

Up- and down-regulation by steroid hormones

Similarly to GnRH, progesterone treatment led to either inhibition or stimulation of promoter activity in gonadotrope versus placental cells, respectively (Cheng et al., 2001b). A progesterone binding site located at −535 to −521 has been shown to mediate, at least partially, both the inhibitory and stimulatory action of progesterone. Overexpression of the human progesterone receptor A and B isoforms increased the negative effect of progesterone in αT3-1 cells, whereas only B isoform mediated its positive action in JEG-3 placental cells. It is important to point out that the A isoform mediated inhibitory action in both cell lines, suggesting that the balance in the expression of A and B isoforms may be critical for GnRHR expression in the pituitary. The involvement of the progesterone receptor in binding the −535/−521 motif has been further substantiated by gel-shift and antibody super-shift assay.

In OVCAR3 ovarian carcinoma and MCF7 breast carcinoma cell lines, E_2-induced repression of *Gnrhr* promoter activity through an E_2 receptor α (ERα)-mediated mechanism (Cheng et al., 2003). This occurred in a dose- and time-dependent manner, the maximal effect being obtained at 10^{-8} M E_2 after a 48 h-long treatment (80% reduction of promoter activity). Repression occurred *via* an AP1-like element located at position −130/−124. This element was able to bind c-FOS and c-JUN but not ERα as demonstrated by EMSA. DNA binding by ERα was not needed for the E_2 repression of *Gnrhr* promoter activity. Further experiments strongly suggested that recruitment of AP1 and ERα to CREB binding protein (CBP) was mutually exclusive leading to inhibition of AP1-stimulated promoter activity by E_2.

IN VIVO ANALYSIS OF THE MOUSE, OVINE, AND RAT PROMOTERS IN TRANSGENIC MICE

Since *in vitro* studies of promoter functions often suffer from limitation of the cellular models used in transient transfection analyses, the next and complementary approach consists in analyzing promoter activity in an *in vivo* context through the generation of transgenic mice.

Several studies have been published that use this procedure. The initial study by McCue et al. (1997) demonstrated the homologous up-regulation of *Gnrhr* promoter activity by GnRH. A 1900-bp fragment corresponding the mouse *Gnrhr* promoter fused to the luciferase reporter gene has been microinjected in mouse embryos and mice harboring the transgene were selected. Analysis of luciferase activity in various tissues showed that the fusion gene was expressed essentially in the pituitary gland, to a 10-fold lower level in the brain and to a limited extend in the testis. These data are in agreement with those deduced from autoradiographic studies using ^{125}I-labeled GnRH or *in situ* hybridization (Jennes et al., 1988, 1995; Leblanc et al., 1988; Ban et al., 1990; see review in Jennes et al., 1997). Surprisingly, the expression of the transgene was not detected in the ovary contrasting with a number of studies reporting the presence of GnRHR in this tissue, specifically in granulosa cells of atretic follicles. Using an antibody directed against GnRH, the authors further showed a decrease in transgene expression in the pituitary gland but not in the brain or testis. The GnRH antibody inhibitory action could be reversed by a GnRH agonist treatment. As expected from *in vitro* studies, the 1900-bp promoter contains essential GnRH response elements. However, E_2 treatment of these transgenic mice did not alter the activity of the transgene. This diverges with a number of reports demonstrating that, *in vivo*, E_2 increases GnRHR number and steady-state level of *Gnrhr* mRNA in the pituitary (Hamernik et al., 1995; Turzillo et al., 1995; Kirkpatrick et al., 1998).

The same group has thus reinvestigated this regulation with novel lines of transgenic mice harboring a fusion construct containing the ovine receptor gene promoter linked to the luciferase reporter gene (Duval et al., 2000). Using either a 9.1 or a 2.7 kb promoter, they first showed that the ovine transgene displayed the same tissue-specific expression as the mouse promoter. The ovine transgene was indeed consistently expressed in the pituitary, brain, and gonads across the three analyzed transgenic lines. Pituitary expression was higher in females than in males whereas ovarian expression was significantly lower than the testicular one. In agreement with results obtained with the mouse promoter, immunoneutralization of GnRH reduced pituitary-specific expression of the luciferase reporter gene in ovariectomized mice, expression that could be restored by E_2 treatment. Similar results were observed in castrated, male transgenic mice. Finally, combined treatments with GnRH agonist and E_2 increased pituitary expression of the luciferase fusion gene to an extent greater than the sum of each individual treatment, suggesting synergistic activation of the ovine promoter.

The third study involving transgenic mice was different in at least two facets. Firstly, in this case, the reporter gene was the simian virus 40 (SV40) large T antigen and, secondly, the mouse promoter was the shortest used since it was 1.2-kb long only (Albarracin et al., 1999). With this fusion construct, the resulting heterozygote transgenic female mice were infertile preventing the generation of homozygote animals. Interestingly, all transgenic animals developed large intracranial tumors by 4–5 months of age that were of pituitary origin. As evidenced by *in situ* hybridization, these tumors expressed the marker genes of the gonadotrope phenotype, i.e., GnRHR, glycoprotein hormone α-subunit as well as FSHβ and LHβ subunits. The large T antigen was also expressed in the pituitary tumors but neither in the gonads or in the brain. This may indicate that the 1.2-kb, as compared with the 1.9-kb promoter fragment, is not able to direct transgene expression to sites other than the pituitary, notably brain and gonads. Surprisingly, the expression of the SV40 large T antigen transgene driven by the GnRHR gene promoter results in female-specific infertility due to disruption of gonadotropin production and secretion even before tumor development (Jeong et al., 2009).

In our laboratory, the 3.2 kb rat promoter was placed upstream of the human placental alkaline phosphatase reporter gene (*ALPP*) and inserted into the mouse genome. The resulting transgenic mice expressed the ALPP exclusively in gonadotropes within the pituitary gland (Granger et al., 2004). Transgene expression was detected within the developing pituitary at E13.5 in some of the cells that also expressed the *Cga*. It showed that *Gnrhr* is the earliest marker of gonadotrope cell differentiation, before SF1 that is detected at E14.5. At E15.5, ALPP expression was localized in LHX3- and ISL1-immunoreactive positive cells in agreement with *in vitro* data showing that these LIM-HD proteins are involved in rat and mouse promoter activity. Importantly, the 3.2 kb promoter was also able to direct *ALPP* expression to several brain areas, in particular the hippocampus and the lateral septum, in agreement with previous data (Jennes et al., 1988, 1995; Leblanc et al., 1988; Ban et al., 1990; see review in Jennes et al., 1997). In contrast with the pituitary gland, transgene activity in the hippocampus was detected only after birth, increasing gradually until 14–20 days after birth and then remaining at constant level until 60 days after birth (Schang et al., 2011b). This occurred simultaneously in fibers extending from the hippocampus to the lateral septum, suggesting that GnRHR may be involved in post-natal maturation of the septo-hippocampal system. The same time course was observed by measuring *Gnrhr* mRNA in rat hippocampus by quantitative RT-PCR, indicating that transgene expression directed by the rat promoter recapitulates rat endogenous *Gnrhr* expression in a mouse context. Further experiments using transient transfection of *Gnrhr* promoter luciferase fusion constructs in primary culture of rat hippocampus cell revealed that a RE1-silencing transcription factor (REST also known as NRSF)-like element located at −2.5 kb may be involved in the inhibition of *Gnrhr* gene expression before birth. Finally, GnRH treatment of rat hippocampus primary cell culture led to stimulation of several markers of neurogenesis such as EGR1, synaptophysin, and spinophilin. Using this transgenic mouse model, several additional sites of transgene expression were detected, notably in the oculomotor pathway (Schang et al., 2011a). Interestingly, transgene expression was also detected in two functionally and evolutionary related organs, the pineal gland and the retina. Again, the onset of transgene expression was specific to these tissues, being detected at E13.5 and E17.5 in the pineal gland and retina, respectively (Schang et al., 2012a). In the pineal gland, transgene expression persisted until adulthood whereas it strongly decreased in the retina. During development, transgene expression was the strongest in the neuroblast cell layer of the retina and less marked in the ganglion cell layer. In the pineal gland, transgene expression was constantly observed in approximately 50% of the cells whatever the developmental stage. Finally, transgene expression was strongly detected in the testes of transgenic mice in some Leydig cells (Schang et al., 2011a).

Recent studies involving functional genomic approaches have shown that regulatory domains may be located within the gene locus at several kilobases, either 5′ upstream or 3′ downstream as well as within intronic regions. This is well demonstrated particularly for genes coding for transcription factors, notably SF1 (Shima et al., 2012 and references therein), or genes encoding for factors involved in early developmental processes such as the LIM-HD proteins LHX3 and ISL1 (Kappen and Salbaum, 2009; Mullen et al., 2012). Conversely, other studies have shown that the most important genetic regulation may be contained within only 1 kb 5′ upstream of the transcription start site, including informations regarding epigenetic modifications such as pattern of DNA methylation (Lienert et al., 2011). Furthermore, species-specific informations would be encoded into DNA sequence and appears to prevail over species-specific cellular environment. A human chromosome introduced into a mouse cell line directs genetic and epigenetic modifications as it does in a human cell context and thus differently from its mouse counterpart (Wilson et al., 2008). Therefore, data obtained using transgenic mice as well as those described above must be considered bearing in mind the fact that all regulatory sequences are not necessarily contained within the 5′ upstream region of the gene only, even if relatively short 5′ upstream sequences may contain master regulatory informations. This could explain why the human *GNRHR* promoter responded negatively while mouse or rat promoters are stimulated by GnRH.

To overcome these limitations, a double knock-in mice model was recently developed. In this binary genetic approach, the Cre-recombinase was inserted into the *Gnrhr* locus whereas the YFP reporter gene, preceded by a floxed stop signal, was inserted into the ubiquitously expressed ROSA26 locus. The Cre-mediated excision of the stop signal led to a constitutive YFP expression in about 15% of the cells in the male anterior pituitary. Furthermore, the fluorescent signal was only colocalized with LHβ and/or FSHβ subunits as demonstrated by immunohistochemistry. These YFP mice have allowed single-cell analysis on living cells which have revealed unexpected heterogeneity in the resting properties of gonadotrope cells as well as in their secretory, electrophysiological, and calcium responses to GnRH (Wen et al., 2008).

SF1, A PAN-SPECIES TRANSCRIPTION FACTOR CRITICAL FOR GONADOTROPE-SPECIFIC EXPRESSION

An obvious conclusion that emerges from this overview of the mechanisms involved in *Gnrhr* expression is the important role of the orphan nuclear receptor SF1. It is undoubtedly involved in the tissue-specific expression of the human, mouse, and rat *GnRHR*. It is also likely involved in the tissue-specific expression of the ovine gene since the promoter is strongly homologous to its human counterpart. SF1 is crucial not only for tissue-specific expression but also for the regulation by extracellular signals as evidenced by PACAP and PKA-dependent regulations of the rat promoter. This may be related to the other important functions of SF1 in the tissue-specific and regulated expression of *Cga* and *Lhb* genes, two other markers of the gonadotrope lineage. Consistent with these data, the SF1 knockout mice exhibit impaired expression of LHβ, FSHβ, and GnRHR in pituitary gonadotropes in addition to other major defects such as agenesis of the ventro-medial hypothalamus, complete adrenal and gonadal agenesis and male-to-female sex reversal with persistence of Müllerian structures in male (Ingraham et al., 1994; Ikeda et al., 1995; Luo et al., 1995). To bypass the influence of hypothalamic deficiencies inherent to this transgenic model, SF1 has been inactivated specifically in the anterior pituitary using the Cre-loxP system (Zhao et al., 2001). These pituitary-specific SF1 knockout mice are sterile and never mature sexually. Consistent with a direct role of SF1 at the pituitary level, FSH and LH are markedly decreased in the pituitary-specific SF1 knockout mice as well as are gonadotropin β-subunit and *Gnrhr* mRNAs as assessed by semi-quantitative RT-PCR.

The important role of SF1 has been further confirmed in humans by the discovery of a heterozygous missense mutation in the DNA binding domain of SF1 in a patient with complete sex reversal, testicular dysgenesis, and adrenal failure (Achermann et al., 1999). However, this patient displayed a relative preservation of gonadotrope function. This may be due either to its heterozygous genotype or to a relative autonomy of the gonadotrope function with respect to SF1. In agreement with the latest hypothesis, GnRH treatment can restore LH and FSH secretion in SF1 knockout mice (Ikeda et al., 1995), suggesting that SF1 is not required for the emergence and maintenance of gonadotrope function. Furthermore, some tissues known to express GnRHR such as amygdala and hippocampus are deprived of SF1 (Schang et al., 2011b). This suggests that other factor(s) than SF1 are needed for the tissue-specific transcriptional onset of the *Gnrhr*. To identify this (or these) factor(s), several parameters must be considered. From an ontogenetic point of view, the date of appearance of the *Gnrhr* transcripts must be correlated with the presence of the factor in the fetal pituitary or in fetal tissues that will express the GnRHR in the adult. For instance, binding sites for GnRH have been detected as early as 12–13 days of gestation in the rat developing pituitary and GnRHR mRNA at 14.5 and 15.5 days post-conception in testis and ovary from rat fetuses (Aubert et al., 1985; Jennes, 1990; Botté et al., 1998). This factor should also be able to activate the promoter of the *Gnrhr* in an SF1-independent manner in transient transfection assays.

CONCLUSIONS AND PERSPECTIVES

An increasing number of studies on gene regulations and promoter activities aim to demonstrate the existence of specific regulatory units that bring together several response elements. From one tissue to another, the same elements may bind different factors resulting in tissue- or cell-specific modulations of gene expression. This ability to bind different factors is likely facilitated by sequence degeneracy of the response elements that lie within these regulatory units. Consequently, the degenerated response elements may be less efficient than their canonical counterparts when they are isolated from their promoter context. Efficiency is recovered in the original promoter context through synergistic interactions with other transcription factors belonging to the regulatory unit. Interestingly, this synergy may be attenuated if the wild-type degenerated element is artificially replaced by its canonical counterpart (Ito et al., 2000). In the *Gnrhr* promoters, several elements display such characteristics. In particular, the SF1 binding site and the proximal CRE in the rat and mouse promoter differ from the consensus sequence (TGACGTTT instead of TGACGTCA for the later). In gel-shift experiment, both the SF1 element and the CRE display an apparent weaker affinity for their cognate transcription factors than the SF1 binding site from the rat aromatase gene or the canonical CRE sequence (Pincas et al., 2001a,b). PACAP- and PKA-dependent regulations of the rat promoter are mediated by these two elements that may thus be considered as a cAMP regulatory unit (Roesler, 2000). The SURG-1 and SURG-2 elements establish another functional regulatory unit since they are both required for the GnRH up-regulation of the mouse promoter. The distal GnSE together with the proximal domain containing the SF1 binding site also form a regulatory unit for the tissue-specific activity of the rat promoter. Different regulatory units may also bind different combinations of factors depending on the tissue or the cell type that expresses the *Gnrhr*. We have recently demonstrated that OTX2 interacted with two distinct partners depending on the cell context (Schang et al., 2012a).

In a gonadotrope cell context, OTX2 interacted with PROP1 on two adjacent response elements located between −388 and −357, each of them encompassing a core TAAT motif. In a neutral cell context, OTX2 acted in synergy with CREB and formed a regulatory unit that involved CRE, an AP1 response element together with a new OTX2 binding site containing a TAAT core motif located at −163/−160. This motif is thus located 50 bp upstream of the CRE and 180 bp downstream of the AP1 element establishing a regulatory unit extending over 200 bp within the proximal promoter, markedly larger than the PROP1/OTX2 regulatory unit (Schang et al., 2012a). Whether such difference in size of these regulatory units as well as the other cited above is functionally relevant remains to be determined. In this respect, an important point that must be considered is the chromatin structure that depends on epigenetic modifications. At least, two histone H3 modifications are predominantly involved in transcriptional regulation: tri-methylation of Lys 4 of histone H3 (H3K4me3) and tri-methylation of Lys 27 of histone H3 (H3K27me3; see review in Greer and Shi, 2012). They are linked to gene activity and gene silencing, respectively. H3K4me3 is catalyzed by trithorax group (trxG) proteins, whereas H3K27me3 is catalyzed by polycomb-group (PcG) proteins (Schuettengruber et al., 2007; Ku et al., 2008). PcG proteins reside in two main complexes, termed Polycomb repressive complexes 1 and 2 (PRC1 and PRC2). PRC2 catalyzes H3K27me3 and components of PRC1 are recruited to the modified histone leading to ubiquitinylation of histone H2A at lysine 119 which in turn prohibits RNA polymerase II elongation (Simon and Kingston, 2009). This results in stable transcriptional repression. Analysis of H3K4me3 and H3K27me3 modifications by ChIP assay showed that in gonadotrope cell lines, the *Gnrhr* promoter preferentially displayed the active mark whereas in lactosomatotrope or corticotrope cell lines, it displayed preferentially the repressive mark (unpublished data). This is well correlated with *Gnrhr* mRNA levels that are not detected in lactosomatotrope and corticotrope cell lines. Constitutive *Gnrhr* transcription is thus likely controlled by mechanisms involving trxG proteins in gonadotrope cells whereas in other pituitary cells, PcG proteins stably repress *Gnrhr* expression. In mammals, composition of trxG and PcG protein complexes displays broad diversity depending on the considered family of genes. A critical point would be to determine what are the main actors involved in histone methyltransferase and demethylase activity regarding the *Gnrhr*. Furthermore, PcG complexes are known to be clustered into subnuclear structures that look like nuclear foci termed polycomb bodies (Pirrotta and Li, 2012). Conversely, active genes are preferentially located in different subnuclear structures referred to as transcription factories that contain active RNA polymerase II or interchromatin granule clusters (also termed nuclear speckles) that contain histone-modifying enzymes, transcription elongation factors, and splicing machinery (Meldi and Brickner, 2011; Spector and Lamond, 2011). In the developing pituitary gland, lineage specification likely requires relocation of marker genes like the *Gnrhr* into these subnuclear structures (Yang et al., 2011). The elucidation of the mechanisms underlying this reorganization would permit to shed new light on *Gnrhr* expression, on gonadotrope cell lineage specification and differentiation, and more generally on organ development.

ACKNOWLEDGMENTS

This study was supported by grants from the Centre National de la Recherche Scientifique, the Paris 7 University, and the Agence Nationale pour la Recherche (ANR-08-CES-011-03). Anne-Laure Schang is supported by a fellowship from the Ministère de l'Education Nationale, de la Recherche et de la Technologie (MENRT).

REFERENCES

Achermann, J. C., Ito, M., Ito, M., Hindmarsh, P. C., and Jameson, J. L. (1999). A mutation in the gene encoding steroidogenic factor-1 causes XY sex reversal and adrenal failure in humans. *Nat. Genet.* 22, 125–126.

Achermann, J. C., Weiss, J., Lee, E. J., and Jameson, J. L. (2001). Inherited disorders of the gonadotropin hormones. *Mol. Cell. Endocrinol.* 179, 89–96.

Alarid, E. T., Windle, J. J., Whyte, D. B., and Mellon, P. L. (1996). Immortalization of pituitary cells at discrete stages of development by directed oncogenesis in transgenic mice. *Development* 122, 3319–3329.

Albarracin, C. T., Frosch, M. P., and Chin, W. W. (1999). The gonadotropin-releasing hormone receptor gene promoter directs pituitary-specific oncogene expression in transgenic mice. *Endocrinology* 140, 2415–2421.

Albarracin, C. T., Kaiser, U. B., and Chin, W. W. (1994). Isolation and characterization of the 5′-flanking region of the mouse gonadotropin-releasing hormone receptor gene. *Endocrinology* 135, 2300–2306.

Anderson, L. (1996). Intracellular mechanisms triggering gonadotrophin secretion. *Rev. Reprod.* 1, 193–202.

Aubert, M. L., Begeot, M., Winiger, B. P., Morel, G., Sizonenko, P. C., and Dubois, P. M. (1985). Ontogeny of hypothalamic luteinizing hormone-releasing hormone (GnRH) and pituitary GnRHRs in fetal and neonatal rats. *Endocrinology* 116, 1565–1576.

Bachir, L. K., Garrel, G., Lozach, A., Laverrière, J. N., and Counis, R. (2003). The rat pituitary promoter of the neuronal nitric oxide synthase gene contains an Sp1-, LIM homeodomain-dependent enhancer and a distinct bipartite gonadotropin-releasing hormone-responsive region. *Endocrinology* 144, 3995–4007.

Bachir, L. K., Laverrière, J. N., and Counis, R. (2001). Isolation and characterization of a rat nitric oxide synthase type I gene promoter that confers expression and regulation in pituitary gonadotrope cells. *Endocrinology* 142, 4631–4642.

Ban, E., Crumeyrolle-Arias, M., Latouche, J., Leblanc, P., Heurtier, J. F., Drieu, K., et al. (1990). GnRHRs in rat brain, pituitary and testis; modulation following surgical and gonadotropin-releasing hormone agonist-induced castration. *Mol. Cell. Endocrinol.* 70, 99–107.

Bliss, S. P., Miller, A., Navratil, A. M., Xie, J., McDonough, S. P., Fisher, P. J., et al. (2009). ERK signaling in the pituitary is required for female but not male fertility. *Mol. Endocrinol.* 23, 1092–1101.

Bodner, M., Castrillo, J. L, Theill, L. E., Deerinck, T., Ellisman, M., and Karin, M. (1988). The pituitary-specific transcription factor GHF-1 is a homeobox-containing protein. *Cell* 55, 505–518.

Botté, M. C., Chamagne, A. M., Carre, M. C., Counis, R., and Kottler, M. L. (1998). Fetal expression of GnRH and Gnrhrs in rat testis and ovary. *J. Endocrinol.* 159, 179–189.

Braden, T. D., and Conn, P. M. (1992). Activin-A stimulates the synthesis of gonadotropin-releasing hormone receptors. *Endocrinology* 130, 2101–2105.

Brown, P., and McNeilly, A. S. (1999). Transcriptional regulation of pituitary gonadotrophin subunit genes. *Rev. Reprod.* 4, 117–124.

Cheng, C. K., and Leung, P. C. (2005). Molecular biology of gonadotropin-releasing hormone (GnRH)-I, GnRH-II, and their receptors in humans. *Endocr. Rev.* 26, 283–306.

Cheng, C. K., Chow, B. K., and Leung, P. C. (2003). An activator protein 1-like motif mediates 17β-estradiol repression of gonadotropin-releasing hormone receptor promoter via an estrogen receptor alpha-dependent mechanism in ovarian and breast cancer cells. *Mol. Endocrinol.* 17, 2613–2629.

Cheng, C. K., Yeung, C. M., Chow, B. K., and Leung, P. C. (2002a).

Characterization of a new upstream GnRH receptor promoter in human ovarian granulosa-luteal cells. *Mol. Endocrinol.* 16, 1552–1564.

Cheng, C. K., Yeung, C. M., Hoo, R. L., Chow, B. K., and Leung, P. C. (2002b). Oct-1 is involved in the transcriptional repression of the gonadotropin-releasing hormone receptor gene. *Endocrinology* 143, 4693–4701.

Cheng, K. W., and Leung, P. C. (2001). Human gonadotropin-releasing hormone receptor gene transcription: up-regulation by 3′,5′-cyclic adenosine monophosphate/protein kinase A pathway. *Mol. Cell. Endocrinol.* 181, 15–26.

Cheng, K. W., Chow, B. K., and Leung, P. C. (2001a). Functional mapping of a placenta-specific upstream promoter for human gonadotropin-releasing hormone receptor gene. *Endocrinology* 142, 1506–1516.

Cheng, K. W., Cheng, C. K., and Leung, P. C. (2001b). Differential role of PR-A and -B isoforms in transcription regulation of human Gnrhr. *Mol. Endocrinol.* 15, 2078–2092.

Cheng, K. W., Ngan, E. S., Kang, S. K., Chow, B. K., and Leung, P. C. (2000). Transcriptional down-regulation of human gonadotropin-releasing hormone (GnRH) receptor gene by GnRH: role of protein kinase C and activating protein 1. *Endocrinology* 141, 3611–3622.

Cherrington, B. D., Bailey, J. S., Diaz, A. L., and Mellon, P. L. (2008). NeuroD1 and Mash1 temporally regulate GnRH receptor gene expression in immortalized mouse gonadotrope cells. *Mol. Cell. Endocrinol.* 295, 106–114.

Cherrington, B. D., Farmerie, T. A., and Clay, C. M. (2006). A specific helical orientation underlies the functional contribution of the activin responsive unit to transcriptional activity of the murine gonadotropin-releasing hormone receptor gene promoter. *Endocrine* 29, 425–433.

Cherrington, B. D., Farmerie, T. A., Lents, C. A., Cantlon, J. D., Roberson, M. S., and Clay, C. M. (2005). Activin responsiveness of the murine gonadotropin-releasing hormone receptor gene is mediated by a composite enhancer containing spatially distinct regulatory elements. *Mol. Endocrinol.* 19, 898–912.

Chevrier, L., Guimiot, F., and de Roux, N. (2011). GnRH receptor mutations in isolated gonadotropic deficiency. *Mol. Cell. Endocrinol.* 346, 21–28.

Clay, C. M., Nelson, S. E., Digregorio, G. B., Campion, C. E., Wiedemann, A. L., and Nett, R. J. (1995). Cell-specific expression of the mouse gonadotropin-releasing hormone (GnRH) receptor gene is conferred by elements residing within 500 bp of proximal 5′ flanking region. *Endocrine* 3, 615–622.

Connor, E. E., Ashwell, M. S., Kappes, S. M., and Dahl, G. E. (1999). Mapping of the bovine growth hormone-releasing hormone receptor (GHRH-R) gene to chromosome 4 by linkage analysis using a novel PCR-RFLP. *J. Anim. Sci.* 77, 793–794.

de Roux, N., and Milgrom, E. (2001). Inherited disorders of GnRH and gonadotropin receptors. *Mol. Cell. Endocrinol.* 179, 83–87.

de Roux, N., Young, J., Misrahi, M., Genet, R., Chanson, P., Schaison, G., et al. (1997). A family with hypogonadotropic hypogonadism and mutations in the gonadotropin-releasing hormone receptor. *N. Engl. J. Med.* 337, 1597–1602.

Delahaye, R., Manna, P. R., Berault, A., Berreur-Bonnenfant, J., Berreur, P., and Counis R. (1997). Rat gonadotropin-releasing hormone receptor expressed in insect cells induces activation of adenylyl cyclase. *Mol. Cell. Endocrinol.* 135, 119–127.

Drouin, J., Lamolet, B., Lamonerie, T., Lanctôt, C., and Tremblay, J. J. (1998). The PTX family of homeodomain transcription factors during pituitary developments. *Mol. Cell. Endocrinol.* 140, 31–36.

Duan, W. R., Ito, M., Park, Y., Maizels, E. T., Hunzicker-Dunn, M., and Jameson, J. L. (2002). GnRH regulates early growth response protein 1 transcription through multiple promoter elements. *Mol. Endocrinol.* 16, 221–233.

Duval, D. L., Ellsworth, B. S., and Clay, C. M. (1999). Is gonadotrope expression of the gonadotropin releasing hormone receptor gene mediated by autocrine/paracrine stimulation of an activin response element? *Endocrinology* 140, 1949–1952.

Duval, D. L., Farris, A. R., Quirk, C. C., Nett, T. M., Hamernik, D. L., and Clay C. M. (2000). Responsiveness of the ovine gonadotropin-releasing hormone receptor gene to estradiol and gonadotropin-releasing hormone is not detectable *in vitro* but is revealed in transgenic mice. *Endocrinology* 141, 1001–1010.

Duval, D. L., Nelson, S. E., and Clay, C. M. (1997a). A binding site for steroidogenic factor-1 is part of a complex enhancer that mediates expression of the murine gonadotropin-releasing hormone receptor gene. *Biol. Reprod.* 56, 160–168.

Duval, D. L., Nelson, S. E., and Clay, C. M. (1997b). The tripartite basal enhancer of the gonadotropin-releasing hormone (GnRH) receptor gene promoter regulates cell-specific expression through a novel GnRHR activating sequence. *Mol. Endocrinol.* 11, 1814–1821.

Ellsworth, B. S., Burns, A. T., Escudero, K. W., Duval, D. L., Nelson, S. E., and Clay, C. M. (2003a). The gonadotropin releasing hormone (GnRH) receptor activating sequence (GRAS) is a composite regulatory element that interacts with multiple classes of transcription factors including Smads, AP-1 and a forkhead DNA binding protein. *Mol. Cell. Endocrinol.* 206, 93–111.

Ellsworth, B. S., White, B. R., Burns, A. T., Cherrington, B. D., Otis, A. M., and Clay, C. M. (2003b). c-JunN-terminal kinase activation of activator protein-1 underlies homologous regulation of the gonadotropin-releasing hormone receptor gene in alpha T3-1cells. *Endocrinology* 144, 839–849.

Ericson, J., Norlin, S., Jessell, T. M., and Edlund, T. (1998). Integrated FGF and BMP signaling controls the progression of progenitor cell differentiation and the emergence of pattern in the embryonic anterior pituitary. *Development* 125, 1005–1015.

Fan, N. C., Jeung, E. B., Peng, C., Olofsson, J. I., Krisinger, J., and Leung, P. C. (1994). The human gonadotropin-releasing hormone (GnRH) receptor gene: cloning, genomic organization and chromosomal assignment. *Mol. Cell. Endocrinol.* 103, R1–R6.

Fan, N. C., Peng, C., Krisinger, J., and Leung, P. C. (1995). The human gonadotropin-releasing hormone receptor gene: complete structure including multiple promoters, transcription initiation sites, and polyadenylation signals. *Mol. Cell. Endocrinol.* 107, R1–R8.

Fernandez-Vazquez, G., Kaiser, U. B., Albarracin, C. T., and Chin, W. W. (1996). Transcriptional activation of the gonadotropin-releasing hormone receptor gene by activin A. *Mol. Endocrinol.* 10, 356–366.

Garrel, G., Delahaye, R., Hemmings, B. A., and Counis, R. (1995). Modulation of regulatory and catalytic subunit levels of cAMP-dependent protein kinase A in anterior pituitary cells in response to direct activation of protein kinases A and C or after GnRH stimulation. *Neuroendocrinology* 62, 514–522.

Garrel, G., Lerrant, Y., Siriostis, C., Berault, A., Magre, S., Bouchaud, C., et al. (1998). Evidence that gonadotropin-releasing hormone stimulates gene expression and levels of active nitric oxide synthase type I in pituitary gonadotrophs, a process altered by desensitization and, indirectly, by gonadal steroids. *Endocrinology* 139, 2163–2170.

Garrel, G., McArdle, C. A., Hemmings, B. A., and Counis, R. (1997). Gonadotropin-releasing hormone and pituitary adenylate cyclase-activating polypeptide affect levels of cyclic adenosine 3′,5′-monophosphate-dependent protein kinase A (PKA) subunits in the clonal gonadotrope alphaT3-1 cells: evidence for cross-talk between PKA and protein kinase C pathways. *Endocrinology* 138, 2259–2266.

Garrel, G., Simon, V., Thieulant, M. L., Cayla, X., Garcia, A., Counis, R., et al. (2010). Sustained gonadotropin-releasing hormone stimulation mobilizes the cAMP/PKA pathway to induce nitric oxide synthase type 1 expression in rat pituitary cells *in vitro* and *in vivo* at proestrus. *Biol. Reprod.* 82, 1170–1179.

Granger, A., Bleux, C., Kottler, M. L., Rhodes, S. J., Counis, R., and Laverrière, J. N. (2006). The LIM-homeodomain proteins Isl-1 and Lhx3 act with steroidogenic factor 1 to enhance gonadotrope-specific activity of the gonadotropin-releasing hormone receptor gene promoter. *Mol. Endocrinol.* 20, 2093–2108.

Granger, A., Ngô-Muller, V., Bleux, C., Guigon, C., Pincas, H., Magre, S., et al. (2004). The promoter of the rat gonadotropin-releasing hormone receptor gene directs the expression of the human placental alkaline phosphatase reporter gene in gonadotrope cells in the anterior pituitary gland as well as in multiple extrapituitary tissues. *Endocrinology* 145, 983–993.

Greer, E. L., and Shi, Y. (2012). Histone methylation: a dynamic mark in health, disease and inheritance. *Nat. Rev. Genet.* 13, 343–357.

Hamernik, D. L., Clay, C. M., Turzillo, A., Van Kirk, E. A., and Moss, G. E. (1995). Estradiol increases amounts of messenger ribonucleic acid for gonadotropin-releasing hormone receptors in sheep. *Biol. Reprod.* 53, 179–185.

Han, X. B., and Conn, P. M. (1999). The role of protein kinases A and C pathways in the regulation of mitogen-activated protein kinase activation in response to gonadotropin-releasing hormone receptor activation. *Endocrinology* 140, 2241–2251.

Hapgood, J. P., Sadie, H., van Biljon, W., and Ronacher, K. (2005). Regulation of expression of mammalian gonadotrophin-releasing hormone receptor genes. *J. Neuroendocrinol.* 17, 619–638.

Hoo, R. L., Ngan, E. S., Leung, P. C., and Chow, B. K. (2003). Two Inr elements are important for mediating the activity of the proximal promoter of the human gonadotropin-releasing hormone receptor gene. *Endocrinology* 144, 518–527.

Ikeda, Y., Luo, X., Abbud, R., Nilson, J. H., and Parker, K. L. (1995). The nuclear receptor steroidogenic factor 1 is essential for the formation of the ventromedial hypothalamic nucleus. *Mol. Endocrinol.* 9, 478–486.

Ingraham, H. A., Chen, R. P., Mangalam, H. J., Elsholtz, H. P., Flynn, S. E., Lin, C. R., et al. (1988). A tissue-specific transcription factor containing a homeodomain specifies a pituitary phenotype. *Cell* 55, 519–529.

Ingraham, H. A., Lala, D. S., Ikeda, Y., Luo, X., Shen, W. H., Nachtigal, M. W., et al. (1994). The nuclear receptor steroidogenic factor 1 acts at multiple levels of the reproductive axis. *Genes Dev.* 8, 2302–2312.

Ito, M., Park, Y., Weck, J., Mayo, K. E., and Jameson, J. L. (2000). Synergistic activation of the inhibin alpha-promoter by steroidogenic factor-1 and cyclic adenosine 3′,5′-monophosphate. *Mol. Endocrinol.* 14, 66–81.

Janovick, J. A., and Conn, P. M. (1994). Gonadotropin-releasing hormone (GnRH)-receptor coupling to inositol phosphate and prolactin production in GH3 cells stably transfected with rat GnRHR complementary deoxyribonucleic acid. *Endocrinology* 135, 2214–2219.

Japón, M.A., Rubinstein, M., Low, M. J. (1994). *In situ* hybridization analysis of anterior pituitary hormone gene expression during fetal mouse development. *J. Histochem. Cytochem.* 42, 1117–1125.

Jennes, L. (1990). Prenatal development of gonadotropin-releasing hormone receptors in the rat anterior pituitary. *Endocrinology* 126, 942–947.

Jennes, L., Brame, B., Centers, A., Janovick, J. A., and Conn, P. M. (1995). Regulation of hippocampal gonadotropin releasing hormone (GnRH) receptor mRNA and GnRH-stimulated inositol phosphate production by gonadal steroid hormones. *Brain Res. Mol. Brain Res.* 33, 104–110.

Jennes, L., Dalati, B., and Conn, P. M. (1988). Distribution of gonadrotropin releasing hormone agonist binding sites in the rat central nervous system. *Brain Res.* 452, 156–164.

Jennes, L., Eyigor, O., Janovick, J. A., and Conn, P. M. (1997). Brain gonadotropin releasing hormone receptors: localization and regulation. *Recent Prog. Horm. Res.* 52, 475–490.

Jeong, K. H., Chin, W. W., and Kaiser, U. B. (2004). Essential role of the homeodomain for pituitary homeobox 1 activation of mouse gonadotropin-releasing hormone receptor gene expression through interactions with c-Jun and DNA. *Mol. Cell. Biol.* 24, 6127–6139.

Jeong, K. H., Gill, J. C., Nosé, V., Parlow, A. F., Carroll, R. S., and Kaiser, U. B. (2009). Expression of a gonadotropin-releasing hormone receptor-simian virus 40 T-antigen transgene has sex-specific effects on the reproductive axis. *Endocrinology* 150, 3383–3391.

Jiang, Z., Gibson, J. P., Archibald, A. L., and Haley, C. S. (2001). The porcine gonadotropin-releasing hormone receptor gene (GNRHR): genomic organization, polymorphisms, and association with the number of corpora lutea. *Genome* 44, 7–12.

Kaiser, U. B., Dushkin, H., Altherr, M. R., Beier, D. R., and Chin, W. W. (1994). Chromosomal localization of the gonadotropin-releasing hormone receptor gene to human chromosome 4q13.1-q21.1 and mouse chromosome 5. *Genomics* 20, 506–508.

Kaiser, U. B., Katzenellenbogen, R. A., Conn, P. M., and Chin, W. W. (1994). Evidence that signalling pathways by which thyrotropin-releasing hormone and gonadotropin-releasing hormone act are both common and distinct. *Mol. Endocrinol.* 8, 1038–1048.

Kakar, S. S. (1997). Molecular structure of the human gonadotropin-releasing hormone receptor gene. *Eur. J. Endocrinol.* 137, 183–192.

Kakar, S. S., and Neill, J. D. (1995). The human gonadotropin-releasing hormone receptor gene (GNRHR) maps to chromosome band 4q13. *Cytogenet. Cell Genet.* 70, 211–214.

Kakar, S. S., Winters, S. J., Zacharias, W., Miller, D. M., and Flynn, S. (2003). Identification of distinct gene expression profiles associated with treatment of LbetaT2 cells with gonadotropin-releasing hormone agonist using microarray analysis. *Gene* 308, 67–77.

Kam, K. Y., Jeong, K. H., Norwitz, E. R., Jorgensen, E. M., and Kaiser, U. B. (2005). Oct-1 and nuclear factor Y bind to the SURG-1 element to direct basal and gonadotropin-releasing hormone (GnRH)-stimulated mouse GnRH receptor gene transcription. *Mol. Endocrinol.* 19, 148–162.

Kang, S. K., Cheng, K. W., Ngan, E. S., Chow, B. K., Choi, K. C., and Leung, P. C. (2000). Differential expression of human gonadotropin-releasing hormone receptor gene in pituitary and ovarian cells. *Mol. Cell. Endocrinol.* 162, 157–166.

Kappen, C., and Salbaum, J. M. (2009). Identification of regulatory elements in the Isl1 gene locus. *Int. J. Dev. Biol.* 53, 935–946.

Kawaminami, M., Etoh, S., Miyaoka, H., Sakai, M., Nishida, M., Kurusu, S., et al. (2002). Annexin 5 messenger ribonucleic acid expression in pituitary gonadotropes is induced by gonadotropin-releasing hormone (GnRH) and modulates GnRH stimulation of gonadotropin release. *Neuroendocrinology* 75, 2–11.

Kirkpatrick, B. L., Esquivel E., Moss, G. E., Hamernik, D. L., and Wise, M. E. (1998). Estradiol and gonadotropin-releasing hormone (GnRH) interact to increase GnRH receptor expression in ovariectomized ewes after hypothalamic-pituitary disconnection. *Endocrine* 8, 225–229.

Kottler, M. L., Lorenzo, F., Bergametti, F., Commercon, P., Souchier, C., and Counis, R. (1995). Subregional mapping of the human gonadotropin-releasing hormone receptor (GnRHR) gene to 4q between the markers D4S392 and D4S409. *Hum. Genet.* 96, 477–480.

Kraus, S., Naor, Z., and Seger, R. (2001). Intracellular signaling pathways mediated by the gonadotropin-releasing hormone (GnRH) receptor. *Arch. Med. Res.* 32, 499–509.

Ku, M., Koche, R. P., Rheinbay, E., Mendenhall, E. M., Endoh, M., Mikkelsen, T. S., et al. (2008). Genomewide analysis of PRC1 and PRC2 occupancy identifies two classes of bivalent domains. *PLoS Genet.* 4:e1000242. doi: 10.1371/journal.pgen.1000242

Larivière, S., Garrel, G., Simon, V., Soh, J. W., Laverrière, J. N., Counis, R., et al. (2007). Gonadotropin-releasing hormone couples to 3′,5′-cyclic adenosine-5′-monophosphate pathway through novel protein kinase Cδ and -ϵ in LβT2 gonadotrope cells. *Endocrinology* 148, 1099–1107.

Larivière, S., Garrel-Lazayres, G., Simon, V., Shintani, N., Baba, A., Counis, R., et al. (2008). Gonadotropin-releasing hormone inhibits pituitary adenylyl cyclase-activating polypeptide coupling to 3′,5′-cyclic adenosine-5′-monophosphate pathway in LβT2 gonadotrope cells through novel protein kinase C isoforms and phosphorylation of pituitary adenylyl cyclase-activating polypeptide type I receptor. *Endocrinology* 149, 6389–6398.

Layman, L. C., Cohen, D. P., Jin, M., Xie, J., Li, Z., Reindollar, R. H., et al. (1998). Mutations in gonadotropin-releasing hormone receptor gene cause hypogonadotropic hypogonadism. *Nat. Genet.* 18, 14–15.

Leblanc, P., Crumeyrolle, M., Latouche, J., Jordan, D., Fillion, G., L'Heritier, A., et al. (1988). Characterization and distribution of receptors for gonadotropin-releasing hormone in the rat hippocampus. *Neuroendocrinology* 48, 482–488.

Lents, C. A., Farmerie, T. A., Cherrington, B. D., and Clay, C. M. (2009). Multiple core homeodomain binding motifs differentially contribute to transcriptional activity of the murine gonadotropin-releasing hormone receptor gene promoter. *Endocrine* 35, 356–364.

Leung, P. C., Squire, J., Peng, C., Fan, N., Hayden, M. R., and Olofsson, J. I. (1995). Mapping of the gonadotropin-releasing hormone (GnRH) receptor gene to human chromosome 4q21.2 by fluorescence in situ hybridization. *Mamm. Genome* 6, 309–310.

Li, J., Liu, Q., Qiu, M., Pan, Y., Li, Y., and Shi, T. (2006). Identification and analysis of the mouse basic/helix-loop-helix transcription factor family. *Biochem. Biophys. Res. Commun.* 350, 648–656.

Li, S., Crenshaw, E. B. III, Rawson, E. J., Simmons, D. M., Swanson, L. W., and Rosenfeld, M. G. (1990). Dwarf locus mutants lacking three pituitary cell types result from mutations in the POU-domain gene Pit-1. *Nature* 347, 528–533.

Lienert, F., Wirbelauer, C., Som, I., Dean, A., Mohn, F., and Schübeler, D. (2011). Identification of genetic elements that autonomously determine DNA methylation states. *Nat. Genet.* 43, 1091–1097.

Lin, X., and Conn, P. M. (1998). Transcriptional activation of gonadotropin-releasing hormone (GnRH) receptor gene by GnRH and cyclic adenosine monophosphate. *Endocrinology* 139, 3896–3902.

Lin, X., and Conn, P. M. (1999). Transcriptional activation of gonadotropin-releasing hormone (GnRH) receptor gene by GnRH: involvement of multiple signal transduction pathways. *Endocrinology* 140, 358–364.

Liu, F., Austin, D. A., Mellon, P. L., Olefsky, J. M., and Webster, N. J. (2002). GnRH activates ERK1/2 leading to the induction of c-fos and LHβ protein expression in LβT2 cells. *Mol. Endocrinol.* 16, 419–434.

Lozach, A., Garrel, G., Lerrant, Y., Berault, A., and Counis, R. (1998). GnRH-dependent up-regulation of nitric oxide synthase I level in pituitary gonadotrophs mediates cGMP elevation during rat proestrus. *Mol. Cell. Endocrinol.* 143, 43–51.

Luo, X., Ikeda, Y., Schlosser, D. A., and Parker, K. L. (1995). Steroidogenic factor 1 is the essential transcript of the mouse Ftz-F1 gene. *Mol. Endocrinol.* 9, 1233–1239.

Maya-Nunez, G., and Conn, P. M. (1999). Transcriptional regulation of the gonadotropin-releasing hormone receptor gene is mediated in part by a putative repressor element and by the cyclic adenosine 3′,5′-monophosphate response element. *Endocrinology* 140, 3452–3458.

Maya-Nunez, G., and Conn, P. M. (2001). Cyclic adenosine 3′,5′-monophosphate (cAMP) and cAMP responsive element-binding protein are involved in the transcriptional regulation of gonadotropin-releasing hormone (GnRH) receptor by GnRH and mitogen-activated protein kinase signal transduction pathway in GGH(3) cells. *Biol. Reprod.* 65, 561–567.

McCue, J. M., Quirk, C. C., Nelson, S. E., Bowen, R. A., and Clay, C. M. (1997). Expression of a murine gonadotropin-releasing hormone receptor-luciferase fusion gene in transgenic mice is diminished by immunoneutralization of gonadotropin-releasing hormone. *Endocrinology* 138, 3154–3160.

McGillivray, S. M., Bailey, J. S., Ramezani, R., Kirkwood, B. J., and Mellon, P. L. (2005). Mouse GnRH receptor gene expression is mediated by the LHX3 homeodomain protein. *Endocrinology* 146, 2180–2185.

Meldi, L., and Brickner, J. H. (2011). Compartmentalization of the nucleus. *Trends Cell Biol.* 21, 701–708.

Montgomery, G. W., Penty, J. M., Lord, E. A., Brooks, J., and McNeilly, A. S. (1995). The gonadotrophin-releasing hormone receptor maps to sheep chromosome 6 outside of the region of the FecB locus. *Mamm. Genome* 6, 436–438.

Morrison, N., Sellar, R. E., Boyd, E., Eidne, K. A., and Connor, J. M. (1994). Assignment of the gene encoding the human gonadotropin-releasing hormone receptor to 4q13.2-13.3 by fluorescence in situ hybridization. *Hum. Genet.* 93, 714–715.

Mullen, R. D., Park, S., and Rhodes, S. J. (2012). A distal modular enhancer complex acts to control pituitary- and nervous system-specific expression of the LHX3 regulatory gene. *Mol. Endocrinol.* 26, 308–319.

Ngan, E. S., Cheng, P. K., Leung, P. C., and Chow, B. K. (1999). Steroidogenic factor-1 interacts with a gonadotrope-specific element within the first exon of the human gonadotropin-releasing hormone receptor gene to mediate gonadotrope-specific expression. *Endocrinology* 140, 2452–2462.

Ngan, E. S., Leung, P. C., and Chow, B. K. (2000). Identification of an upstream promoter in the human gonadotropin-releasing hormone receptor gene. *Biochem. Biophys. Res. Commun.* 270, 766–772.

Ngan, E. S., Leung, P. C., and Chow, B. K. (2001). Interplay of pituitary adenylate cyclase-activating polypeptide with a silencer element to regulate the upstream promoter of the human gonadotropin-releasing hormone receptor gene. *Mol. Cell. Endocrinol.* 176, 135–144.

Ngô, V. M., Laverrière, J. N., and Gourdji, D. (1995). CpG methylation represses the activity of the rat prolactin promoter in rat GH3 pituitary cell lines. *Mol. Cell. Endocrinol.* 108, 95–105.

Noel, S. D., and Kaiser, U. B. (2011). G protein-coupled receptors involved in GnRH regulation: molecular insights from human disease. *Mol. Cell. Endocrinol.* 346, 91–101.

Norwitz, E. R., Cardona, G. R., Jeong, K. H., and Chin, W. W. (1999b). Identification and characterization of the gonadotropin-releasing hormone response elements in the mouse gonadotropin-releasing hormone receptor gene. *J. Biol. Chem.* 274, 867–880.

Norwitz, E. R., Jeong, K. H., and Chin, W. W. (1999a). Molecular mechanisms of gonadotropin-releasing hormone receptor gene regulation. *J. Soc. Gynecol. Investig.* 6, 169–178.

Norwitz, E. R., Xu, S., Jeong, K. H., Bedecarrats, G. Y., Winebrenner, L. D., Chin, W. W., et al. (2002a). Activin A augments GnRH-mediated transcriptional activation of the mouse Gnrhr. *Endocrinology* 143, 985–997.

Norwitz, E. R., Xu, S., Xu, J., Spiryda, L. B., Park, J. S., Jeong, K. H., et al. (2002b). Direct binding of AP-1 (Fos/Jun) proteins to a SMAD binding element facilitates both gonadotropin-releasing hormone (GnRH)- and activin-mediated transcriptional activation of the mouse GnRH receptor gene. *J. Biol. Chem.* 277, 37469–37478.

Pincas, H., Amoyel, K., Counis, R., and Laverriere, J. N. (2001a). Proximal cis-acting elements, including steroidogenic factor 1, mediate the efficiency of a distal enhancer in the promoter of the rat gonadotropin-releasing hormone receptor gene. *Mol. Endocrinol.* 15, 319–337.

Pincas, H., Laverriere, J. N., and Counis, R. (2001b). Pituitary adenylate cyclase-activating polypeptide and cyclic adenosine 3′,5′-monophosphate stimulate the promoter activity of the rat gonadotropin-releasing hormone receptor gene via a bipartite response element in gonadotrope-derived cells. *J. Biol. Chem.* 276, 23562–23571.

Pincas, H., Forrai, Z., Chauvin, S., Laverriere, J. N., and Counis, R. (1998). Multiple elements in the distal part of the 1.2 kb 5′-flanking region of the rat Gnrhr regulate gonadotrope-specific expression conferred by proximal domain. *Mol. Cell. Endocrinol.* 144, 95–108.

Pirrotta, V., and Li, H. B. (2012). A view of nuclear polycomb bodies. *Curr. Opin. Genet. Dev.* 22, 101–109.

Reinhart, J., Xiao, S., Arora, K. K., and Catt, K. J. (1997). Structural organization and characterization of the promoter region of the rat gonadotropin-releasing hormone receptor gene. *Mol. Cell. Endocrinol.* 130, 1–12.

Resuehr, D., Wildemann, U., Sikes, H., and Olcese, J. (2007). E-box regulation of gonadotropin-releasing hormone (GnRH) receptor expression in immortalized gonadotrope cells. *Mol. Cell. Endocrinol.* 278, 36–43.

Roesler, W. J. (2000). What is a cAMP response unit? *Mol. Cell. Endocrinol.* 162, 1–7.

Sadie, H., Styger, G., and Hapgood, J. (2003). Expression of the mouse gonadotropin-releasing hormone receptor gene in alpha T3-1 gonadotrope cells is stimulated by cyclic 3′,5′-adenosine monophosphate and protein kinase A, and is modulated by steroidogenic factor-1 and Nur77. *Endocrinology.* 144, 1958–1971.

Schang, A. L., Bleux, C., Chenut, M. C., Ngô-Muller, V., Quérat, B., Jeanny, J. C., et al. (2012a). Identification and analysis of two novel sites of rat GnRH receptor gene promoter activity: the pineal gland and retina. *Neuroendocrinology.* doi: 10.1159/000337661 [Epub ahead of print].

Schang, A. L., Granger, A., Quérat, B., Bleux, C., Cohen-Tannoudji, J., and Laverrière, J. N. (2012b). GATA2-induced silencing and LIM-homeodomain protein-induced activation are mediated by a bi-functional response element in the rat GnRH receptor gene. *Mol. Endocrinol.* (in press).

Schang, A. L., Counis, R., Magre, S., Bleux, C., Granger, A., Ngô-Muller, V., et al. (2011a). Reporter transgenic mouse models highlight the dual endocrine and neural facet of GnRH receptor function. *Ann. N. Y. Acad. Sci.* 1220, 16–22.

Schang, A. L., Ngô-Muller, V., Bleux, C., Granger, A., Chenut, M. C., Loudes, C., et al. (2011b). GnRH receptor gene expression in the developing rat hippocampus: transcriptional regulation and potential roles in neuronal plasticity. *Endocrinology* 152, 568–580.

Schlosser, G. (2006). Induction and specification of cranial placodes. *Dev. Biol.* 294, 303–351.

Schuettengruber, B., Chourrout, D., Vervoort, M., Leblanc, B., and Cavalli, G. (2007). Genome regulation by polycomb and trithorax proteins. *Cell* 128, 735–745.

Scully, K. M., and Rosenfeld, M. G. (2002). Pituitary development: regulatory codes in mammalian organogenesis. *Science* 295, 2231–2235.

Shima, Y., Miyabayashi, K., Baba, T., Otake, H., Oka, S., Zubair, M., et al. (2012). Identification of an enhancer in the Ad4BP/SF-1 gene specific for fetal Leydig cells. *Endocrinology* 153, 417–425.

Silveira, L. F., Stewart, P. M., Thomas, M., Clark, D. A., Bouloux, P. M., and MacColl, G. S. (2002). Novel homozygous splice acceptor site GnRHR (GnRHR) mutation: human GnRHR "knockout." *J. Clin. Endocrinol. Metab.* 87, 2973–2977.

Simon, J. A., and Kingston, R. E. (2009). Mechanisms of polycomb gene silencing: knowns and unknowns. *Nat. Rev. Mol. Cell Biol.* 10, 697–708.

Sosnowski, R., Mellon, P. L., and Lawson, M. A. (2000). Activation of translation in pituitary gonadotrope cells by gonadotropin-releasing hormone. *Mol. Endocrinol.* 14, 1811–1819.

Spector, D. L., and Lamond, A. I. (2011). Nuclear speckles. *Cold Spring Harb. Perspect. Biol.* 3, a000646.

Stanislaus, D., Arora, V., Awara, W. M., and Conn, P. M. (1996). Biphasic action of cyclic adenosine 3′,5′-monophosphate in gonadotropin-releasing hormone (GnRH) analog-stimulated hormone release from GH3 cells stably transfected with GnRHR complementary deoxyribonucleic acid. *Endocrinology* 137, 1025–1031.

Stanislaus, D., Janovick, J. A., Jennes, L., Kaiser, U. B., Chin, W. W., and Conn, P. M. (1994). Functional and morphological characterization of four cell lines derived from GH3 cells stably transfected with gonadotropin-releasing hormone receptor complementary deoxyribonucleic acid. *Endocrinology* 135, 2220–2227.

Stewart, A. J., Katz, A. A., Millar, R. P., and Morgan, K. (2009). Retention and silencing of prepro-GnRH-II and type II GnRH receptor genes in mammals. *Neuroendocrinology* 90, 416–432.

Stojilkovic, S. S., Reinhart, J., and Catt, K. J. (1994). Gonadotropin-releasing hormone receptors: structure and signal transduction pathways. *Endocr. Rev.* 15, 462–499.

Stopa, M., Anhuf, D., Terstegen, L., Gatsios, P., Gressner, A. M., and Dooley, S. (2000). Participation of Smad2, Smad3, and Smad4 in transforming growth factor beta (TGF-beta)-induced activation of Smad7. The TGF-beta response element of the promoter requires functional Smad binding element and E-box sequences for transcriptional regulation. *J. Biol. Chem.* 275, 29308–29317.

Thomas, P., Mellon, P. L., Turgeon, J., and Waring, D. W. (1996). The L beta T2 clonal gonadotrope: a model for single cell studies of endocrine cell secretion. *Endocrinology* 137, 2979–2989.

Turgeon, J. L., Kimura, Y., Waring, D. W., and Mellon, P. L. (1996). Steroid and pulsatile gonadotropin-releasing hormone (GnRH) regulation of luteinizing hormone and GnRH receptor in a novel gonadotrope cell line. *Mol. Endocrinol.* 10, 439–450.

Turzillo, A. M., DiGregorio, G. B., and Nett, T. M. (1995). Messenger ribonucleic acid for gonadotropin-releasing hormone receptor and numbers of gonadotropin releasing hormone receptors in ovariectomized ewes after hypothalamic pituitary disconnection and treatment with estradiol. *J. Anim. Sci.* 73, 1784–1788.

Vazquez-Martinez, R., Shorte, S. L., Boockfor, F. R., and Frawley, L. S. (2001). Synchronized exocytotic bursts from gonadotropin-releasing hormone-expressing cells: dual control by intrinsic cellular pulsatility and gap junctional communication. *Endocrinology* 142, 2095–2101.

Walton, K. L., Makanji, Y., and Harrison, C. A. (2012). New insights into the mechanisms of activin action and inhibition. *Mol. Cell. Endocrinol.* 359, 2–12.

Weiss, J., Crowley, W. F. Jr, Halvorson, L. M., and Jameson, J. L. (1993). Perifusion of rat pituitary cells with gonadotropin-releasing hormone, activin, and inhibin reveals distinct effects on gonadotropin gene expression and secretion. *Endocrinology* 132, 2307–2311.

Wen, S., Schwarz, J. R., Niculescu, D., Dinu, C., Bauer, C. K., Hirdes, W., et al. (2008). Functional characterization of genetically labeled gonadotropes. *Endocrinology* 149, 2701–2711.

White, B. R., Duval, D. L., Mulvaney, J. M., Roberson, M. S., and Clay, C. M. (1999). Homologous regulation of the gonadotropin-releasing hormone receptor gene is partially mediated by protein kinase C activation of an activator protein-1 element. *Mol. Endocrinol.* 13, 566–577.

Wilson, M. D., Barbosa-Morais, N. L., Schmidt, D., Conboy, C. M., Vanes, L., Tybulewicz, V. L., et al. (2008). Species-specific transcription in mice carrying human chromosome 21. *Science* 322, 434–438.

Windle, J. J., Weiner R. I., and Mellon P. L. (1990). Cell lines of the pituitary gonadotrope lineage derived by targeted oncogenesis in transgenic mice. *Mol. Endocrinol.* 4, 597–603.

Yang, L., Lin, C., Liu, W., Zhang, J., Ohgi, K. A., Grinstein, J. D., et al. (2011). ncRNA- and Pc2 methylation-dependent gene relocation between nuclear structures mediates gene activation programs. *Cell* 147, 773–788.

Yeung, C. M., An, B. S., Cheng, C. K., Chow, B. K., and Leung, P. C. (2005). Expression and transcriptional regulation of the GnRH receptor gene in human neuronal cells. *Mol. Hum. Reprod.* 11, 837–842.

Zhao, L., Bakke, M., and Parker, K. L. (2001). Pituitary-specific knockout of steroidogenic factor 1. *Mol. Cell. Endocrinol.* 185, 27–32.

9

Sensitivity of cholecystokinin receptors to membrane cholesterol content

Aditya J. Desai and Laurence J. Miller*

Department of Molecular Pharmacology and Experimental Therapeutics, Mayo Clinic, Scottsdale, AZ, USA

Edited by:
Hubert Vaudry, University of Rouen, France

Reviewed by:
Pedro A. Jose, Georgetown University, USA
Akiyoshi Takahashi, Kitasato University, Japan

Correspondence:
Laurence J. Miller, Department of Molecular Pharmacology and Experimental Therapeutics, Mayo Clinic, 13400 E. Shea Blvd., Scottsdale, AZ 85259, USA.
e-mail: miller@mayo.edu

Cholesterol represents a structurally and functionally important component of the eukaryotic cell membrane, where it increases lipid order, affects permeability, and influences the lateral mobility and conformation of membrane proteins. Several G protein-coupled receptors have been shown to be affected by the cholesterol content of the membrane, with functional impact on their ligand binding and signal transduction characteristics. The effects of cholesterol can be mediated directly by specific molecular interactions with the receptor and/or indirectly by altering the physical properties of the membrane. This review focuses on the importance and differential effects of membrane cholesterol on the activity of cholecystokinin (CCK) receptors. The type 1 CCK receptor is quite sensitive to its cholesterol environment, while the type 2 CCK receptor is not. The possible structural basis for this differential impact is explored and the implications of pathological states, such as metabolic syndrome, in which membrane cholesterol may be increased and CCK1R function may be abnormal are discussed. This is believed to have substantial potential importance for the development of drugs targeting the CCK receptor.

Keywords: cholecystokinin, G protein-coupled receptors, cholesterol

INTRODUCTION

Biological membranes consist of a variety of lipids and proteins that establish diffusional boundaries for the cell and its organelles. An important lipid component of the plasma membrane is cholesterol that may be present in concentrations as high as 20–40 mol%, which is known to have substantial impact on the physical properties of the membrane and on the structure and function of various intrinsic membrane proteins (Mouritsen and Zuckermann, 2004).

The hydrophilic hydroxyl groups of the amphiphilic cholesterol molecules are intercalated into the lipid bilayers, with one cholesterol molecule spanning approximately half of the bilayer (Mouritsen and Zuckermann, 2004). Cholesterol has the unique ability to increase order in such membranes by organizing the arrangement of the surrounding lipids, while maintaining fluidity and lateral diffusion within the membrane. A region of the membrane in which cholesterol is absent typically exhibits disorder and rapid lateral diffusion with randomly packed lipid molecules (Miao et al., 2002; Mouritsen and Zuckermann, 2004). Lowering the temperature can result in a transition from a liquid-disordered phase toward a solid-ordered phase having slower lateral diffusion and greater ordering of the lipid chains. The presence of cholesterol can also induce order in the liquid phase by increasing the density of the packing of fatty acyl chains. This is also identified as a liquid-ordered phase (Ipsen et al., 1987).

Abbreviations: CCK, cholecystokinin; cAMP, cyclic adenosine monophosphate; CCM, cholesterol consensus motif; CRAC, cholesterol recognition/interaction amino acid consensus; DAG, diacylglycerol; FRET, fluorescence resonance energy transfer; GPCRs, guanine nucleotide-binding protein-coupled receptors; MβCD, methyl-beta-cyclodextrin; IP_3, inositol triphosphate.

Cholesterol can also affect the permeability function of the membrane by changing its lateral density fluctuations and structural heterogeneity and thereby regulating its "leakiness." The effect of cholesterol on lipid order also affects the thickness of the bilayer (Ohvo-Rekila et al., 2002; Mouritsen and Zuckermann, 2004). In the presence of low or absent cholesterol, sodium ions are able to passively permeate the lipid bilayer, while such permeability is inhibited in the presence of high (40%) cholesterol (Ohvo-Rekila et al., 2002). Cholesterol can also bind and inhibit some solutes such as ethanol, which become strongly adsorbed as a result of density fluctuations and the heterogeneous composition of the bilayer (Schroeder et al., 1996).

Cholesterol can also contribute to specialized microdomains within the plasma membrane that are known as planar lipid rafts. These are small, low-density regions in the outer leaflet of the bilayer that are enriched in cholesterol and glycosphingolipids. These structures have been identified based on their insolubility in non-ionic detergents at low temperature and their high buoyancy in density gradients (Brown and Rose, 1992). These planar structures may also give rise to caveolae, representing flask-shaped invaginations that can ultimately form free intracellular organelles (Cohen et al., 2004; Shaw, 2006). It is notable that lipid rafts and caveolae can act as organizational platforms for elements involved in signal transduction (Okamoto et al., 1998; Pike, 2003; Cohen et al., 2004; Ostrom and Insel, 2004).

EFFECTS OF MEMBRANE CHOLESTEROL ON G PROTEIN-COUPLED RECEPTORS (GPCRs)

Several GPCRs have been reported to be sensitive to the concentration of cholesterol in the membrane, with different effects observed for different receptors (**Table 1**). Cholesterol can affect receptor conformation, thereby affecting its ligand binding and signaling characteristics. It can affect lateral mobility within the bilayer that is critical for G protein coupling. It can also affect receptor trafficking and sequestration that contribute to desensitization. However, currently there are no well-established rules for which receptors might be influenced by cholesterol and how these receptors might be affected. Two distinct groups of mechanisms have been proposed: (A) direct binding of cholesterol molecules to GPCR molecules, including the possibility of interacting with specific sites or motifs (Albert et al., 1996; Li and Papadopoulos, 1998; Paila et al., 2009) and/or (B) indirect effects of the cholesterol by altering the physical properties of the membrane in which the GPCRs reside (Lee, 2004; Mouritsen and Zuckermann, 2004).

The effects of membrane cholesterol on rhodopsin, the photoreceptor of the retinal rod cells, have been extensively studied. Rhodopsin exists in various conformations known as metarhodopsins. The equilibrium between these conformational states is sensitive to the amount of membrane cholesterol present, with increased cholesterol shifting the equilibrium toward the inactive states of the receptor (Mitchell et al., 1990; Bennett and Mitchell, 2008). The influence of membrane cholesterol on rhodopsin function has been attributed to both direct and indirect mechanisms. Spatial approximation between tryptophan residues of rhodopsin and cholesterol has been demonstrated using fluorescence resonance energy transfer (FRET), with an estimation of one sterol molecule interacting with one rhodopsin molecule (Albert et al., 1996). These observations have been supported by the crystal structure of metarhodopsin I that includes a cholesterol molecule bound between the tryptophan residues of transmembrane segment four of one protomer and transmembrane segments five, six, and seven of the other protomer (Ruprecht et al., 2004). An indirect effect of cholesterol has also been attributed to its effect on the partial free volume of the membrane. The conversion of metarhodopsin I to metarhodopsin II involves an expansion of the protein in the plane of the lipid bilayer (Attwood and Gutfreund, 1980), thereby occupying the partial free volume of the surrounding bilayer. As membrane cholesterol is increased, the formation of metarhodopsin II is decreased by reducing the partial free volume in the membrane (Niu et al., 2002).

Table 1 | List of GPCRs affected by membrane cholesterol.

GPCR	Effect of membrane cholesterol	References
β2-adrenergic	Cholesterol improves stability of the receptor and facilitates its crystallization. It also modulates isolation of the receptor from its signaling components in liquid-ordered lipid nanodomains, and thereby affects signaling.	Ben-Arie et al., 1988; Hanson et al., 2008; Pontier et al., 2008
Cannabinoid	CB1R is dependent on cholesterol concentrated in lipid rafts for ligand binding and signaling and the CRAC motif is responsible for its direct interaction with membrane cholesterol.	Bari et al., 2005a,b; Oddi et al., 2011
Chemokine	Cholesterol is essential for CXCR4 and 5 conformation and function.	Nguyen and Taub, 2002a,b, 2003
Cholecystokinin	Cholesterol interacts at specific sites in the transmembrane segments of the CCK1R (CCKAR), and affects its ligand binding and signaling abilities. CCK2R (CCKBR) is not affected.	Gimpl et al., 1997, 2002; Harikumar et al., 2005b; Potter et al., 2012
Dopamine	D1 receptors in renal cells can associate with caveolin-2 in caveolae, where they activate adenylate cyclase.	Yu et al., 2004; Genedani et al., 2010
Galanin	Membrane cholesterol supports the ligand binding process in a positively co-operative manner.	Pang et al., 1999
Metabotropic glutamate	Enrichment of cholesterol in *Drosophila melanogaster* photoreceptor cell membranes induces receptor association with lipid rafts and shift to the high affinity state.	Eroglu et al., 2003
Muscarinic	Cholesterol promotes cooperativity in binding of antagonists to the M2 muscarinic receptors.	Colozo et al., 2007
Neurokinin	Monomeric neurokinin-1 receptors are localized in the lipid rafts and caveolae. Cholesterol content is directly proportional to the signaling.	Monastyrskaya et al., 2005; Meyer et al., 2006
Opioid	Cholesterol present in lipid rafts and caveolae is important for agonist affinity, where it affects G protein coupling.	Lagane et al., 2000; Xu et al., 2006; Huang et al., 2007
Oxytocin	Amount of cholesterol in the membrane is directly proportional to the ligand binding affinity of the receptor.	Gimpl et al., 1997, 2002; Gimpl and Fahrenholz, 2002
Serotonin	Reduction in cholesterol compromises organization, ligand binding, and G protein coupling at the $5HT_{1A}$ and $5HT_{7A}$ receptors.	Pucadyil and Chattopadhyay, 2004, 2005; Sjogren et al., 2006
Rhodopsin	Elevated cholesterol inhibits the activation of rhodopsin receptor.	Mitchell et al., 1990; Niu et al., 2002; Bennett and Mitchell, 2008

Similarly, cholesterol has been shown to be bound to the β2-adrenergic receptor in its crystal structure (Hanson et al., 2008), and this lipid has been shown to be necessary for ligand binding, G protein interaction, and signal transduction at that receptor (Ben-Arie et al., 1988). Two cholesterol molecules appear to be bound to sites on transmembrane segments one, two, three, and four of a β2-adrenergic receptor molecule (Hanson et al., 2008).

Other examples include the oxytocin receptor, where the amount of cholesterol in the membrane is directly related to the ligand binding affinity of the receptor (Gimpl et al., 1997, 2002; Gimpl and Fahrenholz, 2002) [43% decrease in membrane cholesterol caused a sharp decline in ligand binding (Gimpl et al., 1997)]. This has been shown to be a highly co-operative process where more than six molecules of cholesterol can be bound to one oxytocin receptor molecule (Gimpl et al., 2002). There is clear structural specificity for this interaction, since only cholesterol analogs that are structurally similar to cholesterol are able to reproduce this effect on oxytocin receptor function (Gimpl et al., 1997). Cholesterol is also believed to provide stability against thermal and pH alterations, and to protect some receptors from proteolytic degradation (Gimpl and Fahrenholz, 2002). Similarly, in the case of the galanin-2 receptor, cholesterol affects ligand binding process in a positively co-operative manner (Pang et al., 1999). Only a limited number of cholesterol analogs are able to exhibit similar effects to those of cholesterol, again supporting structural specificity of this interaction (Pang et al., 1999). Other examples of GPCRs affected by membrane cholesterol are listed in **Table 1**.

Some interactions of membrane cholesterol with GPCRs have been attributed to the presence of consensus motifs within these receptors. Several proteins that are known to interact with cholesterol have a characteristic amino acid sequence, termed the cholesterol recognition/interaction amino acid consensus (CRAC) motif, in their transmembrane segments. This is defined by the pattern—L/V-(X)1–5-Y-(X)1–5-R/K-, in which (X)1–5 represents between one and five residues of any amino acid (Li and Papadopoulos, 1998). This sequence is present in rhodopsin, β2-adrenergic, serotonin$_{1A}$, and cholecystokinin (CCK) receptors (Jafurulla et al., 2011; Potter et al., 2012). Another consensus motif, the strict-cholesterol consensus motif (CCM), was described in transmembrane segments by Hanson et al. (2008), and was later expanded by Adamian et al. (2011). This motif [4.39–4.43 (R,K)] [4.50 (W,Y)] [2.45 (S)] [4.46 (I,V,L)] [2.41 (F,Y)] that incorporates the Ballesteros and Weinstein numbering system based on residue position relative to most conserved residues within a given transmembrane segment (Ballesteros and Weinstein, 1992), was recognized from the analysis of the 2.8 Å structure of the human β2-adrenergic receptor and is present in 21% of the class A GPCRs (Hanson et al., 2008). A less-restrictive variant of this motif is also found in 44% of class A GPCRs, where the aromatic residue is absent at the position 2.41. The presence of this motif, suggests that specific sterol binding may be important to the structure and stability of receptors in this family.

CHOLECYSTOKININ (CCK) PEPTIDES AND PHYSIOLOGY

The GPCRs that are responsive to the gastrointestinal and brain peptide, CCK, are the major focus of this review, with one of the CCK receptors affected by cholesterol and the other unaffected. CCK is a polypeptide hormone synthesized in the I-cells of the small intestine (Rehfeld, 1978) that is released in response to protein and fat in the lumen that plays an important role in nutrient homeostasis. CCK was identified based on its ability to stimulate gallbladder contraction, and it was also eventually recognized as being identical to pancreozymin, a hormone that stimulates pancreatic exocrine secretion (Harper and Raper, 1943). CCK also contributes to post-cibal satiety (Kissileff et al., 1981; Smith and Gibbs, 1985; Beglinger et al., 2001), which is a critically important role that could provide the basis of a treatment of obesity. This hormone is also one of the most abundant neuropeptides present in the brain (Miller et al., 1984), and it has been shown to have effects on enteric smooth muscle and nerves at various locations in the peripheral and central nervous system. It also has been described to have direct natriuretic effects on the kidney, and to decrease renal excretion of calcium and magnesium (Duggan et al., 1988; Ladines et al., 2001). CCK is present as a variety of different length peptides that are produced from a single 115-residue preprohormone precursor, all sharing their carboxyl-terminal sequence. These range from 58, 39, 33, and 8 residues, with each containing a sulfated tyrosine residue seven residues from the carboxyl terminus, as well as amidation of the carboxyl-terminal phenylalanine residue (Eysselein et al., 1990; Rehfeld et al., 2001; Miller and Gao, 2008).

CCK RECEPTOR STRUCTURE AND FUNCTION

CCK exerts its physiological functions through the activation of two structurally-related class A GPCRs identified as CCK receptor type 1 (CCK1R) and CCK receptor type 2 (CCK2R) (also known as CCKAR and CCKBR, respectively, related to their prominent presence in "alimentary tract" and "brain") (Dufresne et al., 2006). CCK2R also binds gastrin, another structurally-related polypeptide hormone produced in the gastric antrum (Kopin et al., 1992). In contrast, CCK1R binds gastrin at a very low affinity (by 500-fold). Both these receptors are highly homologous and approximately 50% identical, particularly in the transmembrane regions where they are 70% identical (Miller and Gao, 2008). Although both types of CCK receptors bind and are activated by CCK and gastrin peptides, the molecular basis for peptide binding to these receptors appears to be distinct. The CCK1R requires the carboxyl-terminal CCK heptapeptide-amide that includes the sulfated tyrosine for high affinity binding and biological activity, whereas the CCK2R requires only the carboxyl-terminal tetrapeptide amide that is shared between all CCK and gastrin receptors (Miller and Gao, 2008). The activation of the CCK1R by CCK elicits a broad variety of important physiological functions, such as stimulation of gallbladder contraction and pancreatic exocrine secretion, delay of gastric emptying, relaxation of the sphincter of Oddi, inhibition of gastric acid secretion, and induction of post-cibal satiety (Kerstens et al., 1985; Schmitz et al., 2001). The CCK1R is localized in the human gastric mucosa within D cells (Schmitz et al., 2001) and muscularis propria of human gastric antrum, fundus, and pylorus (Reubi et al., 1997). CCK2R is localized mainly in brain and is also present in the gastric oxyntic mucosa, some enteric smooth muscle, and the kidneys (Noble and Roques, 1999; Von Schrenck et al., 2000). In addition to stimulation of gastric acid secretion, CCK2R also plays a role in anxiety and nociception (Noble and Roques, 1999; Noble, 2007).

The CCK receptors belong to the class A group of GPCRs [see review of CCK receptor structure and pharmacology (Miller and Gao, 2008)]. They share the typical signature sequences of this family, including E/DRY at the intracellular side of transmembrane segment three and NPxxY at the intracellular side of transmembrane segment seven. Both receptors are glycosylated, possess the conserved disulfide bond between extracellular loops one and two (CCK1R also has an extra disulfide bond within the amino-terminal extracellular domain), and include multiple sites for serine and threonine phosphorylation in intracellular loop three and in the carboxyl-terminal tail. The function of phosphorylation is to desensitize the receptor, interfering with its coupling to G proteins (Rao et al., 1997). These receptors also have cysteine residues representing sites of palmitoylation in the intracellular carboxyl-terminal tail, which help to attach an eighth helical segment to the cytosolic face of the bilayer.

A broad range of approaches, including ligand binding and signaling of chimeric and site-specific mutants (Kopin et al., 1995; Miller and Lybrand, 2002), photoaffinity labeling (Ding et al., 2001; Dong et al., 2005, 2007) and fluorescence-based techniques (Harikumar et al., 2004, 2005a, 2006; Harikumar and Miller, 2005) have provided important information regarding the molecular basis of CCK binding to these receptors. Information from these studies has shown that the determinants for CCK binding to the CCK1R are distributed throughout the extracellular loop and amino-terminal tail regions, but not within the predicted transmembrane domain bundle (Miller and Lybrand, 2002; Harikumar et al., 2004). However, a possible difference for CCK binding to these two receptors relates to the position of the carboxyl-terminal end of the peptide. This portion of CCK resides at the surface of the lipid bilayer adjacent to transmembrane segment one for the CCK1R, as directly demonstrated by site-selective photoaffinity labeling (Harikumar et al., 2004), while it may dip into the helical bundle for the CCK2R, although the latter is based on less definitive data coming from site-directed mutagenesis (Harikumar et al., 2006).

Table 2 shows differences in microenvironment-dependent spectral properties of fluorescent CCK ligands docked to CCK1 or CCK2 receptors, supporting the suggested differential binding of the ligands to these two receptors.

Various selective and potent non-natural ligands for the CCK receptor have been developed [see reviews (Herranz, 2003; Kalindjian and McDonald, 2007)]. The most extensively studied in regard to mechanism of binding to CCK receptors is the group of benzodiazepine compounds (Aquino et al., 1996; Darrow et al., 1998; Gao et al., 2008; Cawston et al., 2012). Minor chemical modifications of these compounds have been shown to change receptor subtype selectivity and biological responsiveness (Aquino et al., 1996; Gao et al., 2008; Miller and Gao, 2008). It is now clear, based on receptor mutagenesis, photoaffinity labeling, and pharmacological manipulations, that these ligands bind to an allosteric site within the intramembranous helical bundle that is distinct from the orthosteric CCK peptide-binding site of the CCK1R (Kopin et al., 1994; Hadac et al., 2006; Gao et al., 2008). In fact, using two specific benzodiazepine antagonist ligands, it has been shown that transmembrane segments six and seven [residues 6.51, 6.52, and 7.39 (Ballesteros and Weinstein, 1992)] are most important for binding the CCK1R-selective ligand, whereas residues of transmembrane segments two and seven

Table 2 | Summary of studies demonstrating the differential binding of fluorescent CCK probes to CCK1 and CCK2 receptors.

CCK1R	CCK2R
• CCK-8-based probe had shorter half-life and lower anisotropy (more mobility) in the active than inactive conformation of the receptor.	• CCK-8-based probe had shorter half-life and lower anisotropy (more mobility) in the active than inactive conformation of the receptor. However, when bound, absolute values for lifetime and anisotropy were lower (more exposure to the aqueous milieu) than those in the CCK1R.
• CCK-4-based probe was not tolerated.	• CCK-4-based probe was tolerated. There was less quenching of this probe (reduced exposure to aqueous milieu) than the CCK-8-based probe.
• Fluorophore corresponding to the amino terminus of the CCK (position 24) was more accessible to aqueous milieu in the active than inactive conformations of the receptor.	• Flourophore corresponding to the amino terminus of CCK (position 24) behaved in a similar manner to CCK1R.
• Fluorophore corresponding to the mid-region of the peptide (position 29) was least accessible to the aqueous milieu and unaltered by changes between active and inactive conformations of the receptor.	• Fluorophore corresponding to the mid-region of the peptide (position 29) behaved in a similar manner to the CCK1R.
• Fluorophore corresponding to the carboxyl terminus of the peptide (position 33) was more accessible to aqueous milieu in the active conformation of the receptor.	• The behavior of the fluorophore corresponding to the carboxyl terminus of the peptide (position 33) was less accessible to the aqueous milieu in the active conformation the receptor.

Top, CCK analogs with a fluorescent alexa indicator at the amino terminus of a CCK-8 analog and a CCK-4 analog were used to examine the microenvironment of the fluorophore as docked to CCK1 or CCK2 receptors (Harikumar et al., 2005a).

Bottom, CCK analogs with a fluorescent aladan indicator at the amino terminus, mid-region, or carboxyl-terminus of CCK were used to examine the microenvironment of the fluorophore as docked to CCK1 or CCK2 receptors. Fluorescence quenching, anisotropy and red edge excitation shifts were examined (Harikumar et al., 2006).

(2.61 and 7.39) are most important for binding the CCK2R selective ligand (Cawston et al., 2012).

EFFECTS OF MEMBRANE CHOLESTEROL ON CCK RECEPTOR FUNCTION

The ability of CCK to induce gallbladder contraction has been shown to be reduced in individuals with cholesterol gallstones (Fridhandler et al., 1983; Lamorte et al., 1985; Behar et al., 1989; Chen et al., 1997; Amaral et al., 2001; Kano et al., 2002). Initially, it was shown that high cholesterol diet (1–1.2%) induced cholesterol stone formation in the gallbladders of animals like prairie dogs and ground squirrels (Fridhandler et al., 1983). Gallbladder muscle contraction in these models was impaired in response to CCK, but it was also impaired in response to acetylcholine and the non-hormonal stimulant potassium (Lamorte et al., 1985). Studies using muscle strips from human gallbladders with cholesterol gallstones have also demonstrated reduced contractility in response to CCK (Behar et al., 1989). Similar effects were observed when studying *in vivo* gallbladder contraction in response to CCK in patients with gallbladder disease (Amaral et al., 2001). More specifically, using isolated human gallbladder smooth muscle strips and single muscle cells, it has been shown that specimens with cholesterol stones exhibit lower cAMP responses compared with those in gallbladders with pigment stones. Hence, it was suggested that the muscle defect responsible for this impairment was at the level of the plasma membrane (Chen et al., 1997).

Indeed the plasma membrane can incorporate excessive amounts of cholesterol in the presence of cholesterol-rich environment by diffusion (Nichols and Pagano, 1981). Studies measuring the amount of membrane-bound esterified [^{3}H]cholesterol in the presence of excessive amounts of unesterified [^{3}H]cholesterol, had already confirmed the existence of this phenomenon in cell types such as erythrocytes (Lange and D'Alessandro, 1977) and rat arterial smooth muscle cells (Slotte and Lundberg, 1983). It was suggested from these observations that membrane cholesterol was a key factor in causing the gallbladder muscle impairment. This was confirmed in a study by Yu et al. (1996), in which they measured the cholesterol content of isolated single muscle cells and plasma membranes from gallbladder muscles from prairie dogs, finding an association of elevated cholesterol with reduced muscle contractility. It was reported that after feeding a high cholesterol (1.2%) diet, cholesterol content, and the molar ratio of cholesterol/phospholipid in plasma membranes of gallbladder muscle increased by 90%, with a parallel decrease in muscle contractility by 58% in response to CCK. Similar changes were observed when normal gallbladder muscle cells were incubated with cholesterol-rich liposomes, an effect which was reversed upon incubation with cholesterol-free liposomes (Yu et al., 1996). These observations were also confirmed in human gallbladder muscle from patients with cholesterol gallstones (Chen et al., 1999; Xiao et al., 1999), where the membrane cholesterol content and cholesterol/phospholipid ratio was significantly higher in gallbladders with cholesterol stones than in those with pigment stones. Membrane anisotropy was also higher in gallbladders from patients with pigment gallstones, reflecting lower membrane fluidity in gallbladders from patients with cholesterol gallstones (Chen et al., 1999).

A report studying CCK signaling in isolated single muscle cells from human gallbladders with cholesterol gallstones demonstrated that the production of IP_3 and diacylglycerol (DAG) was reduced when compared with gallbladders from patients with pigment gallstones (by 80–90% and 78%, respectively) (Yu et al., 1995). However, this effect could be circumvented by stimulating the cells with agents acting directly on G proteins. These results suggested that the defect was proximal to the G protein, at the level of the CCK receptor or its coupling with the G protein (Yu et al., 1995). An illustrative clinical report was published in 1995 that described a patient with morbid obesity and cholesterol gallstone disease in whom the CCK1R was misspliced to yield a non-functional variant missing its third exon (Miller et al., 1995). The frequency of such events is likely extremely low based on another study by the same group (Nardone et al., 1995), in which full length sequencing of the cDNA encoding the CCK1R was shown to be entirely normal in 12 patients with cholesterol gallstones undergoing cholecystectomy (Nardone et al., 1995). Despite normal molecular structure, the function of CCK receptors in patients with cholesterol gallstone disease has been directly shown to be abnormal (Xiao et al., 1999). Of particular interest, the apparent affinity of binding was higher than normal, while the ability of this hormone to stimulate a signaling response was decreased. These abnormalities were reversed after extraction of excess cholesterol from the membrane by incubation with cholesterol-free liposomes (Xiao et al., 1999).

Indeed the impact of membrane cholesterol on this receptor was further explored in manipulatable model systems in 2005 (Harikumar et al., 2005b). This study included extensive analyses of the CCK1R function in lipid-modified environments and showed that normal CCK1R function is dependent on the content of cholesterol in the membrane. In order to monitor the changes in conformation of the CCK1R in the presence of various levels of cholesterol, the study used two different fluorescence-based approaches by measuring anisotropy and lifetimes of a fluorescent full agonist ligand, which shows a decrease in both of these parameters when occupying a receptor in active conformation (Harikumar et al., 2002). Cholesterol depletion from CCK1R-bearing cells using chemical (MβCD chelator) or metabolic (lipoprotein deficient serum supplemented with hydroxymethylglutaryl-CoA reductase inhibitor) methods increased the movement of the label as reflected by decreased anisotropy and reduced lifetime, whereas cholesterol enrichment had the opposite effect. The fluorescence changes in the presence of increased cholesterol were similar to those observed in the presence of a non-hydrolyzable GTP analog which is known to shift the receptor into an inactive, G protein-uncoupled state (Harikumar et al., 2002).

The changes in the conformation of the CCK1R in response to varying amounts of membrane cholesterol are reflected in its ligand binding characteristics and in its biological activity (Harikumar et al., 2005b). Cholesterol depletion was shown to be associated with a reduction in CCK binding affinity, while augmentation of membrane cholesterol content actually increased CCK binding affinity. However, the higher binding in the presence of increased cholesterol was non-productive, resulting in lower biological responsiveness, like the membranes depleted in cholesterol. Notably, the defective intracellular calcium responses to CCK after cholesterol depletion were reversed upon cholesterol repletion. These observations support a defective coupling of the CCK receptor to its G protein in the presence of abnormal membrane cholesterol content (Chen et al., 1997; Xiao et al., 1999).

Other properties such as clathrin-mediated receptor internalization after agonist occupation, and receptor recycling were unaffected by modulation of the membrane cholesterol content, although these regulatory processes have been described to be abnormal after modification of membrane sphingolipid content. This indicates that two different lipid components by themselves or in combination with other lipid components of the plasma membrane probably induce different conformational changes to the CCK1R which can lead to either defective G protein coupling (in case of cholesterol), or disruption in the internalization and recycling pathways (sphingolipid) of the CCK1R. These are reflected by the differences in the observed effects on binding, signaling, and receptor internalization (Harikumar et al., 2005b). However, it is still unclear whether these effects of modification of cholesterol and sphingolipids reflect events occurring in the bulk phase of the plasma membrane or within rafts. Nevertheless, these insights have added a new dimension to our understanding of CCK receptor biology.

POSSIBLE STRUCTURAL BASIS FOR THE DIFFERENTIAL SENSITIVITY OF CCK RECEPTORS TO CHOLESTEROL

In contrast, the other subtype of CCK receptor, the CCK2R, is not sensitive to alterations in membrane cholesterol (Potter et al., 2012). As noted earlier, these receptors are highly homologous and, in fact, share all of the predicted cholesterol binding motifs (**Figure 1**). The key structural determinant for cholesterol sensitivity appears to reside in the third exon of the CCK1R which encodes most of the transmembrane segment three and four, including one CRAC motif and one CCM motif (Potter et al., 2012). It should be noted that the CCK1R and CCK2R do not contain the entire four-component strict-CCM, but a less restrictive CCM motif that is shared by 44% of human class A GPCRs (Hanson et al., 2008). This is due to the absence of an aromatic residue at 2.41. The relevant contributors to this effect were further studied with site-directed mutants (Potter et al., 2012). This suggested that three residues, Y140 (Y3.51), which is a part of the CRAC motif (Li and Papadopoulos, 1998) in transmembrane segment three, W166 (W4.50), which is a part of the CCM (Hanson et al., 2008) in transmembrane segment four and Y237 (Y5.66), which is part of the CRAC motif in transmembrane segment five, are important for the cholesterol sensitivity of the CCK1R. It is noteworthy that mutation of each of the three residues has negative effects on either CCK binding or CCK-induced signaling. Mutation of Y140 to alanine leads to reduced signaling but increased CCK binding affinity and is insensitive to reduction in membrane cholesterol levels. On the other hand, mutation of W166 to alanine leads to decreased CCK binding and signaling ability of the CCK1R, with a further reduction in signaling upon depleting membrane cholesterol. The Y237A mutant displays no change in signaling, but reduced CCK binding affinity, whereas cholesterol reduction results in the reduction of both parameters. Corresponding single residue mutations (Y153A, W179A, Y246A) within the CRAC and the CCM motifs of the CCK2R did not modify receptor function.

It is remarkable that mutation of only Y140 residue within the CRAC motif within transmembrane segment three resulted in loss of cholesterol sensitivity of the CCK1R (Potter et al., 2012). This implies a defective conformation of the receptor, particularly because the mutation alters the conserved (D/E) 3.49-R3.50-Y3.51 motif, and thus its ability to mediate the differential effects of cholesterol in the two structurally related receptors is compromised. However, studies with other class A GPCRs have shown that the mutation of Y3.51 of the D/ERY motif does not affect the ligand binding affinity or receptor trafficking, and has no or marginal effects on receptor signaling (Ohyama et al., 2002; Gaborik et al., 2003; Proulx et al., 2008). So, it appears that probably this residue is specifically responsible for the differential cholesterol sensitivity observed between the CCK receptors. This implies that the transmembrane segment three CRAC cholesterol binding motif could be responsible for the cholesterol sensitivity of the CCK1R, because the transmembrane segment four CCM (W166) and transmembrane segment five CRAC (Y237) mutants are still sensitive to cholesterol. However, the transmembrane segment three CRAC cholesterol-binding motif is essentially the same in both the CCK receptors, differing only in the presence of lysine in CCK1R and an arginine in the CCK2R. Both the residues which are a part of the consensus motif have similar properties.

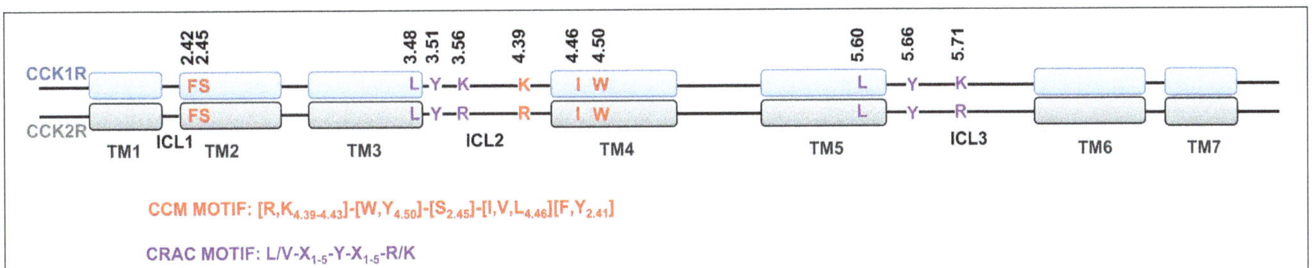

FIGURE 1 | Schematic representation of the alignment of structural segments of the CCK1R and CCK2R. The CCM (red) and the CRAC (violet) are highlighted within the transmembrane segments (rectangles) and intracellular loops (black line) of the CCK1R (top, blue) and CCK2R (bottom, gray).

While the sequence surrounding the motif is largely similar, they do exhibit minor differences between the two receptors that could contribute to the observed difference in the cholesterol sensitivity.

These observations show that the presence of a CRAC or/and CCM motif do not necessarily mean that the receptor is sensitive to cholesterol. At least in the case of the CCK receptors, it appears that the subtype specific conformational changes are conferred by the differences in direct interaction of the membrane cholesterol with the two receptors. It has been shown in the case of the human cannabinoid receptors (CBR), that the type 1 CBR (CB1R) is affected by manipulations in the membrane cholesterol content, in a way similar to the CCK1R exhibiting defective ligand binding and signaling, as well as its localization to membrane rafts (Bari et al., 2005a,b). On the other hand, similar to CCK2R, the type 2 CBR (CB2R) does not share this sensitivity to membrane cholesterol (Bari et al., 2005a,b). In fact it was found that CB1R possesses a CRAC motif in transmembrane segment seven that differs by one residue from that in the CB2R, and the corresponding mutation rendered CB1R insensitive to membrane cholesterol similar to CB2R (Oddi et al., 2011). This explains that cholesterol binding motifs outside of the CCM can have a significant influence on receptor signaling and trafficking.

In addition to this, other possibilities for the differential sensitivity of CCK receptors may be related to the indirect impact of the cholesterol on the processes like mechanism of ligand binding or receptor trafficking. As mentioned earlier, the CCK1R and the CCK2R bind the same CCK peptide ligand differently (Silvente-Poirot and Wank, 1996; Dong et al., 2005; Harikumar et al., 2005a, 2006). The peptide ligand binds to extracellular loops and the amino-terminal tail of the CCK1R, whereas in the CCK2R, the carboxyl-terminal end of the peptide ligand may dip into the helical bundle (Harikumar et al., 2005a, 2006). It can be postulated that in the case of CCK2R the peptide binding within the helical bundle could potentially stabilize it and consequently the intracellular regions as well, and prevent the negative impact of changing membrane cholesterol. On the other hand, the impact of membrane cholesterol cannot be overcome in the case of the CCK1R because the conformational changes affecting the extracellular regions binding the ligand are very different to that conferred to the part of the receptor within the lipid bilayer. So, these differential changes on the domains of the receptors which are physically further away, may dictate the observed effects of cholesterol sensitivity in the CCK1R.

Other processes occurring post ligand binding can also be affected by changes in membrane cholesterol, which can contribute to the observed effects. In the case of CCK1R, the receptor has been described to occupy a unique plasma membrane compartment after CCK stimulation of rat pancreatic acinar cells (Roettger et al., 1995). This was called as a site of "insulation" that is comparatively devoid of G proteins, in which the lateral mobility of the CCK receptor is markedly reduced as another highly specialized cellular mechanism of desensitization (Roettger et al., 1999). Accordingly, it can be postulated that the membrane cholesterol can cause similar changes to the CCK1R, however, there is no information yet about the existence of a similar mechanism for CCK2R. Also, whether the CCK receptors are located in the lipid rafts, and if the cholesterol modulation effects are exclusive to these regions remains to be investigated.

CONCLUSION AND THERAPEUTIC PERSPECTIVES

It is clear that lipid-protein interactions, especially cholesterol-receptor interactions, involved in the function of GPCRs can be extremely important. More specifically, this review has focused on the role of cholesterol in the function of the CCK1R, an important receptor likely to be involved in pathologic states such as obesity and metabolic syndrome. A better understanding of the mechanisms of appetite regulation that contribute to the development of obesity could provide insights into the prevention and more effective treatment of this disorder. The gastrointestinal hormones like CCK play important roles in servomechanisms involved in regulating nutritional homeostasis. The observations showing that elevated membrane cholesterol reduce the effectiveness of stimulus-activity coupling activated by CCK action at the CCK1R provide vital information regarding the pathological phenomenon associated with CCK receptor dysfunction. It is essential and would be very interesting to study the membrane environment of the CCK1R receptor in obese patients, in order to verify these observations in humans. Additionally, it would be very exciting to study whether the mutations affecting the cholesterol sensitivity might also be present in these patients. Overall, the observations so far may suggest that elevated levels of membrane cholesterol described in cholesterol gallstone disease and metabolic syndrome could reduce hormone-stimulated signaling and, thereby, reduce the feedback inhibition of food consumption that is an essential servomechanism. If this is proven true in patients, the CCK1R can become the target for future development of positive allosteric modulators that could "recalibrate," and consequently "normalize" this important regulatory mechanism.

ACKNOWLEDGMENTS

We thank Dr. K. G. Harikumar for critical input on the manuscript and insightful discussions. This work was supported by a grant from the National Institutes of Health (DK32878).

REFERENCES

Adamian, L., Naveed, H., and Liang, J. (2011). Lipid-binding surfaces of membrane proteins: evidence from evolutionary and structural analysis. *Biochim. Biophys. Acta* 1808, 1092–1102.

Albert, A. D., Young, J. E., and Yeagle, P. L. (1996). Rhodopsin-cholesterol interactions in bovine rod outer segment disk membranes. *Biochim. Biophys. Acta* 1285, 47–55.

Amaral, J., Xiao, Z. L., Chen, Q., Yu, P., Biancani, P., and Behar, J. (2001). Gallbladder muscle dysfunction in patients with chronic acalculous disease. *Gastroenterology* 120, 506–511.

Aquino, C. J., Armour, D. R., Berman, J. M., Birkemo, L. S., Carr, R. A., Croom, D. K., et al. (1996). Discovery of 1, 5-benzodiazepines with peripheral cholecystokinin (CCK-A) receptor agonist activity. 1. Optimization of the agonist "trigger". *J. Med. Chem.* 39, 562–569.

Attwood, P. V., and Gutfreund, H. (1980). The application of pressure relaxation to the study of the equilibrium between metarhodopsin I and II from bovine retinas. *FEBS Lett.* 119, 323–326.

Ballesteros, J. A., and Weinstein, H. (1992). Analysis and refinement of criteria for predicting the structure and relative orientations of transmembranal helical domains. *Biophys. J.* 62, 107–109.

Bari, M., Battista, N., Fezza, F., Finazzi-Agro, A., and Maccarrone, M. (2005a). Lipid rafts control signaling of type-1 cannabinoid receptors in neuronal cells. Implications for anandamide-induced apoptosis. *J. Biol. Chem.* 280, 12212–12220.

Bari, M., Paradisi, A., Pasquariello, N., and Maccarrone, M. (2005b). Cholesterol-dependent modulation of type 1 cannabinoid receptors in nerve cells. *J. Neurosci. Res.* 81, 275–283.

Beglinger, C., Degen, L., Matzinger, D., D'Amato, M., and Drewe, J. (2001). Loxiglumide, a CCK-A receptor antagonist, stimulates calorie intake and hunger feelings in humans. *Am. J. Physiol. Regul. Integr. Comp. Physiol.* 280, R1149–R1154.

Behar, J., Lee, K. Y., Thompson, W. R., and Biancani, P. (1989). Gallbladder contraction in patients with pigment and cholesterol stones. *Gastroenterology* 97, 1479–1484.

Ben-Arie, N., Gileadi, C., and Schramm, M. (1988). Interaction of the beta-adrenergic receptor with Gs following delipidation. Specific lipid requirements for Gs activation and GTPase function. *Eur. J. Biochem.* 176, 649–654.

Bennett, M. P., and Mitchell, D. C. (2008). Regulation of membrane proteins by dietary lipids: effects of cholesterol and docosahexaenoic acid acyl chain-containing phospholipids on rhodopsin stability and function. *Biophys. J.* 95, 1206–1216.

Brown, D. A., and Rose, J. K. (1992). Sorting of GPI-anchored proteins to glycolipid-enriched membrane subdomains during transport to the apical cell surface. *Cell* 68, 533–544.

Cawston, E. E., Lam, P. C., Harikumar, K. G., Dong, M., Ball, A. M., Augustine, M. L., et al. (2012). Molecular basis for binding and subtype selectivity of 1, 4-benzodiazepine antagonist ligands of the cholecystokinin receptor. *J. Biol. Chem.* 287, 18618–18635.

Chen, Q., Amaral, J., Biancani, P., and Behar, J. (1999). Excess membrane cholesterol alters human gallbladder muscle contractility and membrane fluidity. *Gastroenterology* 116, 678–685.

Chen, Q., Amaral, J., Oh, S., Biancani, P., and Behar, J. (1997). Gallbladder relaxation in patients with pigment and cholesterol stones. *Gastroenterology* 113, 930–937.

Cohen, A. W., Hnasko, R., Schubert, W., and Lisanti, M. P. (2004). Role of caveolae and caveolins in health and disease. *Physiol. Rev.* 84, 1341–1379.

Colozo, A. T., Park, P. S., Sum, C. S., Pisterzi, L. F., and Wells, J. W. (2007). Cholesterol as a determinant of cooperativity in the M2 muscarinic cholinergic receptor. *Biochem. Pharmacol.* 74, 236–255.

Darrow, J. W., Hadac, E. M., Miller, L. J., and Sugg, E. E. (1998). Structurally similar small molecule photoaffinity CCK-A agonists and antagonists as novel tools for directly probing 7TM receptors-ligand interactions. *Bioorg. Med. Chem. Lett.* 8, 3127–3132.

Ding, X. Q., Dolu, V., Hadac, E. M., Holicky, E. L., Pinon, D. I., Lybrand, T. P., et al. (2001). Refinement of the structure of the ligand-occupied cholecystokinin receptor using a photolabile amino-terminal probe. *J. Biol. Chem.* 276, 4236–4244.

Dong, M., Ding, X. Q., Thomas, S. E., Gao, F., Lam, P. C., Abagyan, R., et al. (2007). Role of lysine187 within the second extracellular loop of the type A cholecystokinin receptor in agonist-induced activation. Use of complementary charge-reversal mutagenesis to define a functionally important interdomain interaction. *Biochemistry* 46, 4522–4531.

Dong, M., Liu, G., Pinon, D. I., and Miller, L. J. (2005). Differential docking of high-affinity peptide ligands to type A and B cholecystokinin receptors demonstrated by photoaffinity labeling. *Biochemistry* 44, 6693–6700.

Dufresne, M., Seva, C., and Fourmy, D. (2006). Cholecystokinin and gastrin receptors. *Physiol. Rev.* 86, 805–847.

Duggan, K. A., Hams, G., and Macdonald, G. J. (1988). Modification of renal and tissue cation transport by cholecystokinin octapeptide in the rabbit. *J. Physiol.* 397, 527–538.

Eroglu, C., Brugger, B., Wieland, F., and Sinning, I. (2003). Glutamate-binding affinity of Drosophila metabotropic glutamate receptor is modulated by association with lipid rafts. *Proc. Natl. Acad. Sci. U.S.A.* 100, 10219–10224.

Eysselein, V. E., Eberlein, G. A., Hesse, W. H., Schaeffer, M., Grandt, D., Williams, R., et al. (1990). Molecular variants of cholecystokinin after endogenous stimulation in humans: a time study. *Am. J. Physiol.* 258, G951–G957.

Fridhandler, T. M., Davison, J. S., and Shaffer, E. A. (1983). Defective gallbladder contractility in the ground squirrel and prairie dog during the early stages of cholesterol gallstone formation. *Gastroenterology* 85, 830–836.

Gaborik, Z., Jagadeesh, G., Zhang, M., Spat, A., Catt, K. J., and Hunyady, L. (2003). The role of a conserved region of the second intracellular loop in AT1 angiotensin receptor activation and signaling. *Endocrinology* 144, 2220–2228.

Gao, F., Sexton, P. M., Christopoulos, A., and Miller, L. J. (2008). Benzodiazepine ligands can act as allosteric modulators of the Type 1 cholecystokinin receptor. *Bioorg. Med. Chem. Lett.* 18, 4401–4404.

Genedani, S., Carone, C., Guidolin, D., Filaferro, M., Marcellino, D., Fuxe, K., et al. (2010). Differential sensitivity of A2A and especially D2 receptor trafficking to cocaine compared with lipid rafts in cotransfected CHO cell lines. Novel actions of cocaine independent of the DA transporter. *J. Mol. Neurosci.* 41, 347–357.

Gimpl, G., Burger, K., and Fahrenholz, F. (1997). Cholesterol as modulator of receptor function. *Biochemistry* 36, 10959–10974.

Gimpl, G., and Fahrenholz, F. (2002). Cholesterol as stabilizer of the oxytocin receptor. *Biochim. Biophys. Acta* 1564, 384–392.

Gimpl, G., Wiegand, V., Burger, K., and Fahrenholz, F. (2002). Cholesterol and steroid hormones: modulators of oxytocin receptor function. *Prog. Brain Res.* 139, 43–55.

Hadac, E. M., Dawson, E. S., Darrow, J. W., Sugg, E. E., Lybrand, T. P., and Miller, L. J. (2006). Novel benzodiazepine photoaffinity probe stereoselectively labels a site deep within the membrane-spanning domain of the cholecystokinin receptor. *J. Med. Chem.* 49, 850–863.

Hanson, M. A., Cherezov, V., Griffith, M. T., Roth, C. B., Jaakola, V. P., Chien, E. Y., et al. (2008). A specific cholesterol binding site is established by the 2.8 A structure of the human beta2-adrenergic receptor. *Structure* 16, 897–905.

Harikumar, K. G., Clain, J., Pinon, D. I., Dong, M., and Miller, L. J. (2005a). Distinct molecular mechanisms for agonist peptide binding to types A and B cholecystokinin receptors demonstrated using fluorescence spectroscopy. *J. Biol. Chem.* 280, 1044–1050.

Harikumar, K. G., Puri, V., Singh, R. D., Hanada, K., Pagano, R. E., and Miller, L. J. (2005b). Differential effects of modification of membrane cholesterol and sphingolipids on the conformation, function, and trafficking of the G protein-coupled cholecystokinin receptor. *J. Biol. Chem.* 280, 2176–2185.

Harikumar, K. G., and Miller, L. J. (2005). Fluorescence resonance energy transfer analysis of the antagonist- and partial agonist-occupied states of the cholecystokinin receptor. *J. Biol. Chem.* 280, 18631–18635.

Harikumar, K. G., Pinon, D. I., and Miller, L. J. (2006). Fluorescent indicators distributed throughout the pharmacophore of cholecystokinin provide insights into distinct modes of binding and activation of type A and B cholecystokinin receptors. *J. Biol. Chem.* 281, 27072–27080.

Harikumar, K. G., Pinon, D. I., Wessels, W. S., Dawson, E. S., Lybrand, T. P., Prendergast, F. G., et al. (2004). Measurement of intermolecular distances for the natural agonist Peptide docked at the cholecystokinin receptor expressed *in situ* using fluorescence resonance energy transfer. *Mol. Pharmacol.* 65, 28–35.

Harikumar, K. G., Pinon, D. I., Wessels, W. S., Prendergast, F. G., and Miller, L. J. (2002). Environment and mobility of a series of fluorescent reporters at the amino terminus of structurally related peptide agonists and antagonists bound to the cholecystokinin receptor. *J. Biol. Chem.* 277, 18552–18560.

Harper, A. A., and Raper, H. S. (1943). Pancreozymin, a stimulant of the secretion of pancreatic enzymes in extracts of the small intestine. *J. Physiol.* 102, 115–125.

Herranz, R. (2003). Cholecystokinin antagonists: pharmacological and therapeutic potential. *Med. Res. Rev.* 23, 559–605.

Huang, P., Xu, W., Yoon, S. I., Chen, C., Chong, P. L., and Liu-Chen, L. Y. (2007). Cholesterol reduction by methyl-beta-cyclodextrin attenuates the delta opioid receptor-mediated signaling in neuronal cells but enhances it in non-neuronal cells. *Biochem. Pharmacol.* 73, 534–549.

Ipsen, J. H., Karlstrom, G., Mouritsen, O. G., Wennerstrom, H., and Zuckermann, M. J. (1987). Phase equilibria in the phosphatidylcholine-cholesterol system. *Biochim. Biophys. Acta* 905, 162–172.

Jafurulla, M., Tiwari, S., and Chattopadhyay, A. (2011). Identification of cholesterol recognition amino acid consensus (CRAC) motif in G-protein coupled receptors. *Biochem. Biophys. Res. Commun.* 404, 569–573.

Kalindjian, S. B., and McDonald, I. M. (2007). Strategies for the design of non-peptide CCK2 receptor agonist and antagonist ligand. *Curr. Top. Med. Chem.* 7, 1195–1204.

Kano, M., Shoda, J., Satoh, S., Kobayashi, M., Matsuzaki, Y., Abei, M., et al. (2002). Increased expression of gallbladder cholecystokinin: a receptor in prairie dogs fed a high-cholesterol diet and its dissociation with decreased contractility in response to cholecystokinin. *J. Lab. Clin. Med.* 139, 285–294.

Kerstens, P. J., Lamers, C. B., Jansen, J. B., De Jong, A. J., Hessels, M., and Hafkenscheid, J. C. (1985). Physiological plasma concentrations of cholecystokinin stimulate pancreatic enzyme secretion and gallbladder contraction in man. *Life Sci.* 36, 565–569.

Kissileff, H. R., Pi-Sunyer, F. X., Thornton, J., and Smith, G. P. (1981). C-terminal octapeptide of cholecystokinin decreases food intake in man. *Am. J. Clin. Nutr.* 34, 154–160.

Kopin, A. S., Beinborn, M., Lee, Y. M., McBride, E. W., and Quinn, S. M. (1994). The CCK-B/gastrin receptor. Identification of amino acids that determine nonpeptide antagonist affinity. *Ann. N.Y. Acad. Sci.* 713, 67–78.

Kopin, A. S., Lee, Y. M., McBride, E. W., Miller, L. J., Lu, M., Lin, H. Y., et al. (1992). Expression cloning and characterization of the canine parietal cell gastrin receptor. *Proc. Natl. Acad. Sci. U.S.A.* 89, 3605–3609.

Kopin, A. S., McBride, E. W., Quinn, S. M., Kolakowski, L. F. Jr., and Beinborn, M. (1995). The role of the cholecystokinin-B/gastrin receptor transmembrane domains in determining affinity for subtype-selective ligands. *J. Biol. Chem.* 270, 5019–5023.

Ladines, C. A., Zeng, C., Asico, L. D., Sun, X., Pocchiari, F., Semeraro, C., et al. (2001). Impaired renal D(1)-like and D(2)-like dopamine receptor interaction in the spontaneously hypertensive rat. *Am. J. Physiol. Regul. Integr. Comp. Physiol.* 281, R1071–R1078.

Lagane, B., Gaibelet, G., Meilhoc, E., Masson, J. M., Cezanne, L., and Lopez, A. (2000). Role of sterols in modulating the human mu-opioid receptor function in *Saccharomyces cerevisiae*. *J. Biol. Chem.* 275, 33197–33200.

Lamorte, W. W., Brotschi, E. A., Scott, T. E., and Williams, L. F. Jr. (1985). Pigment gallstone formation in the cholesterol-fed guinea pig. *Hepatology* 5, 21–27.

Lange, Y., and D'Alessandro, J. S. (1977). Characterization of mechanisms for transfer of cholesterol between human erythrocytes and plasma. *Biochemistry* 16, 4339–4343.

Lee, A. G. (2004). How lipids affect the activities of integral membrane proteins. *Biochim. Biophys. Acta* 1666, 62–87.

Li, H., and Papadopoulos, V. (1998). Peripheral-type benzodiazepine receptor function in cholesterol transport. Identification of a putative cholesterol recognition/interaction amino acid sequence and consensus pattern. *Endocrinology* 139, 4991–4997.

Meyer, B. H., Segura, J. M., Martinez, K. L., Hovius, R., George, N., Johnsson, K., et al. (2006). FRET imaging reveals that functional neurokinin-1 receptors are monomeric and reside in membrane microdomains of live cells. *Proc. Natl. Acad. Sci. U.S.A.* 103, 2138–2143.

Miao, L., Nielsen, M., Thewalt, J., Ipsen, J. H., Bloom, M., Zuckermann, M. J., et al. (2002). From lanosterol to cholesterol: structural evolution and differential effects on lipid bilayers. *Biophys. J.* 82, 1429–1444.

Miller, L. J., and Gao, F. (2008). Structural basis of cholecystokinin receptor binding and regulation. *Pharmacol. Ther.* 119, 83–95.

Miller, L. J., Holicky, E. L., Ulrich, C. D., and Wieben, E. D. (1995). Abnormal processing of the human cholecystokinin receptor gene in association with gallstones and obesity. *Gastroenterology* 109, 1375–1380.

Miller, L. J., Jardine, I., Weissman, E., Go, V. L., and Speicher, D. (1984). Characterization of cholecystokinin from the human brain. *J. Neurochem.* 43, 835–840.

Miller, L. J., and Lybrand, T. P. (2002). Molecular basis of agonist binding to the type A cholecystokinin receptor. *Pharmacol. Toxicol.* 91, 282–285.

Mitchell, D. C., Straume, M., Miller, J. L., and Litman, B. J. (1990). Modulation of metarhodopsin formation by cholesterol-induced ordering of bilayer lipids. *Biochemistry* 29, 9143–9149.

Monastyrskaya, K., Hostettler, A., Buergi, S., and Draeger, A. (2005). The NK1 receptor localizes to the plasma membrane microdomains, and its activation is dependent on lipid raft integrity. *J. Biol. Chem.* 280, 7135–7146.

Mouritsen, O. G., and Zuckermann, M. J. (2004). What's so special about cholesterol? *Lipids* 39, 1101–1113.

Nardone, G., Ferber, I. A., and Miller, L. J. (1995). The integrity of the cholecystokinin receptor gene in gallbladder disease and obesity. *Hepatology* 22, 1751–1753.

Nguyen, D. H., and Taub, D. (2002a). Cholesterol is essential for macrophage inflammatory protein 1 beta binding and conformational integrity of CC chemokine receptor 5. *Blood* 99, 4298–4306.

Nguyen, D. H., and Taub, D. (2002b). CXCR4 function requires membrane cholesterol: implications for HIV infection. *J. Immunol.* 168, 4121–4126.

Nguyen, D. H., and Taub, D. D. (2003). Inhibition of chemokine receptor function by membrane cholesterol oxidation. *Exp. Cell Res.* 291, 36–45.

Nichols, J. W., and Pagano, R. E. (1981). Kinetics of soluble lipid monomer diffusion between vesicles. *Biochemistry* 20, 2783–2789.

Niu, S. L., Mitchell, D. C., and Litman, B. J. (2002). Manipulation of cholesterol levels in rod disk membranes by methyl-beta-cyclodextrin: effects on receptor activation. *J. Biol. Chem.* 277, 20139–20145.

Noble, F. (2007). Pharmacology of CCKRs and SAR studies of peptidic analog ligands. *Curr. Top. Med. Chem.* 7, 1173–1179.

Noble, F., and Roques, B. P. (1999). CCK-B receptor: chemistry, molecular biology, biochemistry and pharmacology. *Prog. Neurobiol.* 58, 349–379.

Oddi, S., Dainese, E., Fezza, F., Lanuti, M., Barcaroli, D., De Laurenzi, V., et al. (2011). Functional characterization of putative cholesterol binding sequence (CRAC) in human type-1 cannabinoid receptor. *J. Neurochem.* 116, 858–865.

Ohvo-Rekila, H., Ramstedt, B., Leppimaki, P., and Slotte, J. P. (2002). Cholesterol interactions with phospholipids in membranes. *Prog. Lipid Res.* 41, 66–97.

Ohyama, K., Yamano, Y., Sano, T., Nakagomi, Y., Wada, M., and Inagami, T. (2002). Role of the conserved DRY motif on G protein activation of rat angiotensin II receptor type 1A. *Biochem. Biophys. Res. Commun.* 292, 362–367.

Okamoto, T., Schlegel, A., Scherer, P. E., and Lisanti, M. P. (1998). Caveolins, a family of scaffolding proteins for organizing "preassembled signaling complexes" at the plasma membrane. *J. Biol. Chem.* 273, 5419–5422.

Ostrom, R. S., and Insel, P. A. (2004). The evolving role of lipid rafts and caveolae in G protein-coupled receptor signaling: implications for molecular pharmacology. *Br. J. Pharmacol.* 143, 235–245.

Paila, Y. D., Tiwari, S., and Chattopadhyay, A. (2009). Are specific nonannular cholesterol binding sites present in G-protein coupled receptors? *Biochim. Biophys. Acta* 1788, 295–302.

Pang, L., Graziano, M., and Wang, S. (1999). Membrane cholesterol modulates galanin-GalR2 interaction. *Biochemistry* 38, 12003–12011.

Pike, L. J. (2003). Lipid rafts: bringing order to chaos. *J. Lipid Res.* 44, 655–667.

Pontier, S. M., Percherancier, Y., Galandrin, S., Breit, A., Gales, C., and Bouvier, M. (2008). Cholesterol-dependent separation of the beta2-adrenergic receptor from its partners determines signaling efficacy: insight into nanoscale organization of signal transduction. *J. Biol. Chem.* 283, 24659–24672.

Potter, R. M., Harikumar, K. G., Wu, S. V., and Miller, L. J. (2012). Differential sensitivity of types 1 and 2 cholecystokinin receptors to membrane cholesterol. *J. Lipid Res.* 53, 137–148.

Proulx, C. D., Holleran, B. J., Boucard, A. A., Escher, E., Guillemette, G., and Leduc, R. (2008). Mutational analysis of the conserved Asp2.50 and ERY motif reveals signaling bias of the urotensin II receptor. *Mol. Pharmacol.* 74, 552–561.

Pucadyil, T. J., and Chattopadhyay, A. (2004). Cholesterol modulates ligand binding and G-protein coupling to serotonin(1A) receptors from bovine hippocampus. *Biochim. Biophys. Acta* 1663, 188–200.

Pucadyil, T. J., and Chattopadhyay, A. (2005). Cholesterol modulates the antagonist-binding function of hippocampal serotonin1A receptors. *Biochim. Biophys. Acta* 1714, 35–42.

Rao, R. V., Roettger, B. F., Hadac, E. M., and Miller, L. J. (1997). Roles of cholecystokinin receptor phosphorylation in agonist-stimulated desensitization of pancreatic acinar cells and receptor-bearing Chinese hamster ovary cholecystokinin receptor cells. *Mol. Pharmacol.* 51, 185–192.

Rehfeld, J. F. (1978). Immunochemical studies on cholecystokinin. II. Distribution and molecular heterogeneity in the central nervous system and small intestine of man and hog. *J. Biol. Chem.* 253, 4022–4030.

Rehfeld, J. F., Sun, G., Christensen, T., and Hillingso, J. G. (2001). The predominant cholecystokinin in human plasma and intestine is cholecystokinin-33. *J. Clin. Endocrinol. Metab.* 86, 251–258.

Reubi, J. C., Waser, B., Laderach, U., Stettler, C., Friess, H., Halter, F., et al. (1997). Localization of cholecystokinin A and cholecystokinin B-gastrin receptors in the human stomach. *Gastroenterology* 112, 1197–1205.

Roettger, B. F., Pinon, D. I., Burghardt, T. P., and Miller, L. J. (1999). Regulation of lateral mobility and cellular trafficking of the CCK receptor by a partial agonist. *Am. J. Physiol.* 276, C539–C547.

Roettger, B. F., Rentsch, R. U., Hadac, E. M., Hellen, E. H., Burghardt, T. P., and Miller, L. J. (1995). Insulation of a G protein-coupled receptor on the plasmalemmal surface of the pancreatic acinar cell. *J. Cell Biol.* 130, 579–590.

Ruprecht, J. J., Mielke, T., Vogel, R., Villa, C., and Schertler, G. F. (2004). Electron crystallography reveals the structure of metarhodopsin I. *EMBO J.* 23, 3609–3620.

Schmitz, F., Goke, M. N., Otte, J. M., Schrader, H., Reimann, B., Kruse, M. L., et al. (2001). Cellular expression of CCK-A and CCK-B/gastrin receptors in human gastric mucosa. *Regul. Pept.* 102, 101–110.

Schroeder, F., Frolov, A. A., Murphy, E. J., Atshaves, B. P., Jefferson, J. R., Pu, L., et al. (1996). Recent advances in membrane cholesterol domain dynamics and intracellular cholesterol trafficking. *Proc. Soc. Exp. Biol. Med.* 213, 150–177.

Shaw, A. S. (2006). Lipid rafts: now you see them, now you don't. *Nat. Immunol.* 7, 1139–1142.

Silvente-Poirot, S., and Wank, S. A. (1996). A segment of five amino acids in the second extracellular loop of the cholecystokinin-B receptor is essential for selectivity of the peptide agonist gastrin. *J. Biol. Chem.* 271, 14698–14706.

Sjogren, B., Hamblin, M. W., and Svenningsson, P. (2006). Cholesterol depletion reduces serotonin binding and signaling via human 5-HT(7(a)) receptors. *Eur. J. Pharmacol.* 552, 1–10.

Slotte, J. P., and Lundberg, B. (1983). Transfer of [3H]cholesterol between lipid vesicles and rat arterial smooth muscle cells *in vitro*. *Biochim. Biophys. Acta* 750, 434–439.

Smith, G. P., and Gibbs, J. (1985). The satiety effect of cholecystokinin. Recent progress and current problems. *Ann. N.Y. Acad. Sci.* 448, 417–423.

Von Schrenck, T., Ahrens, M., De Weerth, A., Bobrowski, C., Wolf, G., Jonas, L., et al. (2000). CCKB/gastrin receptors mediate changes in sodium and potassium absorption in the isolated perfused rat kidney. *Kidney Int* 58, 995–1003.

Xiao, Z. L., Chen, Q., Amaral, J., Biancani, P., Jensen, R. T., and Behar, J. (1999). CCK receptor dysfunction in muscle membranes from human gallbladders with cholesterol stones. *Am. J. Physiol.* 276, G1401–G1407.

Xu, W., Yoon, S. I., Huang, P., Wang, Y., Chen, C., Chong, P. L., et al. (2006). Localization of the kappa opioid receptor in lipid rafts. *J. Pharmacol. Exp. Ther.* 317, 1295–1306.

Yu, P., Chen, Q., Biancani, P., and Behar, J. (1996). Membrane cholesterol alters gallbladder muscle contractility in prairie dogs. *Am. J. Physiol.* 271, G56–G61.

Yu, P., Chen, Q., Harnett, K. M., Amaral, J., Biancani, P., and Behar, J. (1995). Direct G protein activation reverses impaired CCK signaling in human gallbladders with cholesterol stones. *Am. J. Physiol.* 269, G659–G665.

Yu, P., Yang, Z., Jones, J. E., Wang, Z., Owens, S. A., Mueller, S. C., et al. (2004). D1 dopamine receptor signaling involves caveolin-2 in HEK-293 cells. *Kidney Int.* 66, 2167–2180.

10

Desensitization, trafficking, and resensitization of the pituitary thyrotropin-releasing hormone receptor

Patricia M. Hinkle[1]*, Austin U. Gehret[2] and Brian W. Jones[3]

[1] Department of Pharmacology and Physiology, University of Rochester Medical Center, Rochester, NY, USA
[2] Department of Science and Mathematics, National Technical Institute for the Deaf, Rochester Institute of Technology, Rochester, NY, USA
[3] Department of Pharmacology, University of Washington, Seattle, WA, USA

Edited by:
Liliane Schoofs, Catholic University of Leuven, Belgium

Reviewed by:
Perry Barrett, University of Aberdeen, UK
Leo T. Lee, The University of Hong Kong, Hong Kong

***Correspondence:**
Patricia M. Hinkle, Department of Pharmacology and Physiology, University of Rochester Medical Center, 601 Elmwood Avenue Rochester, Rochester, NY 14642, USA.
e-mail: patricia_hinkle@urmc.rochester.edu

The pituitary receptor for thyrotropin-releasing hormone (TRH) is a calcium-mobilizing G protein-coupled receptor (GPCR) that signals through Gq/11, elevating calcium, and activating protein kinase C. TRH receptor signaling is quickly desensitized as a consequence of receptor phosphorylation, arrestin binding, and internalization. Following activation, TRH receptors are phosphorylated at multiple Ser/Thr residues in the cytoplasmic tail. Phosphorylation catalyzed by GPCR kinase 2 (GRK2) takes place rapidly, reaching a maximum within seconds. Arrestins bind to two phosphorylated regions, but only arrestin bound to the proximal region causes desensitization and internalization. Phosphorylation at Thr365 is critical for these responses. TRH receptors internalize in clathrin-coated vesicles with bound arrestin. Following endocytosis, vesicles containing phosphorylated TRH receptors soon merge with rab5-positive vesicles. Over approximately 20 min these form larger endosomes rich in rab4 and rab5, early sorting endosomes. After TRH is removed from the medium, dephosphorylated receptors start to accumulate in rab4-positive, rab5-negative recycling endosomes. The mechanisms responsible for sorting dephosphorylated receptors to recycling endosomes are unknown. TRH receptors from internal pools help repopulate the plasma membrane. Dephosphorylation of TRH receptors begins when TRH is removed from the medium regardless of receptor localization, although dephosphorylation is fastest when the receptor is on the plasma membrane. Protein phosphatase 1 is involved in dephosphorylation but the details of how the enzyme is targeted to the receptor remain obscure. It is likely that future studies will identify biased ligands for the TRH receptor, novel arrestin-dependent signaling pathways, mechanisms responsible for targeting kinases and phosphatases to the receptor, and principles governing receptor trafficking.

Keywords: dephosphorylation, desensitization, internalization, phosphorylation, Rab, thyrotropin-releasing hormone, trafficking, TRH receptor

INTRODUCTION

Thyrotropin-releasing hormone (TRH), a hypothalamic tripeptide, sits atop the hypothalamic/pituitary/thyroid axis, stimulating release of thyrotropin from the anterior pituitary gland. TRH also stimulates prolactin secretion (**Figure 1**). Initially characterized in clonal rat pituitary cell lines, TRH binding sites were later identified in brain membranes (Hinkle and Tashjian, 1973; Burt and Snyder, 1975). The link between TRH receptors and G proteins was made at a time when heterotrimeric G proteins were thought to transduce signals only from receptors coupled to adenylyl cyclase (Hinkle and Kinsella, 1984; Hinkle and Phillips, 1984). It quickly became clear that TRH receptors belong to the G protein-coupled receptor (GPCR) superfamily. A single TRH receptor gene has been found in humans and higher mammals and two genes encoding homologous receptors, TRHR1 and TRHR2, in rodents (Sun et al., 2003). TRHR1 predominates in the anterior pituitary gland while both TRHR1 and TRHR2 are found in rodent CNS (O'Dowd et al., 2000). Thyroid hormones exert powerful feedback inhibition over the TRH response system by inhibiting TRH synthesis and processing in TRH neurons in the paraventricular region of the hypothalamus and decreasing TRH receptors and responses in the pituitary gland (Gershengorn, 1978; Perrone and Hinkle, 1978; Hinkle and Goh, 1982; Segerson et al., 1987; Fekete and Lechan, 2007; Costa and Hollenberg, 2012). Prolonged hypothyroidism leads to a 40-fold increase in TRH receptor mRNA levels in pituitary glands (Costa et al., 2012). In addition, pyroglutamyl peptidase, a highly specific TRH-degrading ectoenzyme, is dramatically increased in hyperthyroid animals (Schomburg and Bauer, 1997; Marsili et al., 2011).

Genetic deletion of either the TRH peptide precursor or TRHR1 results in central hypothyroidism and mild growth retardation in mice, consistent with the established role of TRH in thyroid physiology (Yamada et al., 1997; Rabeler et al., 2004; Zeng et al., 2007). Interestingly, loss of the TRH receptor appears to result in a more severe phenotype than loss of the TRH peptide, possibly because the TRH receptor displays physiologically significant constitutive activity. Mice lacking TRHR1 also exhibit low prolactin and hyperglycemia, as well as increased anxiety and depression. Some of these behavioral effects may be secondary to hypothyroidism. Mice lacking TRHR2 display a subtle phenotype

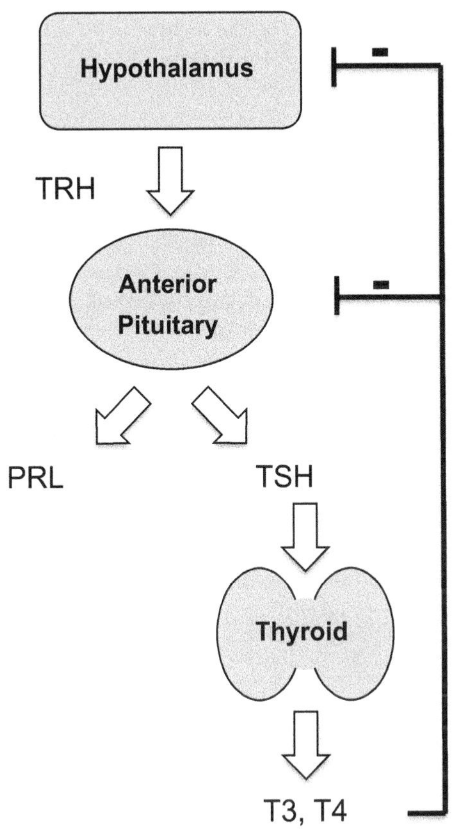

FIGURE 1 | Endocrine role of thyrotropin-releasing hormone. TRH, acting via the type 1 TRH receptor, controls secretion from pituitary thyrotrophs and lactotrophs. Thyroid hormones exert negative feedback control.

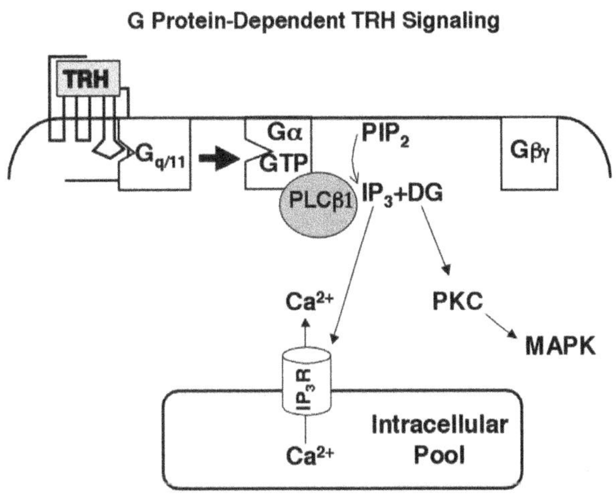

FIGURE 2 | Thyrotropin-releasing hormone signaling. TRH mobilizes intracellular calcium and activates protein kinase C through a well-characterized, Gq/11-dependent pathway. Phospholipase Cβ1, which is activated primarily by Gα-GTP subunits, is the major effector in pituitary cells. Intracellular calcium and protein kinase C initiate multiple responses including activation of MAP kinase and regulation of ion channels.

consistent with depression and decreased anxiety (Sun et al., 2009). In humans, absence of the TRH receptor causes low free T3 and free T4 with thyroid stimulating hormone (TSH) levels inappropriately low for the degree of hypothyroidism (Bonomi et al., 2009). Lack of a TRH receptor does not result in infertility or failure to lactate.

This review focuses on aspects of TRH receptor signaling that have been elucidated in either pituitary cell models expressing endogenous receptors (pituitary tissue, primary cultures of pituitary cells, cell lines derived from pituitary tumors) or generic cell lines expressing transfected TRH receptors (HEK293, CHO, COS, Hela). In rat anterior pituitary tissue, TRH receptor mRNA is found not only in TSH-secreting cells but also in prolactin- and/or growth hormone-secreting cells (Konaka et al., 1997). Although the great majority of pituitary cells that bind rhodamine-labeled TRH and respond to TRH with an increase in intracellular calcium stain for prolactin or TSH-β, responses are occasionally observed in unexpected cell types (Ashworth et al., 1995; Villalobos et al., 1997; Yu et al., 1998). Signal transduction of endogenous TRH receptors has not been characterized in neurons, where no suitable model system has been identified. Even though there is only one TRH receptor in higher mammals, that receptor may be regulated quite differently in pituitary cells and neurons because of different patterns of TRH stimulation and different sets of G protein subunits, effectors, receptors kinases, and phosphatases, arrestins, and downstream targets.

As outlined in **Figure 2**, TRH receptors are textbook calcium-mobilizing receptors: they are coupled to Gq and G11, which activate phospholipase Cβ (PLCβ), hydrolysis of phosphatidylinositol (4,5)bisphosphate, and release of the second messengers inositol (1,4,5)triphosphate (IP3) and diacylglycerol (DG) that in turn mobilize intracellular calcium and activate protein kinase C (Drummond et al., 1984; Drummond, 1985; Gershengorn, 1989). Two of the four forms of phospholipase Cβ (PLCβs 1 and 3) are found in anterior pituitary tissue, and calcium responses to TRH are intact in mice lacking PLCβ3 (Romoser et al., 2001). Thus PLCβ1, which is stimulated by $G\alpha_{q/11}$-GTP but not Gβγ, generates second messengers in response to TRH. Maximal concentrations of intracellular free calcium are attained at concentrations of TRH at least an order of magnitude below the apparent K_d of the receptor and the EC_{50} for IP3 production. These initial events are followed by complex changes that result in depolarization and a sustained influx of extracellular calcium through voltage-gated L-type calcium channels (Hinkle et al., 1996; Barros et al., 1997). When TRH receptors are expressed in embryonic fibroblasts from mice lacking $G\alpha_q$ and $G\alpha_{11}$, TRH does not stimulate any increase in intracellular calcium.

The TRH receptor is a rhodopsin family GPCR with typical features including seven transmembrane domains, several extracellular glycosylation sites, an essential disulfide bond between the first and second extracellular loops, a fairly short third intracellular loop, and a cytoplasmic tail. The receptor has a canonical (D/E)RY at the cytoplasmic end of the third transmembrane segment, the usual NPxxY at the cytoplasmic end of the seventh transmembrane helix, and an intracellular eighth helix anchored by two palmitoylated Cys residues in the carboxyl tail (Du et al., 2005). Except for the most distal region, the cytoplasmic tail of the receptor is conserved among species. The C-terminal amino acids of numerous GPCRs form classical PDZ ligands, sequences that can interact with proteins bearing a PDZ domain; PDZ is an acronym for three proteins containing the domain, PSD98, Dlg1, and zo-1 (Romero et al., 2011). TRH receptors, however, do not contain sequences predicted to interact with PDZ domains. Using a combination of experimental data obtained with receptor mutants, multiple ligands, and molecular modeling, Gershengorn and his colleagues have developed a sequential model for receptor binding and activation in which the TRH tripeptide first interacts weakly with extracellular loops and then moves deeper into the receptor and contacts transmembrane domains to form a high affinity complex. The conformational changes that occur upon receptor activation involve movements in transmembrane helices 5 and 6 and the third intracellular loop that result in G protein coupling (Gershengorn and Osman, 1996).

DESENSITIZATION OF THE TRH RECEPTOR

Thyroid stimulating hormone displays a circadian pattern that is attributed to rhythmic release of hypothalamic TRH. As a consequence, desensitization and resensitization of the TRH signaling pathway are likely to play central roles in regulating TRH actions *in vivo*. TRH rapidly stimulates a large increase in IP3 mass, providing a proximal, easily quantified response. Measurements of IP3 production have established that the TRH receptor undergoes classical desensitization. Continuous application of TRH leads to a transient burst of IP3 that peaks within seconds and falls within a minute, though to levels that remain above baseline (Drummond et al., 1984; Gershengorn and Osman, 1996; Yu and Hinkle, 1997, 1998). When cells are exposed to TRH intermittently, the size of the IP3 response diminishes with successive stimulations. The extent of desensitization depends on the method used to measure it and the cell type under study (Falck-Pedersen et al., 1994). Decoupling the receptor from G proteins contributes to the transient nature of the IP3 elevation, which is more sustained in cells expressing a TRH receptor that lacks most of the cytoplasmic tail and is thereby spared from usual desensitization processes (Yu and Hinkle, 1998; Jones and Hinkle, 2005), as shown in **Figure 3**. Changes further downstream in the signal pathway can also decrease TRH responses by mechanisms including protein kinase C-mediated inhibition of phospholipase Cβ and slow refilling of intracellular calcium stores (Yu and Hinkle, 1997). TRH receptors were the first GPCRs shown to undergo what is now termed homologous downregulation (Hinkle and Tashjian, 1975; Gershengorn, 1978). Incubation with TRH decreases the number of TRH binding sites without changing receptor affinity in pituitary GH3 cells. The molecular basis for downregulation is still not completely understood.

Like many rhodopsin family GPCRs (Bulenger et al., 2005; Milligan, 2009; Lohse, 2010), TRH receptors form oligomers when they are overexpressed in non-native cells (Kroeger et al., 2001; Hanyaloglu et al., 2002; Zhu et al., 2002). Bioluminescence resonance energy transfer (BRET), co-precipitation and biochemical analyses have all been used to document TRH receptor homodimers, and the two rodent TRH receptors (TRHR1 and TRHR2) form heterodimers (Hanyaloglu et al., 2002). TRH increases the apparent fraction of receptors in dimers quantified by all of these techniques, perhaps because TRH causes receptors to concentrate in clathrin-coated pits and endosomes. Truncated receptors that do not recruit arrestin or internalize can form dimers

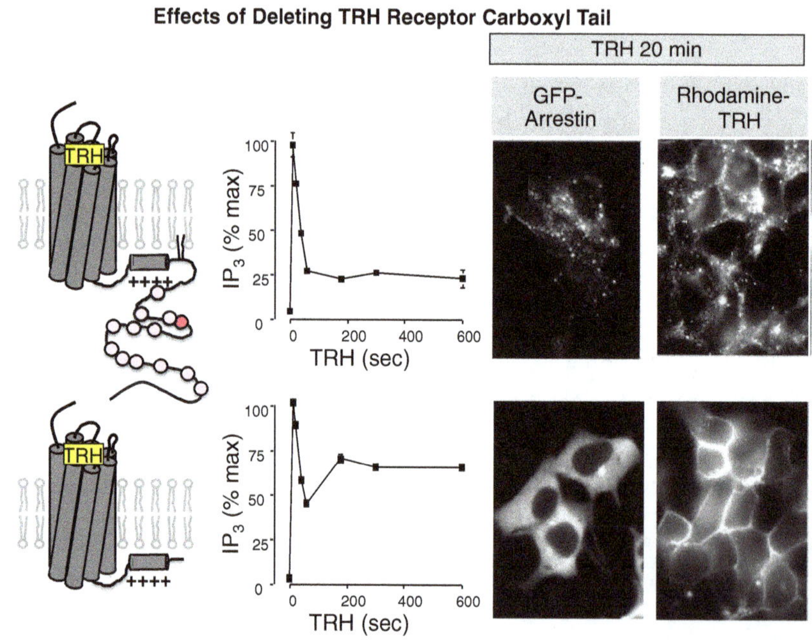

FIGURE 3 | Importance of the TRH receptor carboxyl terminus. Wildtype TRH receptors or receptors deleted at amino acid 334 were incubated with TRH and IP3 mass was measured at intervals (graphs). To visualize arrestin, receptors were expressed with GFP-labeled arrestin3. To visualize receptors, cells were incubated with rhodamine-labeled TRH. GFP-arrestin is recruited to full-length TRH receptors and co-internalizes with them but it does not interact with truncated receptors, which do not internalize.

constitutively but not in response to TRH (Zhu et al., 2002). When receptors are coerced to form oligomers by addition of a chemical dimerizing agent, signaling is not altered but internalization is accelerated and recycling blunted (Song and Hinkle, 2005). It has been difficult to assess the physiological relevance of TRH receptor dimers because no mutations that prevent oligomerization have been identified and available methods are inadequate to characterize endogenous receptors in pituitary cells. Recent studies (Whorton et al., 2007) have provided compelling evidence that at least some rhodopsin family GPCRs can activate G proteins as monomers, yet there are clear examples of receptors that form heterodimers with unique pharmacology (Jordan and Devi, 1999). One possibility is that that only one member of a GPCR pair signals to a single G protein. The TRHR1/TRHR2 heterodimer interacts with arrestins and internalizes in a different pattern from either receptor alone (Pfleger et al., 2004), but the intriguing possibility that the TRH receptor forms heteromers with other GPCRs to impart novel pharmacology has not been explored.

OVERVIEW OF GPCR RECEPTOR DESENSITIZATION

Most GPCRs become phosphorylated after they are activated, and the TRH receptor is no exception. GPCR phosphorylation is catalyzed by members of a family of Ser/Thr protein kinases, GPCR kinases, or GRKs. There are seven GRKs, four of them widely expressed (GRKs 1, 2, 5, and 6; Moore et al., 2007; Gurevich et al., 2012). What sets the GRKs apart from other kinases is their ability to discriminate between GPCRs in inactive versus activated conformations. They act preferentially on agonist-occupied and constitutively active receptors and do not have strict requirements for the amino acid sequence surrounding phosphorylation sites. There are important differences in how different GRKs are recruited to the plasma membrane, however, and examples of GPCRs that are phosphorylated at different sites by different GRKs. GRKs exert a number of kinase-independent effects on GPCR signaling and are known to phosphorylate substrates other than receptors (Moore et al., 2007; Premont and Gainetdinov, 2007; Evron et al., 2012; Gurevich et al., 2012). GPCRs can also be phosphorylated by kinases that become activated in response to signaling such as cAMP-dependent protein kinase and protein kinase C. Phosphorylation carried out by such downstream kinases can influence GPCR-G protein coupling, desensitization, and trafficking.

Once activated and phosphorylated, most GPCRs bind to arrestin, which interrupts the interaction between an activated receptor and its cognate G protein and terminates signaling via the G protein-mediated pathway. Arrestins 2 and 3 (also referred to as β-arrestin1 and β-arrestin2) are ubiquitously expressed. Like G proteins and GRKs, arrestins distinguish between inactive and activated receptor conformations. Arrestins bind preferentially to activated GPCRs; they also contain a positively charged pocket that interacts strongly with negatively charged phosphates (Gurevich and Gurevich, 2006; DeWire et al., 2007; Moore et al., 2007; Premont and Gainetdinov, 2007; DeFea, 2011; Shenoy and Lefkowitz, 2011). The arrestins therefore tend to bind with highest affinity to receptors that are both activated and phosphorylated. When arrestin engages receptor, a buried helical region in the arrestin carboxyl terminus undergoes a major translocation to expose binding sites for AP2 and clathrin, targeting the arrestin-receptor complex to coated pit regions of the membrane destined to pinch off into endosomes in a dynamin-dependent process (Moore et al., 2007; Shenoy and Lefkowitz, 2011).

Arrestin is a scaffolding protein capable of anchoring a wide array of kinases, phosphatases, and other proteins to the arrestin-GPCR complex (Xiao et al., 2007; DeFea, 2011). A rapidly expanding body of literature shows that arrestin-GPCR complexes can initiate alternate signaling pathways, notably those leading to MAP kinase activation (Lefkowitz and Shenoy, 2005; Luttrell and Gesty-Palmer, 2010; Reiter et al., 2012). The Lefkowitz group has proposed that the phosphorylation pattern of a GPCR can act as a barcode in which different phosphosites recruit different arrestins to turn on different signal pathways (Liggett, 2011; Nobles et al., 2011). This model is appealing because it adds tremendous diversity to GPCR signaling, and it is supported by evidence that arrestin2 and arrestin3 bind preferentially to distinct phophosites on several receptors (Ren et al., 2005). There are also many examples of what are termed biased ligands that favor particular pathways (Rajagopal et al., 2010; Reiter et al., 2012). For example, biased ligands may preferentially activate G protein or arrestin cascades, activate one arrestin signaling function but not another (such as kinase activation and internalization), or act as an agonist in one pathway and an antagonist in another. Biased agonists and antagonists open new doors for the development of therapeutically useful GPCR ligands.

G protein-coupled receptors have been broadly divided into two groups based on their interactions with arrestins (Oakley et al., 1999, 2000). Class A receptors bind arrestin 3 more strongly than arrestin 2 or visual arrestin, internalize without associated arrestin, and recycle rapidly. Examples include the well-characterized β2-adrenergic receptor, the μ-opioid receptor and dopamine D1 receptor. Class B receptors bind well to both arrestin 2 and arrestin 3, internalize with arrestin, and traffic to lysosomes where they undergo intracellular degradation or slow recycling. Examples include the V2 vasopressin receptor, type 1a angiotensin II receptor, and the TRH receptor.

PHOSPHORYLATION OF TRH RECEPTORS

Thyrotropin-releasing hormone receptors become phosphorylated rapidly once they are activated. Receptor phosphorylation has been demonstrated by ^{32}P incorporation, an upward mobility shift on gel electrophoresis, and reactivity with phosphosite-specific antibodies (Hanyaloglu et al., 2001; Zhu et al., 2002; Jones and Hinkle, 2005; Jones et al., 2007). All of these changes are reversed by phosphatase treatment. Phosphorylation sites in the TRH receptor have been partially mapped by characterizing ^{32}P incorporation and antibody reactivity of wildtype receptors and receptors lacking various Ser and Thr residues in the cytoplasmic tail. Jones et al. generated antisera against multiply phosphorylated peptides from five different conserved regions of the TRH receptor tail and validated their specificity (Jones and Hinkle, 2008). None of the antibodies recognize TRH receptors from unstimulated cells, but four of them react with receptors from TRH-treated cells. Endogenous TRH receptors in pituitary cells are phosphorylated strongly at residues between amino acids 355 and 365 and less efficiently at two regions farther downstream. Current information about phosphosites in the TRH receptor C-terminus is presented in **Figure 4**. As discussed below, phosphorylation of Thr365 is particularly important for arrestin recruitment, internalization, and desensitization. There is no evidence for phosphorylation at Tyr residues. The distal regions of the TRH receptor are more heavily phosphorylated when the receptor is expressed in HEK293 or CHO cells compared to native receptors. The finding of different site usage in different settings suggests a need for caution when charactering phosphorylation of overexpressed epitope-tagged GPCRs in heterologous cells, an approach that is normally required for analysis by mass spectrometry.

Thyrotropin-releasing hormone receptor phosphorylation does not appear to be hierarchical because the rates of phosphorylation are the same for different phosphosites. TRH does not promote ^{32}P incorporation into receptors truncated before the palmitoylation site and TRH does not alter mobility of truncated receptors, leading to the conclusion that either intracellular loops are not phosphorylated in response to TRH or phosphorylation in the intracellular loops somehow requires the receptor tail. Following TRH addition, nearly all receptors appear to be phosphorylated based on the mobility shift and near quantitative immunoprecipitation with phosphosite-specific antibodies (Jones et al., 2007).

In pituitary cells, endogenous receptors on the plasma membrane are not detectably phosphorylated in the basal state, but they become strongly phosphorylated within 10 s of TRH addition and endocytosis of phospho-receptors is readily apparent by 10 min (**Figure 5**). Interestingly, when rat pituitary tissue from

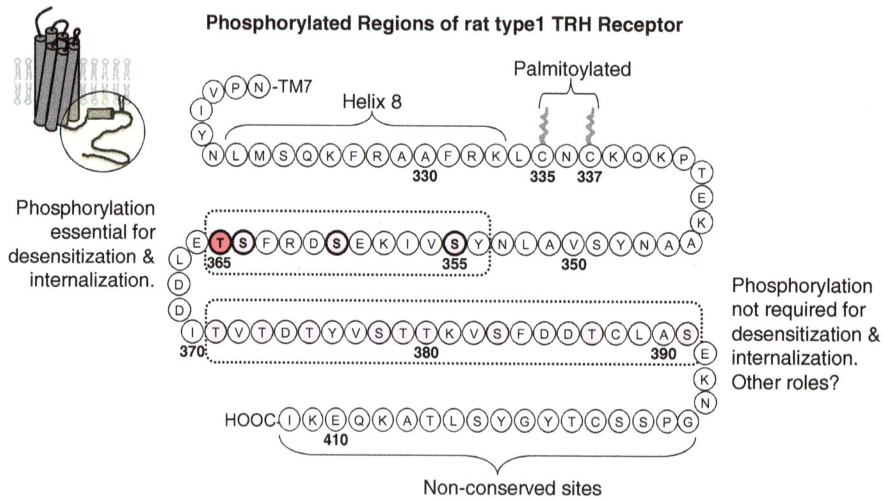

FIGURE 4 | Thyrotropin-releasing hormone receptor phosphorylation sites. The circle outlines the portion of the rat TRH receptor depicted. Ser/Thr residues are shown in pink or red in regions known to undergo TRH-dependent phosphorylation. Phosphorylation at Thr365, in red, is essential for desensitization and internalization, and phosphorylation at other sites between amino acids 355 and 365 has been documented and shown to contribute to these processes. TRH also stimulates phosphorylation at sites from 371 to 391, although the exact phosphosites are not known. Phosphorylation in this region is not essential for desensitization and internalization, but it may be important for different, as yet unidentified signaling functions. Phosphorylation in the non-conserved distal region has not been examined.

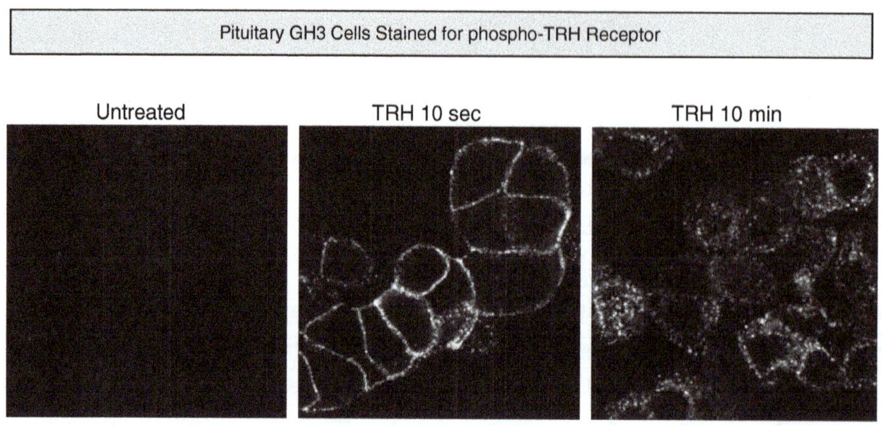

FIGURE 5 | Thyrotropin-releasing hormone-dependent phosphorylation of endogenous TRH receptors. Rat pituitary GH3 cells were stained with affinity-purified antibody specifically recognizing phosphosites at amino acids 355–365 of the TRH receptor before and after TRH exposure.

an untreated animal is examined, phosphorylated TRH receptor is clearly visible. The intensity of the phospho-receptor signal increases greatly minutes after animals are injected with TRH and, as expected, the signal is seen cells that stain for TSH-β and prolactin (Jones et al., 2007).

Thyrotropin-releasing hormone receptor phosphorylation is exceedingly fast, with a half-time of 0.2 min (Jones et al., 2007; Gehret and Hinkle, 2010). This rapid phosphorylation is unusual among GPCRs and marks the TRH receptor as a superior substrate. Rapid phosphorylation is not simply a consequence of the sequence of the receptor tail. The transmembrane helices and intracellular loops of the TRH receptor are likewise important for rapid phosphorylation of the receptor tail even though they are not phosphorylated themselves. A chimeric TRH receptor with the β2-adrenergic receptor tail is phosphorylated at β2-adrenergic receptor GRK sites with kinetics typical of the TRH receptor, not the β2-adrenergic receptor (Gehret and Hinkle, 2010). The rate-limiting step for TRH receptor phosphorylation may be recruitment of GRKs to the activated receptor. In support of this idea, dimerization of a mutant TRH receptor that cannot undergo activation with a truncated TRH receptor that signals well but cannot undergo phosphorylation results in phosphorylation of the signaling-incompetent partner (Song et al., 2007). This is most easily explained if the activatable receptor recruits a kinase that acts on its partner in the receptor dimer. The predicted amphipathic eighth helix between the canonical NPxxY at the end of the seventh transmembrane domain and the palmitoylated Cys-X-Cys motif is not phosphorylated but the positively charged residues in this region are essential for phosphorylation at downstream sites and subsequent internalization (Gehret et al., 2010).

Considerable evidence points toward GRK2 as the kinase responsible for TRH receptor phosphorylation. Phosphorylation is inhibited by dominant negative, kinase dead forms of GRK2 and by siRNAs targeting GRK2 (Jones and Hinkle, 2005; Jones et al., 2007). The effects of siRNA knockdown are seen both in pituitary cells and heterologous cells expressing transfected receptors. In addition, paroxetine, which has recently been recognized as an effective and relatively specific GRK2 inhibitor, delays phosphorylation of the TRH receptor (Thal et al., 2012). In keeping with the rapid rate of TRH receptor phosphorylation, GRK2 translocates to membrane fractions within 10 s of TRH addition (Jones and Hinkle, 2005). All of these experiments implicate GRK2 in TRH receptor phosphorylation, but because GRK2 knockdown and inhibition do not block receptor phosphorylation completely it seems likely that other GRKs are also able to phosphorylate the receptor.

Inhibitor data suggest that casein kinase II, which is predicted to phosphorylate Thr365 and two other downstream sites, may contribute to receptor phosphorylation (Hanyaloglu et al., 2001). Pharmacological activation of conventional protein kinase C isoforms leads to weak phosphorylation of some but not all sites in the TRH receptor tail, but protein kinase C inhibitors do not alter TRH-dependent phosphorylation (Jones et al., 2007). Furthermore, TRH receptor phosphorylation and internalization occur normally in cells lacking $G\alpha_q$ and $G\alpha_{11}$, indicating that calcium- and diacylglycerol-activated kinases are not essential (Yu and Hinkle, 1999; Jones and Hinkle, 2005). Together these results suggest little role for downstream kinases in TRH receptor phosphorylation.

ARRESTIN INTERACTIONS WITH THE TRH RECEPTOR

Arrestin interactions with TRH receptors have been monitored by a variety of approaches including translocation of GFP-arrestin (Groarke et al., 1999, 2001; Oakley et al., 1999, 2000; Yu and Hinkle, 1999; Smith et al., 2001; Hanyaloglu et al., 2002), co-precipitation of arrestin and receptor (Jones et al., 2007), effect of arrestin on agonist affinity (Jones and Hinkle, 2005, 2008), and BRET (Kroeger et al., 2001; Hanyaloglu et al., 2002). GFP-arrestin is diffusely localized in the cytoplasm of cells expressing TRH receptors. When TRH is added, GFP-arrestin2 and GFP-arrestin3 move to the plasma membrane within a minute or two (see **Figure 3**). The ability of TRH receptors to recruit arrestins 2 and 3 places it in the Group B category of GPCRs. Although arrestin translocation is detectable with most GPCRs, arrestin movement seen with the TRH receptor is exceptionally robust (Oakley et al., 2000). GFP-arrestin translocation is not observed in cells expressing TRH receptors lacking palmitoylation sites or truncated before the major phosphorylation sites (Vrecl et al., 1998; Yu and Hinkle, 1998; Hanyaloglu et al., 2001; Smith et al., 2001; Jones and Hinkle, 2005, 2008).

As shown in experiments depicted in **Figure 6**, GFP-arrestin does translocate to receptors with Ala substitutions for the four Ser and Thr residues between 355 and 365, proving that downstream phosphosites are sufficient to bind arrestin (Jones and Hinkle, 2008). This is important because distal phosphosites are not sufficient for desensitization and internalization, as discussed below. Arrestin co-precipitates with activated TRH receptors even if Ser/Thr residues in the 355–365 region are Ala-substituted, again showing that arrestin interacts with at least two regions of the receptor. BRET studies document a close interaction between the type 1 TRH receptor and arrestins 2 and 3 that is lost if the receptor is truncated before the palmitoylation sites (Pfleger et al., 2004). **Figure 7** summarizes current understanding about the importance of different TRH receptor phosphorylation sites.

Because arrestins bind preferentially to activated GPCRs, theoretical considerations dictate that arrestin will increase the affinity of a GPCR for agonists, a prediction borne out by experimental evidence (Gurevich et al., 1997). Consistent with this, the apparent affinity of the potent agonist [^{3}H]MeTRH, measured at room temperature or above in intact cells, is highly dependent on arrestin levels (Jones and Hinkle, 2005, 2008). In arrestin2/3 knockout cells, cotransfection with wildtype arrestin increases the apparent affinity for [^{3}H]MeTRH 14-fold. Arrestin increases the agonist affinity of truncated and Ala-substituted receptors, supporting the concept of multiple arrestin binding sites and raising the possibility of phosphorylation-independent arrestin interactions.

ROLE OF ARRESTIN IN TRH RECEPTOR SIGNALING, DESENSITIZATION AND INTERNALIZATION

Thyrotropin-releasing hormone receptors expressed in arrestin2/3 knockout cells generate strong IP3 responses to TRH. TRH-stimulated IP3 levels are much lower in cells expressing arrestin2, arrestin3, or both, proving that arrestin is important for desensitization and that either arrestin is sufficient for this function.

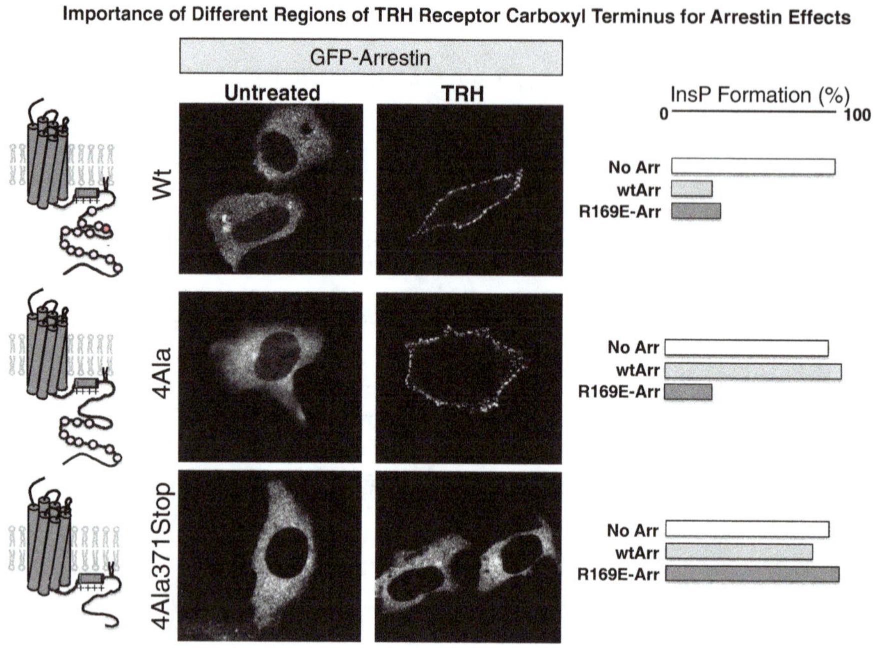

FIGURE 6 | Arrestin recruitment and arrestin-dependent desensitization. Cells expressing the receptors shown were incubated with GFP-arrestin and imaged before or after 3 min exposure to TRH. The right panels show TRH-stimulated IP3 production in arrestin-null cells expressing receptor with no arrestin (No Arr), wildtype arrestin 3 (wtArr), or R169E-Arr, which binds activated GPCRs in a phosphorylation-independent fashion. TRH receptors are: Wt, wildtype; 4Ala, Ala substituted for 4 Ser/Thr residues from amino acids 355 through 365; and 4Ala-371Stop, 4Ala receptor truncated at amino acid 370. Even though arrestin binds robustly to receptors lacking phosphosites at amino acids 355–365, arrestin does not desensitize signaling.

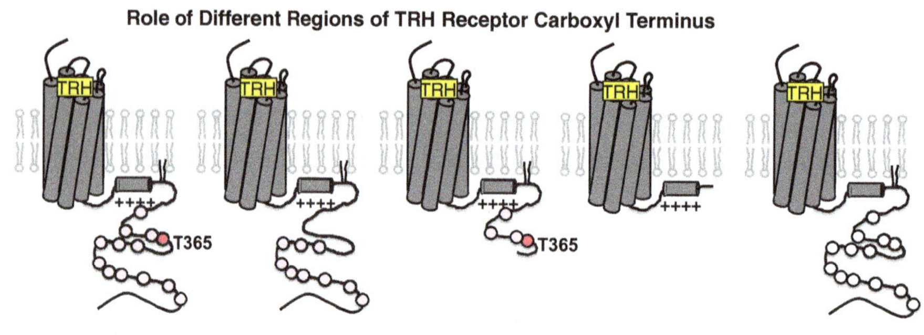

Signaling	+	+	+	+	+
Phosphorylation	+	+	+	--	--
Arrestin binding	+	+	+	--	--
Desensitization	+	--	+	--	--
Internalization	+	--	+	--	--

FIGURE 7 | Importance of different phosphorylated regions of the TRH receptor tail. Pink circles depict Ser/Thr residues in regions known to be phosphorylated, with the critical Thr365 residue shown in red. From left to right, TRH receptors are: wildtype, 4Ala (Ala-substituted for the 4 Ser/Thr residues from amino acids 355 through 365), 371Stop (receptor truncated at amino acid 370), C335Stop (receptor truncated before palmitoylation sites), and receptor with Gln substitutions for 6 Arg/Lys residues between amino acids 326 and 340. White circles depict Ser/Thr residues that are present but weakly phosphorylated.

As expected, arrestins are not required for G protein-dependent signaling. Arrestins do not desensitize IP3 responses if receptors are missing phosphorylation sites between amino acids 355 and 365. Ala substitution of Thr365 severely impairs TRH receptor desensitization and internalization. In contrast, receptors truncated at amino acid 370 are still subject to arrestin-mediated desensitization (Jones et al., 2007; Jones and Hinkle, 2008).

A similar pattern emerges when internalization is examined. Expression of dominant negative arrestin in normal cells or expression of receptors in arrestin-null cells severely restricts the rate and extent of endocytosis (Hanyaloglu et al., 2002; Jones and Hinkle, 2005, 2008). Endogenous arrestin levels control the desensitization and internalization of heterologously expressed TRH receptors; for example, HEK293 and even more so COS-7 cells have lower concentrations of arrestin and correspondingly less desensitization and internalization than pituitary cells (Falck-Pedersen et al., 1994; Vrecl et al., 1998). Arrestin binding to phosphorylated Thr365 and surrounding sites is absolutely required for internalization, but arrestin binding to phosphosites beyond amino acid 370 is not necessary. The TRH receptor is one of several examples where arrestin can bind to a GPCR without leading to internalization (Krasel et al., 2008). Conversely, expression of the R169E arrestin mutant, which binds activated GPCRs in a phosphorylation-independent fashion, restores TRH-dependent internalization to receptors lacking Thr365 and nearby phosphorylation sites (Hanyaloglu et al., 2001; Jones and Hinkle, 2008; see **Figure 6**). Time- and temperature-dependent conversion of receptor-bound radiolabeled peptide to an acid-resistant state has often been taken as a measure of receptor endocytosis. It is worth noting that this is not valid for receptor-bound [^{3}H]MeTRH (Jones and Hinkle, 2008). Acid resistance precedes internalization and occurs at a reduced level with mutant receptors that do not internalize at all and in cells where internalization is blocked. Endocytosis can be documented readily by microscopy or by the TRH-driven loss of surface binding sites for antibodies to an N-terminal epitope tag on the receptor.

One question arising from these observations is whether internalization of TRH receptors contributes to early desensitization. To address this question, TRH responses were quantified in settings where receptor endocytosis was effectively blocked: in the presence of hyperosmolar sucrose, in cells infected with vaccinia virus encoding dominant negative dynamin, and in cells expressing receptors truncated just before the palmitoylation site (Yu and Hinkle, 1998). Signaling was also measured in arrestin-null cells transfected with a mutant arrestin that can bind to receptor but is incapable of interacting with clathrin and AP2 (ΔLIELD/F391A-arrestin) and therefore incapable of promoting internalization (Jones and Hinkle, 2005, 2008). Initial Gq/11-mediated responses and subsequent desensitization of intact receptors were unaffected by the lack of internalization, but the lack of a receptor tail resulted in more persistent elevations in IP3 (Yu and Hinkle, 1998). Together these results confirm the importance of arrestin for both desensitization and internalization and prove that internalization is not the cause of desensitization. In highly sensitive assays, persistent IP1 production can be demonstrated for up to an hour after TRH is washed out in HEK293 cells expressing TRH receptors (Boutin et al., 2012). This sustained response does not depend on internalization. The question of whether there are G protein-independent signaling pathways and if so, whether they persist following receptor endocytosis, has not been answered. For example, TRH activates MAP kinase. A strong early activation depends on protein kinase C-dependent raf phosphorylation but not on internalization of the receptor itself, although it does require an intact endocytic machinery (Ohmichi et al., 1994; Smith et al., 2001). Additional work is needed to establish whether the weak sustained activation of MAP kinase generated by TRH depends on arrestin or continues following internalization in pituitary cells. The known and possible additional roles of arrestin are shown schematically in **Figure 8**.

MECHANISM OF TRH RECEPTOR INTERNALIZATION

Thyrotropin-releasing hormone promotes rapid and extensive internalization of endogenous receptors in pituitary cells (Ashworth et al., 1995). Endocytosis of the activated TRH receptor proceeds via a classical arrestin- and dynamin-dependent pathway and is blocked by pharmacological inhibition of endocytosis and by dominant negative dynamin (Drmota et al., 1998; Yu and Hinkle, 1998). Gq/11-dependent signaling is not required, because internalization occurs normally when TRH receptors are expressed in fibroblasts from mice with genetic deletion of both $G\alpha_q$ and $G\alpha_{11}$, where there is no calcium response (Yu and Hinkle, 1999). Regions of the cytoplasmic receptor tail important for internalization correspond to regions where phosphorylation takes place (Hanyaloglu et al., 2001, 2002; Jones et al., 2007). Endocytosis is much slower although not entirely absent when the TRH receptor is expressed in cells with either no arrestin or dominant negative arrestins (Vrecl et al., 1998; Groarke et al., 2001; Smith et al., 2001; Hanyaloglu et al., 2002; Jones and Hinkle, 2005). The mechanism of the arrestin-independent component is unknown, but TRH receptors appear to be excluded from caveolae (Rudajev et al., 2005).

Ubiquitination is required for endocytosis of several GPCRs (Hanyaloglu and von Zastrow, 2008; Hislop and von Zastrow, 2011) and a fraction of TRH receptors are ubiquitinated, but ubiquitin is not added to receptors on the plasma membrane and ubiquitination does not occur in response to TRH. Furthermore, receptor endocytosis continues at the non-permissive temperature in cells with a temperature-sensitive E1 ubiquitin-activating enzyme (Cook et al., 2003). It is clear, then, that ubiquitination does not tag TRH receptors for internalization, although ubiquitin-mediated degradation serves an important quality control function during TRH receptor biosynthesis.

TRH RECEPTOR TRAFFICKING

Trafficking of TRH receptors fused at the C-terminus to GFP has been characterized by several groups (Drmota et al., 1998; Yu and Hinkle, 1999; Scott et al., 2002). Shortly after TRH addition, receptors cluster on the cell surface, and over the course of about 10 min they internalize in pre-assembled vesicles without transferrin receptors or $G\alpha_q$. These earliest vesicles soon merge with others containing transferrin receptors. Some $G\alpha_q$ is removed from the plasma membrane following TRH receptor activation, but this occurs quite slowly and internalized receptors and $G\alpha_q$ are not colocalized (Drmota et al., 1999; Yu and Hinkle, 1999). After 30 min or longer, GFP-labeled TRH receptors are found in much larger vesicles deep inside the cell. TRH receptors internalize together with arrestin (Groarke et al., 1999; Oakley et al., 2000; Smith et al., 2001; Jones and Hinkle, 2008).

As described above, the TRH receptor follows a familiar pattern of phosphorylation, arrestin binding, desensitization, and endocytosis. Much less is understood about what happens next:

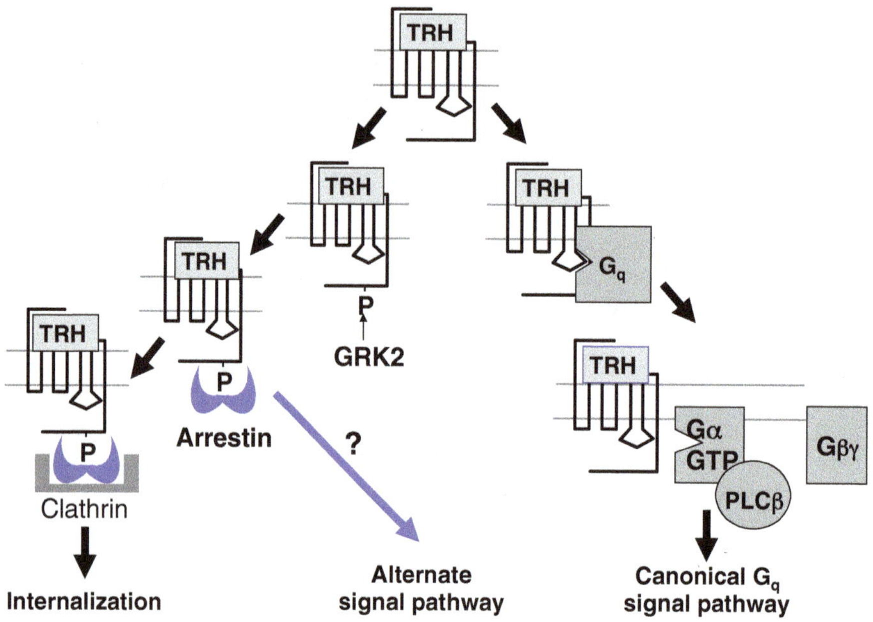

FIGURE 8 | Arrestin effects on TRH receptor signaling. Arrestin binds to phosphorylated receptors, terminating receptor-G protein coupling, and initiating receptor endocytosis. Arrestin is a scaffold for other signaling molecules and it is possible that the arrestin-TRH receptor complex controls as yet unidentified pathways.

how is the TRH receptor (and other GPCRs) dephosphorylated, sorted and trafficked back to the plasma membrane or targeted for degradation? In a study that capitalized on the availability of antibodies specific for phosphorylated TRH receptors, trafficking of phosphorylated, and dephosphorylated TRH receptors was monitored during internalization and recycling. Endosomal compartments were identified with GFP-labeled Rab proteins, and movements of fluorescently labeled arrestin were followed simultaneously (Jones and Hinkle, 2009). Cell surface receptors were selectively labeled with antibody against an HA tag on the extracellular N-terminus of the rat TRH receptor ("antibody feeding") and tracked over time following addition or withdrawal of TRH. Rab5 marks an early endosomal population, and TRH receptors appeared in Rab5-positive vesicles within a few minutes of TRH stimulation. Receptors in these vesicles were almost entirely phosphorylated and associated with arrestin. Over the course of 20 min, receptors moved to vesicles that were both rab4- and rab5-positive, the early sorting endosomes. Both phosphorylated and non-phosphorylated receptors were seen in this pool. Internalized receptors subsequently trafficked to a population of vesicles that were rab4-positive but rab5-negative, typical of rapidly recycling endosomes. These recycling vesicles were enriched in *dephosphorylated* receptors, i.e., receptors that began the experiment on the plasma membrane but were no longer phosphorylated. They were essentially devoid of phosphorylated receptors.

This result raised the question: were receptors able to move into this rab4-positive, rab5-negative "recycling" vesicle population because they were dephosphorylated, or were receptors quickly dephosphorylated once they reached these vesicles? This question was addressed by interrupting normal trafficking with dominant negative rabs. Dominant negative rab5 completely blocked movement of the receptor out of very early endosomes, yet it did not change the rate of receptor dephosphorylation. If dephosphorylation occurred preferentially in a later endosomal population, dominant negative rab5 would have delayed phosphatase action. These results lead to the conclusion that dephosphorylation takes place in sorting endosomes and permits trafficking of the TRH receptor into recycling vesicles.

A small subset of phosphorylated TRH receptors eventually appear in Rab11 vesicles, traditionally viewed as a late recycling compartment, suggesting that the long recycling pathway is taken by some receptors. Rab7 vesicles, which are associated with lysosomes, contained very little TRH receptor. It seems plausible that a fraction of intracellular receptor is degraded with each round of internalization, possibly contributing to the phenomenon of downregulation, but this remains speculative. The trafficking of internalized TRH receptors is summarized in **Figure 9**.

REPOPULATING THE PLASMA MEMBRANE: RECYCLING AND RECRUITMENT

When cells are incubated with TRH to drive internalization and the hormone is removed, receptors reappear at the plasma membrane with a half-time of 20–30 min based on the amount of radioactive TRH able to bind, the amount of epitope-tagged receptor on the membrane determined by FACS or ELISA, or the amount of GFP-labeled receptor at the surface. These results are consistent with receptor recycling, but the story has recently grown more complicated with the discovery that although the total receptor number at the plasma membrane is restored quite quickly, this is largely due to recruitment of new receptors (Cook and Hinkle, 2004; Jones and Hinkle, 2009). An early piece of evidence appeared when the TRH receptor was fused to a derivative of DS-Red dubbed

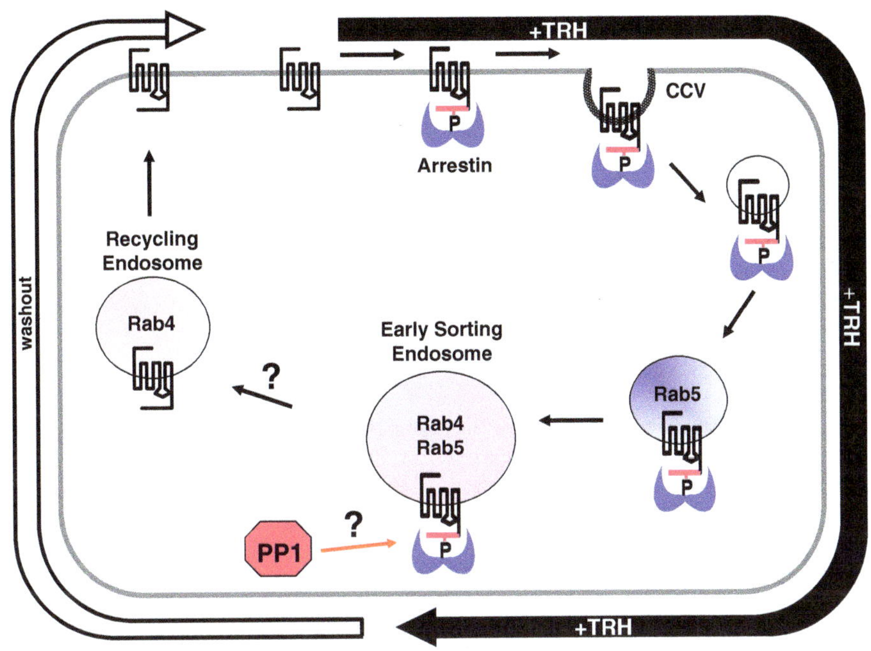

FIGURE 9 | Intracellular trafficking of TRH receptors. TRH activation is rapidly followed by receptor phosphorylation, arrestin binding, and recruitment of the arrestin-phospho-receptor complex to clathrin-coated pits that pinch off in a dynamin-dependent process to form clathrin-coated vesicles (CCVs). Vesicles containing phospho-receptor soon merge with rab5-positive vesicles where they colocalize with transferrin receptors. These vesicles gradually merge with others to form larger endosomes rich in rab4 and rab5, early sorting endosomes. After TRH is removed from the medium, but not before, dephosphorylated receptors start to become detectable in rab4-positive but rab5-negative recycling endosomes. Dephosphorylated receptors then recycle to the plasma membrane. Phosphorylated receptor is rarely seen in these fast recycling vesicles. After long incubations with TRH, small amounts of phospho-receptor are detected in rab11 vesicles, considered to be a slow recycling pool. Protein phosphatase 1 (PP1) acts on the TRH receptor, but it is not known how the removal of extracellular TRH triggers receptor dephosphorylation. The mechanism that permits dephosphorylated receptors to move to recycling endosomes, or alternatively the mechanism that prevents phosphorylated receptors from exiting early sorting vesicles, are also not clear.

"Timer." The unique feature of the Timer protein is that it changes color from red to green with a half-time of 10 h. When TRH was added to drive internalization and then removed to allow recycling, receptors that moved to the plasma membrane were much redder (younger) than those that had been internalized (Cook and Hinkle, 2004). A second approach was an antibody feeding study which showed that intracellular receptors were recruited to the membrane before the internalized receptors had recycled (Jones and Hinkle, 2009). To avoid problems inherent in antibody feeding experiments, TRH receptors were fused at the N-terminus to a 15 amino acid tag that serves as a biotin ligase acceptor. Plasma membrane receptors were selectively labeled with biotin by adding purified bacterial biotin ligase, biotin, and ATP to the medium. TRH receptors on the plasma membrane were essentially the only proteins biotinylated, and biotin-labeled TRH receptor was visualized with fluorescent streptavidin. Again, after TRH-driven endocytosis and several hours of recovery, the surface receptor pool was repopulated initially with recruited rather than recycled (biotin-labeled) receptors (Jones and Hinkle, 2009). Finally, cells were labeled with [^{3}H]TRH (not the higher affinity, slower dissociating [^{3}H]MeTRH), which internalized with the receptor. When [^{3}H]TRH was removed, plasma membrane receptor levels were restored at a time when most [^{3}H]TRH still remained inside the cell. In each of these approaches, most internalized receptors eventually returned to the plasma membrane, but only after an hour or more (Jones and Hinkle, 2009). These results provide another question for future study: How are receptors in an intracellular pool prompted to move to the plasma membrane?

GPCR DEPHOSPHORYLATION

Once a GPCR is activated, phosphorylated, and bound to arrestin, return to its resting state requires dissociation or degradation of the agonist, dissociation of arrestin and dephosphorylation. With rare exceptions, the phosphatases responsible for GPCR dephosphorylation have not been fully characterized. There are many more GPCRs than Ser/Thr phosphatases, necessitating involvement of enzymes with broad substrate specificity. In mammalian cells, the majority of proteins phosphorylated on Ser and Thr residues are dephosphorylated by members of two ubiquitous enzyme families, protein phosphatase 1 (PP1), and protein phosphatase 2A (PP2A; Barford et al., 1998). These protein phosphatases are multisubunit enzymes that achieve specificity by interacting with a wide array of scaffolding and targeting subunits. The catalytic subunits of PP1s can bind directly to substrates through a number of conserved motifs or localize through targeting subunits. Over 150 proteins have been shown to interact with PP1 (Bollen et al., 2010). PP2As are heterotrimers composed of a catalytic subunit, a scaffolding or structural subunit, and a targeting subunit. On the basis of high sensitivity to inhibitors, the PP2A family of phosphatases has been implicated in the dephosphorylation of numerous GPCRs, and PP1, calcineurin (PP2B), and PP2C for others (Croci et al., 2003; Flajolet et al., 2003; Mao et al., 2005).

Pitcher et al. (1995) reported that the β2-adrenergic receptor was dephosphorylated by an endosomal phosphatase in the PP2A family following internalization. This model predicted an essential role for receptor endocytosis: a GPCR had to cycle through endosomal compartments to be dephosphorylated and resensitized. Subsequent work has uncovered many variants on this theme. Many GPCRs can be dephosphorylated while localized on the cell surface. Dephosphorylation of PKA and GRK sites on the β2-adrenergic receptor can take place on the plasma membrane (Iyer et al., 2006). Some sites on the somatostatin 2A receptor are not dephosphorylated until the receptor has internalized, while others can be dephosphorylated regardless of receptor location; different enzymes appear to be involved (Ghosh and Schonbrunn, 2011). Receptors for several peptide hormones cannot recycle until the peptide is degraded in acidified endosomes in a reaction catalyzed by ectopeptidases that cointernalize with the peptide-receptor complex (Roosterman et al., 2008; Cattaruzza et al., 2009). Although the TRH-degrading enzyme is an ectoenzyme present in pituitary tissue, there is no evidence that it plays a role in TRH receptor cycling.

TRH RECEPTOR DEPHOSPHORYLATION

When TRH is removed from the medium or an inverse agonist such as chlordiazepoxide is added, receptor dephosphorylation rapidly ensues (Jones and Hinkle, 2005; Jones et al., 2007; Gehret and Hinkle, 2010, 2012). Once TRH dissociates, receptors return to an inactive conformation, arrestin affinity declines, and arrestin dissociation provides freer access of phosphatases. A number of studies have sought to identify factors controlling the rate of receptor dephosphorylation. The amino acid sequence surrounding the phosphosite does not seem to be a major factor because the rates of TRH receptor dephosphorylation are the same at different phosphosites (Jones et al., 2007). When the β2-adrenergic receptor tail was spliced onto the TRH receptor, the chimeric receptor underwent TRH-dependent phosphorylation at sites that are phosphorylated by GRKs in the β2-adrenergic receptor. The dephosphorylation kinetics of the chimera resembled those of the natural TRH receptor (Gehret and Hinkle, 2010). On the other hand, the location of the TRH receptors is important (Jones et al., 2007; Gehret and Hinkle, 2010). Dephosphorylation occurs more rapidly when receptors are on the plasma membrane than when receptors have undergone endocytosis. In pituitary cells, endogenous receptors are dephosphorylated with a half-time of about 45 s if TRH exposure lasts only a minute (sufficient for complete phosphorylation but not for internalization) but is 3 min if TRH exposure continues for 30 min (when receptors have undergone internalization; Jones et al., 2007). A similar situation holds in heterologous model systems, although dephosphorylation is not nearly as fast.

These data raise an important question: how does removing TRH from the outside of the cell trigger dephosphorylation of receptors in endosomes deep in the cytoplasm? The simplest idea is that some receptors are always at the plasma membrane and as long as TRH is present, they are signaling and somehow maintaining receptor phosphorylation. Removing extracellular TRH terminates signaling and leads to dephosphorylation. If this model is valid, however, the responsible signaling system cannot be traditional Gq/11-mediated activation of PLCβ, because dephosphorylation of internalized receptors is not altered by treatment with an intracellular calcium chelator and protein kinase C inhibitor (Jones et al., 2007).

Recently, the problem of identifying the TRH receptor phosphatase was tackled using an unbiased screen with an siRNA library directed against phosphatase subunits (Gehret and Hinkle, 2012). While this approach had the potential to identify a targeting or scaffolding subunit, only the catalytic subunit of PP1α came up as a bone fide hit in the screen. The results of the screen, which was performed in HEK293 cells, concur with inhibitor effects on dephosphorylation of endogenous TRH receptors in pituitary cells. Dephosphorylation of TRH receptors is powerfully inhibited by calyculin A, which acts on the catalytic subunits of PP1 and PP2A, but insensitive to fostriecin, a highly selective inhibitor of PP2A. Many details, such as the mechanism that targets PP1α to the receptor, remain to be elucidated. The discovery of a specific phosphatase subunit acting on the TRH receptor provides a starting point for dissecting an important aspect of the resensitization process.

FUTURE DIRECTIONS

The TRH receptor has been viewed as a prototypical "calcium-mobilizing" GPCR and the mechanisms of TRH signaling have been the subject of intense investigation for decades. More recently, attention has also been focused on events that turn signaling off. In every instance, the pathways involved have turned out to be more complex than anticipated. This review has sought to review recent work and highlight some of the unknowns pertaining to TRH receptor signaling, desensitization, and trafficking. Once activated by hormone, the TRH receptor is phosphorylated in multiple regions; arrestins bind at different phosphosites with different consequences. It seems likely that the TRH receptor signals via its diverse arrestin interactions in ways that are not yet recognized. The trafficking studies described here show that dephosphorylation must take place before internalized TRH receptors can recycle, yet the nature of the interaction between receptor and phosphatase remains elusive. The recent identification of the protein phosphatase involved opens the door for future studies seeking to describe phosphatase targeting mechanisms. The principles governing receptor trafficking are not well understood, and it is unclear how phosphorylated and desphosphorylated receptors are sorted in endosomes. High throughput screening techniques have aided in the discovery of biased ligands with the capacity to control specific aspects of receptor function, and it is to be hoped that designer ligands for TRH receptors will provide new tools for research or even novel drugs for treating thyroid disease. Finally, long awaited information on the structure of the TRH receptor can be expected in the not too distant future.

ACKNOWLEDGMENTS

Research in the author's laboratory was supported by NIH Grant DK19974.

REFERENCES

Ashworth, R., Yu, R., Nelson, E. J., Dermer, S., Gershengorn, M. C., and Hinkle, P. M. (1995). Visualization of the thyrotropin-releasing hormone receptor and its ligand during endocytosis and recycling. *Proc. Natl. Acad. Sci. U.S.A.* 92, 512–516.

Barford, D., Das, A. K., and Egloff, M. P. (1998). The structure and mechanism of protein phosphatases: insights into catalysis and regulation. *Annu. Rev. Biophys. Biomol. Struct.* 27, 133–164.

Barros, F., del Camino, D., Pardo, L. A., Palomero, T., Giraldez, T., and de la Pena, P. (1997). Demonstration of an inwardly rectifying K+ current component modulated by thyrotropin-releasing hormone and caffeine in GH3 rat anterior pituitary cells. *Pflugers Arch.* 435, 119–129.

Bollen, M., Peti, W., Ragusa, M. J., and Beullens, M. (2010). The extended PP1 toolkit: designed to create specificity. *Trends Biochem. Sci.* 35, 450–458.

Bonomi, M., Busnelli, M., Beck-Peccoz, P., Costanzo, D., Antonica, F., Dolci, C., et al. (2009). A family with complete resistance to thyrotropin-releasing hormone. *N. Engl. J. Med.* 360, 731–734.

Boutin, A., Allen, M. D., Neumann, S., and Gershengorn, M. C. (2012). Persistent signaling by thyrotropin-releasing hormone receptors correlates with G-protein and receptor levels. *FASEB J.* 26, 3473–3482.

Bulenger, S., Marullo, S., and Bouvier, M. (2005). Emerging role of homo- and heterodimerization in G-protein-coupled receptor biosynthesis and maturation. *Trends Pharmacol. Sci.* 26, 131–137.

Burt, D. R., and Snyder, S. H. (1975). Thyrotropin releasing hormone (TRH): apparent receptor binding in rat brain membranes. *Brain Res.* 93, 309–328.

Cattaruzza, F., Cottrell, G. S., Vaksman, N., and Bunnett, N. W. (2009). Endothelin-converting enzyme 1 promotes re-sensitization of neurokinin 1 receptor-dependent neurogenic inflammation. *Br. J. Pharmacol.* 156, 730–739.

Cook, L. B., and Hinkle, P. M. (2004). Fate of internalized thyrotropin-releasing hormone receptors monitored with a timer fusion protein. *Endocrinology* 145, 3095–3100.

Cook, L. B., Zhu, C. C., and Hinkle, P. M. (2003). Thyrotropin-releasing hormone receptor processing: role of ubiquitination and proteasomal degradation. *Mol. Endocrinol.* 17, 1777–1791.

Costa, E. S. R. H., Astapova, I., Ye, F., Wondisford, F. E., and Hollenberg, A. N. (2012). The thyroid axis is regulated by NCoR1 via its actions in the pituitary. *Endocrinology* 153, 5049–5057.

Costa, E. S. R. H., and Hollenberg, A. N. (2012). Minireview: the neural regulation of the hypothalamic-pituitary-thyroid axis. *Endocrinology* 153, 4128–4135.

Croci, C., Sticht, H., Brandstatter, J. H., and Enz, R. (2003). Group I metabotropic glutamate receptors bind to protein phosphatase 1C. Mapping and modeling of interacting sequences. *J. Biol. Chem.* 278, 50682–50690.

DeFea, K. A. (2011). Beta arrestins as regulators of signal termination and transduction: how do they determine what to scaffold? *Cell. Signal.* 23, 621–629.

DeWire, S. M., Ahn, S., Lefkowitz, R. J., and Shenoy, S. K. (2007). Beta-arrestins and cell signaling. *Annu. Rev. Physiol.* 69, 483–510.

Drmota, T., Gould, G. W., and Milligan, G. (1998). Real time visualization of agonist-mediated redistribution and internalization of a green fluorescent protein-tagged form of the thyrotropin-releasing hormone receptor. *J. Biol. Chem.* 273, 24000–24008.

Drmota, T., Novotny, J., Gould, G. W., Svoboda, P., and Milligan, G. (1999). Visualization of distinct patterns of subcellular redistribution of the thyrotropin-releasing hormone receptor-1 and gqalpha/G11alpha induced by agonist stimulation. *Biochem. J.* 340(Pt 2), 529–538.

Drummond, A. H. (1985). Bidirectional control of cytosolic free calcium by thyrotropin-releasing hormone in pituitary cells. *Nature* 315, 752–755.

Drummond, A. H., Bushfield, M., and Macphee, C. H. (1984). Thyrotropin-releasing hormone-stimulated [3H]inositol metabolism in GH3 pituitary tumor cells. Studies with lithium. *Mol. Pharmacol.* 25, 201–208.

Du, D., Raaka, B. M., Grimberg, H., Lupu-Meiri, M., Oron, Y., and Gershengorn, M. C. (2005). Carboxyl tail cysteine mutants of the thyrotropin-releasing hormone receptor type 1 exhibit constitutive signaling: role of palmitoylation. *Mol. Pharmacol.* 68, 204–209.

Evron, T., Daigle, T. L., and Caron, M. G. (2012). GRK2: multiple roles beyond G protein-coupled receptor desensitization. *Trends Pharmacol. Sci.* 33, 154–161.

Falck-Pedersen, E., Heinflink, M., Alvira, M., Nussenzveig, D. R., and Gershengorn, M. C. (1994). Expression of thyrotropin-releasing hormone receptors by adenovirus-mediated gene transfer reveals that thyrotropin-releasing hormone desensitization is cell specific. *Mol. Pharmacol.* 45, 684–689.

Fekete, C., and Lechan, R. M. (2007). Negative feedback regulation of hypophysiotropic thyrotropin-releasing hormone (TRH) synthesizing neurons: role of neuronal afferents and type 2 deiodinase. *Front. Neuroendocrinol.* 28, 97–114.

Flajolet, M., Rakhilin, S., Wang, H., Starkova, N., Nuangchamnong, N., Nairn, A. C., et al. (2003). Protein phosphatase 2C binds selectively to and dephosphorylates metabotropic glutamate receptor 3. *Proc. Natl. Acad. Sci. U.S.A.* 100, 16006–16011.

Gehret, A. U., and Hinkle, P. M. (2010). Importance of regions outside the cytoplasmic tail of G-protein-coupled receptors for phosphorylation and dephosphorylation. *Biochem. J.* 428, 235–245.

Gehret, A. U., and Hinkle, P. M. (2012). Protein Phosphatase 1alpha is involved in the regulation of the thyrotropin-releasing hormone receptor. *FASEB J.* lb180.

Gehret, A. U., Jones, B. W., Tran, P. N., Cook, L. B., Greuber, E. K., and Hinkle, P. M. (2010). Role of helix 8 of the thyrotropin-releasing hormone receptor in phosphorylation by G protein-coupled receptor kinase. *Mol. Pharmacol.* 77, 288–297.

Gershengorn, M. C. (1978). Bihormonal regulation of the thyrotropin-releasing hormone receptor in mouse pituitary thyrotropic tumor cells in culture. *J. Clin. Invest.* 62, 937–943.

Gershengorn, M. C. (1989). Mechanism of signal transduction by TRH. *Ann. N. Y. Acad. Sci.* 553, 191–196.

Gershengorn, M. C., and Osman, R. (1996). Molecular and cellular biology of thyrotropin-releasing hormone receptors. *Physiol. Rev.* 76, 175–191.

Ghosh, M., and Schonbrunn, A. (2011). Differential temporal and spatial regulation of somatostatin receptor phosphorylation and dephosphorylation. *J. Biol. Chem.* 286, 13561–13573.

Groarke, D. A., Drmota, T., Bahia, D. S., Evans, N. A., Wilson, S., and Milligan, G. (2001). Analysis of the C-terminal tail of the rat thyrotropin-releasing hormone receptor-1 in interactions and cointernalization with beta-arrestin 1-green fluorescent protein. *Mol. Pharmacol.* 59, 375–385.

Groarke, D. A., Wilson, S., Krasel, C., and Milligan, G. (1999). Visualization of agonist-induced association and trafficking of green fluorescent protein-tagged forms of both beta-arrestin-1 and the thyrotropin-releasing hormone receptor-1. *J. Biol. Chem.* 274, 23263–23269.

Gurevich, E. V., Tesmer, J. J., Mushegian, A., and Gurevich, V. V. (2012). G protein-coupled receptor kinases: more than just kinases and not only for GPCRs. *Pharmacol. Ther.* 133, 40–69.

Gurevich, V. V., and Gurevich, E. V. (2006). The structural basis of arrestin-mediated regulation of G-protein-coupled receptors. *Pharmacol. Ther.* 110, 465–502.

Gurevich, V. V., Pals-Rylaarsdam, R., Benovic, J. L., Hosey, M. M., and Onorato, J. J. (1997). Agonist-receptor-arrestin, an alternative ternary complex with high agonist affinity. *J. Biol. Chem.* 272, 28849–28852.

Hanyaloglu, A. C., Seeber, R. M., Kohout, T. A., Lefkowitz, R. J., and Eidne, K. A. (2002). Homo- and hetero-oligomerization of thyrotropin-releasing hormone (TRH) receptor subtypes. Differential regulation of beta-arrestins 1 and 2. *J. Biol. Chem.* 277, 50422–50430.

Hanyaloglu, A. C., and von Zastrow, M. (2008). Regulation of GPCRs by endocytic membrane trafficking and its potential implications. *Annu. Rev. Pharmacol. Toxicol.* 48, 537–568.

Hanyaloglu, A. C., Vrecl, M., Kroeger, K. M., Miles, L. E., Qian, H., Thomas, W. G., et al. (2001). Casein kinase II sites in the intracellular C-terminal domain of the thyrotropin-releasing hormone receptor and chimeric gonadotropin-releasing hormone receptors contribute to beta-arrestin-dependent internalization. *J. Biol. Chem.* 276, 18066–18074.

Hinkle, P. M., and Goh, K. B. (1982). Regulation of thyrotropin-releasing hormone receptors and responses by L-triiodothyronine in dispersed rat pituitary cell cultures. *Endocrinology* 110, 1725–1731.

Hinkle, P. M., and Kinsella, P. A. (1984). Regulation of thyrotropin-releasing hormone binding by monovalent cations and guanyl nucleotides. *J. Biol. Chem.* 259, 3445–3449.

Hinkle, P. M., Nelson, E. J., and Ashworth, R. (1996). Characterization of the calcium response to thyrotropin-releasing hormone in lactotrophs and GH cells. *Trends Endocrinol. Metab.* 7, 370–374.

Hinkle, P. M., and Phillips, W. J. (1984). Thyrotropin-releasing hormone stimulates GTP hydrolysis by membranes from GH4C1 rat pituitary tumor cells. *Proc. Natl. Acad. Sci. U.S.A.* 81, 6183–6187.

Hinkle, P. M., and Tashjian, A. H. Jr. (1973). Receptors for thyrotropin-releasing hormone in prolactin producing rat pituitary cells in culture. *J. Biol. Chem.* 248, 6180–6186.

Hinkle, P. M., and Tashjian, A. H. Jr. (1975). Thyrotropin-releasing hormone regulates the number of its own receptors in the GH3 strain of pituitary cells in culture. *Biochemistry* 14, 3845–3851.

Hislop, J. N., and von Zastrow, M. (2011). Role of ubiquitination in endocytic trafficking of G-protein-coupled receptors. *Traffic* 12, 137–148.

Iyer, V., Tran, T. M., Foster, E., Dai, W., Clark, R. B., and Knoll, B. J. (2006). Differential phosphorylation and dephosphorylation of beta2-adrenoceptor sites Ser262 and Ser355,356. *Br. J. Pharmacol.* 147, 249–259.

Jones, B. W., and Hinkle, P. M. (2005). Beta-arrestin mediates desensitization and internalization but does not affect dephosphorylation of the thyrotropin-releasing hormone receptor. *J. Biol. Chem.* 280, 38346–38354.

Jones, B. W., and Hinkle, P. M. (2008). Arrestin binds to different phosphorylated regions of the thyrotropin-releasing hormone receptor with distinct functional consequences. *Mol. Pharmacol.* 74, 195–202.

Jones, B. W., and Hinkle, P. M. (2009). Subcellular trafficking of the TRH receptor: effect of phosphorylation. *Mol. Endocrinol.* 23, 1466–1478.

Jones, B. W., Song, G. J., Greuber, E. K., and Hinkle, P. M. (2007). Phosphorylation of the endogenous thyrotropin-releasing hormone receptor in pituitary GH3 cells and pituitary tissue revealed by phosphosite-specific antibodies. *J. Biol. Chem.* 282, 12893–12906.

Jordan, B. A., and Devi, L. A. (1999). G-protein-coupled receptor heterodimerization modulates receptor function. *Nature* 399, 697–700.

Konaka, S., Yamada, M., Satoh, T., Ozawa, H., Watanabe, E., Takata, K., et al. (1997). Expression of thyrotropin-releasing hormone (TRH) receptor mRNA in somatotrophs in the rat anterior pituitary. *Endocrinology* 138, 827–830.

Krasel, C., Zabel, U., Lorenz, K., Reiner, S., Al-Sabah, S., and Lohse, M. J. (2008). Dual role of the beta2-adrenergic receptor C terminus for the binding of beta-arrestin and receptor internalization. *J. Biol. Chem.* 283, 31840–31848.

Kroeger, K. M., Hanyaloglu, A. C., Seeber, R. M., Miles, L. E., and Eidne, K. A. (2001). Constitutive and agonist-dependent homo-oligomerization of the thyrotropin-releasing hormone receptor. Detection in living cells using bioluminescence resonance energy transfer. *J. Biol. Chem.* 276, 12736–12743.

Lefkowitz, R. J., and Shenoy, S. K. (2005). Transduction of receptor signals by beta-arrestins. *Science* 308, 512–517.

Liggett, S. B. (2011). Phosphorylation barcoding as a mechanism of directing GPCR signaling. *Sci. Signal.* 4, pe36.

Lohse, M. J. (2010). Dimerization in GPCR mobility and signaling. *Curr. Opin. Pharmacol.* 10, 53–58.

Luttrell, L. M., and Gesty-Palmer, D. (2010). Beyond desensitization: physiological relevance of arrestin-dependent signaling. *Pharmacol. Rev.* 62, 305–330.

Mao, L., Yang, L., Arora, A., Choe, E. S., Zhang, G., Liu, Z., et al. (2005). Role of protein phosphatase 2A in mGluR5-regulated MEK/ERK phosphorylation in neurons. *J. Biol. Chem.* 280, 12602–12610.

Marsili, A., Sanchez, E., Singru, P., Harney, J. W., Zavacki, A. M., Lechan, R. M., et al. (2011). Thyroxine-induced expression of pyroglutamyl peptidase II and inhibition of TSH release precedes suppression of TRH mRNA and requires type 2 deiodinase. *J. Endocrinol.* 211, 73–78.

Milligan, G. (2009). G protein-coupled receptor hetero-dimerization: contribution to pharmacology and function. *Br. J. Pharmacol.* 158, 5–14.

Moore, C. A., Milano, S. K., and Benovic, J. L. (2007). Regulation of receptor trafficking by GRKs and arrestins. *Annu. Rev. Physiol.* 69, 451–482.

Nobles, K. N., Xiao, K., Ahn, S., Shukla, A. K., Lam, C. M., Rajagopal, S., et al. (2011). Distinct phosphorylation sites on the beta(2)-adrenergic receptor establish a barcode that encodes differential functions of beta-arrestin. *Sci. Signal.* 4, ra51.

Oakley, R. H., Laporte, S. A., Holt, J. A., Barak, L. S., and Caron, M. G. (1999). Association of beta-arrestin with G protein-coupled receptors during clathrin-mediated endocytosis dictates the profile of receptor resensitization. *J. Biol. Chem.* 274, 32248–32257.

Oakley, R. H., Laporte, S. A., Holt, J. A., Caron, M. G., and Barak, L. S. (2000). Differential affinities of visual arrestin, beta arrestin1, and beta arrestin2 for G protein-coupled receptors delineate two major classes of receptors. *J. Biol. Chem.* 275, 17201–17210.

O'Dowd, B. F., Lee, D. K., Huang, W., Nguyen, T., Cheng, R., Liu, Y., et al. (2000). TRH-R2 exhibits similar binding and acute signaling but distinct regulation and anatomic distribution compared with TRH-R1. *Mol. Endocrinol.* 14, 183–193.

Ohmichi, M., Sawada, T., Kanda, Y., Koike, K., Hirota, K., Miyake, A., et al. (1994). Thyrotropin-releasing hormone stimulates MAP kinase activity in GH3 cells by divergent pathways. Evidence of a role for early tyrosine phosphorylation. *J. Biol. Chem.* 269, 3783–3788.

Perrone, M. H., and Hinkle, P. M. (1978). Regulation of pituitary receptors for thyrotropin-releasing hormone by thyroid hormones. *J. Biol. Chem.* 253, 5168–5173.

Pfleger, K. D., Kroeger, K. M., and Eidne, K. A. (2004). Receptors for hypothalamic releasing hormones TRH and GnRH: oligomerization and interactions with intracellular proteins. *Semin. Cell Dev. Biol.* 15, 269–280.

Pitcher, J. A., Payne, E. S., Csortos, C., DePaoli-Roach, A. A., and Lefkowitz, R. J. (1995). The G-protein-coupled receptor phosphatase: a protein phosphatase type 2A with a distinct subcellular distribution and substrate specificity. *Proc. Natl. Acad. Sci. U.S.A.* 92, 8343–8347.

Premont, R. T., and Gainetdinov, R. R. (2007). Physiological roles of G protein-coupled receptor kinases and arrestins. *Annu. Rev. Physiol.* 69, 511–534.

Rabeler, R., Mittag, J., Geffers, L., Ruther, U., Leitges, M., Parlow, A. F., et al. (2004). Generation of thyrotropin-releasing hormone receptor 1-deficient mice as an animal model of central hypothyroidism. *Mol. Endocrinol.* 18, 1450–1460.

Rajagopal, S., Rajagopal, K., and Lefkowitz, R. J. (2010). Teaching old receptors new tricks: biasing seven-transmembrane receptors. *Nat. Rev. Drug Discov.* 9, 373–386.

Reiter, E., Ahn, S., Shukla, A. K., and Lefkowitz, R. J. (2012). Molecular mechanism of beta-arrestin-biased agonism at seven-transmembrane receptors. *Annu. Rev. Pharmacol. Toxicol.* 52, 179–197.

Ren, X. R., Reiter, E., Ahn, S., Kim, J., Chen, W., and Lefkowitz, R. J. (2005). Different G protein-coupled receptor kinases govern G protein and beta-arrestin-mediated signaling of V2 vasopressin receptor. *Proc. Natl. Acad. Sci. U.S.A.* 102, 1448–1453.

Romero, G., von Zastrow, M., and Friedman, P. A. (2011). Role of PDZ proteins in regulating trafficking, signaling, and function of GPCRs: means, motif, and opportunity. *Adv. Pharmacol.* 62, 279–314.

Romoser, V. A., Graves, T. K., Wu, D., Jiang, H., and Hinkle, P. M. (2001). Calcium responses to thyrotropin-releasing hormone, gonadotropin-releasing hormone and somatostatin in phospholipase css3 knockout mice. *Mol. Endocrinol.* 15, 125–135.

Roosterman, D., Kempkes, C., Cottrell, G. S., Padilla, B. E., Bunnett, N. W., Turck, C. W., et al. (2008). Endothelin-converting enzyme-1 degrades internalized somatostatin-14. *Endocrinology* 149, 2200–2207.

Rudajev, V., Novotny, J., Hejnova, L., Milligan, G., and Svoboda, P. (2005). Dominant portion of thyrotropin-releasing hormone receptor is excluded from lipid domains. Detergent-resistant and detergent-sensitive pools of TRH receptor and Gqalpha/G11alpha protein. *J. Biochem.* 138, 111–125.

Schomburg, L., and Bauer, K. (1997). Regulation of the adenohypophyseal thyrotropin-releasing hormone-degrading ectoenzyme by estradiol. *Endocrinology* 138, 3587–3593.

Scott, M. G., Benmerah, A., Muntaner, O., and Marullo, S. (2002). Recruitment of activated G protein-coupled receptors to pre-existing clathrin-coated pits in living cells. *J. Biol. Chem.* 277, 3552–3559.

Segerson, T. P., Kauer, J., Wolfe, H. C., Mobtaker, H., Wu, P., Jackson, I. M., et al. (1987). Thyroid hormone regulates TRH biosynthesis in the paraventricular nucleus of the rat hypothalamus. *Science* 238, 78–80.

Shenoy, S. K., and Lefkowitz, R. J. (2011). β-Arrestin-mediated receptor trafficking and signal transduction. *Trends Pharmacol. Sci.* 32, 521–533.

Smith, J., Yu, R., and Hinkle, P. M. (2001). Activation of MAPK by TRH requires clathrin-dependent endocytosis and PKC but not receptor interaction with beta-arrestin or receptor endocytosis. *Mol. Endocrinol.* 15, 1539–1548.

Song, G. J., and Hinkle, P. M. (2005). Regulated dimerization of the thyrotropin-releasing hormone receptor affects receptor trafficking but not signaling. *Mol. Endocrinol.* 19, 2859–2870.

Song, G. J., Jones, B. W., and Hinkle, P. M. (2007). Dimerization of the thyrotropin-releasing hormone receptor potentiates hormone-dependent receptor phosphorylation. *Proc. Natl. Acad. Sci. U.S.A.* 104, 18303–18308.

Sun, Y., Lu, X., and Gershengorn, M. C. (2003). Thyrotropin-releasing hormone receptors – similarities and differences. *J. Mol. Endocrinol.* 30, 87–97.

Sun, Y., Zupan, B., Raaka, B. M., Toth, M., and Gershengorn, M. C. (2009). TRH-receptor-type-2-deficient mice are euthyroid and exhibit increased depression and reduced anxiety phenotypes. *Neuropsychopharmacology* 34, 1601–1608.

Thal, D. M., Homan, K. T., Chen, J., Wu, E. K., Hinkle, P. M., Huang, Z. M., et al. (2012). Paroxetine is a direct inhibitor of G protein-coupled receptor kinase 2 and increases myocardial contractility. *ACS Chem. Biol.* 7, 1830–1839.

Villalobos, C., Nunez, L., Frawley, L. S., Garcia-Sancho, J., and Sanchez, A. (1997). Multi-responsiveness of single anterior pituitary cells to hypothalamic-releasing hormones: a cellular basis for paradoxical secretion. *Proc. Natl. Acad. Sci. U.S.A.* 94, 14132–14137.

Vrecl, M., Anderson, L., Hanyaloglu, A., McGregor, A. M., Groarke, A. D., Milligan, G., et al. (1998). Agonist-induced endocytosis and recycling of the gonadotropin-releasing hormone receptor: effect of beta-arrestin on internalization kinetics. *Mol. Endocrinol.* 12, 1818–1829.

Whorton, M. R., Bokoch, M. P., Rasmussen, S. G., Huang, B., Zare, R. N., Kobilka, B., et al. (2007). A monomeric G protein-coupled receptor isolated in a high-density lipoprotein particle efficiently activates its G protein. *Proc. Natl. Acad. Sci. U.S.A.* 104, 7682–7687.

Xiao, K., McClatchy, D. B., Shukla, A. K., Zhao, Y., Chen, M., Shenoy, S. K., et al. (2007). Functional specialization of beta-arrestin interactions revealed by proteomic analysis. *Proc. Natl. Acad. Sci. U.S.A.* 104, 12011–12016.

Yamada, M., Saga, Y., Shibusawa, N., Hirato, J., Murakami, M., Iwasaki, T., et al. (1997). Tertiary hypothyroidism and hyperglycemia in mice with targeted disruption of the thyrotropin-releasing hormone gene. *Proc. Natl. Acad. Sci. U.S.A.* 94, 10862–10867.

Yu, R., Ashworth, R., and Hinkle, P. M. (1998). Receptors for thyrotropin-releasing hormone on rat lactotropes and thyrotropes. *Thyroid* 8, 887–894.

Yu, R., and Hinkle, P. M. (1997). Desensitization of thyrotropin-releasing hormone receptor-mediated responses involves multiple steps. *J. Biol. Chem.* 272, 28301–28307.

Yu, R., and Hinkle, P. M. (1998). Signal transduction, desensitization, and recovery of responses to thyrotropin-releasing hormone after inhibition of receptor internalization. *Mol. Endocrinol.* 12, 737–749.

Yu, R., and Hinkle, P. M. (1999). Signal transduction and hormone-dependent internalization of the thyrotropin-releasing hormone receptor in cells lacking Gq and G11. *J. Biol. Chem.* 274, 15745–15750.

Zeng, H., Schimpf, B. A., Rohde, A. D., Pavlova, M. N., Gragerov, A., and Bergmann, J. E. (2007). Thyrotropin-releasing hormone receptor 1-deficient mice display increased depression and anxiety-like behavior. *Mol. Endocrinol.* 21, 2795–2804.

Zhu, C. C., Cook, L. B., and Hinkle, P. M. (2002). Dimerization and phosphorylation of thyrotropin-releasing hormone receptors are modulated by agonist stimulation. *J. Biol. Chem.* 277, 28228–28237.

11

Relaxin-3/RXFP3 signaling and neuroendocrine function – a perspective on extrinsic hypothalamic control

Despina E. Ganella[1,2], Sherie Ma[1] and Andrew L. Gundlach[1,3,4]*

[1] The Florey Institute of Neuroscience and Mental Health, The University of Melbourne, Melbourne, VIC, Australia
[2] Department of Biochemistry and Molecular Biology, The University of Melbourne, Melbourne, VIC, Australia
[3] Florey Department of Neuroscience and Mental Health, The University of Melbourne, Melbourne, VIC, Australia
[4] Department of Anatomy and Neuroscience, The University of Melbourne, Melbourne, VIC, Australia

Edited by:
Hubert Vaudry, University of Rouen, France

Reviewed by:
Michiru Hirasawa, Memorial University, Canada
Barbara McGowan, Guys and St. Thomas Hospital, UK

***Correspondence:**
Andrew L. Gundlach, The Florey Institute of Neuroscience and Mental Health, 30 Royal Parade, Parkville, VIC 3052, Australia
e-mail: andrew.gundlach@florey.edu.au

Complex neural circuits within the hypothalamus that govern essential autonomic processes and associated behaviors signal using amino acid and monoamine transmitters and a variety of neuropeptide (hormone) modulators, often via G-protein coupled receptors (GPCRs) and associated cellular pathways. Relaxin-3 is a recently identified neuropeptide that is highly conserved throughout evolution. Neurons expressing relaxin-3 are located in the brainstem, but broadly innervate the entire limbic system including the hypothalamus. Extensive anatomical data in rodents and non-human primate, and recent regulatory and functional data, suggest relaxin-3 signaling via its cognate GPCR, RXFP3, has a broad range of effects on neuroendocrine function associated with stress responses, feeding and metabolism, motivation and reward, and possibly sexual behavior and reproduction. Therefore, this article aims to highlight the growing appreciation of the relaxin-3/RXFP3 system as an important "extrinsic" regulator of the neuroendocrine axis by reviewing its neuroanatomy and its putative roles in arousal-, stress-, and feeding-related behaviors and links to associated neural substrates and signaling networks. Current evidence identifies RXFP3 as a potential therapeutic target for treatment of neuroendocrine disorders and related behavioral dysfunction.

Keywords: relaxin-3, oxytocin, arginine vasopressin, CRH, feeding, metabolism, stress, reproduction

INTRODUCTION

Precise regulation of complex neural circuits in the hypothalamus governs essential autonomic processes *and* associated behaviors, such as metabolism, growth, and feeding; stress responses, arousal, and locomotor activity; as well as reproduction and social/sexual behavior (1–7). These intrinsic and often interacting neural circuits utilize various neuroendocrine peptides/hormones, such as thyrotropin-releasing hormone (TRH), growth hormone-releasing hormone (GHRH), somatostatin, orexins, melanin-concentrating hormone (MCH), agouti-related peptide (AgRP), pro-opiomelanocortin (POMC) gene products [alpha-melanocyte-stimulating hormone (α-MSH)], neuropeptide Y (NPY), corticotropin-releasing hormone (CRH) and urocortins, gonadotropin-releasing hormone (GnRH), arginine vasopressin (AVP), and oxytocin (8–16). The majority of these peptides and hormones signal via G-protein coupled receptors (GPCRs) and often multiple receptors exist for different members of a peptide family or for the same peptide modulator [e.g., Ref. (17–19)].

This combination of a large number of ligands and multiple receptors results in a vast diversity in the potential regulation of different populations of hypothalamic neurons. For example, a recent survey revealed more than 300 different GPCRs are expressed by the heterogeneous neurons in the paraventricular (PVN) and supraoptic nuclei (SON) alone (20). This diversity of potential functional regulation provides a challenge for neuroscientists and neuroendocrinologists to document the anatomical distribution and dissect the primary and integrative actions of different signaling systems, both within hypothalamic circuits and via their descending and ascending inputs. Importantly, modern experimental approaches including conventional and viral-based tract-tracing (21) and other viral-based methods, such as optogenetics and DREADD technology (22–25), combined with molecular genetics and complementary methods for measuring changes in physiology and behavior, are successfully dissecting the role of individual neuron populations and the key mediators involved. In turn, this is allowing a reappraisal of the "dogma" related to the function of several established neural transmitter and hormone networks in the hypothalamus and the integration of new "chemical players" into the existing circuitry.

Just over a decade ago, the final member of the relaxin and insulin-like peptide superfamily was discovered and named H3 relaxin (human) or relaxin-3 (rodents), in line with the prior discovery and characterization of two other relaxin genes in humans (26). However, unlike its related peptide, H2 relaxin or relaxin, which is widely distributed within the brain *and* peripheral tissues [see Ref. (27, 28) for review], relaxin-3 was found to be most highly expressed in brain (26, 29). In 2003, GPCR135 (now known as RXFP3) was identified as the cognate relaxin-3 receptor (30, 31) and was shown to be highly localized in various rat brain areas (30, 32), which were later confirmed to contain relaxin-3-positive axonal projections and terminations (33). A similar central distribution of relaxin-3 neurons and projections to that reported in the rat was subsequently observed in the mouse [Ref. (34); Allen Brain Atlas[1]] and macaque brain (35, 36), suggesting that this neuropeptide system has been highly conserved throughout evolution. Indeed, bioinformatic studies revealed that a relaxin-3-like ancestral peptide gave rise to the relaxin and insulin-like peptide superfamily and its sequence has been highly conserved by strong purifying selection, consistent with a highly conserved function in the central nervous system (37, 38).

After their discovery, characterization of the neuroanatomical distribution of relaxin-3- and RXFP3-expressing neurons provided insights into putative functions of relaxin-3; and a growing number of experimental studies have subsequently confirmed roles for relaxin-3/RXFP3 signaling in arousal, feeding, stress responses, and cognition [see Ref. (39) for review]. Several of these actions of relaxin-3 likely involve effects on RXFP3-positive hypothalamic neuron populations. Therefore, in this article we will provide a summary of the hypothalamic distribution of RXFP3 mRNA and protein, and relaxin-3 projections, a concise review of experimental data indicating that this neuropeptide/receptor system is a modulator of hypothalamic function, and a perspective on the future studies required to better understand this system and to exploit its therapeutic potential.

[1] www.brain-map.org

NEUROANATOMY OF THE RELAXIN-3/RXFP3 SYSTEM

Relaxin-3 is a 5 kDa peptide that shares common structural features with all relaxin and insulin-like peptide family members – an A- and B-chain held together by three disulfide bonds (26, 40, 41). The native peptide is synthesized as a pre-prohormone that is subsequently cleaved by proteolytic processing of the signal and C-peptides to form the mature peptide [see e.g., Ref. (42, 43)]. Early *in situ* hybridization studies revealed that relaxin-3 mRNA was highly expressed by a cluster of neurons in the rat pontine central gray, identified as the *ventromedial dorsal tegmental area* (29), more commonly known as the *nucleus incertus* [NI; (44, 45)]. Smaller dispersed populations were also identified in the medial periaqueductal gray (PAG), pontine raphe (PR), and a region dorsal of the substantia nigra (dSN) in the rat (33, 46), mouse (34), and macaque (36) (**Figure 1**).

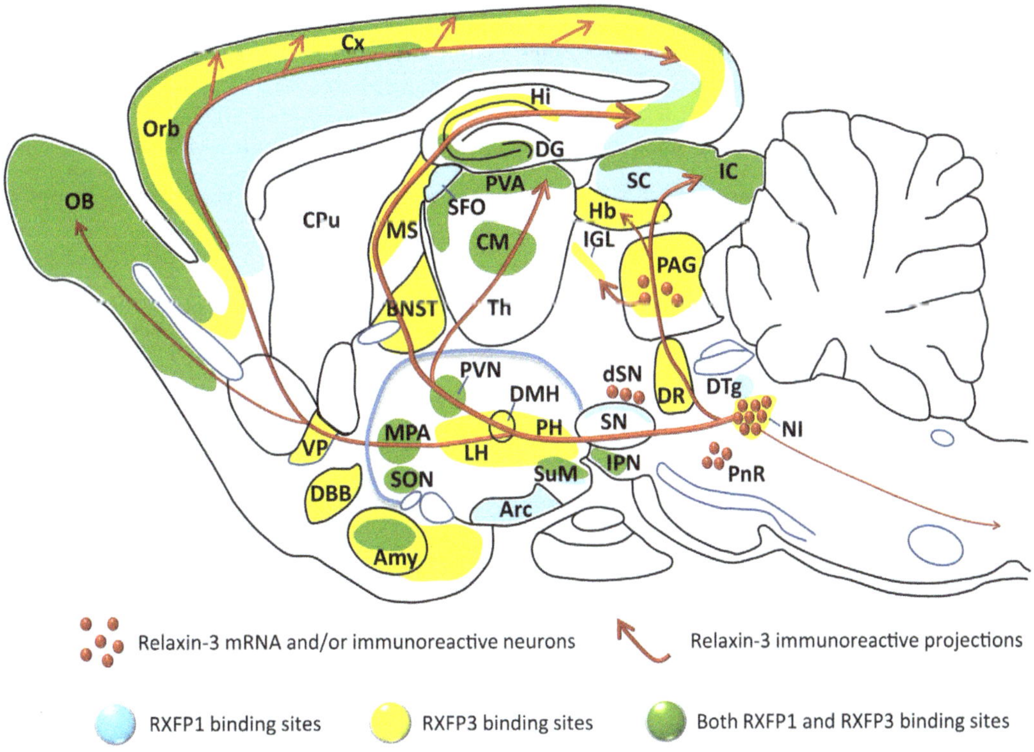

FIGURE 1 | Distribution of the relaxin-3 neural network and RXFP3 in relation to RXFP1, illustrated on a schematic parasagittal profile of the rodent brain. Relaxin-3 immunoreactive fibers (red), RXFP3 binding sites (yellow), RXFP1 binding sites (blue), and regions that contain both RXFP1 and RXFP3 binding sites (green) are illustrated [see (32–34, 46, 62) and (28)]. Amy, amygdala; Arc, arcuate nucleus; BNST, bed nucleus of the stria terminalis; CM, centromedial thalamic nucleus; CPu, caudate putamen; Cx, cerebral cortex; DBB, diagonal band of Broca; DG, dentate gyrus; DMH, dorsomedial nucleus of hypothalamus; DR, dorsal raphe nucleus; DTg, dorsal tegmental nucleus; Hb, habenula; Hi, hippocampus; IC, inferior colliculus; IGL, intergeniculate leaflet; IPN, interpeduncular nucleus; LH, lateral hypothalamus; MPA, medial preoptic area; MS, medial septum; NI, nucleus incertus; OB, olfactory bulb; Orb, orbitofrontal cortex; PAG, periaqueductal gray; PH, posterior hypothalamus; PnR, pontine raphe; PVA, paraventricular thalamic area; PVN, paraventricular nucleus of hypothalamus; SC, superior colliculus; SFO, subfornical organ; SON, supraoptic nucleus; SN, substantia nigra; SuM, supramammillary nucleus; Th, thalamus; VP, ventral pallidum. Adapted from a figure kindly provided by Dr. Craig Smith (The Florey Institute of Neuroscience and Mental Health, Melbourne, Australia).

Ultrastructural analysis of relaxin-3 immunoreactivity in the rat NI identified the peptide in the rough endoplasmic reticulum and Golgi apparatus in the cell soma and within dense-core vesicles adjacent to synapses in nerve terminals of distant target regions such as the lateral hypothalamus (46) and medial septum (47), indicating that relaxin-3 is processed and released as a transmitter.

The efferent and afferent connections of the rat NI have been characterized (44, 45, 48–50) and many NI projection target regions, including the hypothalamus, contain relaxin-3 immunoreactive fibers and terminals, and neurons expressing RXFP3 (33, 50) (**Figure 1**; **Table 1**), suggesting many of these areas are innervated by NI relaxin-3 neurons. Not surprisingly, NI relaxin-3 neurons have been the focus of the majority of functional studies to date, which indicate they are highly responsive to neurogenic stressors and CRH (46, 51–53).

Less is known about the connections, regulation and function of other relaxin-3 neuron populations, but a recent study demonstrated that PAG relaxin-3 neurons strongly innervate and modulate neuronal activity in the intergeniculate leaflet [IGL; (46, 54, 55)], a region that is known to contribute to the regulation of arousal and circadian activity (56–58). In brain slice studies, patch-clamp recordings of IGL neurons, revealed that activation of RXFP3 by bath application of the agonist peptide, R3/I5, produced depolarization of identified NPY-containing neurons (55), which are known to project to the suprachiasmatic nucleus via the geniculohypothalamic tract (56, 58). Neurons in the IGL also project to a number of other hypothalamic areas, including the anterior and lateral hypothalamic areas, and the dorsomedial nucleus (58).

There are, however, several brain regions like the aforementioned IGL and the amygdala that contain dense relaxin-3 immunoreactivity and/or RXFP3, but sparse NI projections; suggesting they are also more strongly innervated by other relaxin-3 populations. In fact, there is anatomical evidence, chiefly from neural tract-tracing studies, to suggest the various RXFP3-positive regions in the hypothalamus are also innervated by relaxin-3 neurons in the NI *and* other relaxin-3 groups. For example, a recent study of brainstem inputs to the PVN and surrounding area in the rat (59) revealed projections from the medial PAG, PR, and "dorsal to substantia nigra" regions, which contain relaxin-3 neurons.

RXFP3 has been localized in various subregions of the hypothalamus in the rat (32, 33) mouse (34, 60) (**Table 1**), and macaque (36). The highest densities are present in the PVN, SON and adjacent medial (MPO) and lateral preoptic (LPO) nuclei, but there are RXFP3-positive neurons in other hypothalamic areas, including the periventricular nucleus (33, 34) (**Table 1**), which is consistent with a putative role of relaxin-3/RXFP3 signaling in the control of a range of homeostatic and autonomic behaviors via modulation of related hypothalamic networks.

RELAXIN-3 RECEPTOR BINDING AND ACTIVATION IN BRAIN

Effects of endogenous relaxin-3 are predicted to be mediated by its cognate receptor, RXFP3, but relaxin-3 is also an agonist at the relaxin-family receptors, RXFP1 and RXFP4, when administered at pharmacological doses, albeit with lower potency than at RXFP3

Table 1 | Comparative distribution of relaxin-3 and its receptor, RXFP3, in hypothalamic regions of rat and mouse brain.

Hypothalamic area/nucleus	RLN3-LI		RXFP3 mRNA		RXFP3 binding sites	
	Mouse	Rat	Mouse	Rat	Mouse	Rat
Anterior hypothalamic n.	−/+	++	+	++	−/+	+
Arcuate n.	−	+	+	+	−	−/+
Dorsomedial hypothalamic n.	+	+++	+	+++	+	n.r.
Lateral hypothalamic area	+++	+++	++	++	+	+
Lateral mammillary n.	++	+	−/+	−/+	−	−
Lateroanterior hypothalamic n.	−/+	++	+	++	−	n.r.
Medial mammillary n.	+	++	−	+	−	−
Paraventricular hypothalamic n.	+	++	+++	+++	+++	+++
Periventricular hypothalamic n.	−/+	+	+++	++	++	++
Posterior hypothalamic area	+++	+++	++	+	+	n.r.
Premammillary n.	+	++	+	+	+	n.r.
Preoptic area, lateral	++	+++	++	++	++	+
Preoptic area, medial	−/+	++	+	+++	−/+	−/+
Suprachiasmatic n.	+	−/+	+	−/+	−	−
Supramammillary n.	+++	+++	++	++	−/+	−
Supraoptic n.	+++	++	+++	+++	++	+++
Tuberomammillary n.	+	+++	+	+++	+	n.r.
Ventromedial hypothalamic n.	+/++	++	+	++	+	n.r.

Relative abundance values are given: − not detectable, + low density, ++ moderate density, +++ high density, n.r. not reported). Adapted from Ma et al. (33), Smith et al. (34), Sutton et al. (32), Tanaka et al. (46), Allen Brain Institute Brain Atlas (http://mouse.brain-map.org/experiment/show/71358555). RLN3-LI, relaxin-3 like immunoreactivity.

(30, 61). RXFP1 and RXFP4 are likely expressed in the human brain, along with RXFP3, but based on animal studies these receptors and the peptides which bind and activate them (relaxin, insulin-like peptide 5, and relaxin-3, respectively) are expressed in quite distinct regions of the brain and at very different levels [e.g., Ref. (26, 29, 30, 33, 46, 62)], so a current working hypothesis that can be tested is that these receptors mediate distinct functional effects in the brain, which modulate different homeostatic processes and behaviors.

Cell signaling events associated with the relaxin-family receptors have been studied in different cell lines transfected with the human receptors (28, 63) and activation of RXFP1 and RXFP3/4 by H3 relaxin leads to different intracellular responses *in vitro*. In Chinese hamster ovary (CHO) cells, RXFP3 and RXFP4 couple to the inhibitory $G_{\alpha i}/G_{\alpha o}$-protein system and receptor activation leads to sequestration of these G-proteins and inhibition of adenylate cyclase (AC), and subsequent cAMP accumulation (30, 64). The intracellular signaling pathway of the relaxin-3-RXFP3 interaction has also been studied in the SN56 neuronal-like cell line, in which the $G_{\alpha i}/G_{\alpha o}$ pathway was recruited, suggesting an inhibitory intracellular pathway may be activated *in vivo* when relaxin-3 binds to RXFP3-expressing neurons within the brain (63), an idea that can be tested in different functional networks [see Ref. (54, 55)]. In contrast, RXFP1 activation by either relaxin or relaxin-3 in mammalian cell expression systems initiates a downstream accumulation of cAMP, as it is predominantly coupled to the stimulatory G_s-protein. These *in vitro* studies suggest activation of different receptors may lead to different downstream effects in neurons *in vivo*. Little is known, however, about the native intracellular signaling of any of the relaxin family of receptors (RXFP1–RXFP4) in specific neuronal populations, apart from a recent *in vitro* study that revealed activation of RXFP3 by the agonist peptide, R3/I5 (65), produced depolarization of identified NPY-containing neurons and hyperpolarization of adjacent non-NPY neurons (55).

Although there is no definitive evidence that major biological effects mediated by relaxin-3 are caused by activation of either RXFP1 and/or RXFP4, the ability of relaxin-3 to activate RXFP1 and RXFP4 as well as RXFP3 must be considered as a confounding factor when using pharmacological doses of peptides *in vivo*, in attempts to study neuropeptide function in the rodent. From a practical viewpoint, the rat is suited to studies of the neurobiology of relaxin-3/RXFP3 signaling, since RXFP4 is a pseudogene in this species, and so not a "confound." However, *in situ* hybridization and radioligand binding site studies indicate RXFP1 is expressed in the rat brain in a number of regions positive for RXFP3, including the cerebral cortex, amygdala, thalamus, and hypothalamus (32, 33, 62). Consequently RXFP1 activity must be considered in studies of exogenous relaxin-3 peptide administration [e.g., Ref. (40, 66–70)]. The relative degree to which RXFP1 activation has impacted outcomes in studies of relaxin-3 actions within the hypothalamus and other brain areas is hard to gage, although in some cases comparative effects of relaxin were reported [see Ref. (71) below]. Fortunately, the development more recently of agonist and antagonist peptides which selectively activate or inhibit RXFP3 [e.g., Ref. (65, 72–74)] has facilitated investigations of the behavioral and physiological effects of specific relaxin-3/RXFP3 interactions. Indeed, several studies have used these peptides to assess relaxin-3/RXFP3 related functions associated with the hypothalamus, although their use is not as widespread as it might be [e.g., Ref. (69, 70)], particularly in light of the availability of a chemically less-complex, single-chain peptide antagonist for RXFP3 (73).

ACTIONS OF THE RELAXIN-3/RXFP3 SYSTEM – FOCUS ON HYPOTHALAMUS

FEEDING AND ENERGY BALANCE

The PVN and arcuate nucleus (ARC) are two hypothalamic nuclei which tightly regulate food intake and energy homeostasis [e.g., Ref. (3, 4, 12, 15, 75)]. Relaxin-3 immunoreactivity and RXFP3 mRNA and binding sites have been identified in the PVN and ARC (30, 32, 33) (**Table 1**) and extensive research has demonstrated that H3 relaxin can alter feeding and appetite in rats [see Ref. (76)]. Central (icv) administration of H3 relaxin caused hyperphagia in satiated male Wistar rats in the first hour after treatment in both the light and the dark phase, while equivalent doses of H2 relaxin did not produce a similar effect (66). The doses of H3 relaxin administered icv (180 pmol) or directly into the PVN (18 pmol) at which a significant increase in feeding was observed (see below) were similar to doses of other "feeding" peptides which elicit an increased feeding response upon similar administration [e.g., NPY ~80 pmol iPVN; (77)], consistent with a physiological role for relaxin-3/RXFP3 signaling in modulating appetite and feeding behavior. Importantly, icv administration of the selective agonist, R3/I5, produced an increase in first-hour food intake and this effect was inhibited by co-administration of the selective antagonist, ΔR3/I5 (72), further suggesting RXFP3 involvement. In these feeding studies, the food intake was monitored for only 24 h post-injection, as it was predicted the injected peptide would be quite rapidly degraded by proteolysis. In a study of longer term effects of relaxin-3 on feeding and body weight, H3 relaxin (600 pmol/day) was infused icv into rats for 14 days via osmotic mini-pump, which produced a significant increase in food intake and body weight gain, and plasma leptin and insulin levels, compared to vehicle (78). This data indicated that the relaxin-3 induced increase in food intake could be sustained and lead to an increase in body weight and associated biochemical changes in the rat.

Given the primary role of the hypothalamus in energy balance, the effect on feeding of local hypothalamic injections of relaxin-3 was assessed. Acute H3 relaxin injection into the PVN (iPVN) increased food intake over the first hour (67). Sub-chronic iPVN H3 relaxin administration in *ad libitum* fed rats also produced an increase in food intake and cumulative body weight gain *c.f.* vehicle (67). These authors also used "Fos-activation" mapping after icv administration of H3 relaxin to identify activated hypothalamic nuclei. In addition to the PVN, the SON, ARC, and anterior preoptic area displayed increased Fos staining (79). When injected directly into these and other hypothalamic nuclei H3 relaxin stimulated a significant increase in food intake within the first hour, relative to control (79), suggesting multiple hypothalamic nuclei may mediate these potent orexigenic effects. Unfortunately the potential involvement of RXFP1 activation in the observed effects cannot be reliably excluded, as RXFP3-selective peptides were not utilized. It is also possible the injected peptide is able to diffuse from the injection site to adjacent areas that are primarily involved in the activation of feeding, although some targeted sites were not associated with feeding (79).

In order to circumvent issues associated with acute peptide administration and cross-reactivity of H3 relaxin at RXFP1, we used a viral strategy to investigate the effect of chronic R3/I5 mediated RXFP3 activation within the hypothalamic PVN (43). Using a recombinant adeno-associated virus (rAAV) engineered to locally secrete bioactive R3/I5 (rAAV-R3/I5), we demonstrated an increase in food intake in the R3/I5 expressing rats (~5.2 g/day more than control) which was sustained for up to 2 months, leading to an ~23% increase in cumulative body weight gain (43). In an attempt to identify targets of RXFP3 activation within the hypothalamus, levels of mRNA for a number of genes were also assessed in dissected hypothalamic tissue blocks using quantitative reverse transcription PCR. Notably, no major differences were identified in expression of some "major" feeding peptide genes (NPY, AgRP, POMC) between rAAV-R3/I5 and rAAV-control treated groups, whereas the levels of oxytocin and AVP mRNA were altered. This is, however, consistent with the strong expression of RXFP3 by neurons in the PVN and SON (30, 32, 33) (**Table 1**), which contain oxytocin- and AVP-containing magnocellular neurons. Chronic viral-mediated expression of R3/I5 in the hypothalamus for up to ~14 weeks led to a marked reduction in oxytocin mRNA expression in PVN (~50%) and a smaller reduction in AVP (~25%), compared to control expression (43). These data suggest the acute orexigenic effect of RXFP3 activation may be mediated by changes in oxytocin release (and perhaps AVP) [see Ref. (80)], an idea that can be tested experimentally. Furthermore, there is a substantial literature relating to oxytocin as a satiety factor that also supports this putative acute and chronic mechanism of action.

INTERACTION WITH OXYTOCIN AND ARGININE VASOPRESSIN SYSTEMS IN THE PVN

Oxytocin is a peptide hormone highly expressed in magnocellular and some parvocellular neurons of the hypothalamic PVN and SON (81–83). Oxytocin is classically known as a reproductive hormone with roles in parturition, lactation, sexual behavior, and pair bonding and attachment [see Ref. (84, 85) for review]. However, early studies revealed that central administration of oxytocin dose-dependently reduced food consumption and time spent eating and increased the latency to the first meal in pre-fasted rats; an effect prevented by co-administration of an oxytocin receptor antagonist (86). A number of studies have since confirmed central oxytocin administration inhibits food intake, strengthening the hypothesis that oxytocin serves a key role in appetite control (87–89). More recent data is consistent with this view, as oxytocin null mutation mice display enhanced intake of sweet and non-sweet carbohydrate solutions (90, 91) and develop late-onset obesity (92).

The magnitude of the increase in feeding and body weight gain observed in our hypothalamic R3/I5 expression studies (43) was modest relative to those seen after similar viral-mediated NPY and AgRP over-expression, consistent with actions independent of direct effects on these neurons. The down-regulation of oxytocin and AVP mRNA expression observed (43), suggests the R3/I5 agonist peptide is activating RXFP3 on oxytocin- and AVP-containing neurons, which results in downstream effects on the transcription of oxytocin and AVP mRNA in these neurons (e.g., Ref. (93, 94)] and subsequent effects on production and release of this anorexigenic hormone. If RXFP3 associated cell signaling in these neurons is similar to effects reported *in vitro*, this could be associated with reduction in cellular cAMP levels (via inhibitory G_i-protein coupling) and inhibition or hyperpolarization of target neurons – a possibility that can be assessed experimentally using *in vitro* or *in vivo* electrophysiological and biochemical methods [e.g., Ref. (55, 95)].

It is also necessary to establish whether it is the proposed reduction in oxytocin production and release which produces the observed increase in food intake in AAV-R3/I5-treated rats, or whether the chronic increase in food intake caused by hypothalamic RXFP3 activation over time leads to down-regulation of oxytocin mRNA via a distinct mechanism. This could be explored by conducting acute peptide administration studies or shorter time course viral infusion studies, and assessing oxytocin mRNA, peptide and release levels, before any marked changes in body weight have occurred.

Indeed, a recent study examined the effect of icv H3 relaxin on anxiety-like behavior in rats and observed an anxiolytic effect in the elevated plus maze test and the shock probe-burying test (70), consistent with our studies demonstrating that icv administration of a selective RXFP3 agonist peptide reduced anxiety-like behavior in the light-dark box and elevated plus maze (96). Notably, these authors used microarray and peptidomics approaches to identify associated downstream signaling targets in the hypothalamus altered by icv H3 relaxin and detected a relatively acute (6–24 h) and quite specific *increase* in the level of hypothalamic oxytocin mRNA and peptide levels (70). This data is, however, more consistent with the ability of H3 relaxin to *activate* neurons via RXFP1 [see e.g., Ref. (40, 67, 68)] rather than via RXFP3, which based on predicted signaling (28, 63) might be expected to decrease oxytocin neuron activity (and mRNA and peptide levels), as seen in our study (43). Therefore, further studies are required to identify specific effects of RXFP3 (and RXFP1) activation in hypothalamus and other areas in altered feeding and metabolism and anxiety-like behavior (76, 96).

Further evidence for an association of a down-regulation/inhibition of PVN oxytocin activity with a hyperphagic phenotype was reported recently. Optogenetic electrophysiological studies revealed that GABA/AgRP neurons in the ARC project to a population of oxytocin neurons in the PVN and strongly inhibit their activity, and this suppression of oxytocin neurons by AgRP neuronal activation drives evoked feeding (23). This study also demonstrated that increased food seeking and consumption in response to GABA/AgRP neuron activation is similarly induced by suppressing the activity of the PVN neurons that (selectively) express the *single-minded 1* (SIM1) transcription factor (23, 97).

Importantly from a clinical perspective, a number of disease states in which hyperphagia is a symptom are associated with hypothalamic oxytocin dysregulation. A small population of PVN oxytocin neurons is selectively lost in Prader–Willi syndrome, which is a condition involving insatiable hunger (98); and disruption of synaptic release of hypothalamic oxytocin results in overeating (99). Oxytocin deficits in SIM1 haploinsufficient mice and mutations in the SIM1 gene in humans lead to hyperphagic obesity (97, 100, 101). In the mouse model, an ~80% reduction in oxytocin and ~30% reduction in AVP was observed (97). These studies illustrate that modulation of relaxin-3 signaling and associated alterations in oxytocin neuron activity may be a fruitful area to explore for treating disease states associated with eating disorders. For example, a recent clinical cross-sectional study reported that female patients with anorexia nervosa, characterized by food restriction, low weight, and hypoleptinemia, had higher mean circulating oxytocin levels than healthy controls at all times assessed (102). The severity of disease psychopathology was also positively associated with circulating oxytocin levels (102).

HYPOTHALAMIC-PITUITARY-ADRENAL AXIS AND STRESS RESPONSES

Integration of the stress response via the hypothalamic-pituitary-adrenal (HPA) axis occurs via interaction between brain areas which are sensitive to stress and neuroendocrine neurons of the hypothalamic PVN, particularly those in the parvocellular region producing CRH [see Ref. (1, 6, 103) for review]. CRH stimulates the secretion and synthesis of adrenocorticotropin hormone (ACTH) from the pituitary and is the main regulator of HPA axis activity during stress.

Early regulatory studies revealed that neurons in the NI and specifically relaxin-3 expressing neurons respond to stress and CRH (46, 104), and that relaxin-3-containing neurons in the NI express CRH type 1 receptors (CRH-R1) (46). Upon icv administration of CRH, 65% of relaxin-3-positive neurons underwent activation (detected using Fos-immunostaining 2 h post-infusion) (46). Electrophysiological characterization of NI neurons revealed that a significant population increased firing following icv administration of CRH, of which the majority were relaxin-3-positive, though an almost equal number of non-relaxin-3 neurons exhibited a decrease in firing in the anesthetized rat (53). These findings are consistent with semi-quantitative immunohistochemical studies of the NI revealing this heterogeneous neuron population consists of relaxin-3 neurons that all co-express CRH-R1, though not all CRH-R1 contain relaxin-3, in addition to a significant population that are CRH-R1 negative (53). Rats tested in a water immersion-restraint stress paradigm, displayed increased Fos-immunostaining and an up-regulation of relaxin-3 mRNA in NI neurons (46). Subsequently, the effect of a repeat forced swim on relaxin-3 expression in the NI was examined and led to a rapid increase in relaxin-3 mRNA expression (51). This increase was largely mediated by CRH activation of CRH-R1 located on NI neurons, as pre-treatment with the CRH antagonist, antalarmin, reduced the increase in relaxin-3 mRNA expression by 70–80%. Levels of relaxin-3 heteronuclear (hn) RNA were also increased in NI neurons after the repeat forced swim (51). Changes in hnRNA are a measure of transcriptional activity and are thought to reflect the level of encoded peptide synthesis (105), suggesting in this case, an increase in relaxin-3 utilization.

Initial insights into the hypothalamic action of relaxin-3 in relation to the stress response have been obtained by monitoring the effect of icv administration of relaxin-3 in male rats (69). Increased Fos staining in the PVN and SON was observed 1 h post-administration and levels of c-*fos* and CRH mRNA in the PVN were also increased 2 h after H3 relaxin administration. Central H3 relaxin administration also elicited an increase in circulating plasma ACTH (69). These data *suggest* a role for relaxin-3 in the acute hypothalamus-pituitary CRH-ACTH system response, but these studies did not directly identify the presence of RXFP3 on CRH neurons or measure the direct acute excitatory or inhibitory effect of RXFP3 activation on these neurons [see Ref. (55)].

Notably, a recent report also suggests sex-specific regulation of CRH and relaxin-3 systems in response to combined stressors. Chronically stressed and repeatedly food-restricted female rats consumed more standard chow during recovery and had an increased bodyweight relative to controls, whereas male rats exposed to this regime had a reduction in bodyweight (106). Stressed/food-restricted female rats had elevated plasma corticosterone and low PVN CRH mRNA levels. CRH neurons in the medial preoptic area were identified as a source of increased CRH production/release during stress in female brain, i.e., CRH mRNA levels in this area were – higher in female than male rats, increased by chronic stress, and increased in female, not male, rats after repeated food restriction (106).

Further studies are now required to determine precisely how the robust, consistently observed stress and CRH-induced activation of NI and relaxin-3 neurons (46, 51, 53, 106) directly or indirectly activates (or possibly inhibits) the PVN and the main components of the HPA axis; and whether and how these processes are regulated by steroid and other hormones under different conditions.

EFFECTS ON REPRODUCTIVE NEUROENDOCRINE SYSTEMS

Preliminary studies have indicated a putative role for relaxin-3 in reproductive physiology. Following injection into the PVN and surrounds, H3 relaxin increased levels of marker hormones of the hypothalamic-pituitary-gonadal (HPG) axis (71, 107); and anatomical studies have identified RXFP3 in many areas in the hypothalamus relevant to reproductive neuroendocrinology, including the preoptic area and the PVN and SON (33). H3 relaxin administered icv or iPVN significantly increased plasma luteinizing hormone (LH) levels 30 min post-injection in male Wistar rats, an effect blocked by peripheral pre-treatment with a GnRH antagonist, consistent with increased central GnRH release (71). In these initial studies, H2 relaxin administration via the same routes produced a small, non-significant increase in LH, suggesting a stronger relaxin-3/RXFP3-mediated effect (71). Activity of the endogenous peptide at RXFP1 cannot be completely excluded from an involvement in these effects, however, as RXFP1 is expressed in the anterior hypothalamus and PVN of the rat (62). If so, high levels of endogenous relaxin-3 may act via RXFP1 to stimulate the HPG axis, an idea that could be tested experimentally. It would also be of interest to observe the effects of icv or iPVN administration of RXFP3-selective peptides (65, 72–74) on the HPG axis in female rats to check for similar hormone changes to those observed in male rats.

Notably, treatment of mouse hypothalamic neuron-like (GT1–7) cells or hypothalamic explants with synthetic H3 relaxin, produced a dose-dependent increase in secretion of GnRH (71). However, it is again unclear if this is an RXFP3-mediated effect, as GT1–7 cells and hypothalamic explants also express RXFP1; and H3 relaxin binds and activates these receptors. As these cells express both RXFP1 and RXFP3, the relaxin-3 mediated secretion of GnRH should be assessed for sensitivity to blockade with an RXFP3 antagonist (71–73).

In our recent study, we assessed the effect of chronic (~14 weeks) viral-mediated expression of R3/I5 in the hypothalamus on GnRH mRNA levels (43). Although the difference between groups was not statistically significant, there was a trend for increased GnRH mRNA levels in AAV-R3/I5-treated compared to control rats, with considerable variability in individual values. Given the dispersed nature of GnRH expressing neurons in the hypothalamus, the variability observed suggests that different numbers (populations) of GnRH expressing neurons may have been dissected in these assays and/or there may be a genuine increase in GnRH transcription as a result of the treatment. This important question needs to be further investigated using suitable quantitative methods, in conjunction with further assessments of relaxin3/RXFP3 indices relative to GnRH and other reproductive peptides and receptors during different stages of pregnancy, birth and lactation.

OTHER HYPOTHALAMIC SITES OF RELAXIN-3/RXFP3 ACTION

The relaxin-3/RXFP3 system may have actions in other hypothalamic nuclei, demonstrated by the presence of both relaxin-3 immunoreactive fibers and RXFP3 mRNA/protein in the lateral and medial preoptic areas, anterior, posterior, dorsomedial, and ventromedial regions, and the adjacent supramammillary nucleus (SuM) (33) (**Table 1**). The functions of these regions will be briefly reviewed, in view of the postulated role of relaxin-3 in arousal, feeding, behavioral state, and cognition (39).

The SuM receives a moderate relaxin-3 innervation in the rat (33) and the mouse (34), and this nucleus represents a major target of the peptide network in the macaque brain (35). In contrast to other "hypothalamic" regions, this nucleus is best characterized as a key input to and modulator of the hippocampus and hippocampal theta rhythm (108, 109), a synchronous activity between 4 and 12 Hz associated with active waking behavior and REM sleep (110), mnemonic processing (111, 112), spatial navigation and exploration (113), and sensorimotor integration (114, 115). There is growing evidence that the NI is a key player in mediating brainstem-elicited theta rhythm (47, 53, 116). In addition to projections to the SuM, there are strong relaxin-3-containing NI projections to other regions subserving theta rhythm generation, such as medial septum (48–50), *reticularis pontine oralis*, and the hippocampus, as well as the median raphe, which is involved in theta desynchronization [see (52) for review]. In fact, relaxin-3 projections to the medial septum have been shown to promote hippocampal theta rhythm and are necessary for normal spatial navigation of rats in a spontaneous alternation task (47). Thus, the SuM is likely a further node at which this neuropeptide system acts to regulate hippocampal theta activity and associated cognitive/autonomic processes.

The lateral and medial preoptic areas of hypothalamus are also rich in relaxin-3 projections and RXFP3. The LPO area contains populations of neurons that have identified roles in thermoregulation (117, 118) and sleep-wakefulness (ventrolateral neurons) (119), so it will be of interest, to assess the precise topography of RXFP3 in these areas and to assess the effects of RXFP3 activation/inhibition in these regions on these physiological parameters, particularly as our laboratory has anatomical and functional data consistent with effects of relaxin-3 on sleep-wake activity in mice (34, 120). Similarly, as discussed, the role of relaxin-3/RXFP3 signaling in the medial preoptic area may be important in stress responses in female rats and the possible regulation of CRH neurons in the area (106).

RELAXIN-3/RXFP3 IN MOUSE HYPOTHALAMUS – SPECIES DIFFERENCES

The distribution of relaxin-3 neurons and projections, as well as the distribution of RXFP3 mRNA and binding sites in the mouse brain, is regionally similar to that in the rat both generally throughout the forebrain and within the hypothalamus (33, 34). Furthermore, the distribution of Rxfp3 mRNA in the C57BL6/J mouse detailed in the Allen Brain Institute Brain Atlas (see text footnote 1) using a digoxigenin-labeled RNA probe is similar to that observed in our studies using radioactively labeled oligonucleotides (34) (**Table 1**). However, a more detailed analysis is required to determine whether identical populations of neurons are targeted within key hypothalamus areas, such as the arcuate, periventricular, PVN, and SON of rat and mouse to assess whether relaxin-3 signaling might regulate similar neuroendocrine processes in these species.

We have conducted several studies to assess the possible role of relaxin-3/RXFP3 in food intake in mice (121). After the administration of similar or higher levels of relaxin-3 or various RXFP3-selective agonists (R3/I5, RXFP3-A2) used in studies on rats [see (76) for review], we did not observe an increase in food intake of satiated C57BL/6J mice. In more recent studies, we have observed that the icv administration of the RXFP3 antagonist, R3(B1–22)R (73) produced a reduction in the robust feeding that occurred in mice offered access to regular chow after a 4 h period of isolated housing in a novel cage without bedding and in the absence of food (Smith and Gundlach, unpublished data). These particular conditions are presumed to induce a level of stress, hypothermia, and energy deficiency in the mice, which motivates their feeding; and suggests that relaxin-3/RXFP3 signaling in mice may not influence feeding significantly under basal conditions, but may play a role under altered stress conditions. These possibilities are currently being explored experimentally.

Consistent with these pharmacological studies, however, there is no genotypic difference between relaxin-3 KO and wild type littermates in bodyweight, total food consumption, or circadian rhythm of food consumption (120, 122). These findings are in contrast to data obtained by Sutton et al. (123) in a separately derived colony of relaxin-3 KO mice on a mixed C57BL6/J/SV129 background, which displayed a markedly reduced body weight relative to wild type mice when both genotypes were fed a diet with a moderately elevated fat content. However, subsequent studies of a null mutation Rxfp3 KO mouse strain revealed no body weight-related phenotype, but did reveal an identical circadian hypoactivity phenotype to the relaxin-3 KO mouse (120, 124, 125). This suggests the relaxin-3 KO phenotype reported by Sutton et al. (123) was associated with genetic differences independent of relaxin-3/RXFP3 [see (39)].

With regard to the specificity of pharmacological studies of RXFP3 signaling in the mouse, while the presence of insulin-like peptide 5 (INSL5) and RXFP4 in the mouse brain has been reported (126), these findings have not been independently validated; and in a separate study, the presence of INSL5-sensitive receptor binding sites could not be identified (127). Furthermore, the ligand/receptor expression profile suggests the INSL5/RXFP4 system acts primarily within the gastrointestinal tract and large intestine (28, 128). While it is possible that peripheral INSL5 signaling may alter central (hypothalamic) function, at this stage no such data is available.

CONCLUSION AND PERSPECTIVES

A decade of research has revealed the basic structural framework of central relaxin-3/RXFP3 networks and their likely functional importance in mammalian brain (27, 39, 76); and several studies have highlighted the interaction between hypothalamic homeostatic systems and relaxin-3/RXFP3 signaling, predominantly in pharmacological and regulatory studies in the rat. Together, these studies point to a role for relaxin-3/RXFP3 in regulating hypothalamic activity, with evidence suggesting it does so via interactions with oxytocin, AVP, and/or CRH, to modulate neuroendocrine function associated with stress, feeding, and metabolism, and motivation and reward. Further studies are now required to clarify the nature of these various effects and how they are coordinated and regulated by hormonal and transmitter inputs onto relaxin-3 neurons and integrated signaling at the level of hypothalamic loops (e.g., HPA, HPG axes). Recent research strongly suggests the relaxin-3/RXFP3 system is an important regulator of the neuroendocrine axis, with potential as a novel therapeutic target for the treatment of neuroendocrine disorders and associated behavioral dysfunction.

ACKNOWLEDGMENTS

Research in the authors' laboratory is supported by grants from the National Health and Medical Research Council (NHMRC) of Australia (Andrew L. Gundlach, Sherie Ma), the Besen Family and Pratt Foundations (Andrew L. Gundlach), and by the Victorian Government Operational Infrastructure Support Program. Despina E. Ganella was the recipient of a Commonwealth Australian Postgraduate Award. Andrew L. Gundlach is the recipient of an NHMRC (Australia) Research Fellowship.

REFERENCES

1. Herman JP, Cullinan WE, Ziegler DR, Tasker JG. Role of the paraventricular nucleus microenvironment in stress integration. *Eur J Neurosci* (2002) **16**:381–5. doi:10.1046/j.1460-9568.2002.02133.x
2. Small CJ, Stanley SA, Bloom SR. Appetite control and reproduction: leptin and beyond. *Semin Reprod Med* (2002) **20**:389–98. doi:10.1055/s-2002-36712
3. Morton GJ, Cummings DE, Baskin DG, Barsh GS, Schwartz MW. Central nervous system control of food intake and body weight. *Nature* (2006) **443**:289–95. doi:10.1038/nature05026
4. Gao Q, Horvath TL. Neurobiology of feeding and energy expenditure. *Annu Rev Neurosci* (2007) **30**:367–98. doi:10.1146/annurev.neuro.30.051606.094324
5. Adamantidis A, de Lecea L. Physiological arousal: a role for hypothalamic systems. *Cell Mol Life Sci* (2008) **65**:1475–88. doi:10.1007/s00018-008-7521-8
6. Ulrich-Lai YM, Herman JP. Neural regulation of endocrine and autonomic stress responses. *Nat Rev Neurosci* (2009) **10**:397–409. doi:10.1038/nrn2647
7. Zeltser LM, Seeley RJ, Tschöp MH. Synaptic plasticity in neuronal circuits regulating energy balance. *Nat Neurosci* (2012) **15**:1336–42. doi:10.1038/nn.3219
8. Lantos TA, Görcs TJ, Palkovits M. Immunohistochemical mapping of neuropeptides in the premamillary region of the hypothalamus in rats. *Brain Res Rev* (1995) **20**:209–49. doi:10.1016/0165-0173(94)00013-F
9. Broberger C, De Lecea L, Sutcliffe JG, Hokfelt T. Hypocretin/orexin- and melanin-concentrating hormone-expressing cells form distinct populations in the rodent lateral hypothalamus: relationship to the neuropeptide Y and agouti gene-related protein systems. *J Comp Neurol* (1998) **402**:460–74. doi:10.1002/(SICI)1096-9861(19981228)402:4<460::AID-CNE3>3.3.CO;2-J
10. Carlin KM, Vale WW, Bale TL. Vital functions of corticotropin-releasing factor (CRF) pathways in maintenance and regulation of energy homeostasis. *Proc Natl Acad Sci U S A* (2006) **103**:3462–7. doi:10.1073/pnas.0511320103
11. Lechan RM, Fekete C. The TRH neuron: a hypothalamic integrator of energy metabolism. *Prog Brain Res* (2006) **153**:209–35. doi:10.1016/S0079-6123(06)53012-2
12. Meister B. Neurotransmitters in key neurons of the hypothalamus that regulate feeding behavior and body weight. *Physiol Behav* (2007) **92**:263–71. doi:10.1016/j.physbeh.2007.05.021
13. Sakurai T. The neural circuit of orexin (hypocretin): maintaining sleep and wakefulness. *Nat Rev Neurosci* (2007) **8**:171–81. doi:10.1038/nrn2092
14. Saito Y, Nagasaki H. The melanin-concentrating hormone system and its physiological functions. *Results Probl Cell Differ* (2008) **46**:159–79. doi:10.1007/400_2007_052
15. Williams KW, Elmquist JK. Lighting up the hypothalamus: coordinated control of feeding behavior. *Nat Neurosci* (2011) **14**:277–8. doi:10.1038/nn0311-277
16. Parker JA, Bloom SR. Hypothalamic neuropeptides and the regulation of appetite. *Neuropharmacology* (2012) **63**:18–30. doi:10.1016/j.neuropharm.2012.02.004
17. Michel MC, Beck-Sickinger A, Cox H, Doods HN, Herzog H, Larhammar D, et al. XVI. International Union of Pharmacology recommendations for the nomenclature of neuropeptide Y, peptide YY, and pancreatic polypeptide receptors. *Pharmacol Rev* (1998) **50**:143–50.
18. Bale TL, Vale WW. CRF and CRF receptors: role in stress responsivity and other behaviors. *Annu Rev Pharmacol Toxicol* (2004) **44**:525–57. doi:10.1146/annurev.pharmtox.44.101802.121410
19. Alexander SP, Mathie A, Peters JA. Guide to receptors and channels (GRAC), 5th edition. *Br J Pharmacol* (2011) **164**(Suppl 1):S1–324. doi:10.1111/j.1476-5381.2011.01649_1.x
20. Hazell GG, Hindmarch CC, Pope GR, Roper JA, Lightman SL, Murphy D, et al. G protein-coupled receptors in the hypothalamic paraventricular and supraoptic nuclei – serpentine gateways to neuroendocrine homeostasis. *Front Neuroendocrinol* (2012) **33**:45–66. doi:10.1016/j.yfrne.2011.07.002
21. Knobloch HS, Charlet A, Hoffmann LC, Eliava M, Khrulev S, Cetin AH, et al. Evoked axonal oxytocin release in the central amygdala attenuates fear response. *Neuron* (2012) **73**:553–66. doi:10.1016/j.neuron.2011.11.030
22. Krashes MJ, Koda S, Ye CP, Rogan SC, Adams AC, Cusher DS, et al. Rapid, reversible activation of AgRP neurons drives feeding behavior in mice. *J Clin Invest* (2011) **121**:1424–8. doi:10.1172/JCI46229
23. Atasoy D, Betley JN, Su HH, Sternson SM. Deconstruction of a neural circuit for hunger. *Nature* (2012) **488**:172–7. doi:10.1038/nature11270
24. de Lecea L, Carter ME, Adamantidis A. Shining light on wakefulness and arousal. *Biol Psychiatry* (2012) **71**:1046–52. doi:10.1016/j.biopsych.2012.01.032
25. Zhan C, Zhou JF, Feng QR, Zhang JE, Lin SL, Bao JH, et al. Acute and long-term suppression of feeding behavior by POMC neurons in the brainstem and hypothalamus, respectively. *J Neurosci* (2013) **33**:3624–32. doi:10.1523/JNEUROSCI.2742-12.2013
26. Bathgate RAD, Samuel CS, Burazin TCD, Layfield S, Claasz AA, Reytomas IGT, et al. Human relaxin gene 3 (H3) and the equivalent mouse relaxin (M3) gene: novel members of the relaxin peptide family. *J Biol Chem* (2002) **277**:1148–57. doi:10.1074/jbc.M107882200
27. Ma S, Gundlach AL. Relaxin-family peptide and receptor systems in brain: insights from recent anatomical and functional studies. *Adv Exp Med Biol* (2007) **612**:119–37. doi:10.1007/978-0-387-74672-2_9

28. Bathgate RAD, Halls ML, van der Westhuizen ET, Callander GE, Kocan M, Summers RJ. Relaxin family peptides and their receptors. *Physiol Rev* (2013) **93**:405–80. doi:10.1152/physrev.00001.2012
29. Burazin TCD, Bathgate RAD, Macris M, Layfield S, Gundlach AL, Tregear GW. Restricted, but abundant, expression of the novel rat gene-3 (R3) relaxin in the dorsal tegmental region of brain. *J Neurochem* (2002) **82**:1553–7. doi:10.1046/j.1471-4159.2002.01114.x
30. Liu C, Eriste E, Sutton S, Chen J, Roland B, Kuei C, et al. Identification of relaxin-3/INSL7 as an endogenous ligand for the orphan G-protein coupled receptor GPCR135. *J Biol Chem* (2003) **278**:50754–64. doi:10.1074/jbc.M308995200
31. Bathgate RAD, Ivell R, Sanborn BM, Sherwood OD, Summers RJ. International Union of Pharmacology LVII: recommendations for the nomenclature of receptors for relaxin family peptides. *Pharmacol Rev* (2006) **58**:7–31. doi:10.1124/pr.58.1.9
32. Sutton SW, Bonaventure P, Kuei C, Roland B, Chen J, Nepomuceno D, et al. Distribution of G-protein-coupled receptor (GPCR)135 binding sites and receptor mRNA in the rat brain suggests a role for relaxin-3 in neuroendocrine and sensory processing. *Neuroendocrinology* (2004) **80**:298–307. doi:10.1159/000083656
33. Ma S, Bonaventure P, Ferraro T, Shen PJ, Burazin TCD, Bathgate RAD, et al. Relaxin-3 in GABA projection neurons of nucleus incertus suggests widespread influence on forebrain circuits via G-protein-coupled receptor-135 in the rat. *Neuroscience* (2007) **144**:165–90. doi:10.1016/j.neuroscience.2006.08.072
34. Smith CM, Shen PJ, Banerjee A, Bonaventure P, Ma S, Bathgate RAD, et al. Distribution of relaxin-3 and RXFP3 within arousal, stress, affective, and cognitive circuits of mouse brain. *J Comp Neurol* (2010) **518**:4016–45. doi:10.1002/cne.22442
35. Ma S, Sang Q, Lanciego JL, Gundlach AL. Localization of relaxin-3 in brain of *Macaca fascicularis* – identification of nucleus incertus in primate. *J Comp Neurol* (2009) **517**:856–72. doi:10.1002/cne.22197
36. Ma S, Shen P-J, Sang Q, Lanciego JL, Gundlach AL. Distribution of relaxin-3 mRNA and immunoreactivity, and RXFP3 binding sites in the brain of the macaque, *Macaca fascicularis*. *Ann N Y Acad Sci* (2009) **1160**:256–8. doi:10.1111/j.1749-6632.2009.03954.x
37. Hsu SYT. New insights into the evolution of the relaxin-LGR signaling system. *Trends Endocrinol Metab* (2003) **14**:303–9. doi:10.1016/S1043-2760(03)00106-1
38. Wilkinson TN, Speed TP, Tregear GW, Bathgate RAD. Evolution of the relaxin-like peptide family. *BMC Evol Biol* (2005) **5**:14. doi:10.1186/1471-2148-5-14
39. Smith CM, Ryan PJ, Hosken IT, Ma S, Gundlach AL. Relaxin-3 systems in the brain – the first 10 years. *J Chem Neuroanat* (2011) **42**:262–75. doi:10.1016/j.jchemneu.2011.05.013
40. Bathgate RAD, Lin F, Hanson NF, Otvos LJ, Guidolin A, Giannakis C, et al. Relaxin-3: improved synthesis strategy and demonstration of its high-affinity interaction with the relaxin receptor LGR7 both in vitro and in vivo. *Biochemistry* (2006) **45**:1043–53. doi:10.1021/bi052233e
41. Hossain MA, Smith CM, Ryan PJ, Büchler E, Bathgate RAD, Gundlach AL, et al. Chemical synthesis and orexigenic activity of rat/mouse relaxin-3. *Amino Acids* (2013) **44**:1529–36. doi:10.1007/s00726-013-1478-0
42. Sherwood OD. Relaxin's physiological roles and other diverse actions. *Endocr Rev* (2004) **25**:205–34. doi:10.1210/er.2003-0013
43. Ganella DE, Callander GE, Ma S, Bye CR, Gundlach AL, Bathgate RAD. Modulation of feeding by chronic rAAV expression of a relaxin-3 peptide agonist in rat hypothalamus. *Gene Ther* (2013) **20**:703–16. doi:10.1038/gt.2012.83
44. Goto M, Swanson LW, Canteras NS. Connections of the nucleus incertus. *J Comp Neurol* (2001) **438**:86–122. doi:10.1002/cne.1303
45. Olucha-Bordonau FE, Teruel V, Barcia-Gonzalez J, Ruiz-Torner A, Valverde-Navarro AA, Martinez-Soriano F. Cytoarchitecture and efferent projections of the nucleus incertus of the rat. *J Comp Neurol* (2003) **464**:62–97. doi:10.1002/cne.10774
46. Tanaka M, Iijima N, Miyamoto Y, Fukusumi S, Itoh Y, Ozawa H, et al. Neurons expressing relaxin 3/INSL7 in the nucleus incertus respond to stress. *Eur J Neurosci* (2005) **21**:1659–70. doi:10.1111/j.1460-9568.2005.03980.x
47. Ma S, Olucha-Bordonau FE, Hossain MA, Lin F, Kuei C, Liu C, et al. Modulation of hippocampal theta oscillations and spatial memory by relaxin-3 neurons of the nucleus incertus. *Learn Mem* (2009) **16**:730–42. doi:10.1101/lm.1438109
48. Teruel-Marti V, Cervera-Ferri A, Nunez A, Valverde-Navarro AA, Olucha-Bordonau FE, Ruiz-Torner A. Anatomical evidence for a ponto-septal pathway via the nucleus incertus in the rat. *Brain Res* (2008) **1218**:87–96. doi:10.1016/j.brainres.2008.04.022
49. Cervera-Ferri A, Rahmani Y, Martínez-Bellver S, Teruel-Martí V, Martínez-Ricós J. Glutamatergic projection from the nucleus incertus to the septohippocampal system. *Neurosci Lett* (2012) **517**:71–6. doi:10.1016/j.neulet.2012.04.014
50. Olucha-Bordonau FE, Otero-García M, Sánchez-Pérez AM, Núñez A, Ma S, Gundlach AL. Distribution and targets of the relaxin-3 innervation of the septal area in the rat. *J Comp Neurol* (2012) **520**:1903–39. doi:10.1002/cne.23018
51. Banerjee A, Shen PJ, Ma S, Bathgate RAD, Gundlach AL. Swim stress excitation of nucleus incertus and rapid induction of relaxin-3 expression via CRF_1 activation. *Neuropharmacology* (2010) **58**:145–55. doi:10.1016/j.neuropharm.2009.06.019
52. Ryan PJ, Ma S, Olucha-Bordonau FE, Gundlach AL. Nucleus incertus – an emerging modulatory role in arousal, stress and memory. *Neurosci Biobehav Rev* (2011) **35**:1326–41. doi:10.1016/j.neubiorev.2011.02.004
53. Ma S, Blasiak A, Olucha-Bordonau FE, Verberne AJM, Gundlach AL. Heterogeneous responses of nucleus incertus neurons to corticotropin-releasing factor and coherent activity with hippocampal theta rhythm. *J Physiol* (2013) **591**:3981–4001. doi:10.1113/jphysiol.2013.254300
54. Blasiak A, Blasiak T, Hossain MA, Wade JD, Gundlach AL. Relaxin-3 innervation and modulation of the intergeniculate leaflet of the rat thalamus. *Neuropeptides* (2009) **43**:430.
55. Blasiak A, Blasiak T, Lewandowski MH, Hossain MA, Wade JD, Gundlach AL. Relaxin-3 innervation of the intergeniculate leaflet of the rat thalamus – neuronal tract-tracing and *in vitro* electrophysiological studies. *Eur J Neurosci* (2013) **37**:1284–94. doi:10.1111/ejn.12155
56. Morin LP, Allen CN. The circadian visual system, 2005. *Brain Res Rev* (2006) **51**:1–60. doi:10.1016/j.brainresrev.2005.08.003
57. Delogu A, Sellers K, Zagoraiou L, Bocianowska-Zbrog A, Mandal S, Guimera J, et al. Subcortical visual shell nuclei targeted by ipRGCs develop from a Sox14+-GABAergic progenitor and require Sox14 to regulate daily activity rhythms. *Neuron* (2012) **75**:648–62. doi:10.1016/j.neuron.2012.06.013
58. Morin LP. Neuroanatomy of the extended circadian rhythm system. *Exp Neurol* (2013) **243**:4–20. doi:10.1016/j.expneurol.2012.06.026
59. Ziegler DR, Edwards MR, Ulrich-Lai YM, Herman JP, Cullinan WE. Brainstem origins of glutamatergic innervation of the rat hypothalamic paraventricular nucleus. *J Comp Neurol* (2012) **520**:2369–94. doi:10.1002/cne.23043
60. Boels K, Hermans-Borgmeyer I, Schaller HC. Identification of a mouse orthologue of the G-protein-coupled receptor SALPR and its expression in adult mouse brain and during development. *Dev Brain Res* (2004) **152**:265–8. doi:10.1016/j.devbrainres.2004.06.002
61. Sudo S, Kumagai J, Nishi S, Layfield S, Ferraro T, Bathgate RA, et al. H3 Relaxin is a specific ligand for LGR7 and activates the receptor by interacting with both the ectodomain and the exoloop 2. *J Biol Chem* (2003) **278**:7855–62. doi:10.1074/jbc.M212457200
62. Ma S, Shen P-J, Burazin TCD, Tregear GW, Gundlach AL. Comparative localization of leucine-rich repeat-containing G-protein-coupled receptor-7 (RXFP1) mRNA and [^{33}P]-relaxin binding sites in rat brain: restricted somatic co-expression a clue to relaxin action? *Neuroscience* (2006) **141**:329–44. doi:10.1016/j.neuroscience.2006.03.076
63. van der Westhuizen ET, Werry TD, Sexton PM, Summers RJ. The relaxin family peptide receptor 3 activates extracellular signal-regulated kinase 1/2 through a protein kinase C-dependent mechanism. *Mol Pharmacol* (2007) **71**:1618–29. doi:10.1124/mol.106.032763

64. Liu C, Chen J, Sutton S, Roland B, Kuei C, Farmer N, et al. Identification of relaxin-3/INSL7 as a ligand for GPCR142. *J Biol Chem* (2003) **278**:50765–70. doi: 10.1074/jbc.M308996200
65. Liu C, Chen J, Kuei C, Sutton S, Nepomuceno D, Bonaventure P, et al. Relaxin-3/Insulin-like peptide 5 chimeric peptide, a selective ligand for G protein-coupled receptor (GPCR)135 and GPCR142 over leucine-rich repeat-containing G protein-coupled receptor 7. *Mol Pharmacol* (2005) **67**:231–40. doi: 10.1124/mol.104.006700
66. McGowan BM, Stanley SA, Smith KL, White NE, Connolly MM, Thompson EL, et al. Central relaxin-3 administration causes hyperphagia in male wistar rats. *Endocrinology* (2005) **146**:3295–300. doi:10.1210/en.2004-1532
67. McGowan BM, Stanley SA, Smith KL, Minnion JS, Donovan J, Thompson EL, et al. Effects of acute and chronic relaxin-3 on food intake and energy expenditure in rats. *Regul Pept* (2006) **136**:72–7. doi:10.1016/j.regpep.2006.04.009
68. Otsubo H, Onaka T, Suzuki H, Katoh A, Ohbuchi T, Todoroki M, et al. Centrally administered relaxin-3 induces Fos expression in the osmosensitive areas in rat brain and facilitates water intake. *Peptides* (2010) **31**:1124–30. doi: 10.1016/j.peptides.2010.02.020
69. Watanabe Y, Miyamoto Y, Matsuda T, Tanaka M. Relaxin-3/INSL7 regulates the stress-response system in the rat hypothalamus. *J Mol Neurosci* (2011) **43**:169–74. doi:10.1007/s12031-010-9468-0
70. Nakazawa C, Shikata K, Uesugi M, Katayama H, Aoshima K, Tahara K, et al. Prediction of relaxin-3-induced downstream pathway resulting in anxiolytic-like behaviors in rats based on a microarray and peptidome analysis. *J Recept Signal Transduct Res* (2013) **33**:224–33. doi:10.3109/10799893.2012.756895
71. McGowan BM, Stanley SA, Donovan J, Thompson EL, Patterson M, Semjonous NM, et al. Relaxin-3 stimulates the hypothalamic-pituitary-gonadal axis. *Am J Physiol Endocrinol Metab* (2008) **295**:E278–86. doi:10.1152/ajpendo.00028.2008
72. Kuei C, Sutton S, Bonaventure P, Pudiak C, Shelton J, Zhu J, et al. R3(Bδ23-27)R/I5 chimeric peptide, a selective antagonist for GPCR135 and GPCR142 over relaxin receptor LGR7: in vitro and in vivo characterization. *J Biol Chem* (2007) **282**:25425–35. doi: 10.1074/jbc.M701416200
73. Haugaard-Kedstrom LM, Shabanpoor F, Hossain MA, Clark RJ, Ryan PJ, Craik DJ, et al. Design, synthesis, and characterization of a single-chain peptide antagonist for the relaxin-3 receptor RXFP3. *J Am Chem Soc* (2011) **133**:4965–74. doi:10.1021/ja110567j
74. Shabanpoor F, Hossain MA, Ryan PJ, Belgi A, Layfield S, Kocan M, et al. Minimization of human relaxin-3 leading to high-affinity analogues with increased selectivity for relaxin-family peptide 3 receptor (RXFP3) over RXFP1. *J Med Chem* (2012) **55**:1671–81. doi: 10.1021/jm201505p
75. Dietrich MO, Horvath TL. Feeding signals and brain circuitry. *Eur J Neurosci* (2009) **30**:1688–96. doi:10.1111/j.1460-9568.2009.06963.x
76. Ganella DE, Ryan PJ, Bathgate RAD, Gundlach AL. Increased feeding and body weight gain after acute/chronic hypothalamic activation of RXFP3 by relaxin-3 and receptor-selective synthetic and rAAV-driven agonist peptides: functional and therapeutic implications. *Behav Pharmacol* (2012) **23**:516–25. doi:10.1097/FBP.0b013e3283576999
77. Stanley BG, Daniel DR, Chin AS, Leibowitz SF. Paraventricular nucleus injections of peptide-YY and neuropeptide-Y preferentially enhance carbohydrate ingestion. *Peptides* (1985) **6**:1205–11. doi:10.1016/0196-9781(85)90452-8
78. Hida T, Takahashi E, Shikata K, Hirohashi T, Sawai T, Seiki T, et al. Chronic intracerebroventricular administration of relaxin-3 increases body weight in rats. *J Recept Signal Transduct Res* (2006) **26**:147–58. doi:10.1080/10799890600623373
79. McGowan BM, Stanley SA, White NE, Spangeus A, Patterson M, Thompson EL, et al. Hypothalamic mapping of orexigenic action and Fos-like immunoreactivity following relaxin-3 administration in male Wistar rats. *Am J Physiol Endocrinol Metab* (2007) **292**:E913–9. doi:10.1152/ajpendo.00346.2006
80. Landgraf R, Neumann ID. Vasopressin and oxytocin release within the brain: a dynamic concept of multiple and variable modes of neuropeptide communication. *Front Neuroendocrinol* (2004) **25**:150–76. doi:10.1016/j.yfrne.2004.05.001
81. Swaab DF, Nijveldt F, Pool CW. Distribution of oxytocin and vasopressin in the rat supraoptic and paraventricular nucleus. *J Endocrinol* (1975) **67**:461–2. doi: 10.1677/joe.0.0670461
82. Poulain DA, Wakerley JB. Electrophysiology of hypothalamic magnocellular neurons secreting oxytocin and vasopressin. *Neuroscience* (1982) **7**:773–808. doi:10.1016/0306-4522(82)90044-6
83. Buijs RM, De Vries G, Van Leeuwen FW, Swaab DF. Vasopressin and oxytocin: distribution and putative functions in the brain. *Prog Brain Res* (1983) **60**:115–22. doi:10.1016/S0079-6123(08)64379-4
84. Neumann ID. Brain oxytocin: a key regulator of emotional and social behaviours in both females and males. *J Neuroendocrinol* (2008) **20**:858–65. doi:10.1111/j.1365-2826.2008.01726.x
85. Onaka T, Takayanagi Y, Yoshida M. Roles of oxytocin neurones in the control of stress, energy metabolism, and social behaviour. *J Neuroendocrinol* (2012) **24**:587–98. doi:10.1111/j.1365-2826.2012.02300.x
86. Arletti R, Benelli A, Bertolini A. Influence of oxytocin on feeding-behaviour in the rat. *Peptides* (1989) **10**:89–93. doi:10.1016/0196-9781(89)90082-X
87. Olson BR, Drutarosky MD, Chow MS, Hruby VJ, Stricker EM, Verbalis JG. Oxytocin and an oxytocin agonist administered centrally decrease food-intake in rats. *Peptides* (1991) **12**:113–8. doi:10.1016/0196-9781(91)90176-P
88. Olson BR, Drutarosky MD, Stricker EM, Verbalis JG. Brain oxytocin receptor antagonism blunts the effects of anorexigenic treatment in rats – evidence for central oxytocin inhibition of food-intake. *Endocrinology* (1991) **129**:785–91. doi:10.1210/endo-129-2-785
89. Olszewski PK, Klockars A, Schiöth HB, Levine AS. Oxytocin as feeding inhibitor: maintaining homeostasis in consummatory behavior. *Pharmacol Biochem Behav* (2010) **97**:47–54. doi:10.1016/j.pbb.2010.05.026
90. Amico JA, Vollmer RR, Cai H-M, Miedlar JA, Rinaman L. Enhanced initial and sustained intake of sucrose solution in mice with an oxytocin gene deletion. *Am J Physiol Regul Integr Comp Physiol* (2005) **289**:R1798–806. doi:10.1152/ajpregu.00558.2005
91. Sclafani A, Rinaman L, Vollmer RR, Amico JA. Oxytocin knockout mice demonstrate enhanced intake of sweet and nonsweet carbohydrate solutions. *Am J Physiol Regul Integr Comp Physiol* (2007) **292**:R1828–33. doi:10.1152/ajpregu.00826.2006
92. Camerino C. Low sympathetic tone and obese phenotype in oxytocin-deficient mice. *Obesity* (2009) **17**:980–4. doi:10.1038/oby.2009.12
93. Douglas AJ, Meeren HK, Johnstone LE, Pfaff DW, Russell JA, Brooks PJ. Stimulation of expression of the oxytocin gene in rat supraoptic neurons at parturition. *Brain Res* (1998) **782**:167–74. doi: 10.1016/S0006-8993(97)01275-4
94. Gundlach AL, Burazin TCD, Larm JA. Distribution, regulation and role of hypothalamic galanin systems: renewed interest in a pleiotropic peptide family. *Clin Exp Pharmacol Physiol* (2001) **28**:100–5. doi:10.1046/j.1440-1681.2001.03411.x
95. Ebner K, Bosch OJ, Kramer SA, Singewald N, Neumann ID. Release of oxytocin in the rat central amygdala modulates stress-coping behavior and the release of excitatory amino acids. *Neuropsychopharmacology* (2004) **30**:223–30. doi:10.1038/sj.npp.1300607
96. Ryan PJ, Büchler E, Shabanpoor F, Hossain MA, Wade JD, Lawrence AJ, et al. Central relaxin-3 receptor (RXFP3) activation decreases anxiety- and depressive-like behaviours in the rat. *Behav Brain Res* (2013) **244**:142–51. doi: 10.1016/j.bbr.2013.01.034
97. Kublaoui BM, Gemelli T, Tolson KP, Wang Y, Zinn AR. Oxytocin deficiency mediates hyperphagic obesity of Sim1 haploinsufficient mice. *Mol Endocrinol* (2008) **22**:1723–34. doi:10.1210/me.2008-0067
98. Swaab DF, Purba JS, Hofman MA. Alterations in the hypothalamic paraventricular nucleus and its oxytocin neurons (putative satiety cells) in Prader-Willi-Syndrome – a study of 5 cases. *J Clin Endocrinol Metab* (1995) **80**:573–9. doi:10.1210/jc.80.2.573
99. Zhang G, Bai H, Zhang H, Dean C, Wu Q, Li J, et al. Neuropeptide exocytosis involving synaptotagmin-4 and oxytocin in hypothalamic

programming of body weight and energy balance. *Neuron* (2011) **69**:523–35. doi:10.1016/j.neuron.2010.12.036
100. Holder JL, Butte NF, Zinn AR. Profound obesity associated with a balanced translocation that disrupts the SIM1 gene. *Hum Mol Genet* (2000) **9**:101–8. doi:10.1093/hmg/9.1.101
101. Traurig M, Mack J, Hanson RL, Ghoussaini M, Meyre D, Knowler WC, et al. Common variation in SIM1 is reproducibly associated with BMI in pima Indians. *Diabetes* (2009) **58**:1682–9. doi:10.2337/db09-0028
102. Lawson EA, Holsen LM, Santin M, Meenaghan E, Eddy KT, Becker AE, et al. Oxytocin secretion is associated with severity of disordered eating psychopathology and insular cortex hypoactivation in anorexia nervosa. *J Clin Endocrinol Metab* (2012) **97**:E1898–908. doi:10.1210/jc.2012-1702
103. Herman JP, Cullinan WE. Neurocircuitry of stress: central control of the hypothalamo-pituitary-adrenocortical axis. *Trends Neurosci* (1997) **20**:78–84. doi:10.1016/S0166-2236(96)10069-2
104. Bittencourt JC, Sawchenko PE. Do centrally administered neuropeptides access cognate receptors? An analysis in the central corticotropin-releasing factor system. *J Neurosci* (2000) **20**:1142–56.
105. Torres G, Horowitz JM, Laflamme N, Rivest S. Fluoxetine induces the transcription of genes encoding c-fos, corticotropin-releasing factor and its type 1 receptor in rat brain. *Neuroscience* (1998) **87**:463–77. doi:10.1016/S0306-4522(98)00147-X
106. Lenglos C, Mitra A, Guèvremont G, Timofeeva E. Sex differences in the effects of chronic stress and food restriction on body weight gain and brain expression of CRF and relaxin-3 in rats. *Genes Brain Behav* (2013) **12**:370–87. doi:10.1111/gbb.12028
107. McGowan BM, Stanley SA, Ghatei MA, Bloom SR. Relaxin-3 and its role in neuroendocrine function. *Ann N Y Acad Sci* (2009) **1160**:250–5. doi:10.1111/j.1749-6632.2008.03796.x
108. Vertes RP, Kocsis B. Brainstem-diencephalo-septohippocampal systems controlling the theta rhythm of the hippocampus. *Neuroscience* (1997) **81**:893–926.
109. Pan WX, McNaughton N. The role of the medial supramammillary nucleus in the control of hippocampal theta activity and behaviour in rats. *Eur J Neurosci* (2002) **16**:1797–809. doi:10.1046/j.1460-9568.2002.02267.x
110. Buzsaki G. Theta oscillations in the hippocampus. *Neuron* (2002) **33**:325–40. doi:10.1016/S0896-6273(02)00586-X
111. Hasselmo ME. What is the function of hippocampal theta rhythm? Linking behavioral data to phasic properties of field potential and unit recording data. *Hippocampus* (2005) **15**:936–49. doi:10.1002/hipo.20116
112. Vertes RP. Hippocampal theta rhythm: a tag for short-term memory. *Hippocampus* (2005) **15**:923–35. doi:10.1002/hipo.20118
113. Kahana MJ, Sekuler R, Caplan JB, Kirschen M, Madsen JR. Human theta oscillations exhibit task dependence during virtual maze navigation. *Nature* (1999) **399**:781–4. doi:10.1038/21645
114. Bland BH, Oddie SD. Theta band oscillation and synchrony in the hippocampal formation and associated structures: the case for its role in sensorimotor integration. *Behav Brain Res* (2001) **127**:119–36. doi:10.1016/S0166-4328(01)00358-8
115. Cruikshank LC, Singhal A, Hueppelsheuser M, Caplan JB. Theta oscillations reflect a putative neural mechanism for human sensorimotor integration. *J Neurophysiol* (2012) **107**:65–77. doi:10.1152/jn.00893.2010
116. Nunez A, Cervera-Ferri A, Olucha-Bordonau FE, Ruiz-Torner A, Teruel V. Nucleus incertus contribution to hippocampal theta rhythm generation. *Eur J Neurosci* (2006) **23**:2731–8. doi:10.1111/j.1460-9568.2006.04797.x
117. Nakamura K. Central circuitries for body temperature regulation and fever. *Am J Physiol Regul Integr Comp Physiol* (2011) **301**:R1207–28. doi:10.1152/ajpregu.00109.2011
118. Mallick HN, Kumar VM. Basal forebrain thermoregulatory mechanism modulates auto-regulated sleep. *Front Neurol* (2012) **3**:102. doi:10.3389/fneur.2012.00102
119. Saper CB, Scammell TE, Lu J. Hypothalamic regulation of sleep and circadian rhythms. *Nature* (2005) **437**:1257–63. doi:10.1038/nature04284
120. Smith CM, Hosken IT, Sutton SW, Lawrence AJ, Gundlach AL. Relaxin-3 null mutation mice display a circadian hypoactivity phenotype. *Genes Brain Behav* (2012) **11**:94–104. doi:10.1111/j.1601-183X.2011.00730.x
121. Smith CM, Hosken IT, Downer NL, Chua BE, Hossain MA, Wade JD, et al. Pharmacological activation of RXFP3 is not orexigenic in C57BL/6J mice. *Proceedings of 6th International Conference on Relaxin and Related Peptides.* Florence: Florence University Press (Forthcoming 2013).
122. Smith CM, Lawrence AJ, Sutton SW, Gundlach AL. Behavioral phenotyping of mixed background (129S5:B6) relaxin-3 knockout mice. *Ann N Y Acad Sci* (2009) **1160**:236–41. doi:10.1111/j.1749-6632.2009.03953.x
123. Sutton SW, Shelton J, Smith CM, Williams J, Yun S, Motley T, et al. Metabolic and neuroendocrine responses to RXFP3 modulation in the central nervous system. *Ann N Y Acad Sci* (2009) **1160**:242–9. doi:10.1111/j.1749-6632.2008.03812.x
124. Hosken IT, Smith CM, Blasiak A, Gundlach AL. Elimination of RXFP3 signalling causes reduced circadian voluntary wheel running in mice: implications for relaxin-3 networks in arousal and sleep control. *J Sleep Res* (2012) **21**(Suppl 1):120.
125. Hosken IT, Smith CM, Chua BE, Gundlach AL. Consequences of relaxin-3 null mutation in mice on food-entrainable arousal. *Proceedings of 6th International Conference on Relaxin and Related Peptides.* Florence: Florence University Press (Forthcoming 2013).
126. Dun SL, Brailoiu E, Wang Y, Brailoiu GC, Liu-Chen LY, Yang J, et al. Insulin-like peptide 5: expression in the mouse brain and mobilization of calcium. *Endocrinology* (2006) **147**:3243–8. doi:10.1210/en.2006-0237
127. Liu C, Kuei C, Sutton S, Chen J, Bonaventure P, Wu J, et al. INSL5 is a high affinity specific agonist for GPCR142 (GPR100). *J Biol Chem* (2005) **280**:292–300.
128. Mashima H, Ohno H, Yamada Y, Sakai T, Ohnishi H. INSL5 may be a unique marker of colorectal endocrine cells and neuroendocrine tumors. *Biochem Biophys Res Commun* (2013) **432**:586–92. doi:10.1016/j.bbrc.2013.02.042

12

On the existence and function of galanin receptor heteromers in the central nervous system

Kjell Fuxe[1]*, Dasiel O. Borroto-Escuela[1], Wilber Romero-Fernandez[1], Alexander O. Tarakanov[2], Feliciano Calvo[1], Pere Garriga[3], Mercé Tena[3], Manuel Narvaez[4], Carmelo Millón[4], Concepción Parrado[5], Francisco Ciruela[6], Luigi F. Agnati[7,8], José A. Narvaez[4] and Zaida Díaz-Cabiale[4]

[1] Department of Neuroscience, Karolinska Institutet, Stockholm, Sweden
[2] St. Petersburg Institute for Informatics and Automation, Russian Academy of Sciences, Saint Petersburg, Russia
[3] Centre de Biotecnologia Molecular, Departament d'Enginyeria Química, Universitat Politécnica de Catalunya, Barcelona, Spain
[4] Department of Physiology, School of Medicine, University of Málaga, Málaga, Spain
[5] Department of Histology, School of Medicine, University of Málaga, Málaga, Spain
[6] Unitat de Farmacologia, Departament Patologia i Terapéutica Experimental, Universitat de Barcelona, Barcelona, Spain
[7] Department of Biomedical Sciences, University of Modena and Reggio Emilia, Modena, Italy
[8] Istituto di Ricovero e Cura a Carattere Scientifico, Lido Venice, Italy

Edited by:
Hubert Vaudry, University of Rouen, France

Reviewed by:
Wing-Ho Yung, Chinese University of Hong Kong, Hong Kong
Joao C. Cardoso, University of Algarve, Portugal

***Correspondence:**
Kjell Fuxe, Department of Neuroscience, Karolinska Institutet, Retzius väg 8, 17177 Stockholm, Sweden.
e-mail: kjell.fuxe@ki.se

Galanin receptor (GalR) subtypes 1–3 linked to central galanin neurons may form heteromers with each other and other types of G protein-coupled receptors in the central nervous system (CNS). These heteromers may be one molecular mechanism for galanin peptides and their N-terminal fragments (gal 1-15) to modulate the function of different types of glia–neuronal networks in the CNS, especially the emotional and the cardiovascular networks. GalR–5-HT1A heteromers likely exist with antagonistic GalR–5-HT1A receptor–receptor interactions in the ascending midbrain raphe 5-HT neuron systems and their target regions. They represent a novel target for antidepressant drugs. Evidence is given for the existence of GalR1–5-HT1A heteromers in cellular models with trans-inhibition of the protomer signaling. A GalR1–GalR2 heteromer is proposed to be a galanin N-terminal fragment preferring receptor (1-15) in the CNS. Furthermore, a GalR1–GalR2–5-HT1A heterotrimer is postulated to explain why only galanin (1-15) but not galanin (1-29) can antagonistically modulate the 5-HT1A receptors in the dorsal hippocampus rich in gal fragment binding sites. The results underline a putative role of different types of GalR–5-HT1A heteroreceptor complexes in depression. GalR antagonists may also have therapeutic actions in depression by blocking the antagonistic GalR–NPYY1 receptor interactions in putative GalR–NPYY1 receptor heteromers in the CNS resulting in increases in NPYY1 transmission and antidepressant effects. In contrast the galanin fragment receptor (a postulated GalR1–GalR2 heteromer) appears to be linked to the NPYY2 receptor enhancing the affinity of the NPYY2 binding sites in a putative GalR1–GalR2–NPYY2 heterotrimer. Finally, putative GalR–α2-adrenoreceptor heteromers with antagonistic receptor–receptor interactions may be a widespread mechanism in the CNS for integration of galanin and noradrenaline signals also of likely relevance for depression.

Keywords: galanin receptors, heteromers, GPCRs, 5HT1A, NPY receptors, allosteric modulator

INTRODUCTION

Galanin is a neuropeptide (Tatemoto et al., 1983) widely distributed in neurons within the central nervous system (CNS; Jacobowitz et al., 2004). Three Galanin receptor (GalR) subtypes, GalR1–3, have been cloned and belong to the rhodopsin subfamily of G protein-coupled receptor (GPCR; Branchek et al., 2000; Lundstrom et al., 2005; Mitsukawa et al., 2008). GalR1 and GalR2 in particular are found in many regions of the CNS as demonstrated with *in situ* hybridization, radioligand binding, and immunohistochemical studies and have all a high affinity for galanin. GalR1 and GalR3 are coupled to Gi/o leading to inhibition of adenylate cyclase (AC), increases in MAPK activity and opening of G protein-coupled inwardly rectifying K^+ channels. GalR2 is coupled to Gq/11 and its activation leads to increases in phospholipase C with formation of IP3 increasing intracellular calcium levels and of diacylglycerol (DAG) with the subsequent activation of the protein kinase C. These three GalR subtypes are involved in a number of functions in the CNS modulating neuroendocrine, cardiovascular and mood regulation, pain control, food intake, and seizure threshold (Lundstrom et al., 2005; Mitsukawa et al., 2008). Galanin has also been demonstrated to exert neurotrophic and neuroprotective actions. As early as 1988 (Fuxe et al., 1988b) indications for the existence GalR–5-HT1A receptor–receptor interactions were obtained in rat limbic membranes and in 1994 (Mazarati et al., 1994) in a neuropharmacological analysis results were obtained suggesting interactions of GalRs with glutamate receptors in the dorsal striatum.

This review serves to summarize the indications that GalR subtypes may form heteromers with each other and other types of GPCRs in the CNS as a molecular mechanism to modulate the function of different types of glia–neuronal networks in the CNS.

RECEPTOR HETEROMERS AND THEIR ALLOSTERIC RECEPTOR–RECEPTOR INTERACTIONS VIA THE RECEPTOR INTERFACE

We began to test the hypothesis of intramembrane receptor–receptor interactions in 1980–1981 in membrane preparations of various CNS regions and found that neuropeptides could modulate the binding characteristics, especially the affinity of the monoamine receptors, in a receptor subtype specific way (Agnati et al., 1980; Fuxe et al., 1981, 1983). Thus, intramembrane receptor–receptor interactions did exist in addition to indirect actions via phosphorylation and changes in membrane potential. However, it took around 10 years before they began to have an impact in the receptor field. But the good news were that the results were in line with earlier findings by Limbird et al. (1975), showing negative cooperativity in beta-adrenergic receptors, which could be explained by the existence of receptor homodimers leading to receptor–receptor interactions. It was also clear that adapter proteins could be involved in mediating the receptor–receptor interactions in brain membranes. A logical consequence for the indications of direct physical interactions between neuropeptide and monoamine receptors, the term heteromerization was introduced to describe a specific interaction between different types of GPCRs (see Zoli et al., 1993; Fuxe et al., 2012a).

Fluorescence resonance energy transfer (FRET) and bioluminescence resonance energy transfer (BRET) methods gave the evidence needed to demonstrate heteromers among class A GPCRs. In FRET two putative proteins can, e.g., bear a "donor" (CFP or GFP2) or an "acceptor" (YFP). If these two proteins interact then the donor and acceptor fluorophores are likely in proximity (10 nm or less) and energy transfer between donor and acceptor can occur after donor excitation by demonstration of YFP emission. In BRET two putative proteins bear a "donor" (Rluc) or an "acceptor" fluorophore (YFP or GFP2). If these proteins are in proximity they do interact. Then, a donor–acceptor energy transfer can occur after Rluc substrate (h-coelenterazine) oxidation. The bioluminescence formed can activate YFP and YFP emission develops (Fernández-Dueñas et al., 2012; Fuxe et al., 2012a).

More recently, evidence has been presented by means of *in situ* proximity ligation assay (*in situ* PLA) that in HEK293 cells $D_{2L}R$ can form heteromers with $D_{4.7}R$ and especially with $D_{4.2}R$ and $D_{4.4}R$ (Borroto-Escuela et al., 2011). *In situ* PLA have the potential to enable a fuller understanding of GPCR receptor–receptor and could be highly suited to investigate GPCR heteromers in tissue, providing new insights in basic biological mechanisms, heteroreceptor levels and their locations, e.g., in the brain (Borroto-Escuela et al., 2012).

It is clear that allosteric mechanisms make possible the integrative activity taking place intramolecularly in monomers and intermolecularly in homomers and heteromers (see Fuxe et al., 2010b). Allostery is a mode of long distance communication between distal sites in proteins. There may or may not exist a conformational change at the binding site by the allosteric communication. The conformational change is only one of the possible scenarios. We have preferred pathways which vary with given conditions, through which the strain energy is released from the allosteric site following a perturbation event which can pass over the receptor interface into the other protomer of the receptor homomer or heteromer (see Fuxe et al., 2010a). Kenakin (2008) rightly regards "Seven TM receptors as Nature's prototype allosteric protein: de-emphasizing the geography of binding". The allosteric receptor–receptor interactions induced by activation of one receptor protomer can influence the recognition, G protein-coupling and signaling and trafficking of the other protomers in the receptor heteromer.

A high energy strength double arginine-phosphate electrostatic interaction has been found in the $A_{2A}R$–D_2R heteromer by Ciruela et al. (2004) and Woods et al. (2005) which possess a covalent-like stability as demonstrated with mass spectrometry in combination with collision-induced dissociation experiments and confirmed by pull-down techniques. Based on a mathematical approach, Tarakanov and Fuxe (2010) have deduced, based on 48 pairs of receptors that form or not form heterodimers, a set of triplet amino acid homologies that may importantly participate in receptor–receptor interactions with an origin from integrin triplets of marine sponges and toll-like receptor triplets (Tarakanov et al., 2012a,b). We show how such triplets of amino acid residues and their "teams" may be utilized to construct a kind of code that determines (and/or predicts) which receptors should or should not form heterodimers. We propose a "guide-and clasp" manner for receptor–receptor interactions where "adhesive guides" may be the triplet homologies. Ciruela et al. (2004) showed an amazing stability of epitope–epitope electrostatic interaction based on arginine phosphate. Thus, we should note that two main players contain R (Arg): IDR and AAR. Others have distinct relationships to negatively and positively charged amino acids.

The receptor heteromers due to the receptor–receptor interactions (RRI) represent a new target for drugs since they allow *inter alia* a higher selectivity in drug actions. Thus, in principle, it is possible to have not simply drugs acting as agonists, or partial agonists or antagonists on a receptor A that is assembled in a heteromer. Rather it is also possible to modulate receptor A through an action on receptor B which belongs to the same heteromer and interacts, via allosteric RRI, with receptor A (**Figure 1**). Against this background, a new field for pharmacology can be considered. Let us list the possible new opportunities to be investigated in a very simple case that of A–B-receptor heterodimers with the aim to modulate the recognition/decoding processes of receptor A. Due to the RRI in the dimer it could be possible to use: (1) receptor B-agonists, (2) receptor B-partial agonists, (3) receptor B-antagonists, and (4) receptor B allosteric modulators. These treatments could change the recognition/decoding process of:

(a) The complex endogenous ligands/receptor A.
(b) The complexes receptor A-agonist/receptor A, receptor A-partial agonist/receptor A, or receptor A-antagonist/receptor A or receptor A allosteric modulator/receptor A.

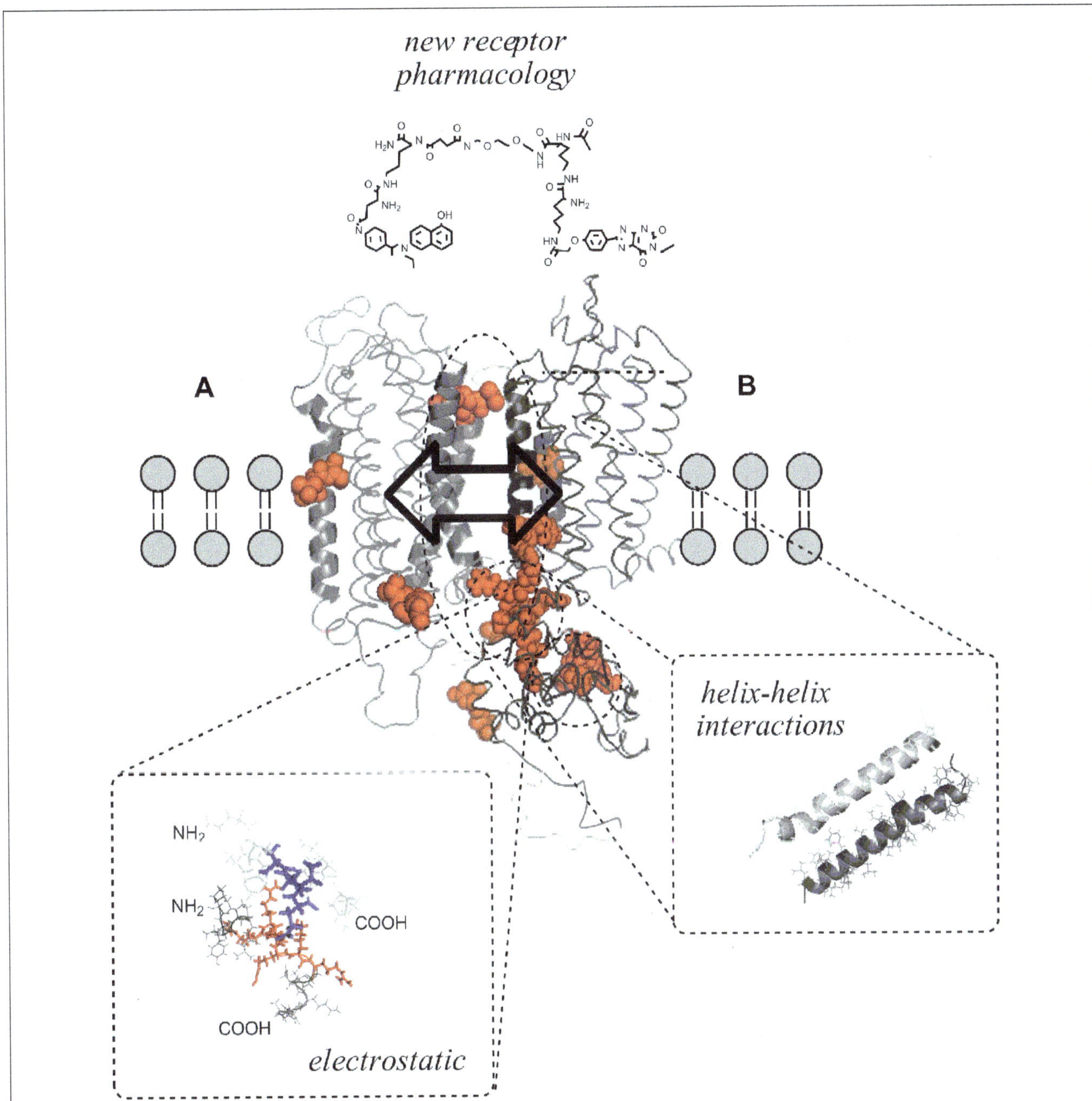

FIGURE 1 | Intermolecular allosteric mechanisms of the GPCR homo/heteromer and their receptor interface making possible molecular integration of transmitter signals. Three-dimensional molecular models of the seven TM regions of two putative GPCR (A and B) were built by means of the homology modeling program Accelrys Discovery Studio 2.5 (San Diego, CA, USA) to show that dimerization of GPCR can result from either covalent and non-covalent unions between receptor protomers. (*Helix–helix interaction*) Seen from a lateral view, representation of the A(TM-IV/)–B(TM-V) interaction in the A–B receptor heterodimer is shown. (*Electrostatic interactions*) Illustration of positively charged arginine-rich epitope (red) in the N-terminal part of the third intracellular loop of receptor A electrostatically interacting with the negatively charged (blue) C-terminal epitopes of the receptor B. These electrostatic interactions may represent important hot spots in the receptor interface of some receptor heteromers like $A_{2A}R$–D_2R, $A_{2A}R$–D_3R, and $A_{2A}R$–D_4R heteromers. Allosteric mechanisms make possible the integrative activity taking place intramolecularly in monomers or intermolecularly in homo/heteromers (arrow with two directions in the interface). Intermolecular allosteric mechanisms take place through the formation of different types of receptor homo/heteromers and receptor/protein complexes which can change the function of an individual receptor protomer present in a homomer or heteromer. One example of the novel pharmacology created by heteromers is the use of heterobivalent ligands containing an A pharmacophore and a B pharmacophore linked through a spacer of variable length which may function as useful molecular probes for targeting the A–B receptor heteromer and in this way counteracting or enhancing the receptor–receptor interactions in these heteromers. Such compounds may have a potential for use in pharmacotherapy of CNS diseases.

In the case of a trimer or even higher order oligomers that is of a receptor mosaic (RM) we should consider especially

(a) Topological organization.
(b) Localization and route of the "Allosteric Pathways" inside the RM.
(c) Possible existence of "Check-Points" along the allosteric pathways.

POTENTIAL EXISTENCE OF GALANINR–5-HT1A HETEROMERS WITH ANTAGONISTIC GalR–5-HT1A RECEPTOR–RECEPTOR INTERACTIONS IN THE ASCENDING MIDBRAIN RAPHE 5-HT NEURON SYSTEMS AND THEIR TARGET REGIONS. A NOVEL TARGET FOR ANTIDEPRESSANT DRUGS

A substantial density of high affinity GalRs was demonstrated in the dorsal raphe by the Jacobowitz group in 1986 (Skofitsch et al., 1986) after having shown the existence of galanin IR cell bodies in the dorsal raphe (DR) after colchicine treatment (Skofitsch and Jacobowitz, 1985). This work inspired the Fuxe group to perform intraventricular (ivt) injections with galanin and evaluate its effects on regional 5-HT levels and metabolism (Fuxe et al., 1988a). In 1986 the coexistence of 5-HT and galanin IR in DR cell bodies was found (Melander et al., 1986) and in 1990 only a proportion of the 5-HT nerve cell bodies in the DR was found to costore galanin and 5-HT IR after colchicine (Fuxe et al., 1990). Intraventricular galanin reduced 5-HT metabolism in ventral limbic cortex, hippocampal formation, and fronto-parietal cortex probably via direct inhibitory actions on DR 5-HT nerve cells reducing their firing rates (Fuxe et al., 1988a). These results for the first time suggested based on the 5-HT hypothesis of depression (see Carlsson et al., 1968) that galanin, via actions on GalRs, mainly GalR in the DR, may contribute to depression by reducing firing in the ascending 5-HT neurons (see also Kehr et al., 2002). Thus, GalR antagonists may represent novel antidepressant drugs.

The same year it was also discovered in limbic membrane preparations that galanin in nanomolar concentrations can reduce the affinity of postjunctional [^{3}H]-5HT1A agonist binding sites suggesting that galanin can reduce 5-HT1A recognition and probably signaling in the limbic system (Fuxe et al., 1988b). This indicates that galanin also via such actions can contribute to development of a state of depression, since postjunctional 5-HT1A receptors likely is one of the 5-HT receptors elevating mood upon activation (see Fuxe et al., 1991). This receptor has also been implicated in the pathophysiology of depression based *inter alia* on analysis of brain samples from depressed suicides (Lowther et al., 1997). These results on GalR modulation of 5-HT1A agonist binding sites gave the first indication that brain GalR/5-HT1A heteromers may exist where GalRs antagonize postjunctional 5-HT1A recognition and signaling via intramembrane receptor–receptor interactions (Fuxe et al., 1990, 1991, 2008; Zoli et al., 1993). The antagonistic GalR/5-HT1A receptor interactions in putative receptor heteromers represented a novel integrative mechanism in 5-HT neurotransmission. The role of galanin in the modulation of 5-HT neurotransmission became, however, more complex with the observations that galanin can increase potassium-induced 5-HT release from synaptosomal preparations (Martire et al., 1991). This gave the first indication there may also exist GalRs that increase 5-HT neurotransmission and thus may be beneficial for treatment of depression. In fact, it has recently been proposed that activation of GalR2 can produce antidepressant actions (Lu et al., 2005; see Lundstrom et al., 2005; Mitsukawa et al., 2008). However, the overall inhibitory influence of GalRs was in dominance (see Fuxe et al., 1988a,b). The relevance of antagonistic GalR/5-HT1A interactions for depression were discussed especially in the frame of the 5-HT isoreceptor disbalance hypothesis of depression (see Fuxe et al., 1977, 1991; Ogren et al., 1979) and the galanin-induced reduction of activity in the ascending 5-HT neurons (Fuxe et al., 1991). GalRs counteract the postjunctional mood elevating 5-HT1A signaling while the signaling over other subtypes of 5-HT receptors like the 5-HT2-like receptors which may be blocked by classical antidepressant drugs (Fuxe et al., 1977, 1991; Ogren et al., 1979) were less affected. A behavioral correlate has been obtained to the postjunctional antagonistic GalR/5-HT1A receptor interactions (Razani et al., 2001). The activation of 5-HT1A receptors in membrane preparations and in brain sections was in contrast found to increase the affinity of the GalRs in diencephalic and telencephalic areas (Hedlund et al., 1991a). Thus, reciprocal intramembrane receptor–receptor interactions may exist in putative GalR/5-HT1A heteromers where an activation of 5-HT1A receptors increases GalR recognition and probably GalR signaling. Thus, if the 5-HT1A receptor is regarded as a hub receptor and the GalR as the accessory receptor in this receptor heteromer, it seems possible that the GalR mediates an inhibitory intramembrane feedback mechanism to dampen overactivity in 5-HT1A receptor signaling (Fuxe et al., 1988b, 1991; Hedlund and Fuxe, 1996). However, it is still unknown which GalR subtype protomers are modulated by the agonist-induced activation of the 5-HT1A protomer in the GalR–5-HT1A heteromers. In other cases, however, the enhancement of the GalR signaling may be the major action, allowing the 5-HT1A protomer to bring down firing in the raphe nuclei further due to increased opening of the GalR regulated GIRK channels leading to increased hyperpolarization (Hedlund et al., 1991b).

GalR–5-HT1A AUTORECEPTOR INTERACTIONS IN THE DORSAL RAPHE 5-HT CELL BODIES/DENDRITES

A time-dependent modulatory action by GalRs exist also on 5-HT1A autoreceptors in the DR nerve cells (Razani et al., 2000). Intraventricular galanin produces first a rapid decrease of the 5-HT1A autoreceptor recognition within 10 min (reduction of affinity) in line with the findings at postjunctional 5-HT1A receptors (Fuxe et al., 1998, 2008). Thus, intramembrane antagonistic GalR/5-HT1A autoreceptor interactions in putative GalR–5-HT1A autoreceptor heteromers can be demonstrated at the soma-dendritic level of the DR 5-HT nerve cells. This will, however, not increase their nerve cell firing since galanin itself causes hyperpolarization (Xu et al., 1998) and it may represent only an intramembrane inhibitory feedback to avoid abnormal inhibition of the DR 5-HT nerve cells.

However, this change in the 5-HT1A autoreceptor is followed after 2 h by a delayed rise in 5-HT1A autoreceptor density probably through reduced internalization of the GalR/5-HT1A receptor heteromers (Razani et al., 2000) and/or a galanin-induced increase in maturation and insertion of these heteromers into the plasma membrane. This was associated with a reduction of galanin mRNA levels and of 5-HT1A mRNA levels in the DR supporting this interpretation. Thus, GalR antagonists may exert antidepressant effects in the DR not only by blockade of GalR signaling but also via blockade of the galanin elicited increase in 5-HT1A autoreceptor density.

A major paper in pointing to a role of raphe GalRs in depression and for the use of GalR antagonists as novel antidepressant drugs was published by Bellido et al. (2002). The discovery was made of an increased density of GalRs in the DR of a genetic rat model of depression based on the use of Flinders Sensitive Line rats. This rise of GalR density was associated with a reduction of galanin IR in the DR and an increase in the immobility time in the forced swimming test. This may represent a primary disturbance contributing to development of human depression by reducing firing in the ascending 5-HT pathways to the limbic system and the diencephalon. These results emphasize the introduction of GalR antagonists targeting the DR in treatment of depression. However, the GalR subtypes appear to have a differential role in depression as demonstrated by Bartfai and colleagues (Bartfai et al., 2004; Lu et al., 2005; Barr et al., 2006). Thus, newly developed non-peptide GalR3 antagonists exert antidepressant like activity in various rodent models of depression (Barr et al., 2006). However, fluoxetine and electroconvulsive shock increase Gal mRNA levels in the DR accompanied by increases in GalR2 receptor binding sites (Lu et al., 2005) giving in contrast an antidepressant potential to GalR2 agonists. In fact, GalR2 may be the GalR involved in releasing 5-HT from synaptosomal preparations (Martire et al., 1991). Based on the available information it therefore seems that general GalR and GalR3 antagonists have antidepressant properties while GalR2 antagonists may reduce mood.

EVIDENCE FOR THE EXISTENCE OF GalR1–5-HT1A HETEROMERS IN CELLULAR MODELS

Previous work has established homodimerization and internalization of GalR1 in living CHO cells using FRET and time lapse confocal imaging (Wirz et al., 2005). Thus, GalR1 can exist as a dimer in the plasma membrane which may undergo desensitization and internalization upon agonist activation with Gal1-29.

We have examined the possible existence of GalR–5-HT1A heteromers in HEK-293 cells co-transfected with GFP2-tagged 5-HT1A receptor and YFP-tagged GalR1 receptor using a proximity-based FRET assay (Borroto-Escuela et al., 2010). In addition, a novel bioinformatic approach to predict receptor–receptor interface interactions was used (Tarakanov and Fuxe, 2010) together with an analysis of signaling.

Upon co-expression of the 5-HT1A-GFP2 and GalR1-YFP cDNA, a significantly higher FRET signal was observed in comparison to the FRET signal obtained from a mixture of cells individually expressing one of the two receptors. It represented a constitutive heteromers since the observed FRET ratios were unaltered by agonist treatments. In cells co-expressing 5-HT1A-GFP2 and GalR1-YFP the two receptors became clearly co-distributed in the plasma membrane at 48 h. And the specificity of this heteromer is indicated by the observation that expression of GalR2 does not block the FRET signal from developing in the 5-HT1A-GFP2 and GalR1-YFP heteromer. Instead, the FRET signal is increased. The understanding of the mechanism underlying this increase may unravel whether the formation of a GalR1–GalR2–5-HT1A higher-order heteromer (RM) takes place (Borroto-Escuela et al., 2010).

Using CRE-luciferase and SRE-luciferase reporter assays it was found that signaling by either the MAPK or AC pathways by these heteromers results in a trans-inhibition phenomenon through their interacting interface via allosteric mechanisms that block the development of an excessive activation of Gi/o linked to each of the receptors and an exaggerated inhibition of AC or stimulation of MAPK activity (**Figure 2**; Borroto-Escuela et al., 2010). These receptor heteromers may exist in the ascending raphe 5-HT pathways in view of the demonstration of antagonistic GalR–5-HT1A receptor interactions in the limbic regions and in the raphe reducing the affinity of the 5-HT1A receptors (see above).

Based on a bioinformatics approach, Tarakanov and Fuxe (2010) have deduced a set of triplet homologies that may be responsible for receptor–receptor interactions. This set consists of two non-intersecting subsets: "pro-triplets" and "contra-triplets". Any pro-triplet appears as a homology in at least one heterodimer but does not appear as a homology in any non-heterodimer. The triplets SNS and LAR may have an important role in the GalR–5-HT1A receptor interface. The locations of the triplet SNS in the same transmembrane domains (TM7) of GalR1 and 5-HT1A were shown. The locations of the triplet LAR were found in the cytoplasmic (intracellular) domains of GalR1 (between TM1 and TM2) and 5-HT1A (between TM5 and TM6). These two triplets may therefore participate in the transmembrane and intracellular components of the interface of the GalR1–5-HT1A heteromer.

A GalR1–GalR2 HETEROMER IS PROPOSED TO BE A GALANIN N-TERMINAL FRAGMENT PREFERRING RECEPTOR (1-15) IN THE CNS

The three cloned receptors are known to show a higher affinity for Gal than for galanin N-terminal fragments like Gal (1-15) (Branchek et al., 1998). A substantial further development of this field was the demonstration of specific N-terminal galanin fragment, galanin (1-15) binding sites in the rat brain emphasizing the powerful role of galanin fragments in galanin communication (**Figure 3**), especially in dorsal hippocampus, neocortex, and striatum having few high affinity galanin (1-29) binding sites (Hedlund et al., 1992). Our hypothesis is that these N-terminal Gal fragment preferring sites may be the result of formation of GalR1/GalR2 heteromers leading to conformational changes in their galanin recognition sites converting them into highly specific galanin fragment binding sites with markedly reduced affinity for galanin (1-29) (Fuxe et al., 2008). It is of high interest that gal (1-15) given intraventricularly in the rat has been found to produce marked depression-like behavior in the FST and anxiogenic like effects in the open field (Millon Penuela et al., 2012).

POSTULATED EXISTENCE OF A GalR1–GalR2–5-HT1A HETEROTRIMER

In agreement with above only galanin (1-15) but not galanin (1-29) can antagonistically modulate the 5-HT1A receptors in

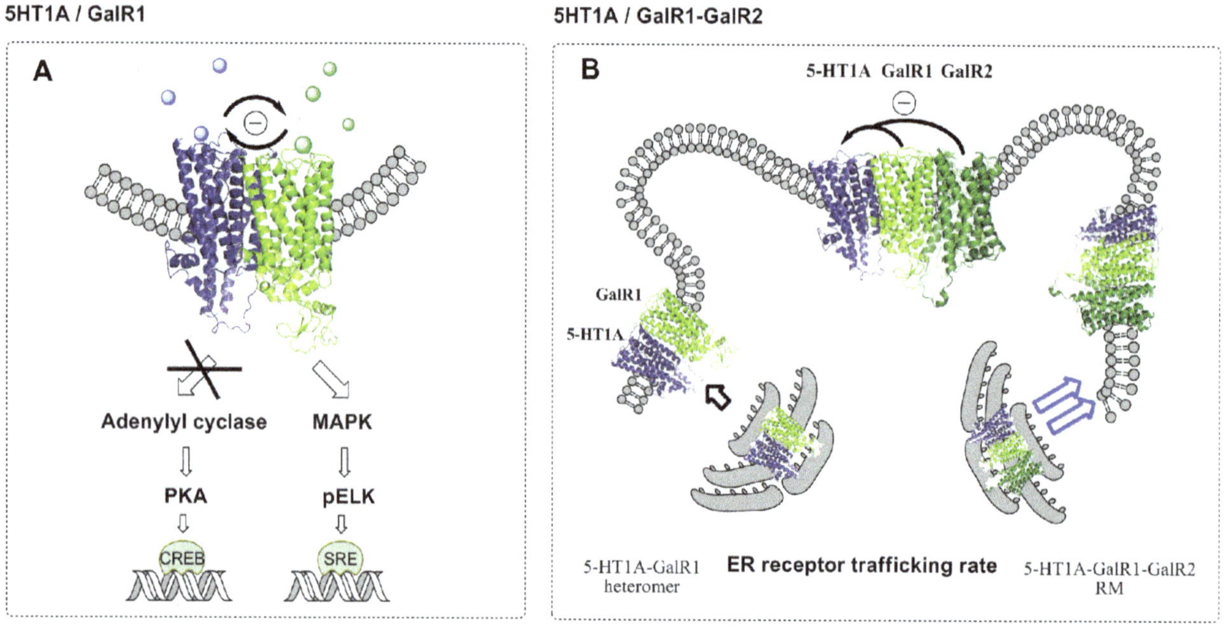

FIGURE 2 | Recognition, signaling, and trafficking pathways and their antagonistic receptor–receptor interactions in serotonin 5-HT1A and galanin receptor (GalR1) heteromers in HEK293 cells and postulated 5-HT1A–GalR1–GalR2 trimers. (A) Schematic representation of the antagonistic interactions observed after co-treatment with 5-HT1A receptor agonist (8-OH-DPAT) and galanin (peptide 1-29) in co-transfected HEK293 cells. Signaling by either the mitogen-activated protein kinase (MAPK) or adenylyl cyclase (AC) pathways by the 5-HT1A–GalR1 heteromers indicates a trans-inhibition phenomenon through their interacting interface via allosteric mechanisms that block the development of an excessive activation of Gi/o with an exaggerated inhibition of AC or stimulation of MAPK activity. **(B)** A study of the subcellular localization of tagged 5-HT1A and tagged GalR1 in the presence of non-tagged GalR2 showed a co-distribution in the plasma membrane of tagged 5-HT1A and tagged GalR1 already at 36 h in comparison to cells expressing tagged 5-HT1A and tagged GalR1 only. In this case, the tagged 5-HT1A receptor showed a more reticular distribution while tagged GalR1 was mainly found in the plasma membrane. In the presence of GalR2 a co-distribution in the plasma membrane of the tagged 5-HT1A and tagged GalR1 is obtained already at 36 h and is maintained at 48 h. A facilitated interaction of the GalR1–5-HT1A heterodimer into the plasma membrane by expression of GalR2 can be explained based on the postulated receptor mosaic (5HT1A–GalR1–GalR2), where the endoplasmic reticulum (ER) trafficking rate is higher than the trafficking rate shown by the 5-HT1A–GalR1 heteromer. Available findings can be explained by postulating that a GalR1–GalR2 heteromer is a galanin fragment preferring receptor which in the postulated trimer with the 5-HT1A receptor exerts a strong antagonistic receptor–receptor interaction with the 5-HT1A protomer at the level of 5-HT1A recognition.

the dorsal hippocampus and this effect may be blocked by a known GalR antagonist M35 (Hedlund et al., 1994). Thus, a RM of GalR1–GalR2/-5-HT1A receptors may exist especially in the dorsal hippocampus, neocortex, the striatum, and the raphe where galanin fragments may effectively antagonize postjunctional and autoreceptor 5-HT1A recognition and may function via activation of the postulated GalR1/GalR2 heteromer (**Figure 2**). Also a cross-inhibition of the GalR1–GalR2 heteromer by the 5-HT1A protomer in the trimer should be considered. The GalR1–GalR2–5-HT1A heterotrimer may have a higher trafficking rate from the endoplasmic reticulum to the plasma membrane than the GalR1–5-HT1A heteromer (**Figure 2**; Borroto-Escuela et al., 2010).

Thus, known GalR antagonists should be putative antidepressant drugs also by blocking galanin fragment preferring sites in addition to galanin binding sites increasing postjunctional 5-HT1A mediated 5-HT signaling and the firing of the ascending 5-HT pathways (Hedlund et al., 1994; Fuxe et al., 1998). Therefore, known GalR antagonists may have multiple targets and it would be of high interest to develop an antagonist for treatment of depression that selectively target the GalR1–GalR2 heteromer postulated to be the galanin N-terminal fragment receptor.

Evidence has been presented that N-terminal galanin fragments can more strongly and more potently reduce postjunctional 5-HT1A receptor recognition also in the ventral limbic cortex where also high affinity GalRs exist (Diaz-Cabiale et al., 2000a). These effects were also blocked by a GalRs antagonist. The galanin fragment preferring receptor may again be formed by the heteromerization of GalR1 and GalR2, since they are known to be present here like in the dorsal hippocampus (O'Donnell et al., 1999). The results underline an important role of different types of GalR–5-HT1A heteroreceptor complexes in depression.

POTENTIAL EXISTENCE OF GalR–NPYY1 RECEPTOR HETEROMERS IN THE NUCLEUS TRACTUS SOLITARIUS (NTS), THE HYPOTHALAMUS AND THE DORSAL RAPHE WITH ANTAGONISTIC GalR–NPYY1 RECEPTOR INTERACTIONS

In a series of papers by Diaz-Cabiale and colleagues (Diaz-Cabiale et al., 2006, 2011; Parrado et al., 2007) evidence has been obtained for an antagonistic GalR modulation of NPY receptor mechanisms suggesting the existence of GALR–NPYY1 interactions involving a likely reduction of NPYY1 receptor agonist affinity probably taking place in GalR/NPYY1 receptor heteromers (**Figure 4A**) in NTS, hypothalamus, and DR (Diaz-Cabiale et al., 2006, 2011; Parrado

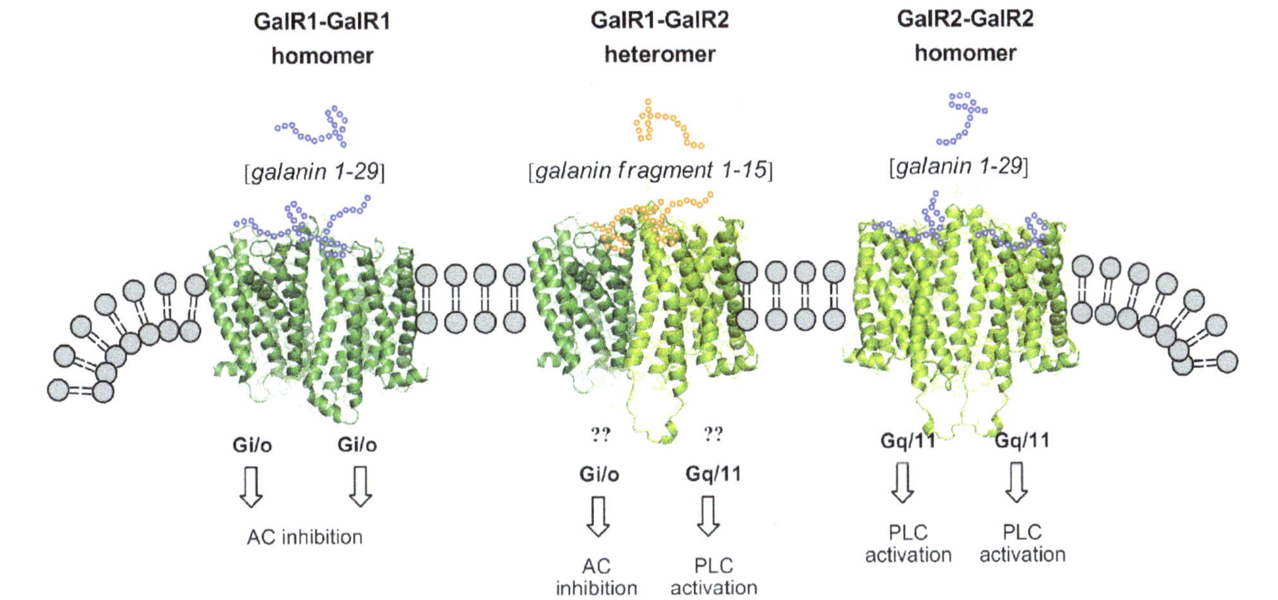

FIGURE 3 | The unknown signaling of the postulated galanin fragment preferring receptor (GalR1–GalR2 heteromer) is compared with the signaling of the GalR1 and GalR2 homomers.

et al., 2007). The results open up the possibility that GalR/NPYY1 receptor–receptor interactions in putative heteromers is a frequent phenomenon in CNS with implications for the integrative functions of galanin and NPY in these regions. Thus, the GalR subtype involved has not been determined. This interaction may be based on a GalR/NPYY1 receptor heteromerization where the galanin induced conformational change in the GalR can cause a conformational change in the NPYY1 receptor via the GalR/NPYY1 interface leading to reduced NPYY1 recognition and G protein coupling and thus to reduced NPYY1 receptor signaling.

In the NTS (Diaz-Cabiale et al., 2006) the results suggest the existence of antagonistic GalR–NPYY1 receptor interactions in cardiovascular regions of this nucleus, reducing NPYY1 signaling and thus vasodepressor activity leading to enhanced vasopressor and tachycardic actions of GalR activation in the NTS.

In the hypothalamus (Parrado et al., 2007) evidence was, for the first time, obtained that GalR activation significantly reduced the NPYY1 receptor agonist binding in the hypothalamus without effects on NPYY2 receptor agonist binding. These GalR–NPYY1 receptor interactions have physiological implications since the food intake induced by the NPYY1 receptor agonist is blocked by galanin. The changes observed on c-Fos expression support the hypothesis that GalR activation modulates the response elicited by the NPYY1 agonist.

In the DR we may postulate, on the basis of the galanin-induced decrease in NPYY1 binding, an inhibitory GalR/NPYY1 receptor–receptor interaction that modulates behavioral functions associated with mood and motivation. Behavioral and neurochemical studies support a role of galanin and NPY in mood disorders and GalR1-3 and NPYY1 receptors have been the receptors implicated in depression with GalR subtype specific antagonists and NPYY1 agonists having an antidepressant role (Lu et al., 2005; Lundstrom et al., 2005; Ishida et al., 2007; Jimenez-Vasquez et al., 2007; Fuxe et al., 2008). The decrease of NPYY1 agonist binding induced by galanin and the demonstrated cross-inhibition of c-Fos expression in the dorsal raphe upon GalR and NPYY1 agonist co-activation provides one possible basis for the use of synergistic interactions of GalR subtype specific antagonists and NPYY1 receptor agonists as a strategy for treatment of depression. Thus, GalR antagonists may also have therapeutic actions in depression by blocking the antagonistic GalR–NPYY1 receptor interactions resulting in increases in NPYY1 transmission and antidepressant effects.

In the amygdala (Parrado et al., 2007) we may instead on the basis of the galanin-induced increase in NPYY1 binding postulate a facilitatory GalR/NPYY1 receptor interaction (**Figure 4B**) that could be expected to produce anxiolytic actions. Behavioral studies support a role of galanin and NPY in reducing anxiety in the amygdala and GalRs, NPYY1, and NPYY5 have been the receptors implicated in this effect (see Moller et al., 1999; Heilig, 2004). The increase of NPYY1 binding induced by galanin in this study provides a possible basis for synergistic interactions of GalR agonists and NPYY1 receptor agonists in counteracting anxiety behavior. The differential modulation of NPYY1 binding by galanin in the hypothalamus and in the amygdala could be explained by *inter alia* the involvement of different GalR subtypes in the interaction with the NPYY1 receptor in the hypothalamus and amygdala, respectively. It may also be that the same GalR subtype and NPY receptor subtypes are involved in the two areas but they may be part of different RMs (cluster of multiple receptors; higher order heteromers) leading to altered GalR/NPYY1 interactions in the two areas due to differences in the multiple receptor–receptor interactions (Rimondini et al., 1999) in discrete RMs (Agnati et al., 1982, 2003; Fuxe et al., 2010a,b). Thus, in this way the GalR may

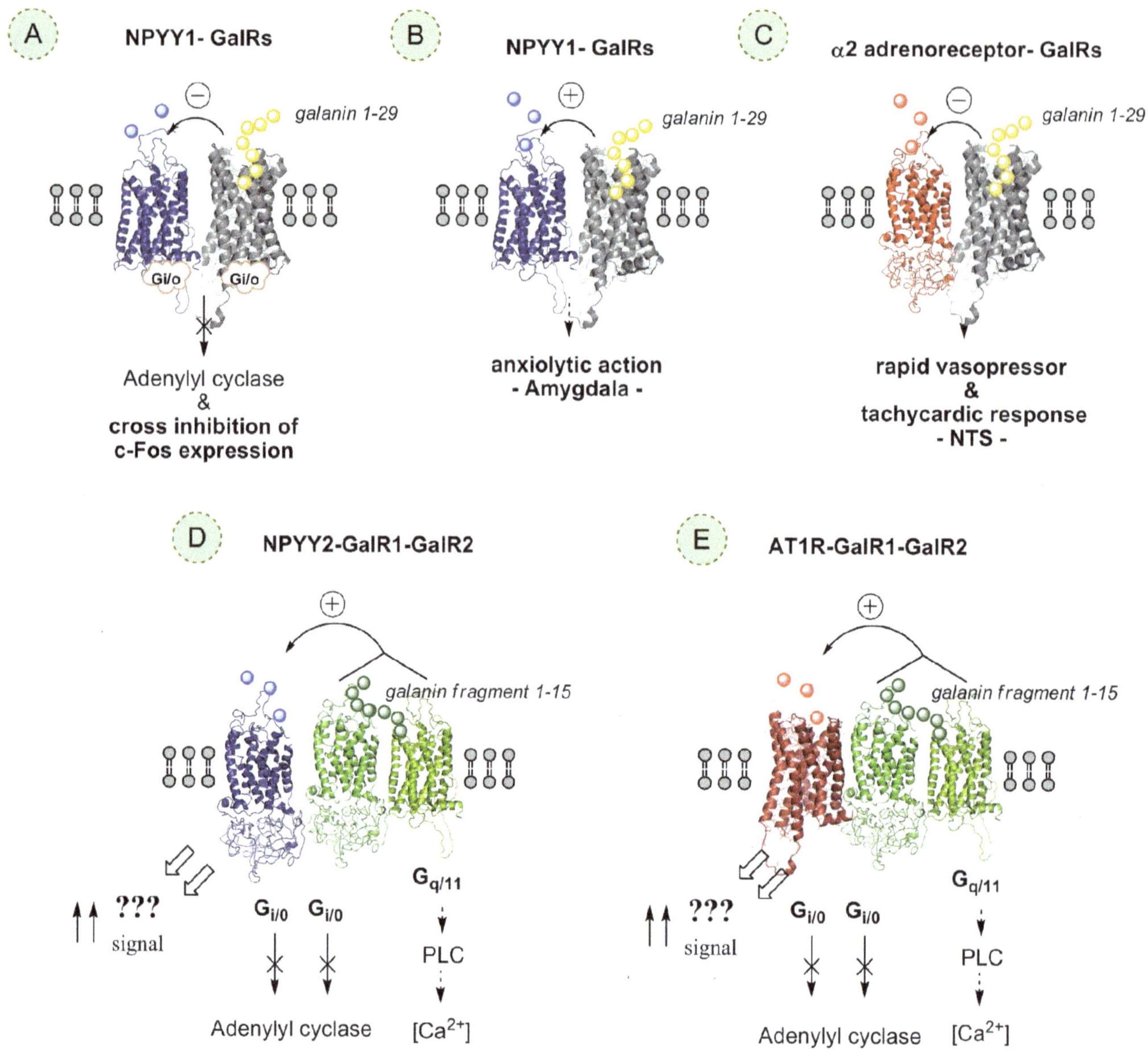

FIGURE 4 | Different types of postulated GalR heteromers and Gal-fragmentR heteromers (postulated heterotrimers) and their allosteric receptor–receptor interactions. Galanin receptor (GalR) subtypes1-3 linked to central galanin neurons may form heteromers with each other and other types of GPCRs in the CNS. These heteromers may be one molecular mechanism for galanin peptides and their N-terminal fragments (galanin 1-15) to modulate the function of different types of glia–neuronal networks in the CNS, especially the emotional and the cardiovascular networks. The allosteric receptor–receptor interactions induced constitutively or by activation of one receptor protomer can influence the recognition, G protein coupling, signaling and trafficking of the other protomers in the receptor heteromer. **(A)** NPYY1–GalRs heteromers likely exist with antagonistic NPYY1–GalR receptor interactions involving a reduction of NPYY1 receptor agonist affinity probably taking place in postulated GalR/NPYY1 receptor heteromers in NTS, hypothalamus, and dorsal raphe. GalR antagonists may also have therapeutic actions in depression by blocking the antagonistic GalR–NPYY1 receptor interactions in putative GalR–NPYY1 receptor heteromers in the CNS resulting in increases in NPYY1 transmission and antidepressant effects. **(B)** In contrast, in the amygdala a facilitatory GalR/NPYY1 receptor interaction, likely involving another GalR subtype than in A, is postulated based on the increase of NPYY1 binding induced by GalR activation in this region expected to produce anxiolytic actions. **(C)** Putative GalR–α2-adrenoreceptor heteromers with antagonistic receptor–receptor interactions reducing α2 function may be a widespread mechanism in the CNS for integration of galanin and noradrenaline signals, also of likely relevance for depression. **(D)** Galanin fragment preferring receptor (a postulated GalR1–GalR2 heteromer) appears to be linked to the NPYY2 receptor enhancing the affinity and signaling of the NPYY2 receptor via unknown signaling pathways in a putative GalR1–GalR2–NPYY2 heterotrimer; a reduction of Gi/o signaling may contribute. **(E)** Furthermore, the postulated GalR1–GalR2 heteromer, a postulated galanin N-terminal fragment preferring receptor (1-15), appears to be linked also to the AT1R in a postulated AT1R–GalR1–GalR2 receptor mosaic enhancing the signaling of the AT1R within the NTS via unknown signaling pathways; a reduction of Gi/o signaling may contribute.

reduce NPYY1 signaling in the hypothalamus and increase it in the amygdala.

POSTULATED EXISTENCE OF A GalR1–GalR2–NPY Y2 HETEROTRIMER IN THE NTS

The presence of specific binding sites for the galanin fragment 1-15 in the nuclei involved in central cardiovascular regulation has been described (Hedlund et al., 1992). In the brainstem a high density of these galanin (1-15) binding sites appears within the NTS, supporting the hypothesis of the existence of a receptor with a higher affinity for the N-terminal fragment than for galanin (Diaz-Cabiale et al., 2005b). We have proposed (see above) that these N-terminal galanin fragment preferring sites may be the result of formation of GalR1/GalR2 heteromers leading to conformational changes in their galanin recognition sites converting them into highly specific galanin fragment binding sites with markedly reduced affinity for galanin (Fuxe et al., 2008). As a matter of fact galanin and N-terminal fragment galanin (1-15) have specific and different roles (hypotensive and vasopressor responses, respectively) in cardiovascular regulation (Diaz-Cabiale et al., 2005b). The N-terminal fragment galanin (1-15) antagonized the cardiovascular effects of galanin (Narvaez et al., 1994) and galanin fragment (1-15) but not galanin decreases baroreceptor reflex sensitivity (Diaz et al., 1996). Galanin and galanin (1-15) also stimulate the expression of c-Fos with different temporal and spatial profiles, especially in the NTS and in the ventrolateral medulla (Marcos et al., 2001). The GalR antagonist M40 is able to block the cardiovascular responses elicited by the N-terminal fragment galanin (1-15) (Narvaez et al., 1994) giving evidence that regular GalR antagonists also can block the galanin fragment preferring receptors (postulated GalR1–GalR2 heteromer).

NPY operates in central cardiovascular regulation through the NPYY1 and Y2 receptor subtypes. Leu31Pro34NPY, a specific NPYY1 receptor agonist, microinjected into the NTS elicits vasodepressor and bradycardic responses (Yang et al., 1993), whereas the injection of the NPY C-terminal fragment (13-36), a specific NPYY2 receptor agonist, leads to vasopressor responses at low doses (Aguirre et al., 1990; Yang et al., 1993). In the study of Diaz-Cabiale et al. (2010) the co-injection of threshold doses of galanin (1-15) and of the NPYY2 agonist resulted in an increase of MAPK of the same magnitude as observed with threshold doses of NPY and galanin (1-15). Galanin (1-15) was also found to specifically increase the NPYY2 agonist binding in the NTS without inducing any effect on NPYY1 agonist binding (Diaz-Cabiale et al., 2010). The increase by galanin (1-15) of the NPYY2 agonist binding may indicate a galanin (1-15)-induced increase of Y2 receptor affinity in the NTS, since the concentration of the NPYY2 agonist used (25 pM) is in the range of the K_d value, where mainly affinity changes affect the binding level. This interaction may be based on GalR1–GalR2–NPYY2 receptor heteromerization (**Figure 4D**) where the galanin (1-15) induced conformational change in the GalR1–GalR2 heteromer via the interface with NPYY2 can cause a conformational change in the NPYY2 receptor leading to increased NPYY2 recognition and switching of G protein coupling likely to Gq and thus to increased novel NPYY2 receptor signaling producing the vasopressor activity (**Figure 4D**; Diaz-Cabiale et al., 2010). These results illustrate the high impact of the allosteric receptor–receptor interactions in heteromers in the integrative mechanisms responsible for the organization of the cardiovascular responses from the local circuit level of the NTS.

POSTULATED EXISTENCE OF GalR1–GalR2–AT1 HETEROTRIMER IN THE NTS

Galanin (1-15)/angiotensin II (Ang II) interactions have also been observed in central cardiovascular control (Diaz-Cabiale et al., 2005a). Thus, intracisternal co-injections of threshold doses of Ang II with galanin (1-15) induce a significant vasopressor response that was maintained during the whole recording period, without any significant effect on heart rate. This response was blocked by the AT1 specific antagonist DuP753 (Diaz-Cabiale et al., 2005a). These data suggest the existence of a synergistic interaction between Ang II and galanin (1-15), in which the AT1 and Gal receptor subtypes participate. It may involve allosteric receptor–receptor interactions in a GalR1–GalR2–AT1 heterotrimer (**Figure 4E**) within the NTS and switching of the AT1R to Gq/11 mediated signaling.

POSTULATED EXISTENCE OF GalR–α2 ADRENORECEPTOR HETEROMERS IN THE CNS

This proposal is *inter alia* based on the effects of galanin on α2-adrenoreceptor activation were evaluated on central cardiovascular regulation in the NTS using also quantitative receptor autoradiography (Diaz-Cabiale et al., 2000b). Central administration of threshold doses of galanin together with an effective vasodepressor dose of the α2-adrenoreceptor agonist clonidine was found to induce a rapid vasopressor and tachycardic response. On the contrary, the co-injection of threshold doses of clonidine and N-terminal galanin fragment (1-15) did not result in any significant cardiovascular change (Diaz-Cabiale et al., 2000b). These functional findings suggest that galanin, but not galanin fragment (1-15), antagonizes α2-adrenoreceptor signaling via a GalR–α2-adrenoreceptor interaction in a postulated heteromer built up of these receptor protomers (**Figure 4C**). The GalR subtypes involved in these heteromers are presently unknown.

Quantitative receptor autoradiography supported this view since galanin decreased the affinity of the α2-adrenoreceptor agonist [^{3}H]p-aminoclonidine in the NTS and also increased significantly the density of the α2-adrenoreceptor agonist binding sites. These effects disappeared in presence of the specific GalR antagonist M35, demonstrating that this action is a direct consequence of GalR activation by galanin (Diaz-Cabiale et al., 2000b, 2005b). Galanin also reduced the affinity of the α2-adrenoreceptor agonist [^{3}H]p-aminoclonidine in the tel- and diencephalon which was also blocked by the specific receptor antagonist M35 (Diaz-Cabiale et al., 2001). Thus, GalR–α2-adrenoreceptor heteromers with antagonistic receptor–receptor interactions may be a widespread mechanism in the CNS for integration of galanin and noradrenaline (NA) signals.

These antagonistic receptor–receptor interactions participate in the regulation of pre- and postjunctional central NA transmission and many antidepressant drugs exert part of their therapeutic effects by increasing NA transmission via blockade of the NA transporter (Carlsson et al., 1966, 1969). Thus, these antagonistic GalR/α2-adrenoreceptor interactions are of relevance for depression and its treatment.

In the NA cell bodies, dendrites and terminal networks the α2-adrenoreceptor function as NA autoreceptors reducing NA cell firing and NA release from the terminal networks. At this level this interaction will therefore favor increases in NA release and thus NA transmission. At the postjunctional level this antagonistic interaction found all over the tel- and diencephalon will change the balance of the pattern of NA isoreceptor activation and favor the increased activation of beta-adrenergic receptor and α1-adrenoreceptor subtypes. In view of the calming influence of α2-adrenoreceptors at the behavioral level (see Fuxe et al., 2012b) the preferential activation of the other adrenergic receptor subtypes by galanin through the antagonistic GalR/α2-adrenoreceptor interaction may result in increased arousal. It will therefore be interesting to explore how this interaction may be altered in the locus coeruleus and in the limbic networks in models of depression.

EXISTENCE OF DopamineR–galaninR HETEROMERS IN THE VENTRAL HIPPOCAMPUS

There exists evidence for the existence of D1R–GalR1 and D5R–GalR1 heteromers in cellular models and D1-like receptors upon agonist-induced activation were shown to enhance the GalR1-induced MAPK signaling (Moreno et al., 2011). D1-like receptor antagonists blocked galanin-induced MAPK activation in the ventral hippocampus and in synaptosomes from this region galanin facilitated acetylcholine release upon co-activation of the D1-like receptors. Thus facilitatory allosteric D1-like-GalR interactions in heteromers may exist in control of hippocampal acetylcholine release and electrophysiological experiments in hippocampal slices using field EPSP recordings suggest a modulatory role of the dopamineR–galaninR heteromers in cholinergic neurotransmission (Moreno et al., 2011).

CONCLUSIONS

GalR subtypes may have a major role in modulating the emotional networks of the brain through heteromerization with 5-HT1A, NPYY1, and α2-adrenoreceptors leading to antagonistic allosteric receptor–receptor interactions producing reductions in 5-HT1A, NPYY1, and α2-adrenoreceptor pre and especially postsynaptic signaling in the central 5-HT and NA neurons. This may be one way in which the activity at certain GalR subtypes and at galanin fragment preferring receptors may contribute to a reduction of mood, which may lead to depression. The GalR heteromers also participate in cardiovascular functions, food intake and regulation of fear and anxiety. The hypothesis is introduced that the galanin fragment preferring receptor is formed by the GalR1–GalR2 heteromer which can mediate the strong depressant actions of Gal 1-15 upon intraventricular injections. Its postulated formation of a trimer with 5-HT1A receptors may represent a novel target for antidepressant drugs.

ACKNOWLEDGMENTS

This work has been supported by grants from *Fundacio la Marato* de TV3, Generalitat de Catalunya, Barcelona, Spain and from the Swedish Research Council (04X-715) to Kjell Fuxe. Karolinska Institutets Forskningsstiftelser 2010 and 2011 to Dasiel O. Borroto-Escuela. Alexander O. Tarakanov has not received any support for this work.

REFERENCES

Agnati, L. F., Ferre, S., Lluis, C., Franco, R., and Fuxe, K. (2003). Molecular mechanisms and therapeutical implications of intramembrane receptor/receptor interactions among heptahelical receptors with examples from the striatopallidal GABA neurons. *Pharmacol. Rev.* 55, 509–550.

Agnati, L. F., Fuxe, K., Zini, I., Lenzi, P., and Hokfelt, T. (1980). Aspects on receptor regulation and isoreceptor identification. *Med. Biol.* 58, 182–187.

Agnati, L. F., Fuxe, K., Zoli, M., Rondanini, C., and Ogren, S. O. (1982). New vistas on synaptic plasticity: the receptor mosaic hypothesis of the engram. *Med. Biol.* 60, 183–190.

Aguirre, J. A., Fuxe, K., Agnati, L. F., and Von Euler, G. (1990). Centrally injected neuropeptide Y (13–36) produces vasopressor effects and antagonizes the vasodepressor action of neuropeptide Y (1–36) in the awake male rat. *Neurosci. Lett.* 118, 5–8.

Barr, A. M., Kinney, J. W., Hill, M. N., Lu, X., Biros, S., Rebek, J. Jr., et al. (2006). A novel, systemically active, selective galanin receptor type-3 ligand exhibits antidepressant-like activity in preclinical tests. *Neurosci. Lett.* 405, 111–115.

Bartfai, T., Lu, X., Badie-Mahdavi, H., Barr, A. M., Mazarati, A., Hua, X. Y., et al. (2004). Galmic, a nonpeptide galanin receptor agonist, affects behaviors in seizure, pain, and forced-swim tests. *Proc. Natl. Acad. Sci. U.S.A.* 101, 10470–10475.

Bellido, I., Diaz-Cabiale, Z., Jimenez-Vasquez, P. A., Andbjer, B., Mathe, A. A., and Fuxe, K. (2002). Increased density of galanin binding sites in the dorsal raphe in a genetic rat model of depression. *Neurosci. Lett.* 317, 101–105.

Borroto-Escuela, D. O., Narvaez, M., Marcellino, D., Parrado, C., Narvaez, J. A., Tarakanov, A. O., et al. (2010). Galanin receptor-1 modulates 5-hydroxtryptamine-1A signaling via heterodimerization. *Biochem. Biophys. Res. Commun.* 393, 767–772.

Borroto-Escuela, D. O., Romero-Fernandez, W., Pérez-Alea, M., Narvaez, M., Tarakanov, A. O., Mudó, G., et al. (2012). The existence of FGFR1-5-HT1A receptor heterocomplexes in midbrain 5-HT neurons of the rat: relevance for neuroplasticity. *J. Neurosci.* 32, 6295–6303.

Borroto-Escuela, D. O., Van Craenenbroeck, K., Romero-Fernandez, W., Guidolin, D., Woods, A. S., Rivera, A., et al. (2011). Dopamine D2 and D4 receptor heteromerization and its allosteric receptor–receptor interactions. *Biochem. Biophys. Res. Commun.* 404, 928–934.

Branchek, T. A., Smith, K. E., Gerald, C., and Walker, M. W. (2000). Galanin receptor subtypes. *Trends Pharmacol. Sci.* 21, 109–117.

Branchek, T., Smith, K. E., and Walker, M. W. (1998). Molecular biology and pharmacology of galanin receptors. *Ann. N. Y. Acad. Sci.* 863, 94–107.

Carlsson, A., Corrodi, H., Fuxe, K., and Hokfelt, T. (1969). Effect of antidepressant drugs on the depletion of intraneuronal brain 5-hydroxytryptamine stores caused by 4-methyl-alpha-ethyl-meta-tyramine. *Eur. J. Pharmacol.* 5, 357–366.

Carlsson, A., Fuxe, K., Hamberger, B., and Lindqvist, M. (1966). Biochemical and histochemical studies on the effects of imipramine-like drugs and (+)-amphetamine on central and peripheral catecholamine neurons. *Acta Physiol. Scand.* 67, 481–497.

Carlsson, A., Fuxe, K., and Ungerstedt, U. (1968). The effect of imipramine on central 5-hydroxytryptamine neurons. *J. Pharm. Pharmacol.* 20, 150–151.

Ciruela, F., Burgueno, J., Casado, V., Canals, M., Marcellino, D., Goldberg, S. R., et al. (2004). Combining mass spectrometry and pull-down techniques for the study of receptor heteromerization. Direct epitope–epitope electrostatic interactions between adenosine A2A and dopamine D2 receptors. *Anal. Chem.* 76, 5354–5363.

Diaz, Z., Narvaez, J. A., Hedlund, P. B., Aguirre, J. A., Gonzalez-Baron, S., and Fuxe, K. (1996). Centrally infused galanin-(1-15) but not galanin-(1-29) reduces the baroreceptor reflex sensitivity in the rat. *Brain Res.* 741, 32–37.

Diaz-Cabiale, Z., Narvaez, J. A., Finnman, U. B., Bellido, I., Ogren, S. O., and Fuxe, K. (2000a). Galanin-(1-16) modulates 5-HT1A receptors in the ventral limbic cortex of the rat. *Neuroreport* 11, 515–519.

Diaz-Cabiale, Z., Narvaez, J. A., Yanaihara, N., Gonzalez-Baron, S., and Fuxe, K. (2000b). Galanin/alpha2-receptor interactions in central cardiovascular control. *Neuropharmacology* 39, 1377–1385.

Diaz-Cabiale, Z., Narvaez, J. A., Garcia-Coronel, M., and Fuxe, K. (2001). Galanin/alpha2-adrenoceptor interactions in telencephalic and diencephalic regions of the rat. *Neuroreport* 12, 151–155.

Diaz-Cabiale, Z., Parrado, C., Narvaez, M., Millon, C., Puigcerver, A., Fuxe, K., et al. (2010). The Galanin N-terminal fragment (1-15) interacts with neuropeptide Y in central cardiovascular control: involvement of the NPY Y2 receptor subtype. *Regul. Pept.* 163, 130–136.

Diaz-Cabiale, Z., Parrado, C., Narvaez, M., Puigcerver, A., Millon, C., Santin, L., et al. (2011). Galanin receptor/Neuropeptide Y receptor interactions in the dorsal raphe nucleus of the rat. *Neuropharmacology* 61, 80–86.

Diaz-Cabiale, Z., Parrado, C., Rivera, A., De La Calle, A., Agnati, L., Fuxe, K., et al. (2006). Galanin-neuropeptide Y (NPY) interactions in central cardiovascular control: involvement of the NPY Y receptor subtype. *Eur. J. Neurosci.* 24, 499–508.

Diaz-Cabiale, Z., Parrado, C., Vela, C., Covenas, R., Yanaihara, N., Fuxe, K., et al. (2005a). Intracisternal galanin/angiotensin II interactions in central cardiovascular control. *Regul. Pept.* 127, 133–140.

Diaz-Cabiale, Z., Parrado, C., Vela, C., Razani, H., Covenas, R., Fuxe, K., et al. (2005b). Role of galanin and galanin(1-15) on central cardiovascular control. *Neuropeptides* 39, 185–190.

Fernández-Dueñas, V., Llorente, J., Gandía, J., Borroto-Escuela, D. O., Agnati, L. F., Tasca, C. I., et al. (2012). Fluorescence resonance energy transfer-based technologies in the study of protein–protein interactions at the cell surface. *Methods* 57, 467–472.

Fuxe, K., Agnati, L. F., Benfenati, F., Celani, M., Zini, I., Zoli, M., et al. (1983). Evidence for the existence of receptor–receptor interactions in the central nervous system. Studies on the regulation of monoamine receptors by neuropeptides. *J. Neural Transm. Suppl.* 18, 165–179.

Fuxe, K., Agnati, L. F., Benfenati, F., Cimmino, M., Algeri, S., Hokfelt, T., et al. (1981). Modulation by cholecystokinins of 3H-spiroperidol binding in rat striatum: evidence for increased affinity and reduction in the number of binding sites. *Acta Physiol. Scand.* 113, 567–569.

Fuxe, K., Agnati, L. F., von Euler, G., Lundgren, K., Zoli, M., Bjelke, B., et al. (1990). "Galanin/5-HTreceptor interactions. A new integrative mechanism in the control of 5-HT neurontransmission in the CNS," in *Serotonin from Cell Biology to Pharmacology and Therapeutics*, eds R. Paoletti and P. M. Vanhoutte (Dordrecht: Kluwer Academic Publisher B.V.), 169–185.

Fuxe, K., Borroto-Escuela, D. O., Marcellino, D., Romero-Fernandez, W., Frankowska, M., Guidolin, D., et al. (2012a). GPCR heteromers and their allosteric receptor–receptor interactions. *Curr. Med. Chem.* 19, 356–363.

Fuxe, K., Borroto-Escuela, D. O., Romero-Fernandez, W., Ciruela, F., Manger, P., Leo, G., et al. (2012b). On the role of volume transmission and receptor–receptor interactions in social behaviour: focus on central catecholamine and oxytocin neurons. *Brain Res.* 1476, 119–131.

Fuxe, K., Hedlund, P., von Euler, G., Lundgren, K., Martire, M., Ogren, S. O., et al. (1991). "Galanin/5-HT interactions in the rat centrral nervous system. Relevance for depression," in *Galanin. A New Multifunctional Peptide in the Neuroendocrine System. Wenner-Gren International Series*, Vol. 58, eds T. Hokfelt, T. Bartfai, D. M. Jacobowitz, and D. Ottoson (London: Macmillan Press), 221–235.

Fuxe, K., Jansson, A., Diaz-Cabiale, Z., Andersson, A., Tinner, B., Finnman, U. B., et al. (1998). Galanin modulates 5-hydroxytryptamine functions. Focus on galanin and galanin fragment/5-hydroxytryptamine1A receptor interactions in the brain. *Ann. N. Y. Acad. Sci.* 863, 274–290.

Fuxe, K., Marcellino, D., Borroto-Escuela, D. O., Frankowska, M., Ferraro, L., Guidolin, D., et al. (2010a). The changing world of G protein-coupled receptors: from monomers to dimers and receptor mosaics with allosteric receptor–receptor interactions. *J. Recept. Signal Transduct. Res.* 30, 272–283.

Fuxe, K., Marcellino, D., Leo, G., and Agnati, L. F. (2010b). Molecular integration via allosteric interactions in receptor heteromers. A working hypothesis. *Curr. Opin. Pharmacol.* 10, 14–22.

Fuxe, K., Marcellino, D., Rivera, A., Diaz-Cabiale, Z., Filip, M., Gago, B., et al. (2008). Receptor–receptor interactions within receptor mosaics. Impact on neuropsychopharmacology. *Brain Res. Rev.* 58, 415–452.

Fuxe, K., Ogren, S. O., Agnati, L., Gustafsson, J. A., and Jonsson, G. (1977). On the mechanism of action of the antidepressant drugs amitriptyline and nortriptyline. Evidence for 5-hydroxytryptamine receptor blocking activity. *Neurosci. Lett.* 6, 339–343.

Fuxe, K., Ogren, S. O., Jansson, A., Cintra, A., Harfstrand, A., and Agnati, L. F. (1988a). Intraventricular injections of galanin reduces 5-HT metabolism in the ventral limbic cortex, the hippocampal formation and the fronto-parietal cortex of the male rat. *Acta Physiol. Scand.* 133, 579–581.

Fuxe, K., Von Euler, G., Agnati, L. F., and Ogren, S. O. (1988b). Galanin selectively modulates 5-hydroxytryptamine 1A receptors in the rat ventral limbic cortex. *Neurosci. Lett.* 85, 163–167.

Hedlund, P., Von Euler, G., and Fuxe, K. (1991a). Activation of 5-hydroxytryptamine1A receptors increases the affinity of galanin receptors in di- and telencephalic areas of the rat. *Brain Res.* 560, 251–259.

Hedlund, P. B., Aguirre, J. A., Narvaez, J. A., and Fuxe, K. (1991b). Centrally coinjected galanin and a 5-HT1A agonist act synergistically to produce vasodepressor responses in the rat. *Eur. J. Pharmacol.* 204, 87–95.

Hedlund, P. B., Finnman, U. B., Yanaihara, N., and Fuxe, K. (1994). Galanin-(1-15), but not galanin-(1-29), modulates 5-HT1A receptors in the dorsal hippocampus of the rat brain: possible existence of galanin receptor subtypes. *Brain Res.* 634, 163–167.

Hedlund, P. B., and Fuxe, K. (1996). Galanin and 5-HT1A receptor interactions as an integrative mechanism in 5-HT neurotransmission in the brain. *Ann. N. Y. Acad. Sci.* 780, 193–212.

Hedlund, P. B., Yanaihara, N., and Fuxe, K. (1992). Evidence for specific N-terminal galanin fragment binding sites in the rat brain. *Eur. J. Pharmacol.* 224, 203–205.

Heilig, M. (2004). The NPY system in stress, anxiety and depression. *Neuropeptides* 38, 213–224.

Ishida, H., Shirayama, Y., Iwata, M., Katayama, S., Yamamoto, A., Kawahara, R., et al. (2007). Infusion of neuropeptide Y into CA3 region of hippocampus produces antidepressant-like effect via Y1 receptor. *Hippocampus* 17, 271–280.

Jacobowitz, D. M., Kresse, A., and Skofitsch, G. (2004). Galanin in the brain: chemoarchitectonics and brain cartography – a historical review. *Peptides* 25, 433–464.

Jimenez-Vasquez, P. A., Diaz-Cabiale, Z., Caberlotto, L., Bellido, I., Overstreet, D., Fuxe, K., et al. (2007). Electroconvulsive stimuli selectively affect behavior and neuropeptide Y (NPY) and NPY Y(1) receptor gene expressions in hippocampus and hypothalamus of Flinders Sensitive Line rat model of depression. *Eur. Neuropsychopharmacol.* 17, 298–308.

Kehr, J., Yoshitake, T., Wang, F. H., Razani, H., Gimenez-Llort, L., Jansson, A., et al. (2002). Galanin is a potent in vivo modulator of mesencephalic serotonergic neurotransmission. *Neuropsychopharmacology* 27, 341–356.

Kenakin, T. P. (2008). Seven transmembrane receptors as nature's prototype allosteric protein: de-emphasizing the geography of binding. *Mol. Pharmacol.* 74, 541–543.

Limbird, L. E., Meyts, P. D., and Lefkowitz, R. J. (1975). Beta-adrenergic receptors: evidence for negative cooperativity. *Biochem. Biophys. Res. Commun.* 64, 1160–1168.

Lowther, S., De Paermentier, F., Cheetham, S. C., Crompton, M. R., Katona, C. L., and Horton, R. W. (1997). 5-HT1A receptor binding sites in post-mortem brain samples from depressed suicides and controls. *J. Affect. Disord.* 42, 199–207.

Lu, X., Barr, A. M., Kinney, J. W., Sanna, P., Conti, B., Behrens, M. M., et al. (2005). A role for galanin in antidepressant actions with a focus on the dorsal raphe nucleus. *Proc. Natl. Acad. Sci. U.S.A.* 102, 874–879.

Lundstrom, L., Elmquist, A., Bartfai, T., and Langel, U. (2005). Galanin and its receptors in neurological disorders. *Neuromol. Med.* 7, 157–180.

Marcos, P., Diaz-Cabiale, Z., Cordon, M. P., Covenas, R., Yanaihara, N., Fuxe, K., et al. (2001). Central galanin and N-terminal galanin fragment induce c-Fos immunoreactivity in the medulla oblongata of the anesthetized rat. *Peptides* 22, 1501–1509.

Martire, M., Fuxe, K., Agnati, L. F., Pistritto, G., and Preziosi, P. (1991). Galanin increases potassium evoked release of [3H]5-hydroxytryptamine from rat hypothalamic synaptosomal preparations. *Neurosci. Lett.* 122, 87–90.

Mazarati, A. M., Telegdi, D., Shandra, A. A., and Godlevskii, L. S. (1994). Interaction of galanin receptors with glutamate receptors in the neostriatum: a neuropharmacological analysis. *Neurophysiology* 26, 230–235.

Melander, T., Hokfelt, T., Rokaeus, A., Cuello, A. C., Oertel, W. H., Verhofstad, A., and Goldstein, M. (1986). Coexistence of galanin-like immunoreactivity with catecholamines, 5-hydroxytryptamine, GABA and neuropeptides in the rat CNS. *J. Neurosci.* 6, 3640–3654.

Millon Penuela, C., Flores, A., Narvaez, M., Parrado, C., Pulgcerver, A., Covenas, R., et al. (2012). "Galanin N-terminal fragment (1-15) produces depressant and anxiogenic like actions in the rat forced swimming test and open field test," in *FENS poster* abstract 936, poster board number F115.

Mitsukawa, K., Lu, X., and Bartfai, T. (2008). Galanin, galanin receptors and drug targets. *Cell. Mol. Life Sci.* 65, 1796–1805.

Moller, C., Sommer, W., Thorsell, A., and Heilig, M. (1999). Anxiogenic-like action of galanin after intra-amygdala administration in the rat. *Neuropsychopharmacology* 21, 507–512.

Moreno, E., Vaz, S. H., Cai, N. S., Ferrada, C., Quiroz, C., Barodia, S. K., et al. (2011). Dopamine–galanin receptor heteromers modulate cholinergic neurotransmission in the rat ventral hippocampus. *J. Neurosci.* 31, 7412–7423.

Narvaez, J. A., Diaz, Z., Aguirre, J. A., Gonzalez-Baron, S., Yanaihara, N., Fuxe, K., et al. (1994). Intracisternally injected galanin-(1-15) modulates the cardiovascular responses of galanin-(1-29) and the 5-HT1A receptor agonist 8-OH-DPAT. *Eur. J. Pharmacol.* 257, 257–265.

O'Donnell, D., Ahmad, S., Wahlestedt, C., and Walker, P. (1999). Expression of the novel galanin receptor subtype GALR2 in the adult rat CNS: distinct distribution from GALR1. *J. Comp. Neurol.* 409, 469–481.

Ogren, S. O., Fuxe, K., Agnati, L. F., Gustafsson, J. A., Jonsson, G., and Holm, A. C. (1979). Reevaluation of the indoleamine hypothesis of depression. Evidence for a reduction of functional activity of central 5-HT systems by antidepressant drugs. *J. Neural Transm.* 46, 85–103.

Parrado, C., Diaz-Cabiale, Z., Garcia-Coronel, M., Agnati, L. F., Covenas, R., Fuxe, K., et al. (2007). Region specific galanin receptor/neuropeptide Y Y1 receptor interactions in the tel- and diencephalon of the rat. Relevance for food consumption. *Neuropharmacology* 52, 684–692.

Razani, H., Diaz-Cabiale, Z., Fuxe, K., and Ogren, S. O. (2000). Intraventricular galanin produces a time-dependent modulation of 5-HT1A receptors in the dorsal raphe of the rat. *Neuroreport* 11, 3943–3948.

Razani, H., Diaz-Cabiale, Z., Misane, I., Wang, F. H., Fuxe, K., and Ogren, S. O. (2001). Prolonged effects of intraventricular galanin on a 5-hydroxytryptamine(1A) receptor mediated function in the rat. *Neurosci. Lett.* 299, 145–149.

Rimondini, R., Fuxe, K., and Ferre, S. (1999). Multiple intramembrane receptor–receptor interactions in the regulation of striatal dopamine D2 receptors. *Neuroreport* 10, 2051–2054.

Skofitsch, G., and Jacobowitz, D. M. (1985). Immunohistochemical mapping of galanin-like neurons in the rat central nervous system. *Peptides* 6, 509–546.

Skofitsch, G., Sills, M. A., and Jacobowitz, D. M. (1986). Autoradiographic distribution of 125I-galanin binding sites in the rat central nervous system. *Peptides* 7, 1029–1042.

Tarakanov, A. O., and Fuxe, K. G. (2010). Triplet puzzle: homologies of receptor heteromers. *J. Mol. Neurosci.* 41, 294–303.

Tarakanov, A. O., Fuxe, K. G., and Borroto-Escuela, D. O. (2012a). Integrin triplets of marine sponges in human D2 receptor heteromers. *J. Recept. Signal Transduct. Res.* 32, 202–208.

Tarakanov, A. O., Fuxe, K. G., and Borroto-Escuela, D. O. (2012b). On the origin of the triplet puzzle of homologies in receptor heteromers: toll-like receptor triplets in different types of receptors. *J. Neural Transm.* 119, 517–523.

Tatemoto, K., Rokaeus, A., Jornvall, H., Mcdonald, T. J., and Mutt, V. (1983). Galanin – a novel biologically active peptide from porcine intestine. *FEBS Lett.* 164, 124–128.

Wirz, S. A., Davis, C. N., Lu, X., Zal, T., and Bartfai, T. (2005). Homodimerization and internalization of galanin type 1 receptor in living CHO cells. *Neuropeptides* 39, 535–546.

Woods, A. S., Ciruela, F., Fuxe, K., Agnati, L. F., Lluis, C., Franco, R., et al. (2005). Role of electrostatic interaction in receptor–receptor heteromerization. *J. Mol. Neurosci.* 26, 125–132.

Xu, Z. Q., Zhang, X., Pieribone, V. A., Grillner, S., and Hokfelt, T. (1998). Galanin-5-hydroxytryptamine interactions: electrophysiological, immunohistochemical and in situ hybridization studies on rat dorsal raphe neurons with a note on galanin R1 and R2 receptors. *Neuroscience* 87, 79–94.

Yang, S. N., Narvaez, J. A., Bjelke, B., Agnati, L. F., and Fuxe, K. (1993). Microinjections of subpicomolar amounts of NPY(13-36) into the nucleus tractus solitarius of the rat counteract the vasodepressor responses of NPY(1-36) and of a NPY Y1 receptor agonist. *Brain Res.* 621, 126–132.

Zoli, M., Agnati, L. F., Hedlund, P. B., Li, X. M., Ferre, S., and Fuxe, K. (1993). Receptor–receptor interactions as an integrative mechanism in nerve cells. *Mol. Neurobiol.* 7, 293–334.

13

Differential roles of orexin receptors in the regulation of sleep/wakefulness

Michihiro Mieda*, Natsuko Tsujino and Takeshi Sakurai*

Department of Molecular Neuroscience and Integrative Physiology, Graduate School of Medical Science, Kanazawa University, Kanazawa, Ishikawa, Japan

Edited by:
Hubert Vaudry, University of Rouen, France

Reviewed by:
Etienne Challet, Centre National de la Recherche Scientifique, France
Christelle Peyron, INSERM U1028, France

***Correspondence:**
Michihiro Mieda and Takeshi Sakurai, Department of Molecular Neuroscience and Integrative Physiology, Graduate School of Medical Science, Kanazawa University, 13-1 Takara-machi, Kanazawa, Ishikawa 920-8640, Japan.
e-mail: mieda@med.kanazawa-u.ac.jp; tsakurai@med.kanazawa-u.ac.jp

Orexin A and orexin B are hypothalamic neuropeptides that play critical roles in the regulation of sleep/wakefulness, as well as in a variety of physiological functions such as emotion, reward, and energy homeostasis. The actions of orexins are mediated by two receptors, orexin 1 (OX1R) and orexin 2 (OX2R) receptors. OX1R and OX2R show partly overlapping but distinct distributions throughout the central nervous system, suggesting their differential roles. This review presents and discusses the current knowledge concerning the physiological roles of each orexin receptor subtype, focusing on the regulation of sleep/wakefulness.

Keywords: orexin, hypothalamus, sleep, monoamine, narcolepsy, arousal

INTRODUCTION

The neuropeptides orexin A and orexin B (also known as hypocretin 1 and hypocretin 2), were originally identified as endogenous ligands for two orphan G-protein-coupled receptors (Sakurai et al., 1998). Both orexin A and orexin B are derived from a common precursor peptide, prepro-orexin. An mRNA encoding the same precursor peptide of hypocretin 1 (corresponding to orexin A) and hypocretin 2 (orexin B) was independently identified by de Lecea et al. (1998) as a hypothalamus-specific transcript.

The actions of orexins are mediated by two receptors, orexin 1 (OX1R) and orexin 2 (OX2R) receptors (also known as HCRTR1 and HCRTR2) (Sakurai et al., 1998). OX1R shows a higher affinity for orexin A than orexin B by one-order, while OX2R binds orexin A and orexin B with similar affinities. Both receptors are coupled to $G_{q/11}$ subclass of G proteins and caused strong excitatory effects on neurons examined thus far (Sakurai and Mieda, 2011). OX2R has also been reported to couple to $G_{i/o}$ in a neuronal cell line when overexpressed (Zhu et al., 2003).

Orexins are produced in a specific population of neurons (orexin neurons) that are located exclusively in the hypothalamus, including the lateral hypothalamic area (LHA), perifornical area, and posterior hypothalamus (PH) (de Lecea et al., 1998; Peyron et al., 1998; Sakurai et al., 1998; Date et al., 1999; Nambu et al., 1999). Orexin neurons project in almost all brain areas with especially dense projections to monoaminergic neurons, which play important roles in the regulation of sleep/wake states. Orexins are thought to be a critical regulator of sleep/wake states. Intracerebroventricular (ICV) administration of orexin A and orexin B increases wakefulness and suppresses both rapid-eye-movement (REM) sleep and non-REM (NREM) sleep (Hagan et al., 1999). More importantly, orexin deficiency causes sleep disorder narcolepsy in humans and animals (Chemelli et al., 1999; Lin et al., 1999; Peyron et al., 2000; Thannickal et al., 2000; Hara et al., 2001). At present, various reports suggest that orexins are involved not only in the sleep/wake regulation but also in other physiological and behavioral processes such as food intake, emotion, stress response, and reward via activation of OX1R and OX2R (Yamanaka et al., 2003; Akiyama et al., 2004; Mieda et al., 2004; Boutrel et al., 2005; Harris et al., 2005; Sakurai et al., 2005; Narita et al., 2006; Yoshida et al., 2006). Recent reports revealed that each orexin receptor has a different function in these processes. Thus, understanding such a difference is important for understanding the function of the orexin system.

This review will discuss the physiological roles of the orexin system in the regulation of sleep/wakefulness, especially focusing on the functions of each orexin receptor.

DISTRIBUTIONS OF OREXIN RECEPTOR mRNA

According to data obtained by *in situ* hybridization histochemistry, many brain regions have been shown to differentially express *OX1R* and *OX2R* mRNAs (Trivedi et al., 1998; Lu et al., 2000; Greco and Shiromani, 2001; Marcus et al., 2001). Consistent with the broad projections of orexin neurons, *OX1R* and *OX2R* show wide distributions within the brain with partly overlapping but distinct and complementary distributions. For example, *OX2R* is expressed in layers 2 and 6 throughout the cerebral cortex, while *OX1R* is expressed in layers 5 and 6, except the cingulate cortex where *OX1R* mRNA is found in layer 3. In the ammon's horn of the hippocampus, CA1 and CA2 express *OX1R*, while CA3 expresses *OX2R*.

In the arcuate nucleus and paraventricular nucleus of the hypothalamus, which are involved in the regulation of feeding, energy homeostasis, autonomic and endocrine systems, *OX2R* is almost exclusively observed. Concerning the nuclei implicated in sleep/wake regulation, the locus ceruleus (LC), laterodorsal tegmental nucleus (LDT), and pedunculopontine tegmental nucleus (PPT) mainly express *OX1R* mRNA, while the tuberomammillary nucleus (TMN) almost exclusively expresses *OX2R* mRNA. The dorsal raphe (DR) and median raphe (MnR) express both subtypes. These distributions suggest partly overlapping and partly distinct roles of these two receptors.

Monoaminergic (i.e., histaminergic, noradrenergic, and serotonergic) and cholinergic neurons in these nuclei have been considered critical for sleep/wakefulness regulation (Pace-Schott and Hobson, 2002; Zeitzer et al., 2006). Our recent work determined precise cellular localization of two orexin receptors in these nuclei (**Figure 1**) (Mieda et al., 2011). All histaminergic neurons in the TMN exclusively expressed *OX2R*, while all noradrenergic neurons in the LC exclusively expressed *OX1R*. In the DR and MnR, approximately 90% of serotonergic neurons expressed *OX1R* and/or *OX2R*. In addition, many non-serotonergic cells in the DR/MnR also expressed *OX1R* or *OX2R* mRNA. At least some populations of these cells were likely to be GABAergic, since a population of *Gad1*-positive cells also expressed detectable *OX1R* or *OX2R* mRNA. In the LDT and PPT, all cholinergic neurons expressed *OX1R* but not *OX2R* mRNA, while many *OX1R*-positive and/or *OX2R*-positive non-cholinergic neurons were intermingled with cholinergic neurons in the area. *Gad1* mRNA staining further revealed that *OX1R*- or *OX2R*-expressing cells included both GABAergic and non-GABAergic cells.

Orexin receptors-positive GABAergic neurons in the DR/MnR and LDT/PPT, which are intermingled with serotonergic and cholinergic neurons, respectively, are intriguing. Since GABAergic neurons are likely to function as local inhibitory interneurons and orexin receptors usually cause excitatory effects on neurons, simultaneous activation of serotonergic/cholinergic neurons with GABAergic interneurons by orexins within a nucleus may inhibit serotonergic/cholinergic neurons. Thus, balance of orexinergic activation between principal neurons and interneurons may be of importance. This point will be further discussed in a later section.

OREXIN AND MONOAMINERGIC/CHOLINERGIC SYSTEMS

Orexin neurons project almost all brain regions with especially dense projections being seen in monoaminergic and cholinergic nuclei involved in the regulation of sleep/wakefulness. Various reports suggested that orexin excites these neurons directly and/or indirectly *in vivo* and *in vitro* (**Figure 1**). This orexinergic regulation may be important to control sleep/wakefulness. Here, we will review *in vitro* and *in vivo* electrophysiological studies of orexin receptors in monoaminergic and cholinergic neurons.

SEROTONERGIC NEURONS OF THE DORSAL RAPHE

In 2001, Brown et al. reported that orexin A strongly excited DR serotonergic neurons in brain slices of rats under the whole-cell patch clamp recording. The depolarization persisted in the presence of the voltage dependent Na^+ channel blocker, tetrodotoxin,

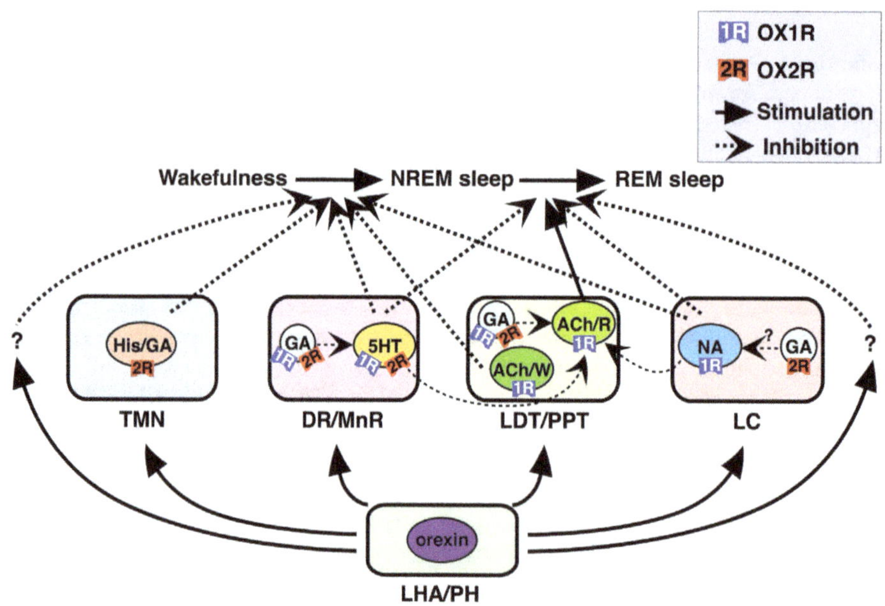

FIGURE 1 | Schematic illustration of presumed pathways underlying orexin actions on NREM and REM sleep (Mieda et al., 2011). Orexins activate histaminergic (His)/GABAergic (GA), serotonergic (5HT), noradrenergic (NA), and cholinergic (ACh) neurons as well as GABAergic putative interneurons in wake-promoting nuclei, including the TMN, DR/MnR, LDT/PPT, and LC. These neurons differentially express OX1R and/or OX2R, and regulate wakefulness/NREM sleep and NREM/REM sleep transitions. OX1R and OX2R may be expressed in the same populations of GABAergic neurons, as shown in the figure, or may be expressed in distinct populations of these neurons in each area. Wake/REM-on cholinergic neurons (ACh/W) are likely to suppress NREM sleep, but REM-on cholinergic neurons (ACh/R), are likely to induce REM sleep. Wake-active serotonergic and noradrenergic neurons in the DR/MnR and LC, respectively, counteract activation of REM-on cholinergic neurons in the LDT/PPT, as well as REM-on neurons in the brainstem reticular formation (Pace-Schott and Hobson, 2002; Sakurai, 2007). Previous reports have suggested contributions of GABAergic interneurons inhibiting PPT cholinergic and raphe serotonergic neurons (Liu et al., 2002; Takakusaki et al., 2005). LHA, lateral hypothalamic area; PH, posterior hypothalamus. Reproduced from Sakurai and Mieda (2011) with permission.

indicating a direct postsynaptic action on the serotonin cells (Brown et al., 2001). Moreover, orexin A and orexin B induced inward currents with similar amplitude and dose-dependency in most serotonergic neurons (Brown et al., 2001; Liu et al., 2002; Soffin et al., 2004) via activation of Na^+/K^+ non-selective cation channels (Liu et al., 2002). These results may suggest that OX2R is mainly involved in the activation of serotonergic neurons, although single-cell PCR, *in situ* hybridization, and immunohistochemical studies revealed that serotonergic neurons express both *OX1R* and *OX2R* (Brown et al., 2001; Liu et al., 2002; Wang et al., 2005; Mieda et al., 2011).

A recent report revealed that orexin A depolarized DR neurons by activating a noisy inward current (Kohlmeier et al., 2004, 2008). This current was through non-selective cation channels that did not contribute to the somatic Ca^{2+} influx. These reports suggested that orexin A has two independent actions: activation of non-selective cation channels and activation of a protein kinase C-dependent enhancement of Ca^{2+} transients mediated by L-type Ca^{2+} channels.

At higher concentrations, orexin also increased spontaneous inhibitory postsynaptic currents in serotonergic neurons indicating orexin excited GABAergic interneurons that project to serotonergic neurons in the DR (Liu et al., 2002). Such a structure of intra-DR circuit may execute a negative feedforward regulation of the activation of serotonergic neurons by orexin neurons.

Regulation of DR neurons by orexin seems to be even more complex. Haj-Dahmane and Shen found that orexin B depresses the evoked glutamate-mediated synaptic currents in DR serotonergic neurons. This effect was mediated by retrograde endocannabinoid release, which depended on the stimulation of postsynaptic orexin receptors and subsequent activation of phospholipase C and DAG lipase enzymatic pathways but not on a rise in postsynaptic intracellular calcium (Haj-Dahmane and Shen, 2005).

In vivo extracellular recording also revealed that application of orexin A increased firing frequency of serotonergic DR neurons in unanesthetized rats during REM sleep or slow-wave sleep, while during wakefulness, a similar amount of orexin A did not increase the firing rate (Takahashi et al., 2005). These reports suggest that orexin excited DR serotonergic neurons in a behavioral state-dependent manner.

NORADRENERGIC SYSTEM

Orexin A and orexin B increased the firing frequency of all LC neurons in the presence of tetrodotoxin in rat brain slices by intracellular recording (Horvath et al., 1999; Soffin et al., 2002). The effects of orexin A are fivefold more potent than orexin B. Moreover, the effect was inhibited by selective orexin 1 receptor antagonist, SB-334867 (Soffin et al., 2002, 2004). These data suggest that orexins directly excited LC noradrenergic neurons via OX1R, which is consistent with exclusive expression of *OX1R* in these neurons demonstrated by *in situ* hybridization (Mieda et al., 2011). The orexin-induced depolarization of LC noradrenergic neurons may be produced by augmentation of the non-selective cationic conductance and suppression of G-protein-coupled inward rectifier (GIRK) channel activity (Hoang et al., 2003; Murai and Akaike, 2005).

In addition to the action of orexins within the LC, orexin A and B also evoked noradrenaline release in the rat cerebrocortical slice, suggesting that orexins act on OX1R on the orexin fibers projecting from the LC in the cerebral cortex (Hirota et al., 2001). Orexin-evoked noradrenaline release was time- and concentration-dependent and partially extracellular Ca^{2+}-dependent (Hirota et al., 2001).

Another report suggested that the orexin modulates LC functions via OX1R by regulating noradrenaline release not only from the axonal terminals, but also from the somatodendritic region of LC noradrenergic neurons (Chen et al., 2008). Application of orexin alone dose-dependently induced somatodendritic noradrenaline release. Orexin A also potentiated *N*-methyl-D-aspartate (NMDA) receptor-mediated somatodendritic noradrenaline release from LC neurons, which was blocked by SB-334867, an OX1R antagonist, or a PKC inhibitor, indicating the involvement of OX1R and PKC. Orexin A enhanced NMDA-induced intracellular Ca^{2+} elevation as well (Chen et al., 2008). Taken together, activation of OX1R of LC noradrenergic neurons regulates not only noradrenergic input to their targets, but also noradrenergic communication in the soma and dendrites.

Excitatory effects of orexin A on LC neurons have been demonstrated also *in vivo* by measuring their firing rates (Bourgin et al., 2000) or noradrenaline release into the hippocampus (Walling et al., 2004). In addition, local administration of orexin A but not orexin B in the LC of rats suppressed REM sleep in a dose-dependent manner and increased wakefulness at the expense of REM sleep and deep slow-wave sleep (Bourgin et al., 2000).

HISTAMINERGIC SYSTEM

Both patch clamp study using freshly isolated neurons and intracellular recording using brain slices revealed that orexin A and orexin B directly and dose-dependently depolarized TMN histaminergic neurons of rats (Bayer et al., 2001; Eriksson et al., 2001; Yamanaka et al., 2002). Orexin A and B showed almost the same potency, indicating that orexin-induced excitation of histaminergic neurons is mediated via OX2R. Consistent with electrophysiological data, *OX2R* was shown to be the principle subtype of orexin receptors by single-cell RT-PCR study, although both receptor mRNAs were detected in most tuberomammillary neurons (Eriksson et al., 2001). Histological studies have demonstrated that TMN histaminergic neurons express *OX2R* almost exclusively (Yamanaka et al., 2002; Mieda et al., 2011).

Orexin-induced depolarization was associated with a small decrease in input resistance. The mechanisms of depolarization of histaminergic neurons are likely to be related to the activation of both the electrogenic Na^+/Ca^{2+} exchanger and Ca^{2+} current (Eriksson et al., 2001), as well as suppression of GIRK channels (Hoang et al., 2003).

On the other hand, a recent *in vitro* optogenetic study demonstrated that postsynaptic currents and rapid increase of firing rates in TMN histaminergic neurons evoked by stimulation of orexin neurons were mediated by glutamate rather than by orexins (orexin neurons are also glutamatergic) (Schone et al., 2012). This suggests a possibility that orexin might play as a modulator of the glutamatergic transmission in these cells.

In vivo application of orexin A to the TMN increased histamine release in both the medial preoptic area and the frontal cortex in a dose-dependent manner (Huang et al., 2001). Moreover, perfusion of orexin A into the TMN of rats through a microdialysis probe promptly increased wakefulness, concomitant with a reduction in REM and NREM sleep (Huang et al., 2001; Yamanaka et al., 2002). These findings indicate that orexins excite TMN histaminergic neurons mainly via OX2R and enhance histamine release from the TMN to maintain wakefulness.

CHOLINERGIC SYSTEM

Laterodorsal tegmental nucleus

Whole-cell recordings revealed that orexin exhibited actions both presynaptically and postsynaptically on LDT cholinergic neurons, as well as in non-cholinergic neurons in the same area. Orexin increased frequency and amplitude of spontaneous EPSCs in these neurons. Postsynaptically, orexin produced an inward current and an increase in membrane current noise, which were accompanied by a conductance increase (Burlet et al., 2002). Being similar to DR serotonergic neurons, orexin A has two independent actions on LDT cholinergic neurons: activation of non-selective cation channels and activation of a protein kinase C-dependent enhancement of Ca^{2+} transients mediated by L-type Ca^{2+} channels (Kohlmeier et al., 2004, 2008).

In a study of *in vivo* extracellular recordings of LDT neurons in rats, the application of orexin A induced long-lasting excitation in five of seven cholinergic neurons (Takahashi et al., 2002). Furthermore, when orexin A was microinjected in the LDT of cats, time spent in wakefulness was significantly increased due to an increase in the duration of wake episodes, and time spent in REM sleep was significantly reduced due to a decrease in the frequency of active sleep episodes (Xi et al., 2001).

Pedunculopontine tegmental nucleus

Whole-cell patch clamp recordings revealed that orexin A and orexin B depolarized PPT cholinergic and non-cholinergic neurons dose-dependently in the presence of tetrodotoxin (Kim et al., 2009a). Approximately 80% of PPT neurons were depolarized by orexin A, and 20% of PPT neurons did not respond to orexin A (Kim et al., 2009b). SB-334867, a selective inhibitor for OX1R, significantly suppressed the orexin A-induced depolarization. These results suggest that orexin depolarized PPT neurons directly through OX1R. This OX1R-mediated depolarization was caused by a decrease of K^+ conductance and an increase of non-selective cationic conductance (Kim et al., 2009a). It was also indicated that it was blocked by D609, a phosphatidylcholine-specific PLC inhibitor, suggesting that the excitatory effects of orexin on PPT neurons are mediated by PLC-dependent pathway (Kim et al., 2009b).

An *in vivo* study demonstrates that orexin inhibited PPT neurons via GABAergic neurons (Takakusaki et al., 2005). In decerebrated cats, an injection of orexin into the PPT increased the intensity of electrical stimulation required at the PPT to induce muscle atonia. The effect of orexin on PPT was abolished by simultaneous injection of bicuculline, a $GABA_A$ receptor antagonist, into the PPT. These results suggest that orexin enhances GABAergic effects on presumably cholinergic PPT neurons *in vivo* to control postural muscle tone.

Cholinergic neurons in these areas include two functionally distinct types of neurons. Some are active during wakefulness and REM sleep (W/REM-on neurons) and others are specifically active during REM sleep (REM-on neurons) (Pace-Schott and Hobson, 2002; Sakurai, 2007). The latter population is likely to play a critical role in REM sleep-related physiological phenomena, including muscle atonia. Orexin A excites both cholinergic and non-cholinergic neurons of the LDT in slice preparations, as described previously (Burlet et al., 2002). Furthermore, orexin A microinjection in the cat LDT increases wakefulness and reduces REM sleep. In addition, as mentioned previously, GABAergic neurons in the PPT mediate suppression of REM sleep and muscle atonia following local injection of orexin A into this area (Takakusaki et al., 2005). Consistent with the actions of orexins on both cholinergic and non-cholinergic neurons, orexin receptors are differentially expressed in cholinergic and GABAergic neurons of the LDT/PPT, shown by a histological study (Mieda et al., 2011). Taken together, these results indicate that in the LDT/PPT, orexin may activate W/REM-on cholinergic neurons through OX1R to facilitate wakefulness. Simultaneously, orexin might activate GABAergic interneurons to inhibit REM-on cholinergic neurons in these nuclei (**Figure 1**).

Basal forebrain

Electrophysiological studies were performed on cultured nucleus basalis neurons from the basal forebrain and on rat brain slice (Eggermann et al., 2001; Hoang et al., 2004). In cultured neurons, orexin A induced a depolarization and increased firing accompanied by a decrease of whole-cell conductance in cholinergic neurons. The mechanism of this neuronal excitation was shown to be accompanied by inhibition of inward rectifier K^+ channel (KirNB) activity (Hoang et al., 2004). In rat brain slices, orexin has a direct excitatory effect on the cholinergic neurons of the contiguous basal forebrain (Eggermann et al., 2001). All cholinergic neurons were excited by orexin A and even more potently by orexin B. This result suggests that the action depends on OX2R. Thus, orexins may excite cholinergic neurons in the basal forebrain via OX2R and contribute to the cortical activation.

The medial septum-diagonal band of Broca (MSDB), via its cholinergic and GABAergic projections to the hippocampus, controls the hippocampal theta rhythm and associated learning and memory functions. MSDB receives a dense innervation of orexin neurons, and neurons of the MSDB express very high levels of OX2R. Septohippocampal cholinergic neurons were excited by orexin A and B with similar EC_{50} in a concentration-dependent manner, mediated via a direct postsynaptic mechanism (Wu et al., 2004). The orexin effect is likely to be mediated by inhibition of a K^+ current, presumably an inward rectifier, and activation of the Na^+–Ca^{2+} exchanger. Thus orexin effects within the septum should increase hippocampal acetylcholine release and thereby promote hippocampal arousal (Wu et al., 2004).

DIFFERENTIAL ROLES OF EACH OREXIN RECEPTOR SUBTYPE IN THE REGULATION OF SLEEP/WAKEFULNESS

MOLECULAR GENETIC STUDIES

Recent studies have established that the orexin (hypocretin) system is one of the most important regulators of sleep/wake states and that its deficiency results in the human sleep disorder narcolepsy (Zeitzer et al., 2006; Sakurai and Mieda, 2011). Narcolepsy is characterized by excessive daytime sleepiness that often results in "sleep attacks" (sudden onset of NREM sleep), cataplexy (sudden bilateral skeletal muscle weakening triggered by emotions without loss of consciousness), hypnagogic hallucinations, and sleep paralysis. These symptoms can be divided into two independent pathological phenomena. One is the inability to maintain a consolidated awake period characterized by abrupt transitions from wakefulness to NREM sleep (i.e., dysregulation of NREM sleep onset). This phenomenon manifests clinically as excessive daytime sleepiness or sleep attacks. The other key phenomenon is the pathological intrusion of REM sleep into wakefulness or at sleep onset (i.e., dysregulation of REM sleep onset). It is during these periods that patients experience cataplexy, hypnagogic hallucinations, and sleep paralysis.

Mice with targeted deletion of the *prepro-orexin* gene (*orexin*$^{-/-}$ mice) display a phenotype strikingly similar to narcolepsy: abrupt behavioral arrests with muscle atonia (cataplexy), fragmented wakefulness (inability to maintain consolidated wakefulness episodes), and direct transitions from wakefulness to REM sleep (Chemelli et al., 1999). In addition, functionally null mutations in the *OX2R* gene were found in two independent lines of familial narcoleptic dogs (Lin et al., 1999).

Based on studies on orexin receptor-deficient mice (*OX1R*$^{-/-}$ and *OX2R*$^{-/-}$ mice), it has been suggested that deletion of *OX1R* produces no measurable effect on sleep/wakefulness states (Sakurai, 2007; Hondo et al., 2010). However, *OX2R*$^{-/-}$ mice have clear characteristics of narcolepsy, although their behavioral and EEG phenotype is less severe than that found in *orexin*$^{-/-}$ mice (Willie et al., 2003). In infrared videophotographic studies in the dark phase, *OX2R*$^{-/-}$ mice showed abrupt behavioral arrests. However, its frequency was much less than in *orexin*$^{-/-}$ mice (31-fold lower frequency in *OX2R*$^{-/-}$ mice as compared to *orexin*$^{-/-}$ mice). Instead, *OX2R*$^{-/-}$ mice showed a distinct variety of behavioral arrests with onsets that were more gradual in nature (gradual arrests). Moreover, *orexin*$^{-/-}$ mice also exhibit gradual arrests with a frequency similar to *OX2R*$^{-/-}$ mice in addition to plenty of abrupt arrests.

In contrast to abrupt arrests, gradual arrests typically began during quiet wakefulness and could be easily distinguished from the normal onset of resting behavior by (i) the absence of stereotypic preparation for sleep (e.g., nesting and/or assumption of a curled or hunched posture with limbs drawn under the body) and (ii) a characteristic ratchet-like "nodding" of the head over a period of several seconds with a transition to a collapsed posture (Willie et al., 2003).

Detailed observations of behaviors during EEG/EMG recordings found that abrupt arrests in *orexin*$^{-/-}$ and *OX2R*$^{-/-}$ mice occurred during direct transitions from wakefulness to REM sleep, whereas EEG/EMG correlates of gradual arrests in both *orexin*$^{-/-}$ and *OX2R*$^{-/-}$ mice invariably revealed the onset of attenuated muscle tone, but not atonia, and an EEG transition from wakefulness to NREM sleep (Chemelli et al., 1999; Willie et al., 2003). Pharmacologically, abrupt arrests in *orexin*$^{-/-}$ mice were suppressed by systemic administration of clomipramine, an anticataplectic agent used for treatment of human narcolepsy. Whereas, administration of caffeine, a psychostimulant used to treat excessive sleepiness in human narcolepsy, tended to produce a mild exacerbation of abrupt arrest frequency. In clear contrast, systemic administration of caffeine dose-dependently suppressed gradual arrests, while administration of an anticataplectic agent clomipramine did not affect the frequency of gradual arrests in both *orexin*$^{-/-}$ and *OX2R*$^{-/-}$ mice. These observations showed strong similarity with those observed in human narcolepsy patients; psychostimulant drugs are effective for the sleepiness, but exacerbate cataplexy, which is treatable with antidepressants. This detailed characterization of behavioral, pharmacological, and electrophysiological features of *orexin*$^{-/-}$ and *OX2R*$^{-/-}$ mice defined abrupt and gradual arrests as the presumptive mouse correlates of cataplexy and sleep attack in human narcolepsy, respectively.

In addition to the gradual behavioral arrests, *OX2R*$^{-/-}$ mice exhibit fragmentation of wakefulness, another sign of sleepiness, to the extent similar to that in *orexin*$^{-/-}$ mice (Willie et al., 2003). *OX1R*$^{-/-}$; *OX2R*$^{-/-}$ mice appear to have the same phenotype with *orexin*$^{-/-}$ mice, implying that these two receptors are sufficient to mediate regulation of sleep/wakefulness by orexins (Sakurai, 2007; Hondo et al., 2010). These results of mouse reverse genetic studies suggest that normal regulation of wake/NREM sleep transitions depends critically on OX2R activation, whereas the profound dysregulation of REM sleep control are unique to narcolepsy from loss of signaling through both OX1R- and OX2R-dependent pathways.

Substantially lower frequency of cataplexy in *OX2R*$^{-/-}$ mice as compared to *orexin*$^{-/-}$ mice appears to be inconsistent with the fact that mutations of *OX2R* gene are solely responsible for an inherited canine model of narcolepsy, which demonstrate frequent occurrence of cataplexy as well as excessive sleepiness (Lin et al., 1999). This may result from species difference (e.g., the precise expression patterns of two orexin receptors). However, even in dogs, the absence of orexin peptides may cause severe narcoleptic symptoms as compared to *OX2R* mutation. Early studies of narcoleptic Dobermans and Labradors found these dogs to be 30- to 80-fold less severely affected with cataplexy than poodles with sporadic narcolepsy that showed literally hundreds of attacks a day (Baker et al., 1982), an effect previously attributed solely to differences in breed and breed size.

As an experiment complementary to the behavioral studies and baseline sleep/wakefulness recordings of *OX1R*$^{-/-}$ and *OX2R*$^{-/-}$ mice, we elucidated that two orexin receptors play distinct and differential roles in the regulation of sleep and wakefulness states by comparing the effects of ICV orexin A administration in wild-type, *OX1R*$^{-/-}$ and *OX2R*$^{-/-}$ mice (Mieda et al., 2011). The effects of orexin A on wakefulness and NREM sleep were significantly attenuated in both knockout mice as compared to wild-type mice, with substantially larger attenuation in *OX2R*$^{-/-}$ mice than in *OX1R*$^{-/-}$ mice. These results suggest that although the OX2R-mediated pathway has a pivotal role in the promotion of wakefulness, OX1R also plays additional roles in promoting arousal.

In contrast, suppression of REM sleep by orexin A administration was slightly and similarly attenuated in both $OX1R^{-/-}$ and $OX2R^{-/-}$ mice, suggesting a comparable contribution of the two receptors to REM sleep suppression (Mieda et al., 2011). In addition, our observations further suggest that orexin A directly suppresses transitions from NREM sleep to REM sleep, and that activation of OX1R is sufficient for this effect. Supplementary role of OX1R in the suppression of NREM sleep is consistent with the fact that $OX2R^{-/-}$ mice on a C57BL/6J genetic background show less fragmented wakefulness when compared to $orexin^{-/-}$ mice and $OX1R^{-/-}$; $OX2R^{-/-}$ mice (but show similarly fragmented wakefulness on a C57BL/6J-129/SvEv mixed background) (Sakurai, 2007; Mochizuki et al., 2011), suggesting that OX1R is indispensable for the maintenance of wakefulness in the absence of OX2R.

Although application of exogenous orexins has been shown to excite many types of neurons (Sakurai and Mieda, 2011), neurons directly downstream to orexin neurons in physiological conditions (i.e., neurons influenced by endogenous orexins that mediate their wake-promoting and REM-suppressing effects), have remained uncertain. Several reports suggested that histaminergic neurons in the TMN play an important role in the arousal-promoting effect of orexin, supported by the facts that the effect of ICV orexin A administration is markedly attenuated by the histamine H1 receptor antagonist pyrilamine (Yamanaka et al., 2002) and is absent in *H1 histamine receptor* knockout mice (Huang et al., 2001) and that the TMN expresses OX2R abundantly (Marcus et al., 2001; Mieda et al., 2011), the subtype whose absence causes narcoleptic phenotype in mice and dogs (Lin et al., 1999; Willie et al., 2003). Mochizuki et al. (2011) produced a mouse model in which a *loxP*-flanked gene cassette disrupts production of the OX2R, but normal OX2R expression can be restored by Cre recombinase. They showed that targeted Cre expression (i.e., focal restoration of OX2R expression), in the TMN and adjacent regions rescues fragmentation of wakefulness in this mouse model, suggesting that the orexin signaling mediated by OX2R in the TMN (and possibly its surrounding area in the PH) is sufficient to prevent sleepiness caused by systemic OX2R deficiency.

On the other hand, this hypothesis is still controversial. Mice lacking both OX1R and histamine H1 receptors demonstrate no abnormality in sleep/wakefulness (Hondo et al., 2010). In addition, a recent optogenetic study showed that orexin-mediated sleep-to-wake transitions do not depend on the TMN histaminergic neurons (Carter et al., 2009). Rather, another optogenetic study suggested the role of LC noradrenergic neurons as a direct downstream pathway of orexin neurons by demonstrating that optogenetic inhibition of LC noradrenergic neurons blocked arousal effects of optogenetic stimulation of orexin neurons (Carter et al., 2012).

PHARMACOLOGICAL STUDIES

Antagonists for orexin receptors are drawing people's attention as novel medications for insomnia (Scammell and Winrow, 2011; Mieda and Sakurai, 2013). Several non-selective (dual) antagonists for orexin receptors, as well as subtype-selective antagonists, have been developed. These drugs are indeed useful also for studying the roles of each subtype in the regulation of sleep/wakefulness without considering any chronic compensatory changes that might complicate the phenotypes of genetically engineered models.

A study reported that an OX2R-selective antagonist JNJ10397049 has a better ability to promote NREM sleep than the dual antagonist almorexant in rats (Dugovic et al., 2009). They suggested that simultaneous inhibition of OX1R attenuates the sleep-promoting effects mediated by selective OX2R blockade, possibly correlated with dopaminergic neurotransmission. In contrast, another recent study led to a different conclusion (Morairty et al., 2012). It reported that an OX1R-selective antagonist SB-334867 produces small increases in REM and NREM sleep, and an OX2R-selective antagonist EMPA produces a significant increase in NREM sleep. But administration of almorexant increases NREM sleep more than these subtype-selective antagonists, leading to the conclusion that dual orexin receptor antagonism is more effective for sleep promotion than subtype-selective antagonism. The difference in these drugs' capabilities of crossing the blood-brain barrier, as well as their pharmacokinetic/pharmacodynamic characters, might influence the effectiveness. The latter view is also consistent with the conclusion derived from studies using subtype-specific knockout mice that OX2R plays a pivotal role, but OX1R has additional effects on promotion of wakefulness (Sakurai, 2007; Mieda et al., 2011).

CONCLUSION

The orexin system is a necessary component for the normal regulation of sleep/wakefulness. Nevertheless, broad expression of orexin receptors throughout the brain makes it difficult to identify neurons and orexin receptor subtypes that are directly regulated by endogenous orexins and mediate their effects on the physiology of interest in a natural context. Future studies using molecular genetic strategies such as brain region/cell type-specific deletions and brain region/cell type-specific rescues of orexin receptors, as well as pharmacological studies of focal administration of subtype-specific orexin agonists/antagonists, would further dissect the differential roles of orexin receptors in the regulation of sleep/wakefulness. Furthermore, the orexin system is also important for the regulation of a variety of physiological functions, such as feeding, reward, and emotions. Thus, precise information of the different roles of the two orexin receptors is beneficial not only for understanding the mechanisms underlying orexinergic regulations of physiology, but also for application of orexin agonists/antagonists as medications for various diseases.

REFERENCES

Akiyama, M., Yuasa, T., Hayasaka, N., Horikawa, K., Sakurai, T., and Shibata, S. (2004). Reduced food anticipatory activity in genetically orexin (hypocretin) neuron-ablated mice. *Eur. J. Neurosci.* 20, 3054–3062.

Baker, T. L., Foutz, A. S., McNerney, V., Mitler, M. M., and Dement, W. C. (1982). Canine model of narcolepsy: genetic and developmental determinants. *Exp. Neurol.* 75, 729–742.

Bayer, L., Eggermann, E., Serafin, M., Saint-Mleux, B., Machard, D., Jones, B., et al. (2001). Orexins (hypocretins) directly excite tuberomammillary neurons. *Eur. J. Neurosci.* 14, 1571–1575.

Bourgin, P., Huitron-Resendiz, S., Spier, A. D., Fabre, V., Morte, B., Criado, J. R., et al. (2000). Hypocretin-1 modulates rapid eye movement sleep through activation of locus coeruleus neurons. *J. Neurosci.* 20, 7760–7765.

Boutrel, B., Kenny, P. J., Specio, S. E., Martin-Fardon, R., Markou, A., Koob, G. F., et al. (2005). Role for hypocretin in mediating stress-induced reinstatement of cocaine-seeking behavior. *Proc. Natl. Acad. Sci. U.S.A.* 102, 19168–19173.

Brown, R. E., Sergeeva, O., Eriksson, K. S., and Haas, H. L. (2001). Orexin A excites serotonergic neurons in the dorsal raphe nucleus of the rat. *Neuropharmacology* 40, 457–459.

Burlet, S., Tyler, C. J., and Leonard, C. S. (2002). Direct and indirect excitation of laterodorsal tegmental neurons by Hypocretin/Orexin peptides: implications for wakefulness and narcolepsy. *J. Neurosci.* 22, 2862–2872.

Carter, M. E., Adamantidis, A., Ohtsu, H., Deisseroth, K., and de Lecea, L. (2009). Sleep homeostasis modulates hypocretin-mediated sleep-to-wake transitions. *J. Neurosci.* 29, 10939–10949.

Carter, M. E., Brill, J., Bonnavion, P., Huguenard, J. R., Huerta, R., and de Lecea, L. (2012). Mechanism for Hypocretin-mediated sleep-to-wake transitions. *Proc. Natl. Acad. Sci. U.S.A.* 109, E2635–E2644.

Chemelli, R. M., Willie, J. T., Sinton, C. M., Elmquist, J. K., Scammell, T., Lee, C., et al. (1999). Narcolepsy in orexin knockout mice: molecular genetics of sleep regulation. *Cell* 98, 437–451.

Chen, X. W., Mu, Y., Huang, H. P., Guo, N., Zhang, B., Fan, S. Y., et al. (2008). Hypocretin-1 potentiates NMDA receptor-mediated somatodendritic secretion from locus ceruleus neurons. *J. Neurosci.* 28, 3202–3208.

Date, Y., Ueta, Y., Yamashita, H., Yamaguchi, H., Matsukura, S., Kangawa, K., et al. (1999). Orexins, orexigenic hypothalamic peptides, interact with autonomic, neuroendocrine and neuroregulatory systems. *Proc. Natl. Acad. Sci. U.S.A.* 96, 748–753.

de Lecea, L., Kilduff, T. S., Peyron, C., Gao, X., Foye, P. E., Danielson, P. E., et al. (1998). The hypocretins: hypothalamus-specific peptides with neuroexcitatory activity. *Proc. Natl. Acad. Sci. U.S.A.* 95, 322–327.

Dugovic, C., Shelton, J. E., Aluisio, L. E., Fraser, I. C., Jiang, X., Sutton, S. W., et al. (2009). Blockade of orexin-1 receptors attenuates orexin-2 receptor antagonism-induced sleep promotion in the rat. *J. Pharmacol. Exp. Ther.* 330, 142–151.

Eggermann, E., Serafin, M., Bayer, L., Machard, D., Saint-Mleux, B., Jones, B. E., et al. (2001). Orexins/hypocretins excite basal forebrain cholinergic neurones. *Neuroscience* 108, 177–181.

Eriksson, K. S., Sergeeva, O., Brown, R. E., and Haas, H. L. (2001). Orexin/hypocretin excites the histaminergic neurons of the tuberomammillary nucleus. *J. Neurosci.* 21, 9273–9279.

Greco, M. A., and Shiromani, P. J. (2001). Hypocretin receptor protein and mRNA expression in the dorsolateral pons of rats. *Brain Res. Mol. Brain Res.* 88, 176–182.

Hagan, J. J., Leslie, R. A., Patel, S., Evans, M. L., Wattam, T. A., Holmes, S., et al. (1999). Orexin A activates locus coeruleus cell firing and increases arousal in the rat. *Proc. Natl. Acad. Sci. U.S.A.* 96, 10911–10916.

Haj-Dahmane, S., and Shen, R. Y. (2005). The wake-promoting peptide orexin-B inhibits glutamatergic transmission to dorsal raphe nucleus serotonin neurons through retrograde endocannabinoid signaling. *J. Neurosci.* 25, 896–905.

Hara, J., Beuckmann, C. T., Nambu, T., Willie, J. T., Chemelli, R. M., Sinton, C. M., et al. (2001). Genetic ablation of orexin neurons in mice results in narcolepsy, hypophagia, and obesity. *Neuron* 30, 345–354.

Harris, G. C., Wimmer, M., and Aston-Jones, G. (2005). A role for lateral hypothalamic orexin neurons in reward seeking. *Nature* 437, 556–559.

Hirota, K., Kushikata, T., Kudo, M., Kudo, T., Lambert, D. G., and Matsuki, A. (2001). Orexin A and B evoke noradrenaline release from rat cerebrocortical slices. *Br. J. Pharmacol.* 134, 1461–1466.

Hoang, Q. V., Bajic, D., Yanagisawa, M., Nakajima, S., and Nakajima, Y. (2003). Effects of orexin (hypocretin) on GIRK channels. *J. Neurophysiol.* 90, 693–702.

Hoang, Q. V., Zhao, P., Nakajima, S., and Nakajima, Y. (2004). Orexin (hypocretin) effects on constitutively active inward rectifier K+ channels in cultured nucleus basalis neurons. *J. Neurophysiol.* 92, 3183–3191.

Hondo, M., Nagai, K., Ohno, K., Kisanuki, Y., Willie, J. T., Watanabe, T., et al. (2010). Histamine-1 receptor is not required as a downstream effector of orexin-2 receptor in maintenance of basal sleep/wake states. *Acta Physiol (Oxf.)* 198, 287–294.

Horvath, T. L., Peyron, C., Diano, S., Ivanov, A., Aston-Jones, G., Kilduff, T. S., et al. (1999). Hypocretin (orexin) activation and synaptic innervation of the locus coeruleus noradrenergic system. *J. Comp. Neurol.* 415, 145–159.

Huang, Z. L., Qu, W. M., Li, W. D., Mochizuki, T., Eguchi, N., Watanabe, T., et al. (2001). Arousal effect of orexin A depends on activation of the histaminergic system. *Proc. Natl. Acad. Sci. U.S.A.* 98, 9965–9970.

Kim, J., Nakajima, K., Oomura, Y., Wayner, M. J., and Sasaki, K. (2009a). Electrophysiological effects of orexins/hypocretins on pedunculopontine tegmental neurons in rats: an in vitro study. *Peptides* 30, 191–209.

Kim, J., Nakajima, K., Oomura, Y., Wayner, M. J., and Sasaki, K. (2009b). Orexin-A and ghrelin depolarize the same pedunculopontine tegmental neurons in rats: an in vitro study. *Peptides* 30, 1328–1335.

Kohlmeier, K. A., Inoue, T., and Leonard, C. S. (2004). Hypocretin/orexin peptide signaling in the ascending arousal system: elevation of intracellular calcium in the mouse dorsal raphe and laterodorsal tegmentum. *J. Neurophysiol.* 92, 221–235.

Kohlmeier, K. A., Watanabe, S., Tyler, C. J., Burlet, S., and Leonard, C. S. (2008). Dual orexin actions on dorsal raphe and laterodorsal tegmentum neurons: noisy cation current activation and selective enhancement of Ca2+ transients mediated by L-type calcium channels. *J. Neurophysiol.* 100, 2265–2281.

Lin, L., Faraco, J., Li, R., Kadotani, H., Rogers, W., Lin, X., et al. (1999). The sleep disorder canine narcolepsy is caused by a mutation in the hypocretin (orexin) receptor 2 gene. *Cell* 98, 365–376.

Liu, R. J., van den Pol, A. N., and Aghajanian, G. K. (2002). Hypocretins (orexins) regulate serotonin neurons in the dorsal raphe nucleus by excitatory direct and inhibitory indirect actions. *J. Neurosci.* 22, 9453–9464.

Lu, X. Y., Bagnol, D., Burke, S., Akil, H., and Watson, S. J. (2000). Differential distribution and regulation of OX1 and OX2 orexin/hypocretin receptor messenger RNA in the brain upon fasting. *Horm. Behav.* 37, 335–344.

Marcus, J. N., Aschkenasi, C. J., Lee, C. E., Chemelli, R. M., Saper, C. B., Yanagisawa, M., et al. (2001). Differential expression of orexin receptors 1 and 2 in the rat brain. *J. Comp. Neurol.* 435, 6–25.

Mieda, M., Hasegawa, E., Kisanuki, Y. Y., Sinton, C. M., Yanagisawa, M., and Sakurai, T. (2011). Differential roles of orexin receptor-1 and -2 in the regulation of non-REM and REM sleep. *J. Neurosci.* 31, 6518–6526.

Mieda, M., and Sakurai, T. (2013). Orexin (hypocretin) receptor agonists and antagonists for treatment of sleep disorders. Rationale for development and current status. *CNS Drugs* 27, 83–90.

Mieda, M., Williams, S. C., Sinton, C. M., Richardson, J. A., Sakurai, T., and Yanagisawa, M. (2004). Orexin neurons function in an efferent pathway of a food-entrainable circadian oscillator in eliciting food-anticipatory activity and wakefulness. *J. Neurosci.* 24, 10493–10501.

Mochizuki, T., Arrigoni, E., Marcus, J. N., Clark, E. L., Yamamoto, M., Honer, M., et al. (2011). Orexin receptor 2 expression in the posterior hypothalamus rescues sleepiness in narcoleptic mice. *Proc. Natl. Acad. Sci. U.S.A.* 108, 4471–4476.

Morairty, S. R., Revel, F. G., Malherbe, P., Moreau, J. L., Valladao, D., Wettstein, J. G., et al. (2012). Dual hypocretin receptor antagonism is more effective for sleep promotion than antagonism of either receptor alone. *PLoS ONE* 7:e39131. doi:10.1371/journal.pone.0039131

Murai, Y., and Akaike, T. (2005). Orexins cause depolarization via nonselective cationic and K+ channels in isolated locus coeruleus neurons. *Neurosci. Res.* 51, 55–65.

Nambu, T., Sakurai, T., Mizukami, K., Hosoya, Y., Yanagisawa, M., and Goto, K. (1999). Distribution of orexin neurons in the adult rat brain. *Brain Res.* 827, 243–260.

Narita, M., Nagumo, Y., Hashimoto, S., Khotib, J., Miyatake, M., Sakurai, T., et al. (2006). Direct involvement of orexinergic systems in the activation of the mesolimbic dopamine pathway and related behaviors induced by morphine. *J. Neurosci.* 26, 398–405.

Pace-Schott, E. F., and Hobson, J. A. (2002). The neurobiology of sleep: genetics, cellular physiology and subcortical networks. *Nat. Rev. Neurosci.* 3, 591–605.

Peyron, C., Faraco, J., Rogers, W., Ripley, B., Overeem, S., Charnay, Y., et al. (2000). A mutation in a case of early onset narcolepsy and a generalized absence of hypocretin peptides in human narcoleptic brains. *Nat. Med.* 6, 991–997.

Peyron, C., Tighe, D. K., van den Pol, A. N., de Lecea, L., Heller, H. C., Sutcliffe, J. G., et al. (1998). Neurons containing hypocretin (orexin) project to multiple neuronal systems. *J. Neurosci.* 18, 9996–10015.

Sakurai, T. (2007). The neural circuit of orexin (hypocretin): maintaining sleep and wakefulness. *Nat. Rev. Neurosci.* 8, 171–181.

Sakurai, T., Amemiya, A., Ishii, M., Matsuzaki, I., Chemelli, R. M., Tanaka, H., et al. (1998). Orexins and orexin receptors: a family of hypothalamic neuropeptides and G protein-coupled receptors that regulate feeding behavior. *Cell* 92, 573–585.

Sakurai, T., and Mieda, M. (2011). Connectomics of orexin-producing neurons: interface of systems of emotion, energy homeostasis and arousal. *Trends Pharmacol. Sci.* 32, 451–462.

Sakurai, T., Nagata, R., Yamanaka, A., Kawamura, H., Tsujino, N., Muraki, Y., et al. (2005). Input of orexin/hypocretin neurons revealed by a genetically encoded tracer in mice. *Neuron* 46, 297–308.

Scammell, T. E., and Winrow, C. J. (2011). Orexin receptors: pharmacology and therapeutic opportunities. *Annu. Rev. Pharmacol. Toxicol.* 51, 243–266.

Schone, C., Cao, Z. F., Apergis-Schoute, J., Adamantidis, A., Sakurai, T., and Burdakov, D. (2012). Optogenetic probing of fast glutamatergic transmission from hypocretin/orexin to histamine neurons in situ. *J. Neurosci.* 32, 12437–12443.

Soffin, E. M., Evans, M. L., Gill, C. H., Harries, M. H., Benham, C. D., and Davies, C. H. (2002). SB-334867-A antagonises orexin mediated excitation in the locus coeruleus. *Neuropharmacology* 42, 127–133.

Soffin, E. M., Gill, C. H., Brough, S. J., Jerman, J. C., and Davies, C. H. (2004). Pharmacological characterisation of the orexin receptor subtype mediating postsynaptic excitation in the rat dorsal raphe nucleus. *Neuropharmacology* 46, 1168–1176.

Takahashi, K., Koyama, Y., Kayama, Y., and Yamamoto, M. (2002). Effects of orexin on the laterodorsal tegmental neurones. *Psychiatry Clin. Neurosci.* 56, 335–336.

Takahashi, K., Wang, Q. P., Guan, J. L., Kayama, Y., Shioda, S., and Koyama, Y. (2005). State-dependent effects of orexins on the serotonergic dorsal raphe neurons in the rat. *Regul. Pept.* 126, 43–47.

Takakusaki, K., Takahashi, K., Saitoh, K., Harada, H., Okumura, T., Kayama, Y., et al. (2005). Orexinergic projections to the cat midbrain mediate alternation of emotional behavioural states from locomotion to cataplexy. *J. Physiol. (Lond.)* 568, 1003–1020.

Thannickal, T. C., Moore, R. Y., Nienhuis, R., Ramanathan, L., Gulyani, S., Aldrich, M., et al. (2000). Reduced number of hypocretin neurons in human narcolepsy. *Neuron* 27, 469–474.

Trivedi, P., Yu, H., MacNeil, D. J., Van der Ploeg, L. H., and Guan, X. M. (1998). Distribution of orexin receptor mRNA in the rat brain. *FEBS Lett.* 438, 71–75.

Walling, S. G., Nutt, D. J., Lalies, M. D., and Harley, C. W. (2004). Orexin-A infusion in the locus ceruleus triggers norepinephrine (NE) release and NE-induced long-term potentiation in the dentate gyrus. *J. Neurosci.* 24, 7421–7426.

Wang, Q. P., Koyama, Y., Guan, J. L., Takahashi, K., Kayama, Y., and Shioda, S. (2005). The orexinergic synaptic innervation of serotonin- and orexin 1-receptor-containing neurons in the dorsal raphe nucleus. *Regul. Pept.* 126, 35–42.

Willie, J. T., Chemelli, R. M., Sinton, C. M., Tokita, S., Williams, S. C., Kisanuki, Y. Y., et al. (2003). Distinct narcolepsy syndromes in Orexin receptor-2 and Orexin null mice: molecular genetic dissection of Non-REM and REM sleep regulatory processes. *Neuron* 38, 715–730.

Wu, M., Zaborszky, L., Hajszan, T., van den Pol, A. N., and Alreja, M. (2004). Hypocretin/orexin innervation and excitation of identified septohippocampal cholinergic neurons. *J. Neurosci.* 24, 3527–3536.

Xi, M. C., Morales, F. R., and Chase, M. H. (2001). Effects on sleep and wakefulness of the injection of hypocretin-1 (orexin-A) into the laterodorsal tegmental nucleus of the cat. *Brain Res.* 901, 259–264.

Yamanaka, A., Beuckmann, C. T., Willie, J. T., Hara, J., Tsujino, N., Mieda, M., et al. (2003). Hypothalamic orexin neurons regulate arousal according to energy balance in mice. *Neuron* 38, 701–713.

Yamanaka, A., Tsujino, N., Funahashi, H., Honda, K., Guan, J. L., Wang, Q. P., et al. (2002). Orexins activate histaminergic neurons via the orexin 2 receptor. *Biochem. Biophys. Res. Commun.* 290, 1237–1245.

Yoshida, K., McCormack, S., Espana, R. A., Crocker, A., and Scammell, T. E. (2006). Afferents to the orexin neurons of the rat brain. *J. Comp. Neurol.* 494, 845–861.

Zeitzer, J. M., Nishino, S., and Mignot, E. (2006). The neurobiology of hypocretins (orexins), narcolepsy and related therapeutic interventions. *Trends Pharmacol. Sci.* 27, 368–374.

Zhu, Y., Miwa, Y., Yamanaka, A., Yada, T., Shibahara, M., Abe, Y., et al. (2003). Orexin receptor type-1 couples exclusively to pertussis toxin-insensitive G-proteins, while orexin receptor type-2 couples to both pertussis toxin-sensitive and -insensitive G-proteins. *J. Pharmacol. Sci.* 92, 259–266.

14

Control of ventricular ciliary beating by the melanin concentrating hormone-expressing neurons of the lateral hypothalamus: A functional imaging survey

Grégory Conductier[1,2†], Agnès O. Martin[3,4,5†], Pierre-Yves Risold[6†], Sonia Jego[7], Raphaël Lavoie[7], Chrystel Lafont[3,4,5], Patrice Mollard[3,4,5‡], Antoine Adamantidis[7‡] and Jean-Louis Nahon[1,2,8 *‡]

[1] UMR7275, Institut de Pharmacologie Moléculaire et Cellulaire, Centre National de la Recherche Scientifique, Valbonne, France
[2] University of Nice Sophia Antipolis, Nice, France
[3] UMR5203, Institut de Génomique Fonctionnelle, Centre National de la Recherche Scientifique, Montpellier, France
[4] U661, INSERM, Montpellier, France
[5] UMR-5203, Universités de Montpellier 1 & 2, Montpellier, France
[6] Laboratoire d'Histologie, IFR 133, Faculté de Médecine et de Pharmacie, Besançon, France
[7] Douglas Mental Health University Institute, Montreal, QC, Canada
[8] Station de Primatologie, UPS 846, Centre National de la Recherche Scientifique, Rousset sur Arc, France

Edited by:
Hubert Vaudry, University of Rouen, France

Reviewed by:
Gert Jansen, Erasmus Medical Centre, Netherlands
Serge H. Luquet, University Paris Diderot, France

***Correspondence:**
Jean-Louis Nahon, UMR7275, Institut de Pharmacologie Moléculaire et Cellulaire, Centre National de la Recherche Scientifique, 660 Route des Lucioles, Sophia Antipolis, Valbonne, France
e-mail: nahonjl@ipmc.cnrs.fr

† Co-Authors
‡ Co-Directors

The cyclic peptide Melanin Concentrating Hormone (MCH) is known to control a large number of brain functions in mammals such as food intake and metabolism, stress response, anxiety, sleep/wake cycle, memory, and reward. Based on neuro-anatomical and electrophysiological studies these functions were attributed to neuronal circuits expressing MCHR1, the single MCH receptor in rodents. In complement to our recently published work (1) we provided here new data regarding the action of MCH on ependymocytes in the mouse brain. First, we establish that MCHR1 mRNA is expressed in the ependymal cells of the third ventricle epithelium. Second, we demonstrated a tonic control of MCH-expressing neurons on ependymal cilia beat frequency using *in vitro* optogenics. Finally, we performed *in vivo* measurements of CSF flow using fluorescent micro-beads in wild-type and MCHR1-knockout mice. Collectively, our results demonstrated that MCH-expressing neurons modulate ciliary beating of ependymal cells at the third ventricle and could contribute to maintain cerebro-spinal fluid homeostasis.

Keywords: MCH, MCHR1, non-neuronal function, cilia, CSF flow

INTRODUCTION

First identified in the early 80s from chum salmon pituitaries, the melanin concentrating hormone (MCH) draw its name from its capability to induced the concentration of melanin in the skin melanophores (2). However, this function seems to be restricted to teleosts [reviewed in Ref. (3)]. In contrast with high MCH structural conservation, the neuronal distribution appears quite different, reflecting evolutionary changes in the prosencephalon across vertebrate species (4). In mammals, this cyclic peptide is mainly expressed in neurons of the lateral hypothalamic area (LHA), projecting widely throughout the brain (5); reviewed in Ref. (6). Accordingly, MCH is involved in a broad spectrum of cerebral functions [for recent reviews, see Ref. (7, 8)]. Nevertheless, all of these seem to converge to the adaptation of global physiologic state to metabolic needs by promoting memory processes and reward pathways activation on one hand and by decreasing arousal and thermogenesis on the other hand. Activation of these cognitive and neuroendocrine networks leads to an increase in food intake and energy storage, respectively [reviewed in Ref. (9, 10)].

The structure of the *Pmch* gene locus appears to be complex and sense/antisense transcripts could generate different protein-derivatives. Indeed, the precursor ppMCH may be processed mainly, but not exclusively, in two different peptides (MCH and NEI) in the brain and in several intermediates, including the dipeptide MCH-NEI, in peripheral organs (11–14). An additional protein, named MGOP, may be produced by an alternative splicing of the *Pmch* gene primary transcript in all cells producing MCH (15, 16). Finally a set of proteins, involved in DNA repair, may be synthesized by expression of the *AROM/PARI* gene located on the complementary strand overlapping the *Pmch* gene (8, 17). Based on this disparity in gene-products expression, it is quite difficult to associate a single molecular substrate responsible to the wide phenotypic changes observed in *Pmch* gene KO mice in which the full exon-intron sequences of the *Pmch* gene as well as the 3′UTR region of spliced AROM/PARI gene transcripts were deleted. Meanwhile, the issue of developmental compensation (or adaptation) in these genetic models of *Pmch* gene inactivation should also be considered [see Ref. (9) for discussion of this point].

Efforts to identify the MCH receptor initially led to the discovery of a spliced variant of the seven-transmembrane G-coupled protein named SLC-1 (18) as a cognate MCH receptor and thereafter referred to as MCHR1 (19–23). MCHR1 is widely localized in brain regions involved in the control of neuroendocrine, reward, motivational, and cognitive aspects of feeding behavior (9, 10, 24–26). Interestingly, MCHR1-deficient mice are lean due to hyperactivity and increased metabolism (27). A second MCH receptor, named here MCHR2, was identified and characterized in human tissues and cell lines (27–33). This MCH receptor displayed a brain distribution that overlapped partially with that of MCHR1 in the primate and fish brain (32, 34). However, MCHR2 is lacking in rat and mouse genomes (35). Furthermore, in contrast to MCHR1 that signals to either Gai or Gaq, depending on the transfected or native cell systems, MCHR2 signaling operates apparently exclusively through Gaq protein [our unpublished data; reviewed in Ref. (35–37)].

Based on neuro-anatomical mapping and electrophysiological data, it was assumed that synaptic transmission represents the main mode of action of MCH in the brain. However, non-neuronal intercellular communication or "volume" transmission may also be involved but evidence were lacking. In a recently published study (1), we mapped numerous MCH fibers in close vicinity to MCHR1 expressed into ependymocytes of the ventral part of the third ventricle (3V). Developing new techniques to measure and analyze the ependymal cilia beat frequency (CBF) in acute mouse brain slice preparations, we also showed that the CBF is increased by MCH application or LHA stimulation, an effect blocked by a selective MCHR1 antagonist and absent in MCHR1-knockout (MCHR1-KO) mice. In addition, using *in vivo* brain MRI, we demonstrated that the volume of both the lateral and third ventricles is increased in MCHR1-KO mice compared to their wild-type (WT) littermates. Thus, our study revealed a previously unknown function of the MCH/MCHR1 signaling system in non-neuronal cells. Here, we first demonstrated MCH mRNA expression in the ventral 3V ependymal cells isolated by laser-capture and *in situ* hybridization. We then extended our previous work, by using *in vitro* optogenetic activation or inhibition of MCH neurons. Finally, we investigated *in vivo* tracking of fluorescent micro-beads through the 3V in WT and MCHR1-KO mice. Collectively, we demonstrate a dynamic control of MCH neurons on spontaneous CBF of MCHR1 mRNA-expressing ependymal cells and discuss the current strategies for measuring CSF flows in small animal models.

MATERIALS AND METHODS

ANIMALS

The experiments were conducted with male C57BL/6J mice (for laser-captured cell mapping, *in situ* hybridization and cellular optogenetic measurements) and female KO MCHR1 mice (*in vivo* CSF flow experiments) of 10–12 weeks of age. The animals were obtained from heterozygous breeding in the local animal facilities and maintained on a 12-h dark/light cycle (7 a.m./7 p.m.) with food and water *ad libitum*. The MCHR1-KO mice were established as previously described (38).

All the protocols were carried out in accordance with French ethical guidelines for laboratory animals (Agreement N°75–178, 05/16/2000) and were approved by the IPMC care committee. Attention was paid to use only the number of animals requested and necessary to generate reproducible results.

LASER MICRO-DISSECTION OF THIRD VENTRICLE EPITHELIUM

After decapitation, each brain ($n = 2$) was dissected out in <2 min and immediately frozen at −80°C using a Snapfrost (Alphelys, France). Sections (10 μm thick) were cut on a cryostat (Microm HM 560; object holder and chamber were kept at −21°C). Eight sections passing through the posterior hypothalamus were collected on pen membrane slides. Slides, continuously maintained on dry ice, were dehydrated in three baths of increasing ethanol baths (70, 95, and 100%) and two baths of fresh xylene (Roth, France) for 5 min each. Sections were air dried and kept in the vacuum of a dessicator until dissection.

Dissections were performed using a PixCell® (Arcturus Engineering) with CapSure® HS LCM caps. The dissection time never exceeded 20 min/slide, starting from when the slide was removed from the dessicator. Laser parameters were calibrated for each dissection by measuring the impact of shots on the membrane of the slide adjacent to the tissue. The area of interest was then dissected and laser-captured using UV laser to cut the tissue and IR laser to capture the sample. Four samples were collected per cap (micro-dissection of two slides in <40 min in total) and only one cap per brain. As soon as the fourth sample was obtained, the cap was examined under the microscope to ensure the absence of unwanted debris. The sample lysis and the RNA extraction were performed using the RNAqueous®-Micro Kit (Ambion, France) following the manufacturer's instructions. The quality of the samples was finally evaluated with the Agilent 2100 Bioanalyzer (Agilent Technology). A rin of 6.1 was twice obtained.

After reverse transcription (Superscript III, Invitrogen), cDNA corresponding to 1 ng of RNA was used as input in a PCR reaction (GoTaq Green MasterMix, Promega, Charbonnières, France) for MCHR1 and HPRT as positive control (MCHR1 F: 5′-GCTCTATGCCAGGCTTATCC-3′, MCHR1 R: CAGCTGTCTGAGCATTGCTG-3′, amplicon size: 494 bp; HPRT F: CTCCGGAAAGCAGTGAGGTAAG, HPRT R: GGAGGGAGAAAAATGCGGAGTG, amplicon size: 306 bp). Sample for which reverse transcriptase was omitted was used as negative control. PCR protocol used was designed as follow: initial denaturation: 95°C, 5 min follow by 40 cycles composed of 95°C, 30 s, 58°C, 30 s, 72°C, 1 min, and a final elongation for 7 min at 72°C.

IN SITU HYBRIDIZATION

Frozen sections were post-fixed in 4% paraformaldehyde in 0.1 M phosphate buffer and digested with proteinase K (1 μg/mL, Roche) for 30 min at 37°C. Slides were incubated for 8 min in 0.1 M triethanolamine (TEA), pH 8.0, and then for 5 min at room temperature in 100 mL 0.1 M TEA + 500 μL acetic anhydride followed by a decarboxylation in active diethyl pyrocarbonate (DEPC).

Sections were then rinsed briefly with 5× standard citrate sodium (SSC) buffer then incubated for 2 h in prehybridization buffer at 56°C. After rinsing in 0.2× SSC, the sections were incubated overnight at 56°C, in humid chambers, with 50 μL hybridization buffer containing 5% Denhardt's and 50 ng labeled RNA probes. After rinsing with 5× SSC, sections were incubated successively in 2× SSC at 56°C (1 h 30 min) and 0.2× at room temperature (5 min). They were incubated in anti-DIG Fab fragments conjugated to alkaline phosphatase (1/1300, overnight) and revealed with enzyme substrate NBT-BCIP (overnight, at room temperature).

Two MCHR1 RNA probes were used; one probe was kindly provided by Drs Civelli and Chung (University of California, Irvine,

CA, USA) and one made by reverse transcription/polymerase chain reaction from mouse genomic DNA. Control hybridization, including hybridization with sense DIG-labeled riboprobes was realized and did not reveal any signal.

MEASURES OF CILIA BEAT FREQUENCY USING MCH NEURON-SPECIFIC OPTOGENETIC EXCITATION OR INHIBITION

We have previously shown that electrical stimulation of the LHA induced an increase in the CBF in the 3V (1). To further extend and improve the specificity of the response, we used new models allowing the optogenetic control of MCH neurons activity. All procedures and controls were previously published in (39). Briefly, using cre-dependent Ef1a-DIO-ChETA-EYFP AAV mediated transduction, the fast mutant of the light-activated Channel rhodopsin-2 (ChETA) or the chloride pump halorhodopsin (NpHR) was specifically expressed in MCH neurons of two different groups of 3 week-old mice. Four weeks after stereotactic injection of the AAV vectors in the LHA (AP: −1.45 mm, ML: ±1 mm, DV: −5.5 mm), brain slices were made and recordings were made in CBF as described elsewhere (1) before, during, and after stimulation of ChETA-expressing MCH neurons (473 nm, stimulation frequency: 1, 5, 10, 20, and 40 Hz, pulse length: 10 ms, total stimulation duration: 3 min) or NpHR (590 nm, continuous stimulation during 8.5 s each 10 s, 5 min). For each slice and area of recording, the instantaneous CBF was calculated. All samples in which basal CBF was out of a range comprised between 5 and 20 Hz (considered as the natural basal frequency in healthy slices) were not included. The mean of the basal frequency during the first 5 min of recordings were used as a baseline for normalization of the experimental values. Results are expressed as the percentile variation of this baseline.

MEASURE OF CSF FLOW INDEX USING FLUORESCENT MICRO-BEADS

Littermate controls and female MCHR1-KO mice (aged 12 weeks old) were anesthetized by intraperitoneal injection of ketamine hydrochloride 50 mg/kg and xylazine 10 mg/kg and placed in a stereotaxic frame tip of a 26 gage needle was brought to the following coordinates relative to the bregma: 1.75 mm posterior, 2.5 mm ventral, and 0 mm right and left. About 10 μL of polystyrene beads (diameter 3 μm (sigma L4530) dilution 1:4 in 0.09% NaCl) was injected in the third ventricle.

Fibered confocal fluorescence microscopy (FCFM) (CellviZio; Mauna Kea Technologies, Paris, France) imaging was used to visualize the *in vivo* movement of the polystyrene beads in the CSF flux. FCFM provides an easy access to these regions of interest with low disturbance of brain structure (40, 41). Small-diameter fiber-optic probe consisting of tens of thousands of fibers was implanted in the brain of the mice and connected to a Laser scanning unit LSU-488 (FibroScan) that uses a laser source with a wavelength of 488 nm. We used a MiniZ probe of 300 μm diameter with a working distance of 70 μm. The probe was stereotaxically lowered in the third ventricle at 2.5 mm ventral. Sensitive, single-pixel detection of fluorescence stimulated by the photodiode laser pulse through each fiber element, combined with the high scan rate allows the visualization of beads movements. Four acquisition sessions of at least 10 min was recorded for each animal at a frame rate of 11 frames/s.

STATISTICS

Variation in the CBF

Statistics were performed using Prism software (Graphpad Inc., La Jolla, CA, USA). The global mean for grouped time points (baseline, stimulation, and recovery) were compared Using One way ANOVA followed by Bonferroni's multiple comparison test (BMCT). N = number of mice, n = number of slices, n = number of cells considered. p Value <0.05 were considered significant.

Measure of CSF flow index using fluorescent micro-beads

Movies were visualized on ImageCell™ viewer. The speed of the beads was analyzed by tracking 10 beads/10 min films. The mean speed for an animal was the mean of the four films speeds. The movies displaying significant modifications of the speed over time were excluded as probably corresponding to pressure due to probe positioning or blood clot.

RESULTS

LASER MICRO-DISSECTION OF THIRD VENTRICLE EPITHELIUM AND *IN SITU* HYBRIDIZATION

As illustrated in **Figures 1A,B**; ependymal cell layer was carefully dissected and used for RNA extraction. RT-PCR results indicate that mRNA coding for MCHR1 were present in the 3V epithelium (**Figure 1C**). This was further confirmed by *in situ* hybridization with two specific probes recognizing MCHR1 mRNA. Indeed, numerous (but not all; see open arrowhead) ependymocytes were labeled with antisense probe (**Figure 1D**), within the cytoplasm (**Figure 1E**), while sense probe did not stain any cell types (**Figure 1F**). These results are in agreement with our immunohistochemical study (1) and recent data from Maratos-Flier's lab using a *MCHR1-cre/tdTomato* mouse strain (26).

MCH NEURON-SPECIFIC OPTOGENETIC TOOLS

The ChETA-NpHR system was used to dissect MCH neuronal circuitry reaching 3V ependymal cells and controlling CBF.

The stimulation of ChETA-expressing MCH neurons in the LHA induces an increase in the CBF reaching 134% of the basal value (**Figures 2A,B**; 1 Hz, N = 5, n = 7, n = 10, $F_{5.069, 29} = 0.0131$, BMCT: baseline vs. ChETA $t = 2.896$, $p < 0.05$). After 10 min recovery, the subsequent stimulation at 5 Hz tended to increase the CBF but did not reach the significance level (**Figure 2B**; 5 Hz, N = 5, n = 7, n = 10). For higher frequencies, no effect was observed (not shown, see Discussion). On the other hand, the stimulation of NpHR induced a marked decrease in the CBF reaching 76% of the basal (**Figures 2C,D**; N = 4, n = 8, n = 15, $F_{4.616, 44} = 0.0154$, BMCT: baseline vs. NpHR $t = 3.027$, $p < 0.05$).

MEASURE OF CSF FLOW INDEX USING FLUORESCENT MICRO-BEADS

In order to address the physiological relevance of MCH-driven ciliary beating regulation, we conducted *in vivo* flow measure. FCFM imaging was used to visualize the movement of the polystyrene beads in the CSF flux *in vivo* in groups of WT and KO MCHR1 mice (n = 5 each). The visualization of fluorescent beads movements in the third ventricle allow to approximate the speed of the CSF flux using *in vivo* brain imagery (**Figure 3**).

Overall, no significant statistical difference in the mean speed between the two groups was found. However, 3/5 animals in the

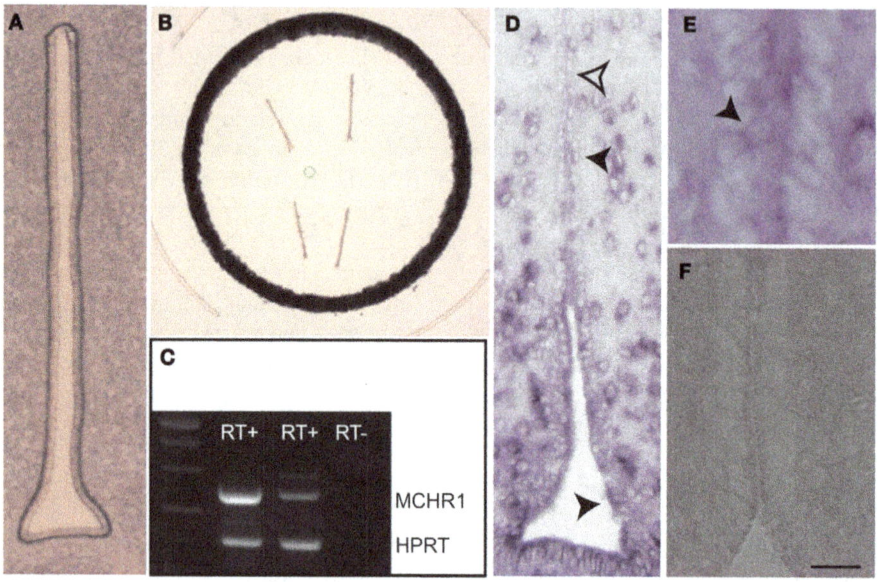

FIGURE 1 | (A) Photomicrograph of the ventricular epithelium before laser micro-dissection. **(B)** Photomicrograph of the ventricular epithelium after laser micro-dissection. **(C)** Illustration of the RT-PCR showing the presence of MCHR1 mRNA in the ventricular epithelium. RT^{+}: after reverse transcription, RT^{-}: negative control of the reverse transcription. HPRT: positive control. **(D)** Photomicrograph to illustrate the distribution of the MCHR1 *in situ* hybridization signal in the periventricular hypothalamus. Ependymocytes expressed the *in situ* signal (black arrowheads), but not all of them were labeled (open arrowhead). **(E)** High magnification to illustrate cytoplasmic expression of MCHR1 mRNA in discrete ependymal cells. **(F)** A negative control using sense MCHR1 gene probe. Scale bar = 25 μm in **(A)**; Scale bar = 20 μm in (D); Scale bar = 10 μm in **(E)** and **(F)**.

KO group displayed a twofold increase in the mean speed by comparison with the WT group (that shows consistently low speed). However, it should be stressed that we are measuring the bulk flow driven by the arterio-venous pressure gradients and arterial pulsations and that the laminar flow (close to the ventricle wall and therefore dependent upon cilia beating) remains too small to be measured. Furthermore, we believe that the technical caveat of the implantation of the probe and beads injection *in vivo* (blood clot, exact position, size of the probe . . .) may induce a methodological bias (see Discussion).

DISCUSSION

The MCH system is involved in a broad spectrum of function through mainly the synaptic release of the peptide(s) and neuronal activity modulation in mammalian brain. However, a growing body of data indicates that MCH may also have non-neuronal function, especially by regulating the activity of more or less specialized peripheral blood mononuclear cells [PBMCs (42)]. The expression of ppMCH and/or MCHR1 genes in pancreatic islets or in adipocytes (43–45) may highlight a metabolism-related function of MCH at the periphery. Nevertheless, such action may not be totally independent of the intracerebral and/or spinal MCH pathway (46). Based on our previous study (1) and the present set of data, we demonstrate a new role for the hypothalamic peptide MCH in modulation of CBF in the ventral part of the third ventricle through activation of ependymal cells.

In combining the laser micro-dissection of ependymal epithelium of the 3V followed by RNA extraction and RT-PCR experiments and *in situ* hybridization data, we demonstrate the presence of MCHR1 transcripts within the epithelium. This is consistent with the data obtained by immunohistochemistry (1) or in a *MCHR1-Cre/tdTomato* mouse model (26).

The optogenetic stimulation of the MCH neurons (through ChETA activation) increased the CBF in the same extend than electrical stimulation did, compared to basal conditions. This confirms also with high temporal precision, the specificity of the response observed in the 3V. Indeed, only ciliated cells lining the ventral 3V that expressed MCHR1 were MCH-sensitive, while those from the dorsal third ventricle or the lateral ventricles were not (1). The spatial specificity of the MCH response adds a new level of complexity to the previously described characteristics of ciliated ependymal cells [orientation, size, beating mode of cilia along the ventricles (47, 48)], and suggests that ciliary beating in cerebral ventricles is fine-tuned to modulate CSF flow in response to metabolic, neurohormonal, and neuroimmune changes. Moreover, our present *in situ* hybridization experiments, previous immunohistochemical data (1) and mapping using *MCHR1-Cre/tdTomato* mouse (26) highly suggested a "cluster-like" distribution of the MCHR1 mRNA and proteins along the 3V. Since adjoining ependymal cells are known to be coupled through GAP junctions (49), it is tempting to speculate that the only few ependymal cells expressing MCHR1 may act as hubs responsible for the effect of MCH neuronal stimulation on the whole epithelium in the 3V.

The results obtained following genetic invalidation and pharmacological inactivation of MCHR1 suggested that the MCH system could exert a tonic positive control on CBF (1). Here, we demonstrate the validity of this hypothesis since the inhibition of MCH neurons activity (through NpHR stimulation) directly

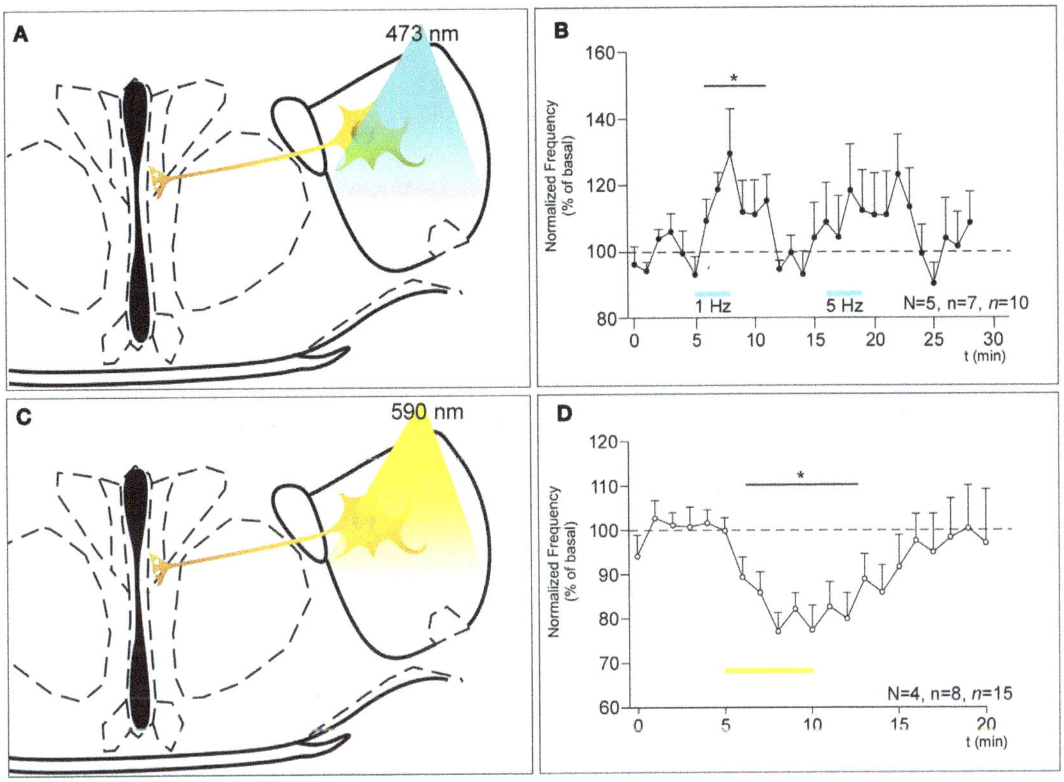

FIGURE 2 | (A,C) Schematics showing the projection of MCH neurons expressing ChETA **(A)** or NpHR **(C)** from the LHA to the ventricular epithelium and their optogenetic stimulation paradigm. **(B)** Consequences of the stimulation of ChETA in MCH neurons, by light pulses of 10 ms at a rate of 1 and 5 Hz as shown by the bars, on the CBF recorded in the ventral 3V expressed as a percentage of the basal frequency. N: number of animals, n: numbers of slices, *n*: number of recording area. **p* < 0.05 **(D)** Consequences of the stimulation of NpHR in MCH neurons as shown by the bars, in MCH neurons on the CBF recorded in the ventral 3V. N: number of animals, n: numbers of slices, *n*: number of recording area.

affects the CBF. To our knowledge, MCH is the only known molecule exerting a tonic positive effect on cilia beating in the brain. Even more interestingly, this tonic control of MCH on the CBF in the 3V does not seem to be compensated through adaptive mechanisms during development, since the basal CBF in MCHR1-KO mice is also reduced (1).

Even if MCH neurons activity seems to be important in the regulation of cilia beating, we have not yet firmly established whether the communication between MCH neurons and ependymal cells involves a true asymmetric synapse or not. With respect to the anatomical distribution of MCH fibers around the v3V, the communication should more likely involve passing fibers "leaking" MCH close to the epithelium basal pole and/or release of the peptide directly into the CSF. Indeed, MCHR1 immunolabeling was observed at both the apex and the basal poles of ciliated ependymal cells as well as MCH fibers crossing the epithelium. The nature of the contacts between ciliated cells and fibers remains to be addressed using a detailed electronic microscopic analysis.

Genetic ablation of MCHR1 results in an increase in the volume of LVs and 3V (both ventral and dorsal) but no change in 4V as reported previously (1). In order to determine the flow of CSF using a non-invasive method, we have tried to transpose clinical tools (CINE-MRI) to mice. Unfortunately, the main limit of such technique is the speed of the flow. Preliminary experiments indicate that this speed is $<10\,\mu m\,s^{-1}$, preventing the use of CINE-MRI in the mouse brain (Kober F., Troalen T., and Viola A. CRMBM. Marseille; personal communication).

The most used methods to study the flow of CSF in rodents consist in the injection of tracers (X-rays or MRI contrast agent) *in vivo* (50), or the use of fluorescent micro-beads or china ink *ex vivo* on dissected epithelia (51). Here, we show that it is possible to follow the migration of fluorescent micro-beads through the v3V. Unexpectedly, our data indicate that, in MCHR1-KO mice, the speed of the CSF flow tends to increase as compared to WT littermates, without reaching the statistical significance level. This paradoxical effect could be explained by the Poiseuille's law which postulates a direct link between the mean speed (V) of a viscous liquid (such as CSF) and the radius (r) of a small cylinder (such as a ventricle) ($V = DP^*\Pi^*r^4/8h \times l$ with h = viscosity, DP = difference of pressure between the extremities of the cylinder, l = length, and r = radius of the cylinder). Indeed, the flow measured at the center of the ventricle would increase when the radius expands. This fits quite well with an enlargement of the ventricle in the KO MCHR1 mice as observed using MRI (1). Another explanation for this discrepancy would be that the optic fiber used for the recording may block the CSF flow in the 3V of WT animals but not in MCHR1-KO

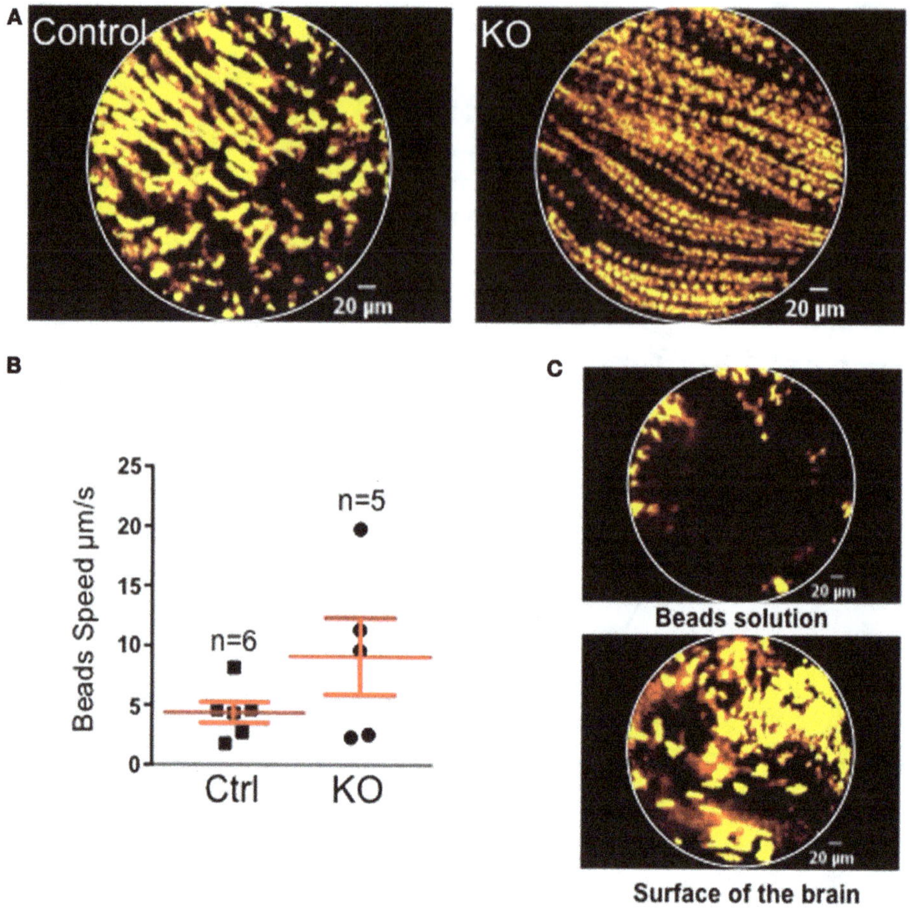

FIGURE 3 | (A) Projections of 10 s acquisition movies illustrating the fluorescent beads movement in the CSF of control (left) and KO MCHR1 (right) animals. In both cases, beads displayed a continuous and orientated movement lasting for at least the recording time. **(B)** Mean speed of the beads in control and KO MCHR1 animals. **(C)** Negative controls. Visualizations of fluorescents beads in solution (top) and at the surface of the living brain (bottom). No orientated movements were detected.

(since the volume of this ventricle is enlarged in these animals). Moreover, an increase in the CSF pressure into the ventricles could not be excluded.

At this point, it seems important to dissociate the global flow of CSF, mainly resulting from cardio-respiratory activity, to the laminar flow imputable to cilia beating. This point is of prime importance since it has been shown that MCHR1-KO mice display an increase in heart and respiratory rate (52). As a consequence, this may be responsible for the increase in global CSF flow. Moreover, because the volume of the ventricle is increased in MCHR1-KO mice, according to the Poiseuille's equation (see above), the speed of the CSF close to the epithelium should be reduced as compared to what is observed in the center of the ventricle. Because of the cilia action, such an effect is reduced and the speed close to epithelial cells is increased. Thus, in MCHR1-KO mice in which the CBF is altered, an increase in the total CSF flow may compensate the local decrease of the flow at the level of cilia. Taking into account all of these parameters, it is not surprising to observe an increase in CSF speed in the 3V.

Our data further suggest that motile ciliated cells of the cerebral ventricles are chemosensory as primary cilia, similar to motile ciliate cells from the airway epithelia (53). Hydrocephalus is one of the features of Bardet–Biedl syndrome (BBS), a genetic disease caused by a mutation in one of several proteins involved in the development of primary cilia, BBS1 being the most frequently affected in humans (54). The characteristics of BBS include ventriculomegaly of the lateral and third ventricles, particularly marked in knockin mice expressing the mutated human BBS1 protein (55). As BBS1 is involved in the trafficking of MCHR1 (54), this ventriculomegaly may be partly due to a defect in MCHR1 expression by ciliated ependymal cells, However, it is worth mentioning that the whole distribution of MCHR1 throughout the brain of BBS mouse models is still lacking. The absence of MCHR1 targeting to primary cilium in BBS models does not seems to affect the ciliogenesis (54). In this context, we found no difference in the morphology of the cilia between WT and MCHR1-KO mice, suggesting that MCHR1 does not play an important role in the development of cilia, but only in the modulation of the CBF, once the cilia are in place (although some compensatory changes could occur during development). This fits quite well with the characterization of MCHR1 mutants in ciliated hREP1 cells and the discovery of a motif in the third intracellular loop that is mandatory for MCHR1 trafficking to the primary cilia but not ciliogenesis. Other GPCR such as, somatostatin 3 receptor (SST3) and serotonin receptor 6 (5-HTR6) are specifically targeted to the primary cilia. Based on the physiological roles of somatostatin, and since new genetically engineered models such as SST3:Cre – cilia GFP mice (56) have been generated, a complete study about SST involvement in CSF and/or CBF regulation should be considered.

In conclusion, this paper and our previous study (1) point to a new role for MCH in maintaining CSF flow and homeostasis in the mouse brain. It is worth noting that the main group of MCH neurons in primitive vertebrates (lampreys) and most fish species (but teleosteans) are located very close (and also projected) to the ventricular surface and could regulate general volume transmission, like in rodents (4, 57). This convergent anatomy could be associated with an ancestral function maintained during evolution. Indeed, MCH neurons could anticipate and initiate the acceleration of CSF circulation, for instance, under conditions of metabolic necessity (glucose withdrawal, fasting, . . .). The strategic location of the ciliated cells innervated by MCH fibers, at the base of the third cerebral ventricle, could allow them to act as a pump to initiate an increase in CSF flow, providing peptides and other messengers to several brain areas and prolonging the effects of these factors in conjunction with neuronal transmission. Moreover, if the same type of CSF flow regulation exists in humans, this work suggests that the chronic administration of brain penetrating MCHR1 antagonists may have long term side effects due to alterations of CSF flows, limiting the probability of their use as therapeutic agents.

AUTHORS CONTRIBUTION

Grégory Conductier conducted and analyzed brain slice imaging experiments (CBF measurements and optogenetics) and participated to writing. Agnès O. Martin, Chrystel Lafont, and Patrice Mollard performed and analyzed the FCFM experiments, and participated in manuscript writing. Pierre-Yves Risold performed laser-captured, RT-PCR and *in situ* hybridization experiments. He participates also to writing. Sonia Jego, Raphaël Lavoie, and Antoine Adamantidis performed vector designing and set up the optogenetics experiments, and participated in manuscript writing. Jean-Louis Nahon acquired funding, designed and analyzed experiments, coordinated collaborations, and participated in manuscript writing and editing.

ACKNOWLEDGMENTS

We warmly thank Dr. Bernard Lakaye of University of Liège (Belgium), for the gift of MCHR1-KO mice and Dr Mounia Annour-Louet for careful reading of the manuscript. We wish to thank Drs Alice Guyon, Frédéric Brau, and Olivier Meste for development and validation of bioinformatics tools, Christophe Houdayer for collecting samples used in laser-captured experiments, Gabrielle Franchi for help in *in situ* hybridization, Veronique Thieffin for animal care, Isabelle Larre for help with immunoassays, and Franck Aguila for excellent artwork. We also thank Mauna Kea Technologies (Paris, France) for providing access to the CellviZio system during the duration of the experiments. Funding sources: this work was funded by the French Government (National Research Agency, ANR) through the "Investments for the Future" LABEX SIGNALIFE:#ANR-11-LABX-0028-01 (Jean-Louis Nahon), ANR-08-MNPS-018-01 (Jean-Louis Nahon), and ANR-2010-BLAN-1415-01 (Patrice Mollard), the Centre National de la Recherche Scientifique (PEPS INSB; Jean-Louis Nahon); the sixth FP EU STREPS/NEST-APES Project no. 28594 (Jean-Louis Nahon), the Fondation de la Recherche Médicale (FRM) (Jean-Louis Nahon), the SFR Biocampus de Montpellier (IPAM platform). Financial support: Gregory Conductier was supported by postdoctoral fellowships from the ANR-08-MNPS-018-01 and the Centre National de la Recherche Scientifique (INSB) and by awards from the "Société Française de Nutrition 2011" and the "Institut Danone 2012."

REFERENCES

1. Conductier G, Brau F, Viola A, Langlet F, Ramkumar N, Dehouck B, et al. Melanin-concentrating hormone regulates beat frequency of ependymal cilia and ventricular volume. *Nat Neurosci* (2013) **16**:845–7. doi:10.1038/nn.3401
2. Rance TA, Baker BI. Possible hypothalamic origin of the teleost melanin-concentrating hormone [proceedings]. *J Endocrinol* (1979) **81**:166.
3. Kawauchi H, Baker BI. Melanin-concentrating hormone signaling systems in fish. *Peptides* (2004) **25**:1577–84. doi:10.1016/j.peptides.2004.03.025
4. Croizier S, Cardot J, Brischoux F, Fellmann D, Griffond B, Risold PY. The vertebrate diencephalic MCH system: a versatile neuronal population in an evolving brain. *Front Neuroendocrinol* (2013) **34**:65–87. doi:10.1016/j.yfrne.2012.10.001
5. Bittencourt JC, Presse F, Arias C, Peto C, Vaughan J, Nahon JL, et al. The melanin-concentrating hormone system of the rat brain: an immuno- and hybridization histochemical characterization. *J Comp Neurol* (1992) **319**:218–45. doi:10.1002/cne.903190204
6. Bittencourt JC. Anatomical organization of the melanin-concentrating hormone peptide family in the mammalian brain. *Gen Comp Endocrinol* (2011) **172**:185–97. doi:10.1016/j.ygcen.2011.03.028
7. Chung S, Parks GS, Lee C, Civelli O. Recent updates on the melanin-concentrating hormone (MCH) and its receptor system: lessons from MCH1R antagonists. *J Mol Neurosci* (2011) **43**:115–21. doi:10.1007/s12031-010-9411-4
8. Presse F, Nahon JL. MCH. In: Kastin AJ, editor. *Handbook of Biologically Active Peptides*. 2nd ed. San Diego, CA: Academic Press (2013). p. 828–37.
9. Pissios P. Animals models of MCH function and what they can tell us about its role in energy balance. *Peptides* (2009) **30**:2040–4. doi:10.1016/j.peptides.2009.05.002
10. Macneil DJ. The role of melanin-concentrating hormone and its receptors in energy homeostasis. *Front Endocrinol (Lausanne)* (2013) **4**:49. doi:10.3389/fendo.2013.00049
11. Nahon JL, Presse F, Bittencourt JC, Sawchenko PE, Vale W. The rat melanin-concentrating hormone messenger ribonucleic acid encodes multiple putative neuropeptides coexpressed in the dorsolateral hypothalamus. *Endocrinology* (1989) **125**:2056–65. doi:10.1210/endo-125-4-2056
12. Viale A, Ortola C, Hervieu G, Furuta M, Barbero P, Steiner DF, et al. Cellular localization and role of prohormone convertases in the processing of pro-melanin concentrating hormone in mammals. *J Biol Chem* (1999) **274**:6536–45. doi:10.1074/jbc.274.10.6536
13. Maulon-Feraille L, Della Zuana O, Suply T, Rovere-Jovene C, Audinot V, Levens N, et al. Appetite-boosting property of pro-melanin-concentrating hormone(131-165) (neuropeptide-glutamic acid-isoleucine) is associated with proteolytic resistance. *J Pharmacol Exp Ther* (2002) **302**:766–73. doi:10.1124/jpet.302.2.766
14. Sandig H, McDonald J, Gilmour J, Arno M, Lee TH, Cousins DJ. Human Th2 cells selectively express the orexigenic peptide, pro-melanin-concentrating hormone. *Proc Natl Acad Sci U S A* (2007) **104**:12440–4. doi:10.1073/pnas.0705457104
15. Toumaniantz G, Bittencourt JC, Nahon JL. The rat melanin-concentrating hormone gene encodes an additional putative protein in a different reading frame. *Endocrinology* (1996) **137**:4518–21. doi:10.1210/en.137.10.4518

16. Allaeys I, Bouyer K, Loudes C, Faivre-Bauman A, Petit F, Ortola C, et al. Characterization of MCH-gene-overprinted-polypeptide-immunoreactive material in hypothalamus reveals an inhibitory role of pro-somatostatin1-64 on somatostatin secretion. *Eur J Neurosci* (2004) **19**:925–36. doi:10.1111/j.0953-816X.2004.03187.x
17. Moldovan GL, Dejsuphong D, Petalcorin MI, Hofmann K, Takeda S, Boulton SJ, et al. Inhibition of homologous recombination by the PCNA-interacting protein PARI. *Mol Cell* (2012) **45**:75–86. doi:10.1016/j.molcel.2011.11.010
18. Kolakowski LF Jr, Jung BP, Nguyen T, Johnson MP, Lynch KR, Cheng R, et al. Characterization of a human gene related to genes encoding somatostatin receptors. *FEBS Lett* (1996) **398**:253–8. doi:10.1016/S0014-5793(96)01160-X
19. Bachner D, Kreienkamp H, Weise C, Buck F, Richter D. Identification of melanin concentrating hormone (MCH) as the natural ligand for the orphan somatostatin-like receptor 1 (SLC-1). *FEBS Lett* (1999) **457**:522–4. doi:10.1016/S0014-5793(99)01092-3
20. Chambers J, Ames RS, Bergsma D, Muir A, Fitzgerald LR, Hervieu G, et al. Melanin-concentrating hormone is the cognate ligand for the orphan G-protein-coupled receptor SLC-1. *Nature* (1999) **400**:261–5. doi:10.1038/22313
21. Lembo PM, Grazzini E, Cao J, Hubatsch DA, Pelletier M, Hoffert C, et al. The receptor for the orexigenic peptide melanin-concentrating hormone is a G-protein-coupled receptor. *Nat Cell Biol* (1999) **1**:267–71. doi:10.1038/12978
22. Saito Y, Nothacker HP, Wang Z, Lin SH, Leslie F, Civelli O. Molecular characterization of the melanin-concentrating-hormone receptor. *Nature* (1999) **400**:265–9. doi:10.1038/22321
23. Shimomura Y, Mori M, Sugo T, Ishibashi Y, Abe M, Kurokawa T, et al. Isolation and identification of melanin-concentrating hormone as the endogenous ligand of the SLC-1 receptor. *Biochem Biophys Res Commun* (1999) **261**:622–6. doi:10.1006/bbrc.1999.1104
24. Kokkotou EG, Tritos NA, Mastaitis JW, Slieker L, Maratos-Flier E. Melanin-concentrating hormone receptor is a target of leptin action in the mouse brain. *Endocrinology* (2001) **142**:680–6. doi:10.1210/en.142.2.680
25. Saito Y, Cheng M, Leslie FM, Civelli O. Expression of the melanin-concentrating hormone (MCH) receptor mRNA in the rat brain. *J Comp Neurol* (2001) **435**:26–40. doi:10.1002/cne.1191
26. Chee MJ, Pissios P, Maratos-Flier E. Neurochemical characterization of neurons expressing melanin-concentrating hormone receptor 1 in the mouse hypothalamus. *J Comp Neurol* (2013) **521**:2208–34. doi:10.1002/cne.23273
27. Marsh DJ, Weingarth DT, Novi DE, Chen HY, Trumbauer ME, Chen AS, et al. Melanin-concentrating hormone 1 receptor-deficient mice are lean, hyperactive, and hyperphagic and have altered metabolism. *Proc Natl Acad Sci U S A* (2002) **99**:3240–5. doi:10.1073/pnas.052706899
28. An S, Cutler G, Zhao JJ, Huang SG, Tian H, Li W, et al. Identification and characterization of a melanin-concentrating hormone receptor. *Proc Natl Acad Sci U S A* (2001) **98**:7576–81. doi:10.1073/pnas.131200698
29. Hill J, Duckworth M, Murdock P, Rennie G, Sabido-David C, Ames RS, et al. Molecular cloning and functional characterization of MCH2, a novel human MCH receptor. *J Biol Chem* (2001) **276**:20125–9. doi:10.1074/jbc.M102068200
30. Mori M, Harada M, Terao Y, Sugo T, Watanabe T, Shimomura Y, et al. Cloning of a novel G protein-coupled receptor, SLT, a subtype of the melanin-concentrating hormone receptor. *Biochem Biophys Res Commun* (2001) **283**:1013–8. doi:10.1006/bbrc.2001.4893
31. Rodriguez M, Beauverger P, Naime I, Rique H, Ouvry C, Souchaud S, et al. Cloning and molecular characterization of the novel human melanin-concentrating hormone receptor MCH2. *Mol Pharmacol* (2001) **60**:632–9.
32. Sailer AW, Sano H, Zeng Z, McDonald TP, Pan J, Pong SS, et al. Identification and characterization of a second melanin-concentrating hormone receptor, MCH-2R. *Proc Natl Acad Sci U S A* (2001) **98**:7564–9. doi:10.1073/pnas.121170598
33. Wang S, Behan J, O'Neill K, Weig B, Fried S, Laz T, et al. Identification and pharmacological characterization of a novel human melanin-concentrating hormone receptor, mch-r2. *J Biol Chem* (2001) **276**:34664–70. doi:10.1074/jbc.M102601200
34. Mizusawa K, Amiya N, Yamaguchi Y, Takabe S, Amano M, Breves JP, et al. Identification of mRNAs coding for mammalian-type melanin-concentrating hormone and its receptors in the scalloped hammerhead shark Sphyrna lewini. *Gen Comp Endocrinol* (2012) **179**:78–87. doi:10.1016/j.ygcen.2012.07.023
35. Tan CP, Sano H, Iwaasa H, Pan J, Sailer AW, Hreniuk DL, et al. Melanin-concentrating hormone receptor subtypes 1 and 2: species-specific gene expression. *Genomics* (2002) **79**:785–92. doi:10.1006/geno.2002.6771
36. Boutin JA, Suply T, Audinot V, Rodriguez M, Beauverger P, Nicolas JP, et al. Melanin-concentrating hormone and its receptors: state of the art. *Can J Physiol Pharmacol* (2002) **80**:388–95. doi:10.1139/y02-056
37. Hervieu G. Melanin-concentrating hormone functions in the nervous system: food intake and stress. *Expert Opin Ther Targets* (2003) **7**:495–511. doi:10.1517/14728222.7.4.495
38. Adamantidis A, Thomas E, Foidart A, Tyhon A, Coumans B, Minet A, et al. Disrupting the melanin-concentrating hormone receptor 1 in mice leads to cognitive deficits and alterations of NMDA receptor function. *Eur J Neurosci* (2005) **21**:2837–44. doi:10.1111/j.1460-9568.2005.04100.x
39. Jego S, Glasgow SD, Herrera CG, Ekstrand M, Reed SJ, Boyce R, et al. Optogenetic identification of a rapid eye movement sleep modulatory circuit in the hypothalamus. *Nat Neurosci* (2013) **16**(11):1637–43. doi:10.1038/nn.3522
40. Vincent P, Maskos U, Charvet I, Bourgeais L, Stoppini L, Leresche N, et al. Live imaging of neural structure and function by fibred fluorescence microscopy. *EMBO Rep* (2006) **7**:1154–61. doi:10.1038/sj.embor.7400801
41. Flusberg BA, Nimmerjahn A, Cocker ED, Mukamel EA, Barretto RP, Ko TH, et al. High-speed, miniaturized fluorescence microscopy in freely moving mice. *Nat Methods* (2008) **5**:935–8. doi:10.1038/nmeth.1256
42. Verlaet M, Adamantidis A, Coumans B, Chanas G, Zorzi W, Heinen E, et al. Human immune cells express ppMCH mRNA and functional MCHR1 receptor. *FEBS Lett* (2002) **527**:205–10. doi:10.1016/S0014-5793(02)03232-5
43. Bradley RL, Kokkotou EG, Maratos-Flier E, Cheatham B. Melanin-concentrating hormone regulates leptin synthesis and secretion in rat adipocytes. *Diabetes* (2000) **49**:1073–7. doi:10.2337/diabetes.49.7.1073
44. Bradley RL, Mansfield JP, Maratos-Flier E, Cheatham B. Melanin-concentrating hormone activates signaling pathways in 3T3-L1 adipocytes. *Am J Physiol Endocrinol Metab* (2002) **283**:E584–92.
45. Pissios P, Ozcan U, Kokkotou E, Okada T, Liew CW, Liu S, et al. Melanin concentrating hormone is a novel regulator of islet function and growth. *Diabetes* (2007) **56**:311–9. doi:10.2337/db06-0708
46. Stanley S, Pinto S, Segal J, Pérez CA, Viale A, DeFalco J, et al. Identification of neuronal subpopulations that project from hypothalamus to both liver and adipose tissue polysynaptically. *Proc Natl Acad Sci U S A* (2010) **107**:7024–9. doi:10.1073/pnas.1002790107
47. Braiman A, Zagoory O, Priel Z. PKA induces Ca2+ release and enhances ciliary beat frequency in a Ca2+-dependent and -independent manner. *Am J Physiol* (1998) **275**:C790–7.
48. Vígh B, Manzano e Silva MJ, Frank CL, Vincze C, Czirok SJ, Szabó A, et al. The system of cerebrospinal fluid-contacting neurons. Its supposed role in the nonsynaptic signal transmission of the brain. *Histol Histopathol* (2004) **19**:607–28.
49. Prochnow N, Dermietzel R. Connexons and cell adhesion: a romantic phase. *Histochem Cell Biol* (2008) **130**:71–7. doi:10.1007/s00418-008-0434-7
50. Sawamoto K, Wichterle H, Gonzalez-Perez O, Cholfin JA, Yamada M, Spassky N, et al. New neurons follow the flow of cerebrospinal fluid in the adult brain. *Science* (2006) **311**:629–32. doi:10.1126/science.1119133
51. Mirzadeh Z, Doetsch F, Sawamoto K, Wichterle H, Alvarez-Buylla A. The subventricular zone en-face: wholemount staining and ependymal flow. *J Vis Exp* (2010). doi:10.3791/1938
52. Astrand A, Bohlooly-Y M, Larsdotter S, Mahlapuu M, Andersén H, Tornell J, et al. Mice lacking melanin-concentrating hormone receptor 1 demonstrate increased heart rate associated with altered autonomic activity. *Am J Physiol Regul Integr Comp Physiol* (2004) **287**:R749–58. doi:10.1152/ajpregu.00134.2004
53. Shah AS, Ben-Shahar Y, Moninger TO, Kline JN, Welsh MJ. Motile cilia of human airway epithelia are chemosensory. *Science* (2009) **325**:1131–4. doi:10.1126/science.1173869
54. Berbari NF, Lewis JS, Bishop GA, Askwith CC, Mykytyn K. Bardet-Biedl syndrome proteins are required for the localization of G protein-coupled receptors to primary cilia. *Proc Natl Acad Sci U S A* (2008) **105**:4242–6. doi:10.1073/pnas.0711027105
55. Davis RE, Swiderski RE, Rahmouni K, Nishimura DY, Mullins RF, Agassandian K, et al. A knockin mouse model of the Bardet-Biedl syndrome 1 M390R mutation has cilia defects, ventriculomegaly, retinopathy, and obesity. *Proc Natl Acad Sci U S A* (2007) **104**:19422–7. doi:10.1073/pnas.0708571104

15

Ghrelin receptors in non-mammalian vertebrates

Hiroyuki Kaiya[1]*, Kenji Kangawa[2] and Mikiya Miyazato[1]

[1] Department of Biochemistry, National Cerebral and Cardiovascular Center Research Institute, Osaka, Japan
[2] National Cerebral and Cardiovascular Center Research Institute, Osaka, Japan

Edited by:
Hubert Vaudry, University of Rouen, France

Reviewed by:
Hélène Volkoff, Memorial University of Newfoundland, Canada
Catharina Olsson, University of Gothenburg, Sweden

***Correspondence:**
Hiroyuki Kaiya, Department of Biochemistry, National Cerebral and Cardiovascular Center Research Institute, 5-7-1 Fujishirodai, Suita, Osaka 565-8565, Japan
e-mail: kaiya@ncvc.go.jp

The growth hormone secretagogue-receptor (GHS-R) was discovered in humans and pigs in 1996. The endogenous ligand, ghrelin, was discovered 3 years later, in 1999, and our understanding of the physiological significance of the ghrelin system in vertebrates has grown steadily since then. Although the ghrelin system in non-mammalian vertebrates is a subject of great interest, protein sequence data for the receptor in non-mammalian vertebrates has been limited until recently, and related biological information has not been well organized. In this review, we summarize current information related to the ghrelin receptor in non-mammalian vertebrates.

Keywords: ghrelin, ghrelin receptor, GHS-R, GHS-R-like receptor, fishes, amphibians, reptiles, birds

GENERAL INTRODUCTION

As implied by their name, growth hormone secretagogues (GHSs), which are artificial derivatives of enkephalin, exhibit growth hormone (GH)-releasing activity (1). Some of these GHSs also stimulate appetite in mammals (2). In 1996, Howard et al. (3) discovered a G-protein-coupled receptor (GPCR) with seven transmembrane domains (TMDs) in humans and pigs, and found that GHSs bound to this receptor and elicited an increase in the intracellular Ca^{2+} concentration of cells in which it was stably expressed. They named this receptor the GHS-receptor type-1a (GHS-R1a); in addition, they found an alternative splice variant of the receptor that lacked the Ca^{2+} signaling capacity and named it GHS-R type-1b (GHS-R1b). The mammalian GHS-R gene (*ghsr*) comprises two exons separated by one intron (4, 5). GHS-R1a comprises 366 amino acids (AAs), where the first exon (exon 1) encodes the first 265 AAs from TMD 1–5, and the second exon (exon 2) encodes the remaining 101 AAs from TMD 6 and 7. In contrast, the alternative splice variant of *ghsr*, GHS-R1b, is formed from the first exon and part of the intron. Thus, the protein sequence of the entire 289-AA GHS-R1b is identical to GHS-R1a from the N-terminal end to TMD 5.

Extensive investigations were performed to identify the endogenous ligand for the orphan GHS-R1a following discovery of the receptor, and reverse pharmacology facilitated the identification of a natural ligand in 1999 by Kojima et al. (6). The peptide ligand, which contains 28 AAs, was isolated from stomach extracts of rats and named "ghrelin." Ghrelin has a unique fatty acid modification on its N-terminal third serine (Ser3), with an *n*-octanoyl group linked to the hydroxyl group of Ser3. This modification is essential for the binding of ghrelin to the receptor (7) and for eliciting various physiological actions. After the discovery of its endogenous ligand, GHS-R1a was found to mediate various physiological functions of ghrelin: neuroendocrine function; appetite regulation; cardiovascular function; gastro-entero-pancreatic function; glucose metabolism; and cell functions including apoptosis, proliferation, and differentiation (8–10).

In non mammalian vertebrates, GHSs affect the regulation of GH release and of appetite in fish and birds (11–14), suggesting the presence of an endogenous ghrelin-like substance and a corresponding receptor system. We first isolated ghrelin from a non-mammalian vertebrate, the bullfrog (15). Subsequently, ghrelin was determined to be present in various non-mammalian vertebrates, and its physiological effects were gradually revealed [for reviews, see Ref. (16, 17)]. However, investigations of non-mammalian ghrelin receptors still lag behind those on mammalian ghrelin receptors. In this review, we summarize our recent work and those of others on ghrelin receptors in non-mammalian vertebrates and provide a comprehensive discussion of their general features.

CLASSIFICATION AND NOMENCLATURE OF GHRELIN RECEPTORS

We begin by describing the nomenclature for the ghrelin receptors in mammals, because the nomenclature for the receptors in non-mammalian vertebrates is more complicated and various names have been used based on the presence of splice variants, paralogs, and different AA lengths. In the first description provided by Howard et al. (3), GHS-R1a was defined as a functional receptor induced by agonist-dependent intracellular Ca^{2+}, and GHS-R1b as a splice variant of unknown function. They classified them simply as "a" and "b" because their sequences and functions differed. Thus the names are based on the sequence and structure: "GHS-R1" refers to the receptor with a "type-1" AA sequence, "a" signifies "activated by ghrelin or GHSs," and "b" indicates "a splice variant of *ghsr*" which contains the first exon and an unspliced intron that continues the coding sequence in the mRNA and terminates at a stop codon within the intron. The International Union of Pharmacology Committee on Receptor Nomenclature and Drug Classification has accepted "GHS-R1a" as the name for the functional ghrelin receptor (18). Hence, two GHS-Rs exist in mammals: GHS-R1a, which is derived from regular splicing of the gene; and GHS-R1b, which originates from alternative splicing of the gene (**Figure 1**). On the basis of these names, we describe the naming of the receptors in non-mammalian vertebrates as follows.

The non-mammalian GHS-Rs are also roughly divided into two types: (i) an isoform that arises from regular splicing of the gene and (ii) an isoform derived from alternative splicing of the gene (**Figure 1**). The former is further classified into two isoforms (**Figure 1**): one denotes an isoform that we designated "GHS-Ra," which has structural properties similar to those of the mammalian GHS-R1a and is activated by ghrelin and GHSs. GHS-Ra is further divided into two paralogs "1a" and "2a," where "GHS-R2a" refers to the receptor with a "type-2" AA sequence distinct from that of GHS-R1a and whose existence is confirmed only in specific fish. The other denotes another isoform that we designated "GHS-R1a-like receptor (GHS-R1a-LR)," which has structural features that differ from those of GHS-Ra and for which intracellular Ca^{2+} increase in response to ghrelin or GHS treatment is either small or not confirmed. This distinction between GHS-Ra and GHS-R1a-LR is evident in the phylogenetic analysis based on the AA sequences of ghrelin receptors (**Figure 2**).

The isoforms derived from alternative splicing of the gene are divided into five types: 1b, 1aV (1c), 1bV, tv, and tv-like receptors. These receptors are formed by different modes of alternative splicing and have distinct structures.

NON-MAMMALIAN VERTEBRATE SPECIES WITH SEQUENCED GHRELIN RECEPTORS

We have summarized the non-mammalian vertebrates for which the cDNA or genes of GHS-R have been identified and made available in public databases in **Table 1** (fish) and **Table 2** (reptiles, amphibians, and birds). The AA sequences of GHS-R1a, 2a; GHS-R1a-LR; and their multiple alignments are shown in **Figure 3**.

Many GHS-Rs have been identified in non-mammalian vertebrates, and the most of the GHS-R types that have been found are present in fish (19 species). With the recent identification of a GHS-R in bullfrog and Japanese tree frog (19), we now know the GHS-Rs for three kinds of frogs, including African clawed frogs. In reptiles, there are no reports about GHS-Rs at present, although the Ensembl genome database search (http://www.ensembl.org/index.html) yields the GHS-R1a gene for the green anole (*Anolis carolinensis*) and painted turtle (*Chrysemys picta bellii*). Very recently, massive numbers of partial nucleotide sequences (approximately 450-bp encoding a 150-AA protein) of GHS-R have been registered for 124 species of *Squamata*, including snakes and Iguanidae, by Wiens et al. (98) at Stony Brook University in the NCBI database. In birds, GHS-Rs have been found in five species.

STRUCTURAL FEATURES OF THE GHRELIN RECEPTOR IN NON-MAMMALIAN VERTEBRATES

Three features are prominent in non-mammalian GHS-Rs: (1) the presence of paralogs in a few species of teleosts; (2) two isoforms, GHS-Ra and GHS-R1a-LR; and (3) avian-specific alternative splice forms of GHS-R (**Figure 1**). Further details are provided below (see also Classification and Nomenclature of Ghrelin Receptors).

PRESENCE OF PARALOGS IN ONLY A FEW SPECIES OF TELEOSTS

The GHS-Ra paralog GHS-R2a is found only in a limited number of teleosts, and little is known about the presence of GHS-R paralogs in other vertebrates. GHS-R2a has an AA sequence that is approximately 70% identical to that of GHS-R1a. At present, this receptor has been identified in Cypriniformes such as goldfish, zebrafish, and carp, and in channel catfish in the order Siluriformes

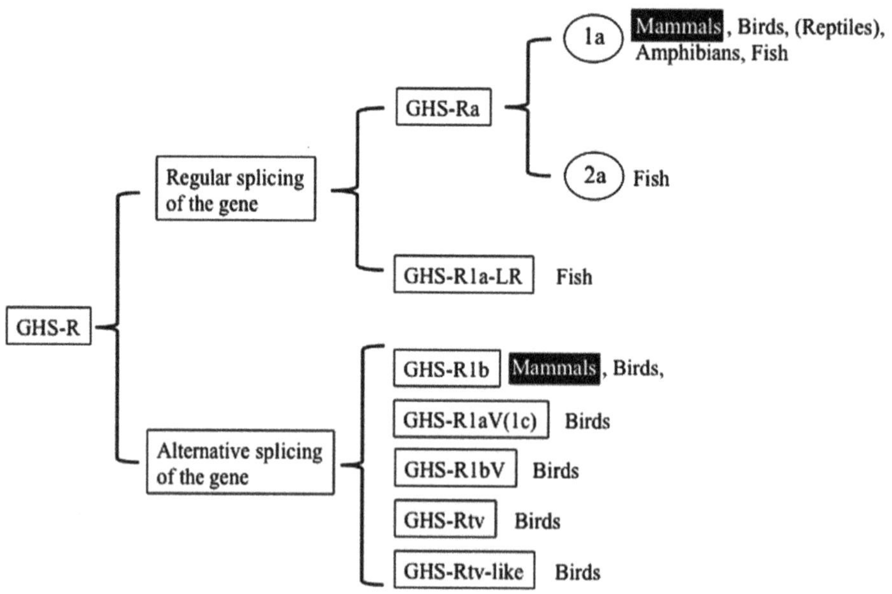

FIGURE 1 | Classification of ghrelin receptors. Receptors that exist in mammals are highlighted.

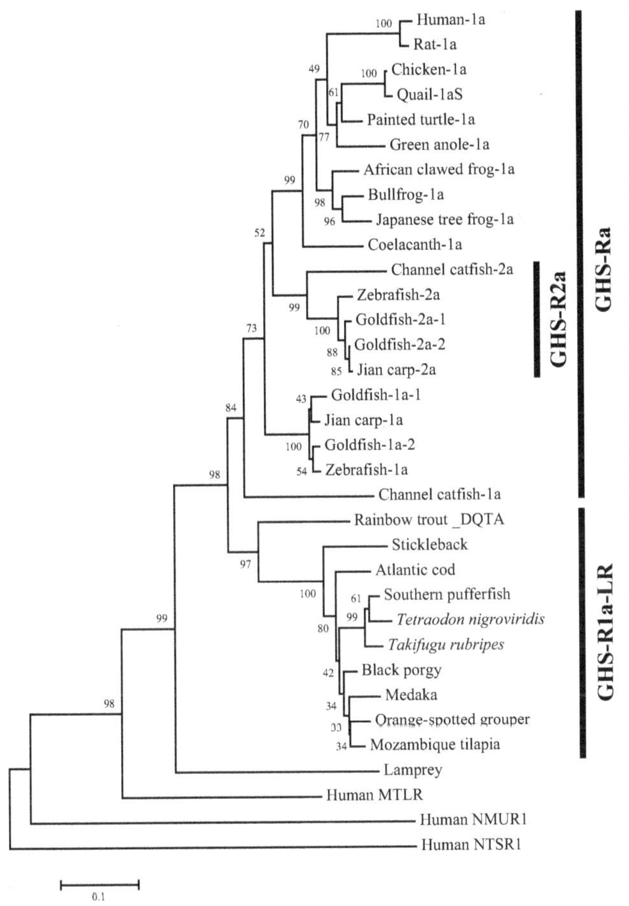

FIGURE 2 | Phylogenetic tree of GHS-Ra and GHS-R1a-LR in non-mammalian vertebrates. The phylogenetic tree was constructed by using the neighbor-joining method with MEGA4 (http://www.megasoftware.net/). The numbers on the branch points are the bootstrap values (as percentages based on 2000 replicates). The scale bar indicates the average number of substitutions per position (a relative measure of evolutionary distance). Receptors for human motilin (MTLR), neuromedin-U (NMUR1), and neurotensin (NTSR1) were used as the outgroup.

(**Figures 2** and **3**). The two isoforms are encoded by different genes (i.e., the zebrafish GHS-R1a and 2a genes are located separately on chromosomes 4 and 24, respectively), which are considered to have diverged via the third round of whole-genome duplication (3R-WGD) that occurred in the ray-finned fish lineage (20, 21).

In addition, isoforms with approximately 95% identity have been found in goldfish (Cypriniformes) and rainbow trout (Salmoniformes). In goldfish, there are two paralogs each for GHS-R1a and 2a: GHS-R1a-1, 1a-2, 2a-1, and 2a-2 (**Figures 2, 3**, and **5**). Each receptor originated from a separate gene demonstrated to have a different intron sequence (22). In the rainbow trout, two paralogous sequences, namely the DQTA/LN-type and ERAT/IS-type, have been identified (23) (**Figure 3**). Their names indicate AA substitutions at D20E, Q32R, T54A, A62T, L168I, and N264S. These two receptor sequences are known to be derived from at least three distinct genes (the DQTA/LN-type derives from two genes and the ERAT/IS-type originates from one gene), on the basis of analyses of an intron sequence of each receptor (23). These paralogs of goldfish and rainbow trout are considered to have originated from polyploidization events that occurred after 3R-WGD (24) and tandem duplication of the genes, which also affected the opsin gene in these species (25). The presence of multiple paralogs may be a peculiar characteristic of *Ostariophysi* and *Protacanthopterygii* in euteleosts (20, 21).

TWO GHRELIN RECEPTOR ISOFORMS: GHS-Ra AND GHS-R1a-LR

As shown in **Figure 1**, there are two isoforms in non-mammalian vertebrates: GHS-Ra and GHS-R1a-LR. GHS-Ra includes GHS-R1a and 2a. Tetrapods including mammals, birds, reptiles, and amphibians have GHS-R1a, whereas some bony fish such as Coelacanthiformes, Cypriniformes (e.g., goldfish, carp, and zebrafish), and Siluriformes (e.g., channel catfish) have both GHS-R1a and 2a. GHS-R1a-LRs show considerable AA identity to GHS-R1a, but have a unique structural feature not found in any tetrapod: the second extracellular loop (ECL2) that connects TMD 4 and 5 is notably longer than that of GHS-R1a (**Figure 4**). In addition, GHS-R1a-LRs have the characteristic that ghrelin or GHS treatment either does not increase intracellular Ca^{2+} (23, 26) or requires pharmacological doses to activate the receptor (27, 28). This type of receptor is seen in a limited number of fish classified as Percomorpha within the superorder *Acanthopterygii*, which is the most evolutionally advanced group of teleosts, including Perciformes such as black porgy and tilapia, Gasterosteiformes such as stickleback and medaka, Tetraodontiformes such as pufferfish, and Salmoniformes such as rainbow trout (**Figure 3**). An exception is the orange-spotted grouper, which belongs to Perciformes but has an ECL2 that is not long (**Figure 3**). These species have some morphological characteristics such as a highly mobilized upper jaw, a respiratory tract not linked to the swim bladder, and a splinter article in their fins. Salmoniformes belong to *Protacanthopterygii*, which contains a number of moderately advanced teleosts. This evolutionary background may be reflected in the molecular evolution and structure of the ghrelin receptor.

A partial sequence similar to that of the ghrelin receptor was found in a database for the sea lamprey (*Petromyzon marinus*). This receptor could not be placed at the branch of GHS-Ra or GHS-R1a-LR in the phylogenetic analysis (**Figure 2**). The sea lamprey belongs to the group Cyclostomata in the class Agnatha, which is a class of fish with the characteristics of ancient basal vertebrates. Therefore, the receptor in the sea lamprey may contain ancestral characteristics of the ghrelin receptor.

AVIAN-SPECIFIC GHS-Rs

Birds have specific alternative spliced forms of GHS-R other than GHS-R1b, i.e., 1aV (or 1c), 1bV, tv, and tv-like receptor (29–32), which are generated by differential modes of splicing from GHS-R1b. GHS-R1aV (30) and GHS-R1c (29) are identical receptors found in chickens. Here, "V" is considered to mean "variant" (30), whereas Geelissen et al. (29) used the designation "c" to indicate an isoform different from "a" or "b." We proposed that GHS-R1c should be referred to as GHS-R1aV because the receptor is identical to GHS-R1a with the exception that it lacks

Table 1 | Ghrelin receptor and ghrelin receptor-like receptor in fish.

Species	Name	type	Accession number	cDNA length (bp)	Number of amino acids	Reference	Remarks
FISH							
Salmo salar	Atlantic salmon	1a	GQ373171	669	220	(65)	Partial sequence
		1b		303	100	(65)	Partial sequence
Acanthopagrus schlegelii	Black porgy	1a	AY151040	1723	385	(28)	
		1b	AY151041	1821	295	(28)	
		GHS-R1 gene	AY151041	1821	-	(28)	
		5′-Flanking region	AY509196	2157	-	(68)	
Ictalurus punctatus	Channel catfish	1a	FJ707319	1632	344	(39)	
		2a	FJ707321	1490	362	(39)	
		1b	FJ707320	1877	307	(39)	
Carassius auratus	Goldfish	1a-1	AB504275	1083	360	(22)	
		1a-2	AB504276	1083	360	(22)	
		2a-1	AB504277	1104	366	(22)	
		2a-2	AB504278	1101	367	(22)	
		GHS-R1-1 gene	AB555555	1722	-	(22)	
		GHS-R1-2 gene	AB555556	2059	-	(22)	
		GHS-R2-1 gene	AB555557	2012	-	(22)	
		GHS-R2-2 gene	AB555558	2859	-	(22)	
Oreochromis mossambicus	Mozambique tilapia	1a-LR	AB361053	1584	384	(23)	
		1a-LR	EU334002	1627	384	(96) (direct submission)	
		GHS-R1-LR gene	AB361055	1815	-	(23)	
		GHS-R1-LR gene	EU910220	3253	-	(97) (direct submission)	
		1b	AB361054, EU334003	897; 1858	298	(23, 96) (direct submission)	
Oreochromis niloticus	Nile tilapia	1a-LR	ENSONIT000 00001069	1158	384	Ensembl Genome Browser	
Oreochromis urolepis	Wami tilapia	1a-LR	EU243664	1646	384	(96) (direct submission)	
		Promotor region	FJ217700	1619		(97) (direct submission)	
		1b	EU243665	1877	298	(96) (direct submission)	
Epinephelus coioides	Orange-spotted grouper	1a-LR	Not deposited	1512	383	(45)	
		1b	Not deposited	1703	303	(45)	
Spheroides nephelus	Pufferfish	78B8 gene	AF082209	1455	374; 313	(27)	
		1b?	AF082209				
Tetraodon nigroviridis	Pufferfish	1a-LR gene	ENSTNIG00000 006665		394	Ensembl Genome Browser	
Takifugu rubripes	Japanese pufferfish	1a-LR			377	Fugu genome project (http://genome.jgi-psf.org/)	
Oncorhynchus mykiss	Rainbow trout	1a-LR (DQTA/LN-rype)	AB362479	1673	387	(23)	
		1a-LR (ERAT/IS-type)	AB362480	1164	387	(23)	
		1b (DQTA/LN-rype)	AB362481	2234	297	(23)	
		1b (DQTA/LN-rype), gene	AB479381		300	(23)	
		1b (ERAT/IS-type), gene	AB362482	1688	297	(23)	

(Continued)

Table 1 | Continued

Species	Name	type	Accession number	cDNA length (bp)	Number of amino acids	Reference	Remarks
Danio rerio	Zebrafish	1a	NM_001146272	1803	360	(93)	
		2a	XM_002666671	1098	365	(16)	
Gadus morhua	Atlantic cod	1a-LR	ENSGNOT000 00014265		377	Ensembl Genome Browser	
Latimeria chalumnae	Coelacanth	1a-LR	ENSLACT000 00015868		363	Ensembl Genome Browser	
Petromyzon marinus	Sea lamprey	1a-LR	ENSMAT000 00007290		344	Ensembl Genome Browser	
Oryzias latipes	Japanese medaka	1a-LR	ENSORLT000 00014679		384	Ensembl Genome Browser	
Xiphophorus maculatus	Southern platyfish	1a-LR	ENSFM005 00000270343		383	Ensembl Genome Browser	
Gasterosteus aculeatus	Three-spined stickleback	1a-LR	ENSGAT000000 14515		381	Ensembl Genome Browser	
Cyprinus carpio jian	Jian carp	1a	HM191491	1083	360	(99) (direct submission)	
		1b	HM191493	1083	360	(99) (direct submission)	
		1a′	HM191492	892	184	(99) (direct submission)	
		1b′	HM191494	892	184	(99) (direct submission)	
		GHS-R1a gene	HM191495	2789		(99) (direct submission)	
		GHS-R2a gene	HQ162474	2064		(99) (direct submission)	
		GHS-R2b gene	HQ162475	2129		(99) (direct submission)	
Cyprinus carpio	Common carp	1b	JN392468	1968	360	(100) (direct submission)	

NCBI (http://www.ncbi.nlm.nih.gov/); NCBI genome database (http://www.ncbi.nlm.nih.gov/genome/); Ensembl Genome Browser (http://www.ensembl.org/index.html).

16 AAs (46 bp) in TMD 6 (16). GHS-R1bV is found in quail. Its C-terminal part differs from that of GHS-R1b, and an AA sequence that differs from 1b is translated from the intermediate intron by a frame-shift due to an 8-bp deletion of the intermediate intron of *ghsr*. GHS-Rtv is found in chickens (31). The signature "tv" was first used by Sirotkin et al. (31), although its meaning is unclear. The composition of GHS-Rtv is complex: two distinct parts of the intermediate intron sequence of *ghsr* lie between the exon 1 and exon 2 sequences of GHS-R1a [see Ref. (33)]. Kitazawa et al. (32) reported a receptor similar to chicken GHS-Rtv in the Japanese quail. Because the composition was different from that of GHS-Rtv, it was designated as a GHS-Rtv-like receptor and considered to be a possible ortholog of GHS-Rtv. The functions of these avian variants are completely unknown.

Kitazawa et al. (32) reported five isoforms of GHS-Rs in the Japanese quail: GHS-R1a-L, 1a-S, 1aV-L, 1b-L, and 1bV-L. The "L" and "S" appended to GHS-R1a signify the long-type (354 AAs) and short-type (347 AAs) receptors for GHS-R1a, respectively. GHS-R1a-S is a receptor that lacks 7 AAs at the N-terminus of GHS-R1a-L. Two ATG initiation codons are present in the cDNA and the functional codon is unknown.

TISSUE EXPRESSION OF GHRELIN RECEPTOR mRNAs AND THEIR ISOFORMS

EXPRESSION OF GHS-Ra AND GHS-R1a-LR

In agreement with a wide range of physiological functions of ghrelin, GHS-R1a transcripts have been detected in human tissues such as the brain, heart, lung, liver, kidney, pancreas, stomach, intestines, and adipose tissue (34, 35). In particular, high expression levels have been detected in the pituitary gland (36), which is consistent with the role of ghrelin in regulating GH release. In the brain, where expression levels are relatively high, GHS-R1a mRNA is widely distributed in regions linked to energy homeostasis such as the arcuate nuclei of the hypothalamus; area postrema; nucleus of the solitary tract; the dorsal motor nucleus of the vagus; hippocampus; dopaminergic neurons in the ventral tegmental area and substantia nigra; parasympathetic preganglionic neurons; the dorsal and medial raphe nuclei; and the dentate gyrus (9, 34, 37, 38).

In non-mammalian vertebrates, GHS-R1a or GHS-R1a-LR transcripts have been found in the central nervous system and various peripheral organs. As in humans, predominant expression occurs in the pituitary in channel catfish (39), chickens (29, 30, 40–43), and ducks (44) for GHS-R1a, as well as in the black porgy (28), orange-spotted grouper (45), and rainbow trout (23)

Table 2 | Ghrelin receptor and ghrelin receptor-like receptor in reptiles, amphibians, and aves.

Species	Name	type	Accession number	cDNA length (bp)	Number of amino acids	Reference	Remarks
REPTILES							
Anolis carolinensis	Green anole	1a	XM_003218148	1038	345		
Chrysemys picta bellii	Western painted turtle	1a	JH584696		358	Ensembl Genome Browser	
124 Species of *Squamata*		1a	JN880998–JN881119				Partial sequence
AMPHIBIAN							
Rana caiesbeiana	Bullfrog	1a	AB626731	1125	374	(19)	
Hylajaponica	Japanese tree frog	1a	AB626732	1116	371	(19)	
Xenopus tropicalis	Tropical clawed toad	1a	XM_002931572	1080	359	NCBI genome database	
AVES							
Gallus gallus	Chicken	1a	NM_204394	1699	347	(29, 30)	
		GHS-R1 gene	AB095994	4121	–	(30)	
		1aV	AB095996	1703	331	(30)	
		1b	AB095997	1351	276	(30)	
		1c	AJ309543	646	215	(29)	Partial sequence
		tv	Not deposited			(31, 33)	
Anas platyrhynchos	Mallard	1a gene	FJ194548	3717	245	(44)	Partial sequence
Coturnix japonica	Japanese quail	1a-L	AB469019	1308	354	(32)	
		1a-S	AB469019	1287	347	(32)	
		1aV-L	AB469020	1260	338	(32)	
		1b-L	AB469022	909	302	(32)	
		1bV-L	AB469021	930	309	(32)	
		tv-like	AB490327	2661	251	(32)	Partial sequence
Meleagris gallopavo	Turkey	1a	NW_003435736	3965	473	NCBI genome database	Partial sequence
Taeniopygia guttata	Zebra finch	1a	XM_002193702	864	287	NCBI genome database	Partial sequence

NCBI (http://www.ncbi.nlm.nih.gov/); NCBI genome database (http://www.ncbi.nlm.nih.gov/genome/); Ensembl Genome Browser (http://wwwensembl.org/index.html).

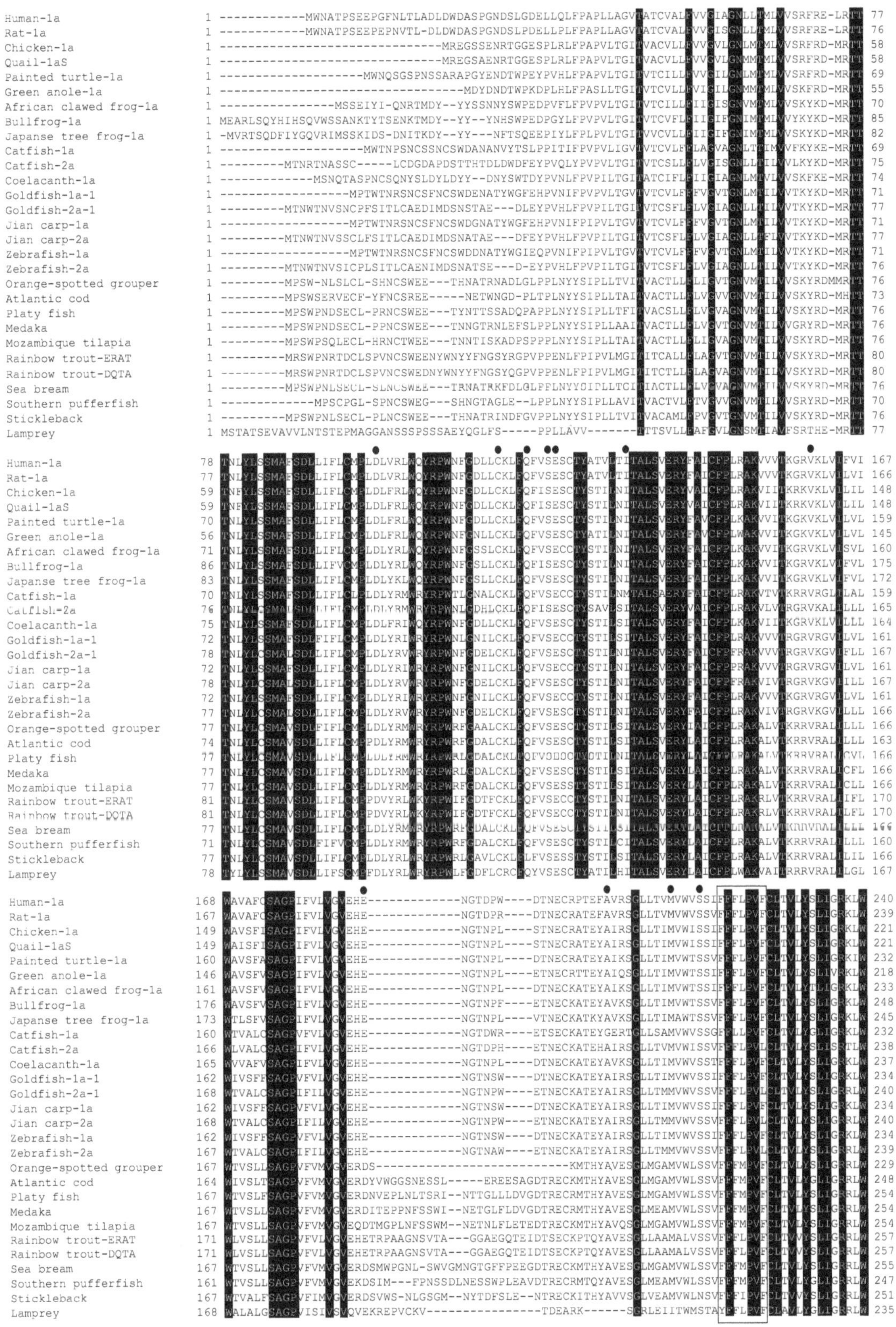

FIGURE 3 | Continued

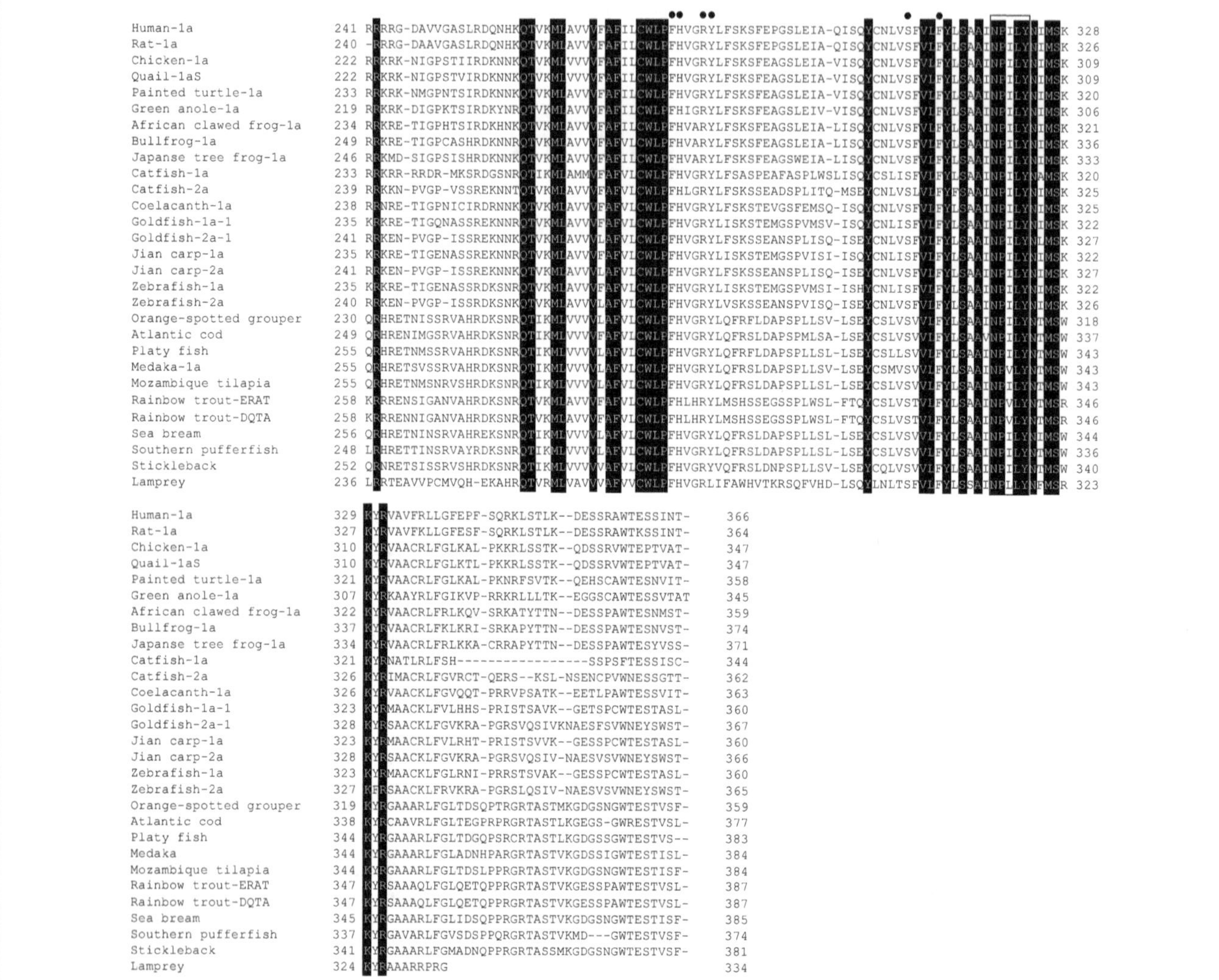

FIGURE 3 | GHS-R1a, 2a and GHS-R1a-LR proteins in non-mammalian vertebrates. Dense shading indicates common amino acids (AAs) in all species. Red letters under black circles represent specific AAs related to ligand binding, selectivity, and constitutive activity of GHS-R1a and 2a. Boxes show the typical motifs of the G-protein-coupled receptor transmembrane domains 5 and 7. Sequences were aligned using GENETYX-Mac version 15.0.1.

for GHS-R1a-LR. However, expression in the pituitary gland is not dominant in all species. In Mozambique tilapia, GHS-R1a-LR mRNA is mainly detected in the brain. The distribution of the ghrelin receptor in other tissues also differs among animal species.

In fish, GHS-R transcripts have been detected in most organs. The genes are expressed in all regions of the brain, including the olfactory bulbs and tracts, telencephalon, diencephalon, optic tectum, vagal lobe, hypothalamus, cerebellum and medulla, and spinal cord. Gene expression has also been detected in the eyes, heart, thymus, liver, stomach, intestine, spleen, gill, gall bladder, muscle, kidney, head kidney, Brockmann bodies, skin, muscle, and gonads (23, 26, 28, 39, 45, 46). In rainbow trout, GHS-R1a-LR mRNA expression has been detected in blood leukocytes and head kidney leukocytes (47). Cypriniformes such as goldfish and zebrafish, as well as Siluriformes such as channel catfish, possess paralogs of GHS-Ra, each of which has different levels and patterns of expression (22, 39, 46).

In amphibians, strong GHS-R1a mRNA expression has been found in brain regions such as the diencephalon and mesencephalon; the stomach and testis; and to a lesser extent in the small and large intestines, adrenal gland, and kidney in the bullfrog (19). In the Japanese tree frog, GHS-R1a transcripts have been detected in almost all tissues examined, although relatively high expression was detected in the duodenum, small and large intestines, and ovary. However, unlike in other animals, pituitary expression was absent in both species (19).

In birds, GHS-R1a mRNA has also been detected in almost all tissues examined. GHS-R1a mRNA is expressed in chicken tissues such as the hypothalamus, telencephalon, cerebrum, cerebellum, optic lobes, brainstem, heart, lung, thymus, liver, spleen, pancreas, proventriculus, gizzard, duodenum, adrenal gland, kidney, gonads, breast muscle, subcutaneous fat, leg muscle, abdominal fat, and uropygial gland (29, 30, 40, 41, 44). Comparing the relative expression levels in these tissues is difficult; nonetheless,

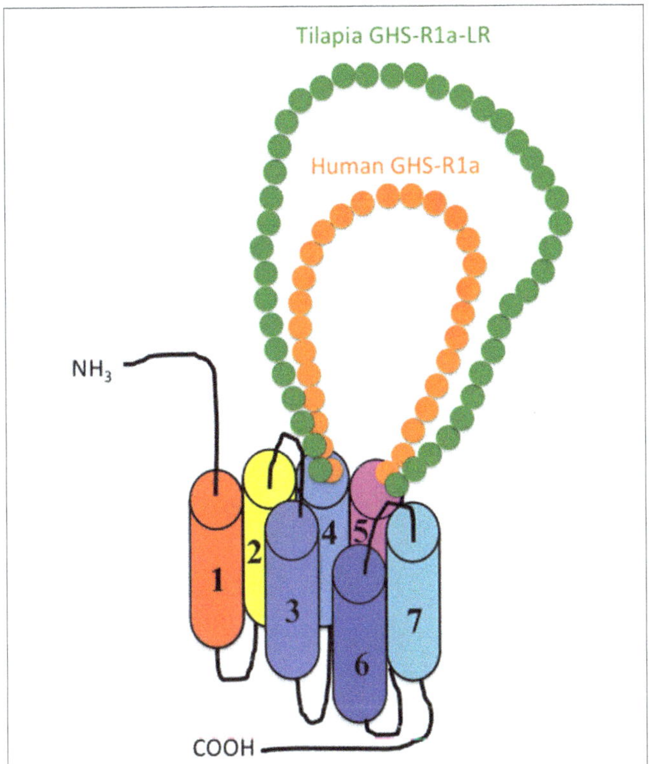

FIGURE 4 | Schematic diagram of the second extracellular loop (ECL2) in the GHS-R1a and GHS-R1a-like receptors. Human GHS-R1a, which has a short ECL2 (orange), and tilapia GHS-R1a-like receptor (GHS-R1a-LR), which has a long ECL2 (green), are shown as representative examples. The length of ECL2 in human GHS-R1a is 28 amino acids (AAs), whereas the ECL2 in tilapia GHS-R1a-LR is 43 AAs. Each receptor is classified in a different branch of the phylogenetic tree (**Figure 2**). GHS-Ra, which includes GHS-R1a or 2a, is found in tetrapods including chickens (birds), mammals, reptiles, and amphibians, as well as some bony fishes such as Coelacanthiformes, Cypriniformes (e.g., goldfish, carp, and zebrafish), and Siluriformes (channel catfish). These animal species have the receptor with the short ECL2. In contrast, GHS-R1a-LR is found only in a fish group that includes Perciformes such as tilapia, Gasterosteiformes such as stickleback and medaka, Tetraodontiformes such as pufferfish, and Salmoniformes such as rainbow trout.

the expression levels in the brain, gastrointestinal tract, liver, and spleen appear to be relatively high compared with other tissues, although strain differences may exist (29, 30, 33). In ducks, mRNA expression has been detected in the subcutaneous fat, hypothalamus, small intestine, testis, cerebellum, and cerebrum (44). In the Japanese quail, GHS-R1a mRNA expression was examined only in the gastrointestinal tract (32), where region-specific expression was detected at relatively high levels in the upper and lower intestines such as the esophagus, crop, and colon, but weak levels in the middle portions of the gastrointestinal tract (e.g., the proventriculus, duodenum, gizzard, jejunum, and ileum).

EXPRESSION OF GHRELIN RECEPTOR ISOFORMS OTHER THAN GHS-Ra AND GHS-R1a-LR

Growth hormone secretagogue-receptor type-1b is a splice variant of the mammalian GHS-R. In humans, its mRNA distribution is more widespread than that of GHS-R1a, and varies spatially and quantitatively from that of GHS-R1a (34). This suggests the possibility that GHS-R1b is involved in specific GHS-R1a-independent physiological activities, although these remain unknown.

In non-mammalian vertebrates, there are a few reports on the mRNA distribution of GHS-R1b. First, GHS-R1b mRNA has been detected in the brain of fish. In the black porgy, the level of expression was highest in the telencephalon, followed by the hypothalamus, pituitary, optic tectum, thalamus, and spinal cord, whereas little was detected in peripheral tissues (28). In Mozambique tilapia, the brain is the site with the highest expression of GHS-R1b mRNA, although transcripts were also detected in the stomach, adipose tissue, gill, liver, intestine, spleen, kidney, and muscle (26). In orange-spotted grouper, the expression levels of GHS-R1b mRNA were high in the pituitary, hypothalamus, cerebellum, medulla, spinal cord, gill filament, spleen, liver, stomach, head kidney, kidney, gonad, red muscle, skin, and fat body (45). In rainbow trout, GHS-R1b mRNA was strongly expressed in the pituitary, whereas weak expression was observed in the hypothalamus, pyloric appendage, middle intestine, spleen, and head kidney (23). In channel catfish, the expression level of GHS-R1b mRNA was highest in the pituitary, but it was approximately 400 times lower in most peripheral tissues compared with the expression level of GHS-R1a (39).

In birds, GHS-R1aV or GHS-Rtv mRNA expression was detected in almost all tissues examined, a pattern almost identical to that of GHS-R1a mRNA expression, although expression levels of each isoform differed (29, 30, 33). GHS-Rtv transcripts were first detected in chicken ovaries (31). In Japanese quail, the expression of the GHS-Rtv-like receptor was detected in the gastrointestinal tract but only in the proventriculus and gizzard (32). The function of these avian variants is entirely unknown.

REGULATION OF GHRELIN RECEPTOR EXPRESSION

Satiation and hunger signals regulate *ghsr* expression. A condition of negative energy balance such as fasting increases GHS-R1a mRNA expression in the hypothalamus and pituitary of rats, while re-feeding restores the increased expression level to a normal level (48, 49). The gene expression of *ghsr* is affected by various hormonal factors, it is stimulated by ghrelin (5, 49–51), GH-releasing hormone (GHRH) (52), thyroid hormone (53), and glucocorticoid (dexamethasone) (54, 55). In contrast, it is inhibited by GH (56–58), leptin (49), glucocorticoid (50), and insulin-like growth factor-I (IGF-I) (59). These are summarized in **Table 3**.

Acute or chronic changes in the energy status or environmental conditions appear to have varying effects on *ghsr* expression in non-mammalian vertebrates (**Table 3**). In Mozambique tilapia, GHS-R1a-LR mRNA levels in the brain are unaffected by fasting, whereas GHS-R1b mRNA expression is increased (60). Peddu et al. (61) reported acute pre- and post-prandial changes in GHS-R1a-LR and GHS-R1b mRNA expression, whereas pre-GHS-R mRNA levels (immature mRNA, hetero-nuclear RNA) did not reflect changes in feeding status. Riley et al. (62) showed that acute increased blood glucose reduced GHS-R1a-LR mRNA levels in the brain and increased gastric ghrelin mRNA expression as well as plasma ghrelin levels. This change in plasma ghrelin levels is

Table 3 | Regulation of ghrelin receptor expression.

Stimulus	Animals (organs)	Receptor, regulation	Reference
Food deprivation	Rats (hypothalamus, pituitary)	1a, ↑	(48, 49)
GHRH	Rats (pituitary)	1a, ↑	(52)
TH	Rats (pituitary)	1a, ↑	(53)
Dexametasone	Rats (hypothalamus, pituitary)	1a, ↑	(54, 55)
L-692,585	Rats (pituitary)	1a, ↓	(52)
GH	Rats (hypothalamus, pituitary)	1a, ↓	(56–58)
Leptin	Rats (hypothalamus)	1a, ↓	(49)
Adrenalectomy	Rats (hypothalamus, pituitary)	1a, ↓	(54, 55)
Glucocorticoids	Humans (recombinant receptor in GH3 cell)	1a, ↓	(50)
IGF-I	Rats (hypothalamus)	1a, ↓	(59)
Food deprivation	Tilapia (brain)	1a-LR, → 1b, ↑ Pre-GHS-R, →	(60)
Pre-prandial Post-prandial	Tilapia (brain)	1a-LR, ↑ 1a-LR, ↓	(60)
Glucose loading	Tilapia (brain)	la-LR, ↓	(62)
14-days starvation	Atlantic salmon (brain)	la-LR, →	(65)
7-days starvation	Goldfish (vagal lobe)	1a-1, ↓ 1a-2, ↓	(22)
10-days starvation	Bullfrog (stomach, ventral skin)	1a, ↑	(19)
10-days dehydration	Japanese tree frog (brain stomach, ventral skin)	1a, ↑	
Catfish GHRL-Gly	Channel catfish (pituitary)	1a, ↑ 2a, →	(39)
	Channel catfish (Brockman bodies)	2a, ↑	
Catfish GHRL-amide	Channel catfish (pituitary)	1a, → 2a, →	
	Channel catfish (Brockman bodies)	2a, ↑	
Goldfish GHRL 12-amide	Zebrafish (brain)	1a, ↑ 2a, ↑	(46)
Rat ghrelin	Orange-spotted grouper (hypothalamus, pituitary)	1a-LR, ↓ 1b, ↓	(45)
Chiken ghrelin	Chickens (pituitary)	1a,↓ 1aV, ↓	(29)
GHRP-6	Black porgy (recombinant in HEK293)	1a-LR, ↑	(68)
Sea bream GH	Orange-spotted grouper (hypothalamus)	1a-LR, →	(45)
	Orange-spotted grouper (pituitary)	1a-LR, ↓	
	Orange-spotted grouper (hypothalamus, pituitary)	1b, ↓	
Bovine GH	Chickens (pituitary)	1a, ↓ 1aV, ↓	(29)
Corticosterone	Chickens (pituitary)	1a, ↓ 1aV, ↓	(29)
Human GHRH 1-29	Chickens (pituitary)	1a, ↓ 1aV, →	(29)

the opposite of that seen in humans or goldfish, where a glucose load decreases plasma ghrelin levels (63, 64). In conditions of chronic negative energy balance, there was no change in the GHS-R1a-LR expression levels in the brains of Atlantic salmon fasted for 14 days (65). In contrast, goldfish GHS-R1a-1 mRNA levels decreased in the vagal lobe and GHS-R1a-2 mRNA levels increased in the liver after 7 days of fasting (22). In bullfrogs, GHS-R1a mRNA expression was up-regulated in the stomach and ventral skin, whereas that in the brain did not change after 10 days of starvation (19). These results suggest that the nutritional condition of the body affects ghrelin receptor expression. Furthermore, GHS-R1a mRNA expression was up-regulated in the brain, stomach, and ventral skin after 10 days of dehydration of tree frog (19). This result may support the view that ghrelin is involved in the regulation of water balance in frogs, as seen in rats (66) and chicks (67).

Hormonal control of *ghsr* expression has been reported. Ghrelin appears to have a stimulatory effect on *ghsr* expression in non-mammalian vertebrates, as it does in mammals. However, the effects differ depending on the ghrelin form, receptor isoform, and target tissue. In channel catfish, the C-terminal structure of ghrelin affects *ghsr* expression (39). In the pituitary, catfish ghrelin-Gly (this is naturally occurring 23-AA ghrelin where Gly is extended at the C-terminus) increased the levels of GHS-R1a mRNA but not of GHS-R2a mRNA. In contrast, catfish ghrelin-amide (22-AA ghrelin with an amide structure at the C-terminus) had no effect on either receptor. In the Brockmann bodies, catfish ghrelin-amide or ghrelin-Gly dramatically increased the GHS-R2a mRNA expression levels with different time courses. In zebrafish, goldfish ghrelin12-amide stimulated the mRNA expression of both GHS-R1a and 2a in the brain, but with different time courses (46). In orange-spotted grouper, rat ghrelin (10^{-5} M) inhibited the expression of GHS-R1a-LR and GHS-R1b mRNA in the hypothalamus and pituitary (45). In chickens, Geelissen et al. (29) reported that ghrelin down-regulated GHS-R1a and GHS-R1aV mRNA expression in the pituitary *in vitro*. In another *in vitro* study, GHRP-6 stimulated the promoter activity of black porgy GHS-R1a-LR expressed in HEK293 cells (68).

The effects of GH or glucocorticoids on non-mammalian *ghsr* expression also vary depending on the GH species used, target tissue, and GHS-R isoform. In orange-spotted grouper, sea bream GH (10^{-7} M) did not affect GHS-R1a-LR levels in the hypothalamus but reduced them in the pituitary, whereas it decreased GHS-R1b mRNA levels in both the hypothalamus and pituitary (45). In chickens, bovine GH and corticosterone decreased mRNA expression of both GHS-R1a and GHS-R1aV, but human GHRH1-29 reduced only GHS-R1a mRNA expression in the pituitary *in vitro* (29).

Yeung et al. (68) analyzed the 5′-flanking region of *ghsr* in black porgy and identified a number of putative binding sites for transcription factors such as AP1, NF-1, Oct-1, and USF. Changes in *ghsr* expression during embryogenesis have been reported in orange-spotted grouper (45) and channel catfish (39). In both species, *ghsr* expression fluctuates depending on the embryonic stage, and the expression levels of GHS-R isoforms are separately regulated.

SIGNALING PATHWAYS OF THE GHRELIN RECEPTOR

Howard et al. (3) observed increases in intracellular Ca^{2+} levels in cells transfected with GHS-R1a. The intracellular signaling of GHS-R1a is mediated by the activation of a G-protein subtype, $G\alpha_{q/11}$, which induces the production of inositol triphosphate (IP3), release of Ca^{2+}, and activation of protein kinase C (PKC) (69). These events are seen in cells transfected with GHS-R1a as well as in somatotrophs (70–74).

In addition, GHS-R1a functions in an agonist-independent manner and causes high basal IP3 production in the absence of agonists, indicating that GHS-R1a is a constitutively active receptor (71, 74, 75). This activity in turn triggers phospholipase C (PLC)–PKC-dependent Ca^{2+} mobilization, which is associated with the L-type voltage-gated calcium channel via PKC. Furthermore, extracellular signal-regulated kinase 1 and 2 (ERK1/2) are activated by GHRP-6. A GHS-R antagonist (D-Lys3)-GHRP-6, was shown to inhibit basal PLC and ERK1/2 activity (76).

When a non-mammalian ghrelin receptor was expressed in mammalian cells, a rise in intracellular Ca^{2+} was observed with ghrelin or GHSs (19, 22, 27, 28, 32, 77, 78). A similar Ca^{2+} mobilization was also induced by ghrelin in the primary culture of goldfish pituitary cells (79, 80), which was important for inducing the release of GH and luteinizing hormone (LH) from goldfish somatotrophs (79) and gonadotrophs (80), respectively. Little is known about the intracellular signaling pathways involved.

In addition to binding ghrelin, non-mammalian ghrelin receptors are capable of binding GHSs such as GHRP-2 and GHRP-6; ipamorelin; and L163,255, L692,585, and L163,540, although the agonistic activity varies according to the receptor present in each animal (19, 22, 27, 28, 32, 77). In addition, a GHS-R1a antagonist (D-Lys3)-GHRP-6, is also capable of inhibiting ghrelin binding to the receptor (22). These results indicate that the structural interactions between the ligand and the AAs of the receptor essential for ligand binding and receptor activation are conserved among vertebrates. However, ligand selectivity has been found in the case of GHRP-6 and hexarelin for goldfish GHS-R1a-1, 1a-2, and 2a-2 (**Figure 5**) (22).

In fish-specific GHS-R1a-LRs, particularly of the pufferfish and black porgy, pharmacological doses of receptor agonists are required in some cases to activate the receptors (27, 28), whereas no reaction was found at all in the receptors in tilapia and rainbow trout, even with homologous ghrelin (23, 26). The reason behind this phenomenon remains to be elucidated.

Receptor functionality has not been examined in the African clawed frog or teleosts such as channel catfish, zebrafish, and Jian carp where GHS-Ra has been identified. We expect that these receptors will be responsive to ghrelin or GHS because of their structural properties, such as the short ECL2 loop (**Figure 4**). However, confirmation of these receptor activities will be required to test this hypothesis in the future.

KEY AMINO ACIDS RELATED TO LIGAND SELECTIVITY AND RECEPTOR FUNCTIONALITY IN THE GHRELIN RECEPTOR STRUCTURE

Feighner et al. (81) reported key AAs that play essential roles in GHS-R1a activation on the basis of the structure of human GHS-R1a and three types of GHSs with different structures, i.e., MK-0677, GHRP-6, and L692,585. Their results showed that D99, C116, E124, M213, S217, and H280 in human GHS-R1a have crucial roles in receptor activation. In particular, M213 is required for the binding of GHRP-6 and L692,585. S217 and H280 are specifically involved with the binding of GHRP-6. In ghrelin receptors identified in non-mammalian vertebrates, all of the AAs listed

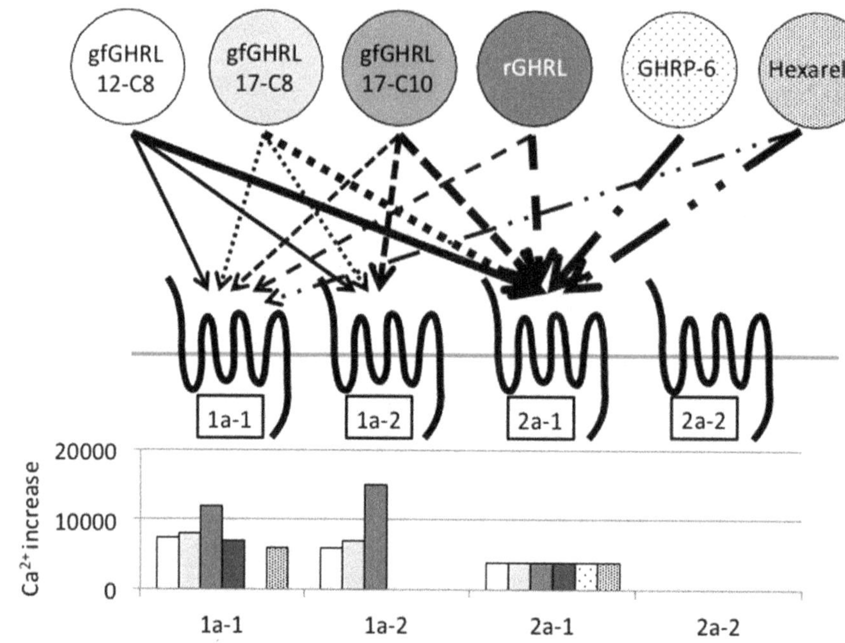

FIGURE 5 | Ligand selectivity and intracellular Ca^{2+} signaling in four goldfish ghrelin receptors. Four goldfish ghrelin receptors exhibited different ligand selectivity. The schematic figures above show the strength of the ligand-receptor affinity based on the thickness of the arrow, while the bar graphs below show the maximum value of the stimulated increase in the intracellular Ca^{2+} signal. Goldfish ghrelin (gfGHRL) 12-C8 (octanoylated ghrelin with 12 amino acids, AAs), 17-C8 (octanoylated ghrelin with 17 AAs), and 17-C10 (decanoylated ghrelin with 17 AAs); rat ghrelin (rGHRL); and two GHSs, GHRP-6 and hexarelin, were used in the experiment. For example, the arrows indicate that the intracellular Ca^{2+} increased in cells expressing GHS-R1a-1 after exposure to gfGHRL12-C8, 17-C8, and 17-C10; rat ghrelin; and hexarelin, but not after exposure to GHRP-6 at a similar dose. The corresponding bar graph shows that gfGHRL17-C10 increased Ca^{2+} much more strongly than the other agonists. Furthermore, although GHS-R2a-2 was capable of binding all of the agonists examined at a low dose, none of the agonists increased the intracellular Ca^{2+} level.

above are conserved, with the exception of an AA that is equivalent to S217 in the stickleback receptor (**Figure 3**). This may suggest that the GHS-Ra and GHS-R1a-LR identified in non-mammalian vertebrates have the ability to bind GHSs. However, as described earlier, goldfish GHS-Ra has ligand selectivity (22). In addition, the GHS-R1a-LR in rainbow trout and tilapia shows no Ca^{2+} response in receptor-expressing mammalian cells (23, 26). Although AAs equivalent to M213, S217, and H280, which are essential for binding of GHRP-6 to the receptor, are all conserved in goldfish GHS-Ra, GHRP-6 does not increase the intracellular Ca^{2+} in HEK 293 cells expressing goldfish GHS-R1a-1 and 1a-2. Thus, the interaction between the ligand and key AAs in the receptor related to ligand binding may be more complicated than anticipated.

Holst et al. (82) found that the ghrelin receptor elicited strong, ligand-independent signaling in transfected COS-7 or HEK293 cells. Independent of ligand selectivity, the relationship between constitutive receptor activity and the AA composition of the receptor has also been examined (83–85). These studies suggest that of the AAs in human GHS-R1a, V160, F279, A204, I134, and A204 are important for controlling constitutive receptor activity (**Figure 3**). These AAs are conserved in the GHS-Ra and GHS-R1a-LR identified in non-mammalian vertebrates (**Figure 3**); therefore, all of them may be constitutively active receptors, although their activity has been confirmed only in the black porgy receptor (86).

PHYSIOLOGICAL FUNCTION OF GHS-Rs

GHS-R1a mediates the information conveyed by ghrelin and elicits its various physiological functions. In addition to its hypophysiotropic effects and regulation of appetite, ghrelin affects many physiological functions, including gastrointestinal motility, cardiovascular performance, cell proliferation, immune function, bone metabolism, sleep, and the promotion of learning and memory (9, 87, 88). Recent evidence suggests that ghrelin functions as a blood glucose regulator (89).

ROLES OF GHS-R1a AND 2a

Growth hormone secretagogue-receptor type-1a or 2a is thought to mediate various physiological functions of ghrelin, although direct evidence in non-mammalian vertebrates remains sparse. Recently, Yahashi et al. (90) reported that the peripheral effects of ghrelin on food intake and locomotor activity in goldfish are mediated via one of the four ghrelin receptor isoforms, GHS-R2a-1. In addition, ghrelin has the ability to stimulate GH and LH release from goldfish pituitary (64, 79, 80, 91). GHS-R1a-2 mRNA shows the most abundant expression in this structure, suggesting that the receptor is involved in the regulation of pituitary hormone release. Changes in GHS-R1a or 2a expression depending on the energy state suggest the involvement of ghrelin in energy homeostasis, as observed in frogs and goldfish (19, 22). However, no change was observed in the case of tilapia (60). In chickens and quails, the distributions of the receptor are consistent with its role in gut contraction (32). However, although the ghrelin receptor is expressed throughout the intestinal tracts of goldfish and rainbow trout, ghrelin has no effects on intestinal motility (92). This result is in contrast to that seen in zebrafish, in which rat and human ghrelin stimulate gut contraction (93). Further studies are necessary to determine the nature of the relationship between ghrelin receptors and physiological function.

ROLES OF GHS-R1b

In contrast with GHS-R1a, little is known about the functions of the GHS-R1b isoform. Mammalian and non-mammalian GHS-R1b show no apparent intracellular Ca^{2+} signaling response to ghrelin or GHSs (32, 86). Co-expression of GHS-R1a and 1b reduces the signaling capacity of GHS-R1a via hetero-dimerization (28, 86, 94), suggesting that GHS-R1b acts as a dominant-negative mutant during signaling via GHS-R1a (86). Intriguingly, GHS-R1b forms heterodimeric associations with other GPCRs such as neurotensin receptor 1 (NTSR1) (95). This heterodimeric receptor binds to peptide hormones other than ghrelin and affects intracellular signaling, i.e., the GHS-R1b/NTSR1 heterodimer binds neuromedin-U and induces cAMP production instead of Ca^{2+} signaling.

Although GHS-R1b exists in the same gene as GHS-R1a, the sites, patterns, levels, and regulation of GHS-R1b expression differ from those of GHS-R1a. Therefore, elucidation of the physiological function of the receptor is awaited.

PERSPECTIVE

In this review, we assembled current knowledge about ghrelin receptors in non-mammalian vertebrates. Many questions remain unanswered because receptor genes have been identified only in a limited number of species. However, the functional importance of the ghrelin system is gradually becoming understood in species where the receptor distribution is clear. Presence of unique GHS-Rs such as GHS-R2a, GHS-R1a-LR, or variants found only in non-mammalian vertebrates are interesting in the divergence of the ghrelin system; therefore, examining the structural relationship and function of non-mammalian GHS-Rs based on comparisons with mammalian GHS-Rs is important for understanding the significance of the ghrelin system in vertebrates. However, the ghrelin system of an animal studied may also need to be considered without preconceptions or making comparisons with mammalian data. Thus, the study of non-mammalian GHS-Rs should be interesting and attract many researchers in the future.

ACKNOWLEDGMENTS

We thank Dr. Christopher A. Loretz (University of Buffalo, Buffalo, NY, USA) for valuable comments on this manuscript. We thank Mrs. Azumi Ooyama for excellent technical assistance. Hiroyuki Kaiya, Mikiya Miyazato, and Kenji Kangawa were supported by a Grant-in-Aid for Scientific Research from the Ministry of Education, Culture, Science, Sports, and Technology (MEXT, KAKENHI) of Japan and by the Takeda Science Foundation.

REFERENCES

1. Tannenbaum GS, Bowers CY. Interactions of growth hormone secretagogues and growth hormone-releasing hormone/somatostatin. *Endocrine* (2001) **14**:21–7. doi:10.1385/ENDO:14:1:021
2. Laferrère B, Abraham C, Russell CD, Bowers CY. Growth hormone releasing peptide-2 (GHRP-2), like ghrelin, increases food intake in healthy men. *J Clin Endocrinol Metab* (2005) **90**:611–4. doi:10.1210/jc.2004-1719
3. Howard AD, Feighner SD, Cully DF, Arena JP, Liberator PA, Rosenblum CI, et al. A receptor in pituitary and hypothalamus that functions in growth hormone release. *Science* (1996) **273**:974–7. doi:10.1126/science.273.5277.974
4. McKee KK, Palyha OC, Feighner SD, Hreniuk DL, Tan CP, Phillips MS, et al. Molecular analysis of rat pituitary and hypothalamic growth hormone secretagogue receptors. *Mol Endocrinol* (1997) **11**:415–23. doi:10.1210/me.11.4.415
5. Petersenn S. Structure and regulation of the growth hormone secretagogue receptor. *Minerva Endocrinol* (2002) **27**:243–56.
6. Kojima M, Hosoda H, Date Y, Nakazato M, Matuso H, Kangawa K. Ghrelin is a growth-hormone-releasing acylated peptide. *Nature* (1999) **402**:656–60. doi:10.1038/45230
7. Großauer J, Kosol S, Schrank E, Zangger K. The peptide hormone ghrelin binds to membrane-mimetics via its octanoyl chain and an adjacent phenylalanine. *Bioorg Med Chem* (2010) **18**:5483–8. doi:10.1016/j.bmc.2010.06.062
8. Hosoda H, Kojima M, Kangawa K. Biological, physiological, and pharmacological aspects of ghrelin. *J Pharmacol Sci* (2006) **100**:398–410. doi:10.1254/jphs.CRJ06002X
9. Chen CY, Asakawa A, Fujimiya M, Lee SD, Inui A. Ghrelin gene products and the regulation of food intake and gut motility. *Pharmacol Rev* (2009) **61**:430–81. doi:10.1124/pr.109.001958
10. Kojima M, Kangawa K. Ghrelin: more than endogenous growth hormone secretagogue. *Ann N Y Acad Sci* (2010) **1200**:140–8. doi:10.1111/j.1749-6632.2010.05516.x
11. Bowers CY, Momany FA, Reynolds GA, Hong A. On the in vitro and in vivo activity of a new synthetic hexapeptide that acts on the pituitary to specifically release growth hormone. *Endocrinology* (1984) **114**:1537–45. doi:10.1210/endo-114-5-1537
12. Geris KL, Hickey GJ, Berghman LR, Visser TJ, Kühn ER, Darras VM. Pituitary and extra-pituitary action sites of the novel nonpeptidyl growth hormone (GH) secretagogue L-692,429 in the chicken. *Gen Comp Endocrinol* (1998) **111**:186–96. doi:10.1006/gcen.1998.7102
13. Geris KL, Hickey GJ, Vanderghote A, Kühn ER, Darras VM. Synthetic growth hormone secretagogues control growth hormone secretion in the chicken at pituitary and hypothalamic levels. *Endocrine* (2001) **14**:67–72. doi:10.1385/ENDO:14:1:067
14. Shepherd BS, Eckert SM, Parhar IS, Vijayan MM, Wakabayashi I, Hirano T, et al. The hexapeptide KP-102 (D-Ala-D-beta-Nal-Ala-Trp-D-Phe-Lys-NH(2)) stimulates growth hormone release in a cichlid fish (*Oreochromis mossambicus*). *J Endocrinol* (2000) **167**:R7–10. doi:10.1677/joe.0.167R007
15. Kaiya H, Kojima M, Hosoda H, Koda A, Yamamoto K, Kitajima Y, et al. Bullfrog ghrelin is modified by *n*-octanoic acid at its third threonine residue. *J Biol Chem* (2001) **276**.40441–8. doi:10.1074/jbc.M105212200
16. Kaiya H, Miyazato M, Kangawa K, Peter RE, Unniappan S. Ghrelin: a multifunctional hormone in non-mammalian vertebrates. *Comp Biochem Physiol A Mol Integr Physiol* (2008) **149**:109–28. doi:10.1016/j.cbpa.2007.12.004
17. Kaiya H, Miyazato M, Kangawa K. Recent advances in the phylogenetic study of ghrelin. *Peptides* (2011) **32**:2155–74. doi:10.1016/j.peptides.2011.04.027
18. Davenport AP, Bonner TI, Foord SM, Harmar AJ, Neubig RR, Pin JP, et al. International Union of Pharmacology. LVI. Ghrelin receptor nomenclature, distribution, and function. *Pharmacol Rev* (2005) **57**:541–6. doi:10.1124/pr.57.4.1
19. Kaiya H, Koizumi Y, Konno N, Yamamoto K, Uchiyama M, Kangawa K, et al. Ghrelin receptor in two species of anuran amphibian, bullfrog (*Rana catesbeiana*), and Japanese tree frog (*Hyla japonica*). *Front Endocrinol (Lausanne)* (2011) **2**:31. doi:10.3389/fendo.2011.00031

20. Meyer A, Schartl M. Gene and genome duplications in vertebrates: the one-to-four (-to-eight in fish) rule and the evolution of novel gene functions. *Curr Opin Cell Biol* (1999) **11**:699–704. doi:10.1016/S0955-0674(99)00039-3
21. Jaillon O, Aury JM, Brunet F, Petit JL, Stange-Thomann N, Mauceli E, et al. Genome duplication in the teleost fish *Tetraodon nigroviridis* reveals the early vertebrate proto-karyotype. *Nature* (2004) **431**:946–57. doi:10.1038/nature03025
22. Kaiya H, Miura T, Matsuda K, Miyazato M, Kangawa K. Two functional growth hormone secretagogue receptor (ghrelin receptor) type 1a and 2a in goldfish, *Carassius auratus*. *Mol Cell Endocrinol* (2010) **327**:25–39. doi:10.1016/j.mce.2010.06.004
23. Kaiya H, Mori T, Miyazato M, Kangawa K. Ghrelin receptor (GHS-R)-like receptor and its genomic organisation in rainbow trout, *Oncorhynchus mykiss*. *Comp Biochem Physiol A Mol Integr Physiol* (2009) **153**:438–50. doi:10.1016/j.cbpa.2009.04.612
24. Leggatt RA, Iwama GK. Occurrence of polyploidy in the fishes. *NULL* (2003) **13**:237–46. doi:10.1023/B:RFBF.0000033049.00668.fe
25. Rennison DJ, Owens GL, Taylor JS. Opsin gene duplication and divergence in ray-finned fish. *Mol Phylogenet Evol* (2012) **62**:986–1008. doi:10.1016/j.ympev.2011.11.030
26. Kaiya H, Riley LG, Janzen W, Hirano T, Grau EG, Miyazato M, et al. Identification and genomic sequence of a ghrelin receptor (GHS-R)-like receptor in the Mozambique tilapia, *Oreochromis mossambicus*. *Zool Sci* (2009) **26**:330–7. doi:10.2108/zsj.26.330
27. Palyha OC, Feighner SD, Tan CP, McKee KK, Hreniuk DL, Gao YD, et al. Ligand activation domain of human orphan growth hormone (GH) secretagogue receptor (GHS-R) conserved from pufferfish to humans. *Mol Endocrinol* (2000) **14**:160–9. doi:10.1210/me.14.1.160
28. Chan CB, Cheng CH. Identification and functional characterization of two alternatively spliced growth hormone secretagogue receptor transcripts from the pituitary of black seabream, *Acanthopagrus schlegeli*. *Mol Cell Endocrinol* (2004) **214**:81–95. doi:10.1016/j.mce.2003.11.020
29. Geelissen SM, Beck IM, Darras VM, Kühn ER, Van der Geyten S. Distribution and regulation of chicken growth hormone secretagogue receptor isoforms. *Gen Comp Endocrinol* (2003) **134**:167–74. doi:10.1016/S0016-6480(03)00250-8
30. Tanaka M, Miyazaki T, Yamamoto I, Nakai N, Ohta Y, Tsushima N, et al. Molecular characterization of chicken growth hormone secretagogue receptor gene. *Gen Comp Endocrinol* (2003) **134**:198–202. doi:10.1016/S0016-6480(03)00247-8
31. Sirotkin AV, Grossmann R, María-Peon MT, Roa J, Tena-Sempere M, Klein S. Novel expression and functional role of ghrelin in chicken ovary. *Mol Cell Endocrinol* (2006) **257–258**:15–25. doi:10.1016/j.mce.2006.06.004
32. Kitazawa T, Maeda Y, Kaiya H. Molecular cloning of growth hormone secretagogue-receptor and effect of quail ghrelin on gastrointestinal motility in Japanese quail. *Regul Pept* (2009) **158**:132–42. doi:10.1016/j.regpep.2009.07.005
33. Richards MP, McMurtry JP. The avian proghrelin system. *Int J Pept* (2010) **2010**:749401. doi:10.1155/2010/749401
34. Gnanapavan S, Kola B, Bustin SA, Morris DG, McGee P, Fairclough P, et al. The tissue distribution of the mRNA of ghrelin and subtypes of its receptor, GHS-R, in humans. *J Clin Endocrinol Metab* (2002) **87**:2988–91. doi:10.1210/jc.87.6.2988
35. Sun Y, Garcia JM, Smith RG. Ghrelin and growth hormone secretagogue receptor expression in mice during aging. *Endocrinology* (2007) **148**:1323–9. doi:10.1210/en.2006-0782
36. Ueberberg B, Unger N, Saeger W, Mann K, Petersenn S. Expression of ghrelin and its receptor in human tissues. *Horm Metab Res* (2009) **1**:814–21. doi:10.1055/s-0029-1233462
37. Guan XM, Yu H, Palyha OC, McKee KK, Feighner SD, Sirinathsinghji DJ, et al. Distribution of mRNA encoding the growth hormone secretagogue receptor in brain and peripheral tissues. *Brain Res Mol Brain Res* (1997) **48**:23–9. doi:10.1016/S0169-328X(97)00071-5
38. Zigman JM, Jones JE, Lee CE, Saper CB, Elmquist JK. Expression of ghrelin receptor mRNA in the rat and the mouse brain. *J Comp Neurol* (2006) **494**:528–48. doi:10.1002/cne.20823
39. Small BC, Quiniou SM, Kaiya H. Sequence, genomic organization and expression of two channel catfish, *Ictalurus punctatus*, ghrelin receptors. *Comp Biochem Physiol A Mol Integr Physiol* (2009) **154**:451–64. doi:10.1016/j.cbpa.2009.07.027
40. Saito E-S, Kaiya H, Tachibana T, Tomonaga S, Denbow DM, Kangawa K, et al. Inhibitory effect of ghrelin on food intake is mediated by the corticotropin-releasing factor system in neonatal chicks. *Regul Pept* (2005) **125**:201–8. doi:10.1016/j.regpep.2004.09.003
41. Richards MP, Poch SM, McMurtry JP. Characterization of turkey and chicken ghrelin genes, and regulation of ghrelin and ghrelin receptor mRNA levels in broiler chickens. *Gen Comp Endocrinol* (2006) **145**:298–310. doi:10.1016/j.ygcen.2005.09.013
42. Yamamoto I, Kaiya H, Tsutsui C, Sakai T, Tsukada A, Miyazato M, et al. Primary structure, tissue distribution, and biological activity of chicken motilin receptor. *Gen Comp Endocrinol* (2008) **156**:509–14. doi:10.1016/j.ygcen.2008.03.007
43. Yamamoto I, Yoshimura Y, Tsukada A, Kansaku N, Tsushima N, Tanaka M. Predominant expression of growth hormone secretagogue receptor in the caudal lobe of chicken pituitary and parallel developmental increase in expression of pituitary GH and proventriculus ghrelin mRNA. *NULL* (2008) **79**:116–21. doi:10.1111/j.1740-0929.2007.00506.x
44. Nie Q, Fang M, Xie L, Peng X, Xu H, Luo C, et al. Molecular characterization of the ghrelin and ghrelin receptor genes and effects on fat deposition in chicken and duck. *J Biomed Biotechnol* (2009) **2009**:567120. doi:10.1155/2009/567120
45. Chen T, Tang Z, Yan A, Li W, Lin H. Molecular cloning and mRNA expression analysis of two GH secretagogue receptor transcripts in orange-spotted grouper (*Epinephelus coioides*). *J Endocrinol* (2008) **199**:253–65. doi:10.1677/JOE-08-0325
46. Cruz SA, Tseng YC, Kaiya H, Hwang PP. Ghrelin affects carbohydrate-glycogen metabolism via insulin inhibition and glucagon stimulation in the zebrafish (*Danio rerio*) brain. *Comp Biochem Physiol A Mol Integr Physiol* (2010) **156**:190–200. doi:10.1016/j.cbpa.2010.01.019
47. Yada T, Kaiya H, Mutoh K, Azuma T, Hyodo S, Kangawa K. Ghrelin stimulates phagocytosis and superoxide production in fish leucocytes. *J Endocrinol* (2006) **189**:57–65. doi:10.1677/joe.1.06187
48. Kim MS, Yoon CY, Park KH, Shin CS, Park KS, Kim SY, et al. Changes in ghrelin and ghrelin receptor expression according to feeding status. *Neuroreport* (2003) **4**:1317–20. doi:10.1097/00001756-200307180-00006
49. Nogueiras R, Tovar S, Mitchell SE, Rayner DV, Archer ZA, Dieguez C, et al. Regulation of growth hormone secretagogue receptor gene expression in the arcuate nuclei of the rat by leptin and ghrelin. *Diabetes* (2004) **53**:2552–8. doi:10.2337/diabetes.53.10.2552
50. Kaji H, Kishimoto M, Kirimura T, Iguchi G, Murata M, Yoshioka S, et al. Hormonal regulation of the human ghrelin receptor gene transcription. *Biochem Biophys Res Commun* (2001) **284**:660–6. doi:10.1006/bbrc.2001.5035
51. Barreiro ML, Suominen JS, Gaytán F, Pinilla L, Chopin LK, Casanueva FF, et al. Developmental, stage-specific, and hormonally regulated expression of growth hormone secretagogue receptor messenger RNA in rat testis. *Biol Reprod* (2003) **68**:1631–40. doi:10.1095/biolreprod.102.008862
52. Kineman RD, Kamegai J, Frohman LA. Growth hormone (GH)-releasing hormone (GHRH) and the GH secretagogue (GHS), L692,585, differentially modulate rat pituitary GHS receptor and GHRH receptor messenger ribonucleic acid levels. *Endocrinology* (1999) **140**:3581–6. doi:10.1210/en.140.8.3581
53. Kamegai J, Tamura H, Ishii S, Sugihara H, Wakabayashi I. Thyroid hormones regulate pituitary growth hormone secretagogue receptor gene expression. *J Neuroendocrinol* (2001) **13**:275–8. doi:10.1046/j.1365-2826.2001.00623.x
54. Tamura H, Kamegai J, Sugihara H, Kineman RD, Frohman LA, Wakabayashi I. Glucocorticoids regulate pituitary growth hormone secretagogue receptor gene expression. *J Neuroendocrinol* (2000)

12:481–5. doi:10.1046/j.1365-2826.2000.00446.x

55. Thomas GB, Bennett PA, Carmignac DF, Robinson IC. Glucocorticoid regulation of growth hormone (GH) secretagogue-induced growth responses and GH secretagogue receptor expression in the rat. *Growth Horm IGF Res* (2000) **10**:45–52. doi:10.1054/ghir.1999.0138
56. Bennett PA, Thomas GB, Howard AD, Feighner SD, van der Ploeg LH, Smith RG, et al. Hypothalamic growth hormone secretagogue-receptor (GHS-R) expression is regulated by growth hormone in the rat. *Endocrinology* (1997) **138**:4552 7. doi:10.1210/en.138.11.4552
57. Kamegai J, Wakabayashi I, Miyamoto K, Unterman TG, Kineman RD, Frohman LA. Growth hormone-dependent regulation of pituitary GH secretagogue receptor (GHS-R) mRNA levels in the spontaneous dwarf rat. *Neuroendocrinology* (1998) **68**:312–8. doi:10.1159/000054379
58. Nass R, Gilrain J, Anderson S, Gaylinn B, Dalkin A, Day R, et al. High plasma growth hormone (GH) levels inhibit expression of GH secretagogue receptor messenger ribonucleic acid levels in the rat pituitary. *Endocrinology* (2000) **141**:2084–9. doi:10.1210/en.141.6.2084
59. Kamegai J, Tamura H, Shimizu T, Ishii S, Sugihara H, Oikawa S. Insulin-like growth factor-I down-regulates ghrelin receptor (growth hormone secretagogue receptor) expression in the rat pituitary. *Regul Pept* (2005) **127**:203–6. doi:10.1016/j.regpep.2004.12.001
60. Riley LG, Fox BK, Breves JP, Kaiya H, Dorough CP, Hirano T, et al. Absence of effects of short-term fasting on plasma ghrelin and brain expression of ghrelin receptors in the tilapia, *Oreochromis mossambicus. Zool Sci* (2008) **25**:821–7. doi:10.2108/zsj.25.821
61. Peddu SC, Breves JP, Kaiya H, Gordon GE, Riley LG Jr. Pre- and postprandial effects on ghrelin signaling in the brain and on the GH/IGF-I axis in the Mozambique tilapia (*Oreochromis mossambicus*). *Gen Comp Endocrinol* (2009) **161**:412–8. doi:10.1016/j.ygcen.2009.02.008
62. Riley LG Jr., Walker AP, Dorough CP, Schwandt SE, Grau EG. Glucose regulates ghrelin, neuropeptide Y, and the GH/IGF-I axis in the tilapia, *Oreochromis mossambicus. Comp Biochem Physiol A Mol Integr Physiol* (2009) **154**:541–6. doi:10.1016/j.cbpa.2009.08.018
63. Shiiya T, Nakazato M, Mizuta M, Date Y, Mondal MS, Tanaka M, et al. Plasma ghrelin levels in lean and obese humans and the effect of glucose on ghrelin secretion. *J Clin Endocrinol Metab* (2002) **87**:240–4. doi:10.1210/jc.87.1.240
64. Unniappan S, Canosa LF, Peter RE. Orexigenic actions of ghrelin in goldfish: feeding-induced changes in brain and gut mRNA expression and serum levels, and responses to central and peripheral injections. *Neuroendocrinology* (2004) **79**:100–8. doi:10.1159/000076634
65. Hevrøy EM, Azpeleta C, Shimizu M, Lanzén A, Kaiya H, Espe M, et al. Effects of short-term starvation on ghrelin, GH-IGF system, and IGF-binding proteins in Atlantic salmon. *Fish Physiol Biochem* (2011) **37**:217–32. doi:10.1007/s10695-010-9434-3
66. Hashimoto H, Ueta Y. Central effects of ghrelin, a unique peptide, on appetite and fluid/water drinking behavior. *Curr Protein Pept Sci* (2011) **12**:280–7. doi:10.2174/138920311795906727
67. Tachibana T, Kaiya H, Denbow DM, Kangawa K, Furuse M. Central ghrelin acts as an anti-dipsogenic peptide in chicks. *Neurosci Lett* (2006) **405**:241–5. doi:10.1016/j.neulet.2006.07.019
68. Yeung CM, Chan CB, Cheng CH. Isolation and characterization of the 5′-flanking region of the growth hormone secretagogue receptor gene from black seabream *Acanthopagrus schlegeli. Mol Cell Endocrinol* (2004) **223**:5–15. doi:10.1016/j.mce.2004.06.005
69. Wettschureck N, Moers A, Wallenwein B, Parlow AF, Maser-Gluth C, Offermanns S. Loss of Gq/11 family G proteins in the nervous system causes pituitary somatotroph hypoplasia and dwarfism in mice. *Mol Cell Biol* (2005) **25**:1942–8. doi:10.1128/MCB.25.5.1942-1948.2005
70. Cheng K, Chan WW, Butler B, Barreto A Jr., Smith RG. Evidence for a role of protein kinase-C in His-D-Trp-Ala-Trp-D-Phe-Lys-NH_2-induced growth hormone release from rat primary pituitary cells. *Endocrinology* (1991) **129**:3337–42. doi:10.1210/endo-129-6-3337
71. Herrington J, Hille B. Growth hormone-releasing hexapeptide elevates intracellular calcium in rat somatotropes by two mechanisms. *Endocrinology* (1994) **135**:1100–8. doi:10.1210/en.135.3.1100
72. Lei T, Buchfelder M, Fahlbusch R, Adams EF. Growth hormone releasing peptide (GHRP-6) stimulates phosphatidylinositol (PI) turnover in human pituitary somatotroph cells. *J Mol Endocrinol* (1995) **14**:135–8. doi:10.1677/jme.0.0140135
73. Bresson-Bépoldin L, Dufy-Barbe L. GHRP6-stimulated hormone secretion in somatotrophs: involvement of intracellular and extracellular calcium sources. *J Neuroendocrinol* (1996) **8**:309–14. doi:10.1046/j.1365-2826.1996.04608.x
74. Lania A, Ballaré E, Corbetta S, Filopanti M, Persani L, Spada A. Growth hormone-releasing hexapeptide (GHRP-6) increases intracellular calcium concentrations in cultured cells from human pituitary adenomas of different types. *Eur J Endocrinol* (1998) **139**:343–8. doi:10.1530/eje.0.1390343
75. Holst B, Brandt E, Bach A, Heding A, Schwartz TW. Nonpeptide and peptide growth hormone secretagogues act both as ghrelin receptor agonist and as positive or negative allosteric modulators of ghrelin signaling. *Mol Endocrinol* (2005) **19**:2400–11. doi:10.1210/me.2005-0059
76. Chu KM, Chow KB, Leung PK, Lau PN, Chan CB, Cheng CH, et al. Over-expression of the truncated ghrelin receptor polypeptide attenuates the constitutive activation of phosphatidylinositol-specific phospholipase C by ghrelin receptors but has no effect on ghrelin-stimulated extracellular signal-regulated kinase 1/2 activity. *Int J Biochem Cell Biol* (2007) **39**:752–64.
77. Chan CB, Leung PK, Wise H, Cheng CH. Signal transduction mechanism of the seabream growth hormone secretagogue receptor. *FEBS Lett* (2004) **577**:147–53. doi:10.1016/j.febslet.2004.08.088
78. Tachibana T, Tanaka M, Kaiya H. Central injection of des-acyl chicken ghrelin does not affect food intake in chicks. *Gen Comp Endocrinol* (2011) **171**:183–8. doi:10.1016/j.ygcen
79. Grey CL, Chang JP. Ghrelin-induced growth hormone release from goldfish pituitary cells involves voltage-sensitive calcium channels. *Gen Comp Endocrinol* (2009) **160**:148–57. doi:10.1016/j.ygcen.2008.11.006
80. Grey CL, Grayfer L, Belosevic M, Chang JP. Ghrelin stimulation of gonadotropins (LH) release from goldfish pituitary cells: presence of the growth hormone secretagogue receptor (GHS-R1a) and involvement of voltage-sensitive Ca^{2+} channels. *Mol Cell Endocrinol* (2010) **317**:64–77. doi:10.1016/j.mce.2009.12.024
81. Feighner SD, Howard AD, Prendergast K, Palyha OC, Hreniuk DL, Nargund R, et al. Structural requirements for the activation of the human growth hormone secretagogue receptor by peptide and nonpeptide secretagogues. *Mol Endocrinol* (1998) **2**:137–45.
82. Holst B, Cygankiewicz A, Jensen TH, Ankersen M, Schwartz TW. High constitutive signaling of the ghrelin receptor – identification of a potent inverse agonist. *Mol Endocrinol* (2003) **217**:2201–10. doi:10.1210/me.2003-0069
83. Holst B, Holliday ND, Bach A, Elling CE, Cox HM, Schwartz TW. Common structural basis for constitutive activity of the ghrelin receptor family. *J Biol Chem* (2004) **279**:53806–17. doi:10.1074/jbc.M407676200
84. Liu G, Fortin JP, Beinborn M, Kopin AS. Four missense mutations in the ghrelin receptor result in distinct pharmacological abnormalities. *J Pharmacol Exp Ther* (2007) **322**:1036–43. doi:10.1124/jpet.107.123141
85. Rediger A, Piechowski CL, Yi CX, Tarnow P, Strotmann R, Grüters A, et al. Mutually opposite signal modulation by hypothalamic heterodimerization of ghrelin and melanocortin-3 receptors. *J Biol Chem* (2011) **86**:39623–31. doi:10.1074/jbc.M111.287607
86. Leung PK, Chow KB, Lau PN, Chu KM, Chan CB, Cheng CH, et al. The truncated ghrelin receptor polypeptide (GHS-R1b) acts as a dominant-negative mutant of the ghrelin receptor. *Cell Signal* (2007) **19**:1011–22. doi:10.1016/j.cellsig.2006.11.011
87. Diano S, Farr SA, Benoit SC, McNay EC, da Silva I, Horvath B, et al. Ghrelin controls hippocampal spine synapse density and memory performance. *Nat Neurosci* (2006) **9**:381–8. doi:10.1038/nn1656
88. Carlini VP, Perez MF, Salde E, Schiöth HB, Ramirez OA, de Barioglio SR. Ghrelin induced

memory facilitation implicates nitric oxide synthase activation and decrease in the threshold to promote LTP in hippocampal dentate gyrus. *Physiol Behav* (2010) **101**:117–23. doi:10.1016/j.physbeh.2010.04.026
89. Verhulst PJ, Depoortere I. Ghrelin's second life: from appetite stimulator to glucose regulator. *World J Gastroenterol* (2012) **18**:3183–95. doi:10.3748/wjg.v18.i25.3183
90. Yahashi S, Kang KS, Kaiya H, Matsuda K. GHRP-6 mimics ghrelin-induced stimulation of food intake and suppression of locomotor activity in goldfish. *Peptides* (2012) **34**:324–8. doi:10.1016/j.peptides.2012.01.025
91. Unniappan S, Peter RE. In vitro and in vivo effects of ghrelin on luteinizing hormone and growth hormone release in goldfish. *Am J Physiol Regul Integr Comp Physiol* (2004) **286**:R1093–101. doi:10.1152/ajpregu.00669.2003
92. Kitazawa T, Itoh K, Yaosaka N, Maruyama K, Matsuda K, Teraoka H, et al. Ghrelin does not affect gastrointestinal contractility in rainbow trout and goldfish in vitro. *Gen Comp Endocrinol* (2012) **178**:539–45. doi:10.1016/j.ygcen
93. Olsson C, Holbrook JD, Bompadre G, Jönsson E, Hoyle CH, Sanger GJ, et al. Identification of genes for the ghrelin and motilin receptors and a novel related gene in fish, and stimulation of intestinal motility in zebrafish (*Danio rerio*) by ghrelin and motilin. *Gen Comp Endocrinol* (2008) **155**:217–26. doi:10.1016/j.ygcen.2007.05.016
94. Chow KB, Sun J, Chu KM, Tai Cheung W, Cheng CH, Wise H. The truncated ghrelin receptor polypeptide (GHS-R1b) is localized in the endoplasmic reticulum where it forms heterodimers with ghrelin receptors (GHS-R1a) to attenuate their cell surface expression. *Mol Cell Endocrinol* (2012) **348**:247–54. doi:10.1016/j.mce.2011.08.034
95. Takahashi K, Furukawa C, Takano A, Ishikawa N, Kato T, Hayama S, et al. The neuromedin U-growth hormone secretagogue receptor 1b/neurotensin receptor 1 oncogenic signaling pathway as a therapeutic target for lung cancer. *Cancer Res* (2006) **66**:9408–19. doi:10.1158/0008-5472.CAN-06-1349
96. Wang H, Gao FY, Huang ZH, Lu MX. Cloning and expression analysis of tilapia growth hormone secretagogue receptor (Unpublished, database only).
97. Wang H, Gao FY, Lu MX, Zhu HP, Huang ZH. Isolation and characterization of the 5′-flanking region of the growth hormone secretagogue receptor gene from O. hornorum. (Unpublished, database only).
98. Wiens JJ, Hutter CR, Mulcahy DG, Noonan BP, Townsend TM, Sites JW Jr., et al. Resolving the phylogeny of lizards and snakes (Squamata) with extensive sampling of genes and species. *Biol Lett* (2012) **8**:1043–6. doi:10.1098/rsbl.2012.0703
99. Yu J. Clone and genetic structure analysis of GHSR genes in Cyprinus carpio jian (Unpublished, database only).
100. Yu HJ. (2011, direct submission, database only).

16

Ancient grandeur of the vertebrate neuropeptide Y system shown by the coelacanth *Latimeria chalumnae*

Dan Larhammar* and Christina A. Bergqvist

Unit of Pharmacology, Department of Neuroscience, Science for Life Laboratory – Uppsala University, Uppsala, Sweden

Edited by:
Jae Young Seong, Korea University, South Korea

Reviewed by:
Hervé Tostivint, Natural History Museum, France
Stacia A. Sower, University of New Hampshire, USA

***Correspondence:**
Dan Larhammar, Unit of Pharmacology, Department of Neuroscience, Science for Life Laboratory – Uppsala University, Box 593, SE-751 24 Uppsala, Sweden.
e-mail: dan.larhammar@neuro.uu.se

The neuropeptide Y (NPY) family receptors and peptides have previously been characterized in several tetrapods, teleost fishes, and in a holocephalan cartilaginous fish. This has shown that the ancestral NPY system in the jawed vertebrates consisted of the peptides NPY and peptide YY (PYY) and seven G-protein-coupled receptors named Y1–Y8 (Y3 does not exist). The different vertebrate lineages have subsequently lost or gained a few receptor genes. For instance, the human genome has lost three of the seven receptors while the zebrafish has lost two and gained two receptor genes. Here we describe the NPY system of a representative of an early diverging lineage among the sarcopterygians, the West Indian Ocean coelacanth *Latimeria chalumnae*. The coelacanth was found to have retained all seven receptors from the ancestral jawed vertebrate. The receptors display the typical characteristics found in other vertebrates. Interestingly, the coelacanth was found to have the local duplicate of the PYY gene, called pancreatic polypeptide, previously only identified in tetrapods. Thus, this duplication took place very early in the sarcopterygian lineage, before the origin of tetrapods. These findings confirm the ancient complexity of the NPY system and show that mammals have lost more NPY receptors than any other vertebrate lineage. The coelacanth has all three peptides found in tetrapods and has retained the ancestral jawed vertebrate receptor repertoire with neither gains or losses.

Keywords: G-protein-coupled receptor, neuropeptide Y, peptide YY, pancreatic polypeptide, coelacanth, *Latimeria chalumnae*

INTRODUCTION

Neuropeptide Y (NPY) and its related peptides named peptide YY (PYY) and pancreatic polypeptide (PP) comprise a system of neuronal and endocrine peptides that act on several G-protein-coupled receptors in vertebrates. They are involved in the regulation of a broad range of functions including appetite/satiety, gut motility, cardiovascular activity, pituitary release of hormones, circadian rhythm, and many more (see Pedrazzini et al., 2003; Brumovsky et al., 2007; Mercer et al., 2011; Zhang et al., 2011 for reviews). NPY and PYY arose by duplication of a common ancestral peptide gene before the vertebrate radiation (Larhammar, 1996). In mammals NPY is almost exclusively neuronal whereas PYY is primarily expressed in endocrine cells in the gastrointestinal tract. In ray finned fishes, PYY too is expressed in the nervous system (Cerdá-Reverter et al., 2000; Söderberg et al., 2000). PP is a local duplicate of PYY (Hort et al., 1995) previously found only in tetrapods (Larhammar, 1996; Cerdá-Reverter and Larhammar, 2000; Conlon, 2002; Sundstrom et al., 2008) and is expressed in pancreatic islets.

Mammals generally possess four receptors for the NPY-family peptides, namely subtypes Y1, Y2, Y4, and Y5 (Larhammar and Salaneck, 2004). Subtype Y3 was postulated from pharmacological experiments but does not exist as a separate gene (Herzog et al., 1993; Jazin et al., 1993). A fifth receptor gene, Y6, is expressed in a few mammals such as mouse and rabbit but is a pseudogene in many others including primates (Matsumoto et al., 1996), pig (Wraith et al., 2000), and guinea-pig (Starbäck et al., 2000). With its three peptides and four receptors, the NPY system in humans and most other mammals displays a degree of complexity resembling many other vertebrate peptide-receptor systems for neuronal and endocrine peptides, for instance the melanocortin system (Dores and Baron, 2011; Liang et al., 2013), the opioid system (Sundstrom et al., 2010), the oxytocin-vasopressin system (Ocampo Daza et al., 2011; Yamaguchi et al., 2012), and the somatostatin-cortistatin system (Tostivint et al., 2008; Ocampo Daza et al., 2012). However, previous evolutionary studies of the NPY receptor family have shown that a larger number of receptors existed in the early stages of vertebrate evolution before the emergence of jawed vertebrates, *Gnathostomata*: by sequence-based phylogenetic analyses and comparison of gene locations on chromosomes, we were able to deduce an ancestral vertebrate set of no less than seven NPY-family receptors (Larhammar and Salaneck, 2004; Larsson et al., 2008), more than for any other known peptide-receptor family. Subsequently, this repertoire was confirmed by our identification of all seven receptor subtypes in a cartilaginous fish (*Chondrichthyes*), the holocephalan elephant shark, or ghost shark, *Callorhinchus milii* (Larsson et al., 2009). Thus, the following evolutionary scenario was corroborated: an ancestral pre-vertebrate chromosome carried the genes for a Y1-like, a Y2-like, and a Y5-like receptor subtype. The two basal vertebrate tetraploidizations (Nakatani et al., 2007; Putnam et al., 2008) quadrupled this chromosome, thereby generating four similar chromosomal regions that probably had as many as 12 (4 × 3) family members, unless some were lost already after the first tetraploidization. In extant

Table 1 | The table lists Ensemble gene ID or NCBI accession number for the coelacanth NPY-family receptor and peptide genes as well as the orthologs genes in human, chicken, zebrafish, and elephant shark.

Species	Receptor	Ensembl gene ID/NCBI accession number	Genome assembly	Comment
Coelacanth	**Y1**	**ENSLACG00000009650**	LatCha1	Manually curated
Human	Y1	NM_000909		
Chicken	Y1	NM_001031535		
Zebrafish	Y1	EU046342		
Elephant shark	Y1	EU637847		
Coelacanth	**Y2**	**ENSLACG00000009115**	LatCha1	Manually curated
Human	Y2	NM_000910		
Chicken	Y2	NM_001031128		
Zebrafish	Y2	XP_001343301		
Zebrafish	Y2-2	XP_001332759		
Elephant shark	Y2	EU637848		
Coelacanth	**Y4**	**Not annotated in database** (JH127692.1: 3,965–4,993)		
Human	Y4	NM_005972		
Chicken	Y4	AF410853		
Zebrafish	Y4	AF037400		
Elephant shark	Y4	EU637849		
Coelacanth	**Y5**	**ABI94072.1**		
Human	Y5	NM_006174		
Chicken	Y5	NM_001031130		
Elephant shark	Y5	EU637850		
Coelacanth	**Y6**	**ABI94073.1**		
Mouse	Y6	ENSMUSG00000038071	GRCm38	
Chicken	Y6	ENSGALG00000021235	WASHUC2	Manually curated
Elephant shark	Y6	EU637851		
Coelacanth	**Y7**	**ENSLACG00000013918**	LatCha1	Manually curated
Chicken	Y7	NP_001032913		
Zebrafish	Y7	AY585098		
Elephant shark	Y7	EU637852		
Coelacanth	**Y8**	**ENSLACG00000008470**	LatCha1	
Zebrafish	Y8a	NM_131437		
Zebrafish	Y8b	AF030245		
Elephant shark	Y8	EU637853		
Human	SSTR1	ENSG00000139874	GRCh37	

For Y6, the mouse sequence is included instead of the human pseudogene. The human somatostatin receptor SSTR1 that was used as outgroup in the phylogenetic tree is also included.
The coelacanth entries are shown in bold.

vertebrate lineages a total of seven family members have been found to remain: four Y1-subfamily genes with one on each of the four chromosomes resulting from the tetraploidizations (Y1, Y4, Y6, and Y8), two Y2-like genes (Y2 linked to Y1, Y7 linked to Y6), and a single surviving Y5 gene (linked to Y1 and Y2) (Larsson et al., 2008, 2009).

Of the vertebrates investigated to date only the elephant shark has maintained all seven of these ancestral vertebrate receptor genes (Larsson et al., 2009). All of the other gnathostome lineages seem to have suffered losses, although some of the genome databases may be incomplete. Among amphibians, the western clawed frog *Silurana (Xenopus) tropicalis* seems to have lost Y6 which appears to be a pseudogene in the frog *Pelophylax esculentus* (previously called *Rana esculenta*; Sundstrom et al., 2012). Amniotes have lost Y8, or possibly this gene was lost independently in birds and mammals (Larsson et al., 2009). The mammalian lineage subsequently lost also Y7. The Y6 gene is a pseudogene in several mammals as mentioned above. In the large and heterogeneous group of rayfinned fishes (*Actinopterygii*), the teleosts are the most carefully studied. In the true teleost species (*Euteleostei*) with sequenced genomes, the receptors Y1, Y2, Y4, Y7, and Y8, as well as a duplicate of Y8 called Y8b, have been identified, albeit only the zebrafish genome contains all of these (Larsson et al., 2008; Salaneck et al., 2008). Thus, the Y8 duplicate seems to be the only surviving copy resulting from the teleost-specific third tetraploidization, 3R (Jaillon et al., 2004). Also, this suggests that Y5 and Y6 are missing in *Euteleostei*. A local duplicate of Y2, named Y2-2, has been found in zebrafish and medaka (Fallmar et al.,

2011). In addition, Y5 and Y6 have been identified in more basally diverging rayfinned fish species, namely a sturgeon and a bichir, as well as an early diverging teleost, the silver arowana, *Osteoglossum bicirrhosum* (Salaneck et al., 2008). Also, we have previously cloned the genes for Y5 and Y6 from the coelacanth *Latimeria chalumnae* (Lch; Larsson et al., 2007). The receptor gene duplication scenario is further supported by findings in lampreys of members of the Y1, Y2, and Y5 lineages (Salaneck et al., 2001; Larsson et al., 2009; Xu et al., 2012). In summary, of all gnathostome species that have been previously investigated only the elephant shark seems to have retained the complete ancestral repertoire of seven NPY receptor genes.

The West Indian Ocean coelacanth, Lch, is an important species for studies of vertebrate evolution as it is one of only two extant and closely related coelacanth species representing a very early *Actinistia* branch among the lobe finned fishes, *Sarcopterygii*. The relationship of coelacanths to lungfishes (Dipnoi) and tetrapods has been difficult to resolve. Recent data suggest that the coelacanths are slightly more closely related to the lungfishes than either of these groups is to tetrapods (Shan and Gras, 2011). The Actinopterygii-Sarcopterygii divergence took place approximately 424 million years ago (Mya) according to a recent estimate based on molecular data (Chen et al., 2012). The coelacanth and tetrapod lineages may have parted only a few tens of millions of years later, well before the split of the amphibian and amniote lineages approximately 350 Mya. Thus, it is of great interest to see which genetic and phenotypic Sarcopterygian characters had already arisen before the coelacanth-tetrapod divergence. In September 2011, a new genome assembly became available for the coelacanth. We present here a genomic analysis of the NPY system in Lch, identifying not only the receptor repertoire but also the genes for the three peptide ligands that bind to these receptors.

MATERIALS AND METHODS

The PreEnsembl sequence database (ENSEMBL LatCha1 released September 2011, database version 69.1) for the West Indian Ocean coelacanth Lch was searched with Blast/Blat using as query sequences the human NPY-family receptors Y1, Y2, and Y4, and the zebrafish receptors Y7 and 8b. Five new receptors were identified, all but Y4 are annotated in Ensembl68. Amino acid sequences for NPY receptors from the following species were used for alignments: human (*Homo sapiens*), chicken (*Gallus gallus*), zebrafish (*Danio rerio*), elephant shark (*C. milii*), mouse (*Mus musculus*), and coelacanth (*L. chalumnae*). A list of genes with corresponding accession numbers is provided in **Table 1** with the coelacanth NPY receptor sequences in bold.

Amino acid alignments were made in Jalview 2.8 version 14.0 (Waterhouse et al., 2009) using the MUSCLE and Clustal W web tool with standard settings. Phylogenetic Neighbor-Joining (NJ; Saitou and Nei, 1987) trees were made by using Clustal X version 2.0.12 (Larkin et al., 2007), standard settings and 1000 bootstrap replicates were applied. The tree shown in **Figure 2** was rooted with the human somatostatin receptor sequence SSTR1. Phylogenetic trees were also made with the Maximum Likelihood (ML) method (Guindon et al., 2010).

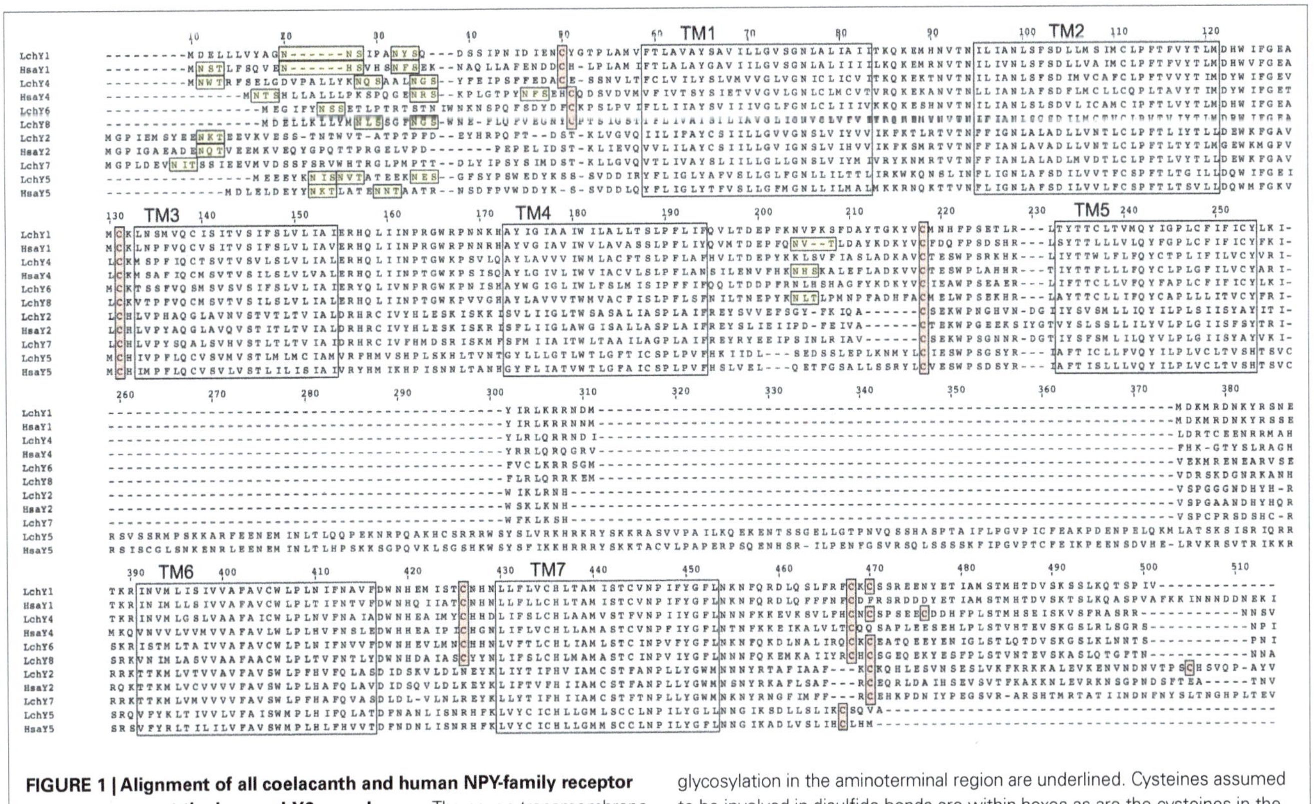

FIGURE 1 | Alignment of all coelacanth and human NPY-family receptor sequences except the human hY6 pseudogene. The seven transmembrane regions are marked with boxes. Consensus sequences for asparagine-linked glycosylation in the aminoterminal region are underlined. Cysteines assumed to be involved in disulfide bonds are within boxes as are the cysteines in the carboxyterminal region that may serve as attachment sites for palmitate.

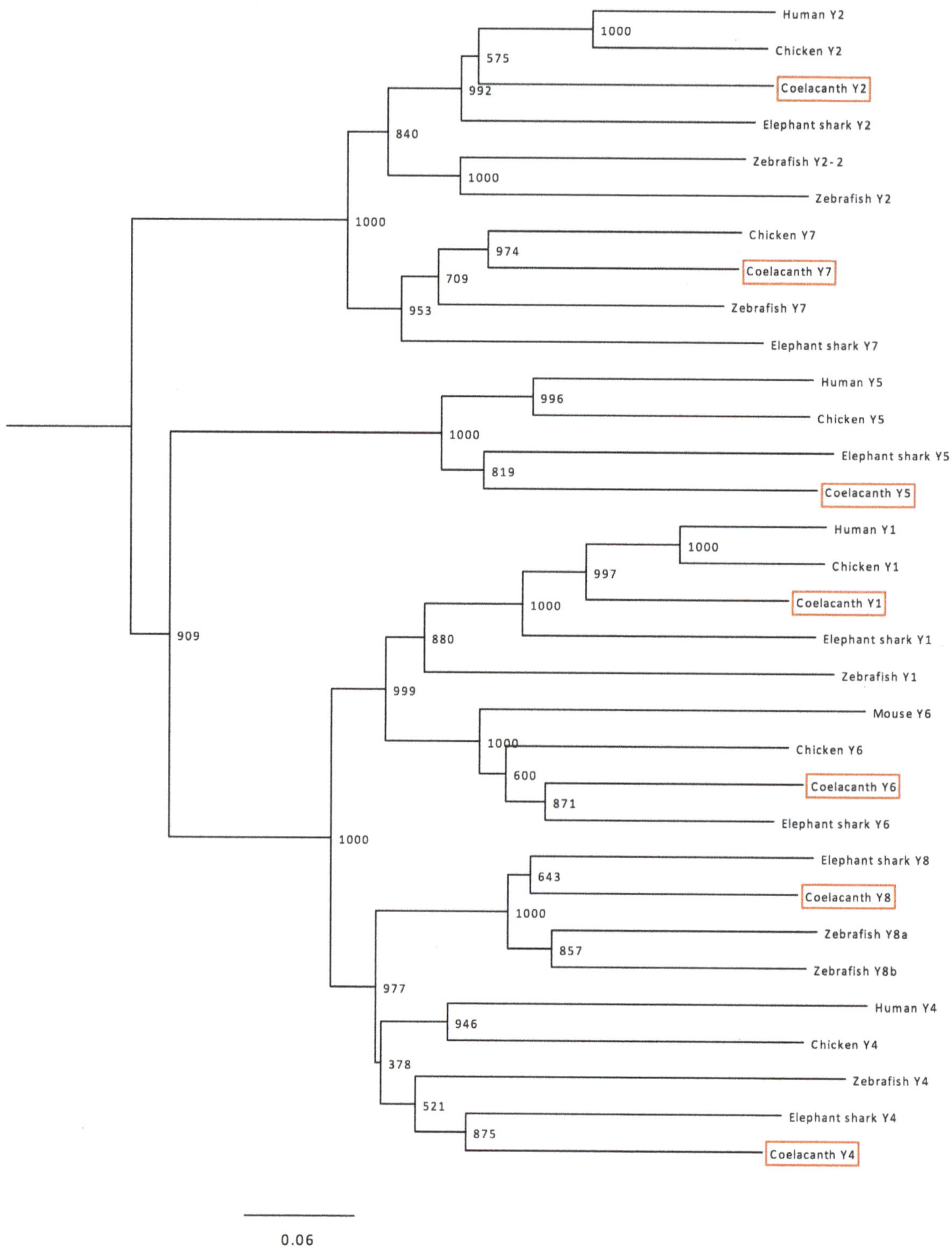

FIGURE 2 | Phylogenetic tree calculated with the Neighbor-Joining method showing the relationships of the NPY-family receptor sequences in coelacanth, human (except Y6 where the mouse sequence is included instead of the human pseudogene), chicken, zebrafish, and elephant shark. The human somatostatin receptor 1 (SSTR1) was used as outgroup to root the tree. The tree was calculated using the complete sequences aligned with Clustal W. Trees were also deduced using the Maximum Likelihood method and both methods were also used to calculate trees based on an alignment generated with MUSCLE. These trees are available from the authors upon request. See text for details.

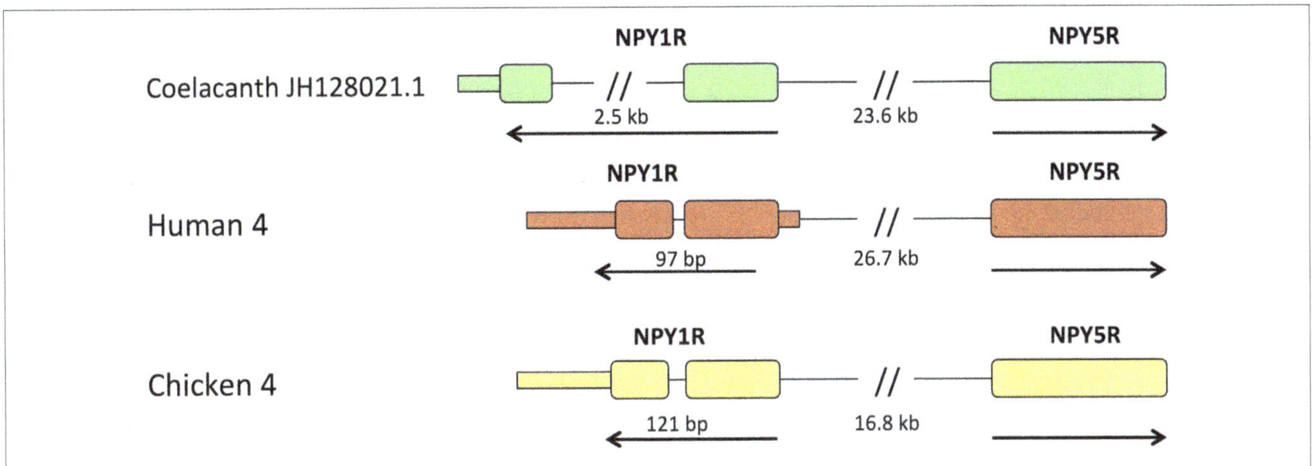

FIGURE 3 | Organization of the Y1 and Y5 genes relative to one another in coelacanth, human, and chicken. Exons are shown as tall boxes for the coding region and low boxes for the 5′- and 3′-untranslated regions where known. The 3′-untranslated region is shown until the position of the first consensus poly(A) signal. The size of the intron in the coding region of Y1 is shown. In all three species, the genes have a "head-to-head" orientation and may share regulatory upstream elements. The distance between the coding regions of the two genes are shown, but it has not yet been fully explored where promoters and any separate 5′-untranslated exons may be located.

RESULTS

LATIMERIA CHALUMNAE NPY-FAMILY RECEPTORS

We have previously reported the coelacanth Y5 and Y6 genes (Larsson et al., 2007). To identify additional NPY-family receptors, we searched the PreEnsemble Lch database with sequences from other species as queries. The identified Lch sequences were aligned with known NPY-family receptors from other vertebrates and subjected to phylogenetic analyses. Some of the sequences had to be manually curated as indicated in **Table 1** which lists all the identified Lch sequences and their Ensemble ID or NCBI accession numbers. The table also lists the sequences for the other species that are included in the alignment and the phylogenetic tree described below. The searches allowed us to identify all the NPY-family receptors known to have arisen before the divergence of the jawed vertebrates, i.e., also Y1, Y2, Y4, Y7, and Y8.

An alignment of all Lch and human NPY-family receptors is shown in **Figure 1**. All of the sequences contain one to three consensus sequences for *N*-linked glycosylation in the aminoterminal region of the receptors, before transmembrane region 1 (TM1), i.e., the sequence NXS/T. The Lch Y6 and Y8 sequences also have a consensus glycosylation sequence in extracellular loop 2 (EL2), as do human Y1 and Y4. All sequences have a cysteine residue in EL1 and one cysteine in EL2 that presumably form a disulfide bond. The four Y1-subfamily sequences Y1, Y4, Y6, and Y8 also have a cysteine in the aminoterminal region and one in EL3, expected to form an additional disulfide bond, as in Y1-subfamily sequences from other species. Finally, one ore more cysteines are present in the cytoplasmic tail after TM7, expected to serve as attachment sites for palmitate to anchor the tail to the inner side of the cytoplasmic membrane. Also many other positions that are known to be highly conserved among NPY-family receptors, either between species or between receptor subtypes (or both), are conserved in the Lch sequences.

Phylogenetic analyses were performed with a more extensive alignment that included also the sequences of the six chicken receptors and the seven elephant shark receptors, plus the mouse Y6 sequence as the human Y6 gene is a pseudogene. The resulting tree is shown in **Figure 2**. The seven Lch sequences could be clearly identified as orthologs to each of the seven previously described receptors in jawed vertebrates. The tree has a few minor deviations from the established order of divergence for the included species, mostly because of higher evolutionary rates for some lineages as explained in the discussion.

Table 2 | The table lists Ensemble gene ID for the coelacanth and human NPY-family peptides NPY, PYY, and PP (pancreatic polypeptide).

Species	Peptide	Ensembl gene ID	Genome assembly	Comment
Coelacanth	NPY	ENSLACG00000001891	LatCha1	
Human	NPY	ENSG00000131096	GRCh37	
Coelacanth	PYY	ENSLACG00000015096	LatCha1	
Human	PYY	ENSG00000131096	GRCh37	
Coelacanth	Pancreatic polypeptide	**Not annotated in database** (JH126680.1:1,154,715–1,154,819)		
Human	Pancreatic polypeptide	ENSG00000108849	GRCh37	

The coelacanth entries are shown in bold.

In all other vertebrates with assembled genomes, the genes for Y1 and Y5 are located close together in a head-to-head orientation, implying that their promoter regions may share some regulatory elements. The distance between the start codons for the human genes is 26.7 kb and for the chicken genes 16.8 kb. In the coelacanth, the distance is 23.6 kb (**Figure 3**). The promoter regions have not been characterized in detail for Y1 and Y5 in any species and furthermore seem to vary between species with

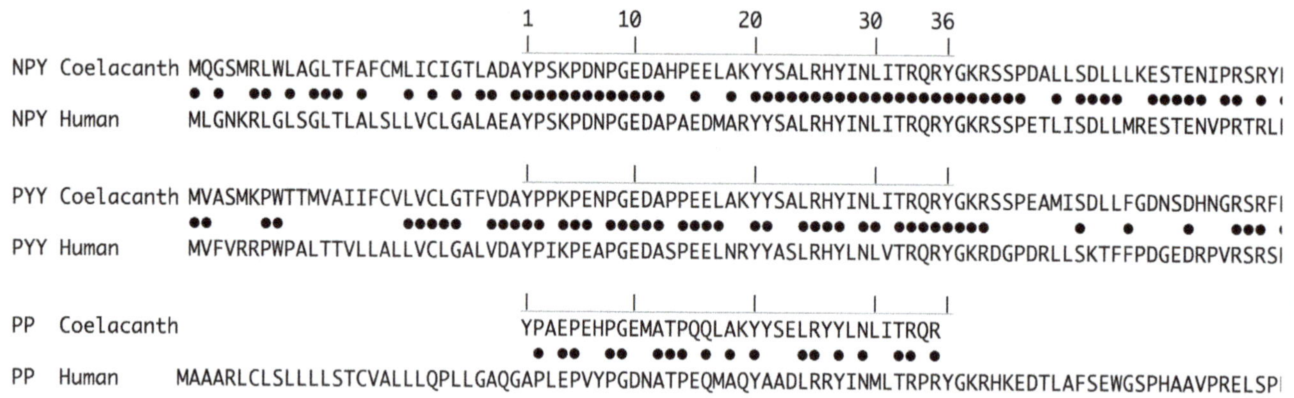

FIGURE 4 | Pairwise prepropeptide sequence alignments between coelacanth and human for NPY, PYY, and PP (pancreatic polypeptide). Identical positions are marked with dots for each pairwise comparison. The mature peptide sequences are marked with the horizontal line and the positions are numbered 1 through 36.

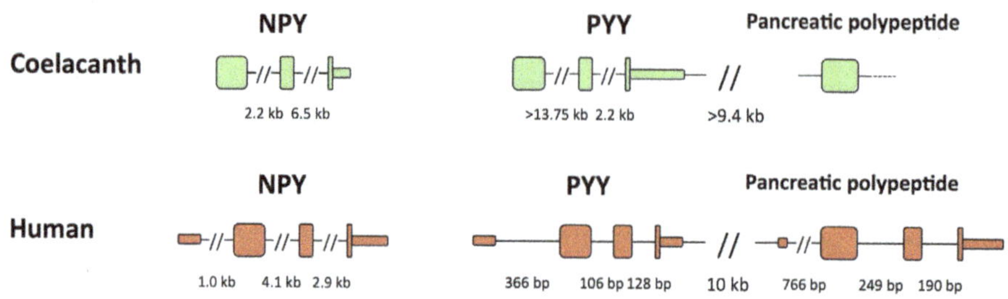

FIGURE 5 | Exon organization of the three coelacanth NPY-family peptide genes and their orthologs human peptide genes. All genes are shown in the 5′-to-3′ direction. PYY and pancreatic polypeptide are located adjacent to each other and have the same orientation on the chromosome, thus a "head-to-tail" orientation. Exons are shown as tall boxes for the coding region and low boxes for the 5′- and 3′-untranslated regions where known. The 3′-untranslated region is shown until the position of the first consensus poly(A) signal. For the coelacanth genes, the separate 5′-untranslated exons are still unknown as are the two 3′ coding exons of the pancreatic polypeptide genes due to incomplete sequence information. Gaps in the genomic sequence of the coelacanth mean that some of its intron sizes and the intergenic distance are minimum estimates.

regard to the possibility of multiple promoters and alternatively spliced 5′UTR exons (Wraith, 1999), why a detailed comparison with Lch is not meaningful at this point. The Y1 gene is the only member of the NPY receptor family that has an intron in the coding region. This intron is very small in mammals (97 bp in the human gene, 110 bp in opossum), chicken (121 bp), anole lizard (698 bp), and the frog *Silurana tropicalis* (92 bp; Sundstrom et al., 2012), but considerably larger in zebrafish with approximately 40 kb (in preparation), a sturgeon (Salaneck et al., 2008), and the two cartilaginous fishes spiny dogfish (Salaneck et al., 2003) and elephant shark (Larsson et al., 2009), the last-mentioned having an intron >3 kb. In the coelacanth, this intron is approximately 2.5 kb (**Figure 3**). Thus, the intron is large both in cartilaginous fishes, a teleost, and the coelacanth. The most parsimonious interpretation is that large size is ancestral and that the intron contracted in the ancestor of tetrapods and has remained small in this lineage.

The synteny groups of the NPY-family receptor genes and their neighboring genes in the same chromosome regions could not be analyzed in the coelacanth due to the small size of the scaffolds as a result of low-coverage sequencing.

LATIMERIA CHALUMNAE NPY-FAMILY PEPTIDES

The coelacanth genome database was searched with the three human members of the NPY peptide family as queries. Hits were found for the most highly conserved parts of both NPY, PYY, and somewhat surprisingly also PP, although this peptide has not previously been identified outside of the tetrapods. Further analyses revealed the presence of the two small 3′ exons encoding the carboxyterminal extensions of the prepropeptides for NPY and PYY. However, for the more rapidly evolving PP, these exons could not be found, most probably because they are missing in the Lch assembly. The Ensemble gene IDs are listed in **Table 2.**

An alignment of the coelacanth and human prepropeptides is shown in **Figure 4**. The mature NPY sequences share 31 och the 36 positions and three of the remaining five are highly conservative replacements, as has been observed for NPY for other vertebrates (Larhammar, 1996; Cerdá-Reverter and Larhammar, 2000). The mature Lch and human PYY sequences share 27 of the 36 positions. The coelacanth PYY sequence is identical to the deduced ancestral vertebrate PYY sequence (not shown), thus the differences are due to divergence of PYY in the lineage leading to humans and other mammals. In contrast, PP has diverged considerably between coelacanth and human and the two species share only 18 of the 36 residues, a degree of identity found also for comparisons between birds or frogs and mammals (Larhammar, 1996; Cerdá-Reverter and Larhammar, 2000; Conlon, 2002). For both NPY and PYY, the differences that exist between coelacanth and human are predominantly located in the middle part of the peptides, suggesting that both ends are kept conserved for functional reasons, presumably interactions with the NPY-family receptors.

The genes for Lch NPY and PYY have the coding region distributed over three exons like in all other vertebrates (**Figure 5**). The introns in the coelacanth PYY gene are much larger, >13.75 and 2.2 kb, respectively, than in the mammalian orthologs, with only 106 and 128 bp in human. The introns in chicken and zebrafish are of intermediate size with 2.2 and 0.3 kb in chicken and similar sizes in zebrafish (Söderberg et al., 2000). For the PP gene, only the exon containing most of the mature PP sequence, preceded by the signal peptide, could be identified. In chicken and mammals, the PYY and PP genes are located in tandem approximately 10 kb apart. The intergenic distance is of a similar magnitude or greater in the coelacanth (the genomic sequence has a gap in the assembly). All three peptide genes have a separate exon for 5′UTR in mammals and this exon has not been identified in any of the coelacanth genes.

DISCUSSION

The seven NPY-family receptor genes identified in the coelacanth genome database display orthology to the subtypes previously deduced to have arisen in the ancestor of the jawed vertebrates, namely subtypes Y1, Y2, Y4, Y5, Y6, Y7, and Y8 (**Figure 3**). Thus, the coelacanth has retained the complete ancestral repertoire like the elephant shark, but in contrast to mammals, chicken, and teleost fishes, all of which has lost one or more of the ancestral receptors. Our findings in the coelacanth corroborate our previous gene duplication scenario for the family of NPY receptors (**Figure 6**), with an ancestral local gene triplication, defining the three subfamilies of Y1, Y2, and Y5, followed by the chromosome quadruplication resulting from the two basal vertebrate tetraploidizations (Larhammar and Salaneck, 2004). Recent studies of other receptor families for neuroendocrine peptide-receptors have also revealed surprising ancestral vertebrate complexity, with six ancient somatostatin receptors (Ocampo Daza et al., 2012), six ancestral oxytocin-vasopressin receptors (Ocampo Daza et al., 2011; Yamaguchi et al., 2012; Ocampo Daza, 2013), and four ancestral GnRH (gonadotropin-releasing hormone) receptors (Kim et al., 2011), followed by losses of genes in mammals as well as other vertebrate lineages.

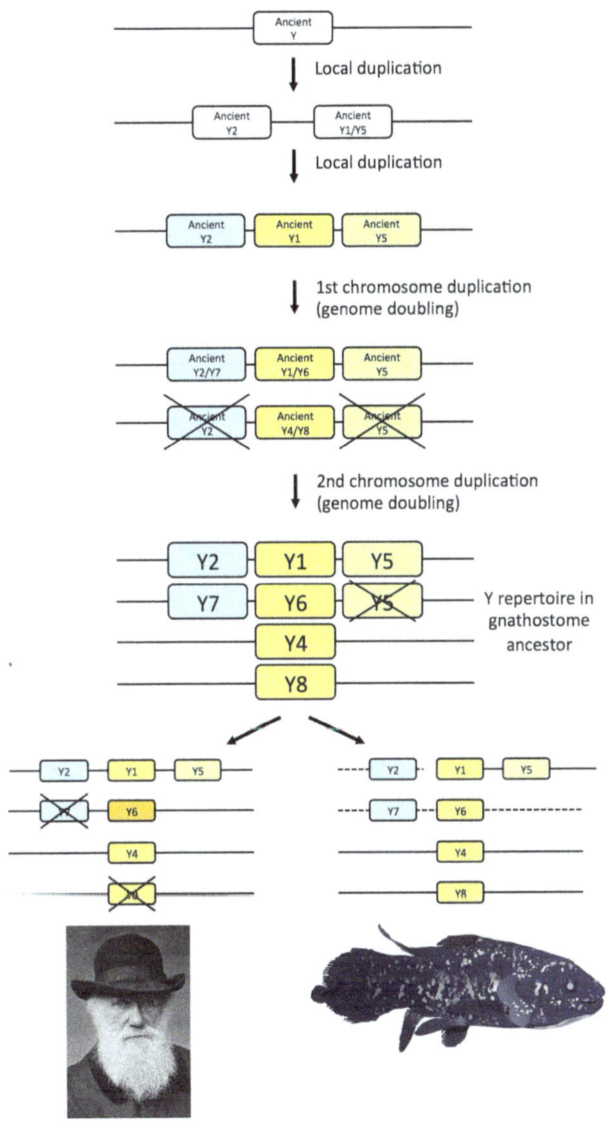

FIGURE 6 | Gene duplication events for the NPY receptor family in early vertebrate evolution including the two basal tetraploidizations. Crosses mark gene losses. The human Y6 gene is a pseudogene, as indicated by orange color. The dashed lines for the coelacanth indicate that it is not known if the genes are syntenic.

The clades in the NJ tree shown in **Figure 2** corresponding to the seven receptor subtypes have high bootstrap support, except for the Y4–Y8 clade which often has been found to display poor resolution (Larsson et al., 2008, 2009) due to faster evolution of the Y4 sequences (Lundell et al., 2002) and the deviating amino acid composition of the zebrafish Y4 receptor, initially named Ya (Starbäck et al., 1999; see Salaneck et al., 2003). Analyses with the ML method give similar topology with this repertoire of species (not shown). Also when additional species are included for NJ and ML, these receptor subtypes fail to form completely separate clades with high bootstrap values, but the orthology relationships between tetrapods and teleosts have been confirmed by conserved synteny for Y4 and Y8 (Larsson et al., 2008). The seven coelacanth receptors can clearly be identified as orthologs of the previously identified seven ancestral vertebrate receptors, as shown by the tree in **Figure 2**.

Within each clade in **Figure 2**, some deviations from the established evolutionary relationships between species can be seen except Y7 which does indeed conform to the conventional species topology. As has been observed for several other gene or protein families, the zebrafish branch is more basal than the elephant shark, namely for Y1 and Y2. This is probably due to a higher evolutionary rate in the teleost fish lineage as compared to cartilaginous fishes and sarcopterygians, as has been observed for conserved non-coding elements (Lee et al., 2011). Also the mouse Y6 branching can probably be accounted for by its higher evolutionary rate. Analyses using the ML method displays similar minor deviations from the species relationships (not shown).

The coelacanth genome project has insufficient coverage for assembly into large scaffolds and therefore does not allow analyses of conserved synteny. Nevertheless, the Y1 and Y5 genes were found to be located close together in a head-to-head orientation like in mammals and chicken, with a similar distance as in human, supporting coregulation of the genes. Y1 and Y5 are known to be coexpressed in brain regions of rat (Parker and Herzog, 1998, 1999; Wolak et al., 2003) and mouse (Naveilhan et al., 1998; Oberto et al., 2007). In the paraventricular region of the hypothalamus, both Y1 and Y5 are known to contribute to the appetite-stimulating effect of NPY as reviewed in Mercer et al. (2011), probably in slightly different ways (Lecklin et al., 2002, 2003). However, the most important promoters and regulatory elements remain to be functionally identified. Indeed, comparison of the pig promoter regions (Wraith, 1999) with those in human (Herzog et al., 1997) suggested that multiple alternative start sites and/or 5′UTR exons exist that may differ even between these mammals, indicating complicated regulation of the two genes.

Based upon previous studies of the highly conserved peptides NPY and PYY, the identification of these in the coelacanth was expected and both of the mature peptides were found to be highly conserved. Indeed, the coelacanth PYY sequence appears to be identical to that of the deduced vertebrate ancestral PYY sequence (Larhammar, 1996), whereas mammalian PYY has undergone a few amino acid replacements. Possibly, the strong conservation of PYY in the coelacanth indicates a broader expression, like in teleost fishes and lamprey where PYY is expressed in both endocrine cells and neurons (Söderberg et al., 1994, 2000; Cerdá-Reverter et al., 2000; Kurokawa and Suzuki, 2002; Montpetit et al., 2005; Murashita et al., 2006, 2009; Wall and Volkoff, 2013), whereas mammalian PYY is almost exclusively expressed in endocrine cells. Broad distribution and/or usage has been found to correlate with higher conservation (Jordan et al., 2005; Khaitovich et al., 2005).

Our finding of PP in the coelacanth genome was unexpected because this peptide has previously only been identified in tetrapods (Larhammar, 1996; Cerdá-Reverter and Larhammar, 2000; Conlon, 2002; Sundstrom et al., 2008). The discovery of PP in the coelacanth could push back its origin by approximately 50 Myr, from a minimum of 340 Myr to a minimum of 390 Myr (Blair and Hedges, 2005). This may even raise the possibility that PP arose before the divergence of lobefinned fishes and rayfinned fishes, and that the PP gene has been lost in the rayfinned fish lineage. The NPY-family peptides so far described in teleosts have been assigned as NPYa, NPYb, PYYa, and PYYb (previously called PY), with the a and b duplicates having resulted from the teleost tetraploidization 3R (Sundstrom et al., 2008). PP in mammals binds to Y4 with higher affinity than either NPY or PYY, showing that partner preference has evolved between PP and Y4 in this lineage (Lundell et al., 1995, 1996; Berglund et al., 2001). In chicken, in contrast, all three peptides bind to Y4 with similar affinities (Lundell et al., 2002). Interestingly, Lch PP does not have the change from the ancestral residue Gln-34 to Pro-34 that is found in all PP sequences, except a few bird sequences that have a histidine at this position and the caecilian *Typhlonectes natans* (an amphibian) which has a serine (Conlon et al., 1998; Conlon, 2002). The coelacanth has retained the ancestral Gln-34 found also in all NPY and PYY sequences. This may indicate that Lch PP has a binding profile that differs from PP in tetrapods with regard to receptor subtype preferences.

Detailed studies of peptide-receptor interactions will require cloning and functional expression of the coelacanth receptors and synthesis of the peptides, especially Lch PP. Hopefully future crystallization of NPY-family receptors will provide good templates for structural modeling of the coelacanth receptors and thereby help explain how this peptide-receptor system has evolved in the vertebrates. Unfortunately, studies of the tissue distribution of the mRNA for the NPY-family peptides and receptors cannot be easily performed with this endangered species.

The large repertoire of NPY-family receptors in the coelacanth may either mean that it has retained the ancestral functions for the seven vertebrate receptors or evolved novel functions for some of them. If ancestral functions are maintained, this might give clues to what functions may have disappeared in mammals with the loss of receptors Y7 and Y8, as well as Y6 in several mammalian lineages. Another possibility is that any such functions are partially or completely mediated by the four to five receptors that still exist in mammals. Information on such scenarios may be obtained from studies of species that represent additional basally diverging lineages, such as lungfishes (which unfortunately have very large genomes, thereby complicating bioinformatic analyses) and basal actinopterygians like the spotted gar whose genome was recently assembled (Amores et al., 2011). This species is especially interesting as it diverged before the third tetraploidization took place in the teleost lineage. Also basal lineages among the teleosts have recently added valuable information on gene family evolution, especially the recently assembled genome for the European eel (Henkel et al., 2012). Clearly considerable genetic complexity arose at an early stage in vertebrate evolution that can be deduced by comparing distantly related vertebrate lineages. An inevitable conclusion is that for several gene families, mammals must be considered to have degenerated by gene loss.

ACKNOWLEDGMENTS

This work was supported by a grant from the Swedish Research Council.

REFERENCES

Amores, A., Catchen, J., Ferrara, A., Fontenot, Q., and Postlethwait, J. H. (2011). Genome evolution and meiotic maps by massively parallel DNA sequencing: spotted gar, an outgroup for the teleost genome duplication. *Genetics* 188, 799–808.

Berglund, M. M., Lundell, I., Eriksson, H., Söll, R., Beck-Sickinger, A. G., and Larhammar, D. (2001). Structure-activity analyses of the neuropeptide Y-family receptor Y4; studies of the human, rat, and the guinea pig receptors using NPY analogues and two distinct radioligands. *Peptides* 22, 351–356.

Blair, J. E., and Hedges, S. B. (2005). Molecular phylogeny and divergence times of deuterostome animals. *Mol. Biol. Evol.* 22, 2275–2284.

Brumovsky, P., Shi, T. S., Landry, M., Villar, M. J., and Hokfelt, T. (2007).

Brumovsky, Neuropeptide tyrosine and pain. *Trends Pharmacol. Sci.* 28, 93–102.

Cerdá-Reverter, J. M., and Larhammar, D. (2000). Neuropeptide Y family of peptides: structure, anatomical expression, function, and molecular evolution. *Biochem. Cell Biol.* 78, 371–392.

Cerdá-Reverter, J. M., Martínez-Rodriguez, G., Anglade, I., Kah, O., and Zanuy, S. (2000). Peptide YY (PYY) and fish pancreatic peptide Y (PY) expression in the brain of the sea bass (Dicentrarchus labrax) as revealed by in situ hybridization. *J. Comp. Neurol.* 426, 197–208.

Chen, M., Zou, M., Yang, L., and He, S. (2012). Basal jawed vertebrate phylogenomics using transcriptomic data from Solexa sequencing. *PLoS ONE* 7:e36256. doi:10.1371/journal.pone.0036256

Conlon, J. M. (2002). The origin and evolution of peptide YY (PYY) and pancreatic polypeptide (PP). *Peptides* 23, 269–278.

Conlon, J. M., Platz, J. E., Chartrel, N., Vaudry, H., and Nielsen, P. F. (1998). Amino acid sequence diversity of pancreatic polypeptide among the amphibia. *Gen. Comp. Endocrinol.* 112, 146–152.

Dores, R. M., and Baron, A. J. (2011). Evolution of POMC: origin, phylogeny, posttranslational processing, and the melanocortins. *Ann. N. Y. Acad. Sci.* 1220, 34–48.

Fallmar, H., Sundstrom, G., Lundell, I., Mohell, N., and Larhammar, D. (2011). Neuropeptide Y/peptide YY receptor Y2 duplicate in zebrafish with unique introns displays distinct peptide binding properties. *Comp. Biochem. Physiol. B Biochem. Mol. Biol.* 160, 166–173.

Guindon, S., Dufayard, J. F., Lefort, V., Anisimova, M., Hordijk, W., and Gascuel, O. (2010). New algorithms and methods to estimate maximum-likelihood phylogenies: assessing the performance of PhyML 3.0. *Syst. Biol.* 59, 307–321.

Henkel, C. V., Burgerhout, E., de Wijze, D. L., Dirks, R. P., Minegishi, Y., Jansen, H. J., et al. (2012). Primitive duplicate Hox clusters in the European eel's genome. *PLoS ONE* 7:e32231. doi:10.1371/journal.pone.0032231

Herzog, H., Darby, K., Ball, H., Hort, Y., Beck-Sickinger, A., and Shine, J. (1997). Overlapping gene structure of the human neuropeptide Y receptor subtypes Y1 and Y5 suggests coordinate transcriptional regulation. *Genomics* 41, 315–319.

Herzog, H., Hort, Y. J., Shine, J., and Selbie, L. A. (1993). Molecular cloning, characterization and localization of the human homolog to the reported bovine NPY Y3 receptor: lack of NPY binding and activation. *DNA Cell Biol.* 12, 465–471.

Hort, Y., Baker, E., Sutherland, G. R., Shine, J., and Herzog, H. (1995). Gene duplication of the human peptide YY gene (PYY) generated the pancreatic polypeptide gene (PPY) on chromosome 17q21.1. *Genomics* 26, 77–83.

Jaillon, O., Aury, J. M., Brunet, F., Petit, J. L., Stange-Thomann, N., Mauceli, E., et al. (2004). Genome duplication in the teleost fish Tetraodon nigroviridis reveals the early vertebrate proto-karyotype. *Nature* 431, 946–957.

Jazin, E. E., Yoo, H., Blomqvist, A. G., Yee, F., Weng, G., Walker, M. W., et al. (1993). A proposed bovine neuropeptide Y (NPY) receptor, or its human homologue, confers neither NPY binding sites nor NPY responsiveness on transfected cells. *Regul. Pept.* 47, 247–258.

Jordan, I. K., Marino-Ramirez, L., and Koonin, E. V. (2005). Evolutionary significance of gene expression divergence. *Gene* 345, 119–126.

Khaitovich, P., Hellmann, I., Enard, W., Nowick, K., Leinweber, M., Franz, H., et al. (2005). Parallel patterns of evolution in the genomes and transcriptomes of humans and chimpanzees. *Science* 309, 1850–1854.

Kim, D. K., Cho, E. B., Moon, M. J., Park, S., Hwang, J. I., Kah, O., et al. (2011). Revisiting the evolution of gonadotropin-releasing hormones and their receptors in vertebrates: secrets hidden in genomes. *Gen. Comp. Endocrinol.* 170, 68–78.

Kurokawa, T., and Suzuki, T. (2002). Development of neuropeptide Y-related peptides in the digestive organs during the larval stage of Japanese flounder, Paralichthys olivaceus. *Gen. Comp. Endocrinol.* 126, 30–38.

Larhammar, D. (1996). Evolution of neuropeptide Y, peptide YY, and pancreatic polypeptide. *Regul. Pept.* 62, 1–11.

Larhammar, D., and Salaneck, E. (2004). Molecular evolution of NPY receptor subtypes. *Neuropeptides* 38, 141–151.

Larkin, M. A., Blackshields, G., Brown, N. P., Chenna, R., McGettigan, P. A., McWilliam, H., et al. (2007). Clustal W and Clustal X version 2.0. *Bioinformatics* 23, 2947–2948.

Larsson, T. A., Larson, E. T., and Larhammar, D. (2007). Cloning and sequence analysis of the neuropeptide Y receptors Y5 and Y6 in the coelacanth Latimeria chalumnae. *Gen. Comp. Endocrinol.* 150, 337–342.

Larsson, T. A., Olsson, F., Sundstrom, G., Lundin, L. G., Brenner, S., Venkatesh, B., et al. (2008). Early vertebrate chromosome duplications and the evolution of the neuropeptide Y receptor gene regions. *BMC Evol. Biol.* 8:184. doi:10.1186/1471-2148-8-184

Larsson, T. A., Tay, B. H., Sundstrom, G., Fredriksson, R., Brenner, S., Larhammar, D., et al. (2009). Neuropeptide Y-family peptides and receptors in the elephant shark, *Callorhinchus milii* confirm gene duplications before the gnathostome radiation. *Genomics* 93, 254–260.

Lecklin, A., Lundell, I., Paananen, L., Wikberg, J. E., Mannistö, P. T., and Larhammar, D. (2002). Receptor subtypes Y1 and Y5 mediate neuropeptide Y induced feeding in the guinea-pig. *Br. J. Pharmacol.* 135, 2029–2037.

Lecklin, A., Lundell, I., Salmela, S., Beck-Sickinger, A. G., and Larhammar, D. (2003). Agonists for neuropeptide Y receptors Y1 and Y5 stimulate different phases of feeding in guinea pigs. *Br. J. Pharmacol.* 139, 1433–1440.

Lee, A. P., Kerk, S. Y., Tan, Y. Y., Brenner, S., and Venkatesh, B. (2011). Ancient vertebrate conserved noncoding elements have been evolving rapidly in teleost fishes. *Mol. Biol. Evol.* 28, 1205–1215.

Liang, L., Reinick, C., Angleson, J. K., and Dores, R. M. (2013). Evolution of melanocortin receptors in cartilaginous fish: melanocortin receptors and the stress axis in elasmobranches. *Gen. Comp. Endocrinol.* 181, 4–9.

Lundell, I., Blomqvist, A. G., Berglund, M. M., Schober, D. A., Johnson, D., Statnick, M. A., et al. (1995). Cloning of a human receptor of the NPY receptor family with high affinity for pancreatic polypeptide and peptide YY. *J. Biol. Chem.* 270, 29123–29128.

Lundell, I., Boswell, T., and Larhammar, D. (2002). Chicken neuropeptide Y-family receptor Y4: a receptor with equal affinity for pancreatic polypeptide, neuropeptide Y and peptide YY. *J. Mol. Endocrinol.* 28, 225–235.

Lundell, I., Statnick, M. A., Johnson, D., Schober, D. A., Starbäck, P., Gehlert, D. R., et al. (1996). The cloned rat pancreatic polypeptide receptor exhibits profound differences to the orthologous human receptor. *Proc. Natl. Acad. Sci. U.S.A.* 93, 5111–5115.

Matsumoto, M., Nomura, T., Momoses, K., Ikeda, Y., Kondou, Y., Akiho, H., et al. (1996). Inactivation of a novel neuropeptide Y/peptide YY receptor gene in primate species. *J. Biol. Chem.* 271, 27217–27220.

Mercer, R. E., Chee, M. J., and Colmers, W. F. (2011). The role of NPY in hypothalamic mediated food intake. *Front. Neuroendocrinol.* 32, 398–415.

Montpetit, C. J., Chatalov, V., Yuk, J., Rasaratnam, I., and Youson, J. H. (2005). "Expression of neuropeptide Y family peptides in the brain and gut during stages of the life cycle of a parasitic lamprey (*Petromyzon marinus*) and a nonparasitic lamprey (*Ichthyomyzon gagei*)," in *Trends in Comparative Endocrinology and Neurobiology*, eds H. Vaudry, E. Roubos, L. Schoofs, G. Flik, and D. Larhammar (New York: The New York Academy of Sciences), 140–149.

Murashita, K., Fukada, H., Hosokawa, H., and Masumoto, T. (2006). Cholecystokinin and peptide Y in yellowtail (Seriola quinqueradiata): molecular cloning, real-time quantitative RT-PCR, and response to feeding and fasting. *Gen. Comp. Endocrinol.* 145, 287–297.

Murashita, K., Kurokawa, T., Nilsen, T. O., and Ronnestad, I. (2009). Ghrelin, cholecystokinin, and peptide YY in Atlantic salmon (Salmo salar): molecular cloning and tissue expression. *Gen. Comp. Endocrinol.* 160, 223–235.

Nakatani, Y., Takeda, H., Kohara, Y., and Morishita, S. (2007). Reconstruction of the vertebrate ancestral genome reveals dynamic genome reorganization in early vertebrates. *Genome Res.* 17, 1254–1265.

Naveilhan, P., Neveu, I., Arenas, E., and Ernfors, P. (1998). Complementary and overlapping expression of Y1, Y2, and Y5 receptors in the developing and adult mouse nervous system. *Neuroscience* 87, 289–302.

Oberto, A., Acquadro, E., Bus, T., Sprengel, R., and Eva, C. (2007). Expression patterns of promoters for NPY Y(1) and Y(5) receptors in Y(5)RitTA and Y(1)RVenus BAC-transgenic mice. *Eur. J. Neurosci.* 26, 155–170.

Ocampo Daza, D. (2013). *Evolution of Vertebrate Endocrine and Neuronal Gene Families: Focus on Pituitary and Retina.* Digital Comprehensive Summaries of Uppsala Dissertations from the Faculty of Medicine. Available at: http://uu.diva-portal.org/smash/record.jsf;jsessionid =

a7e31d1a81174723ce69892e197e?pid=diva2:587276

Ocampo Daza, D., Lewicka, M., and Larhammar, D. (2011). The oxytocin/vasopressin receptor family has at least five members in the gnathostome lineage, inclucing two distinct V2 subtypes. *Gen. Comp. Endocrinol.* 175, 135–143.

Ocampo Daza, D., Sundstrom, G., Bergqvist, C. A., and Larhammar, D. (2012). The evolution of vertebrate somatostatin receptors and their gene regions involves extensive chromosomal rearrangements. *BMC Evol. Biol.* 12:231. doi:10.1186/1471-2148-12-231

Parker, R. M., and Herzog, H. (1998). Comparison of Y-receptor subtype expression in the rat hippocampus. *Regul. Pept.* 75–76, 109–115.

Parker, R. M., and Herzog, H. (1999). Regional distribution of Y-receptor subtype mRNAs in rat brain. *Eur. J. Neurosci.* 11, 1431–1448.

Pedrazzini, T., Pralong, F., and Grouzmann, E. (2003). Neuropeptide Y: the universal soldier. *Cell. Mol. Life Sci.* 60, 350–377.

Putnam, N. H., Butts, T., Ferrier, D. E., Furlong, R. F., Hellsten, U., Kawashima, T., et al. (2008). The amphioxus genome and the evolution of the chordate karyotype. *Nature* 453, 1064–1071.

Saitou, N., and Nei, M. (1987). The neighbor joining method: a new method for reconstructing phylogenetic trees. *Mol. Biol. Evol.* 4, 406–425.

Salaneck, E., Ardell, D., Larson, E. T., and Larhammar, D. (2003). Three neuropeptide Y receptors in the spiny dogfish, *Squalus acanthias*, support chromosome doublings in early vertebrate evolution. *Mol. Biol. Evol.* 20, 1271–1280.

Salaneck, E., Fredriksson, R., Larson, E. T., Conlon, J. M., and Larhammar, D. (2001). A neuropeptide Y receptor Y1-subfamily gene from an agnathan, the European river lamprey. A potential ancestral gene. *Eur. J. Biochem.* 268, 6146–6154.

Salaneck, E., Larsson, T. A., Larson, E. T., and Larhammar, D. (2008). Birth and death of neuropeptide Y receptor genes in relation to the teleost fish tetraploidization. *Gene* 409, 61–71.

Shan, Y., and Gras, R. (2011). 43 genes support the lungfish-coelacanth grouping related to the closest living relative of tetrapods with the Bayesian method under the coalescence model. *BMC Res. Notes* 4:49. doi:10.1186/1756-0500-4-49

Söderberg, C., Pieribone, V. A., Dahlstrand, J., Brodin, L., and Larhammar, D. (1994). Neuropeptide role of both peptide YY and neuropeptide Y in vertebrates suggested by abundant expression of their mRNAs in a cyclostome brain. *J. Neurosci. Res.* 37, 633–640.

Söderberg, C., Wraith, A., Ringvall, M., Yan, Y.-L., Postlethwait, J., Brodin, L., et al. (2000). Zebrafish genes for neuropeptide Y and peptide YY reveal origin by chromosome duplication from an ancestral gene linked to the homeobox cluster. *J. Neurochem.* 75, 908–918.

Starbäck, P., Lundell, I., Fredriksson, R., Berglund, M. M., Yan, Y.-L., Wraith, A., et al. (1999). Neuropeptide Y receptor subtype with unique properties cloned in the zebrafish; the zYa receptor. *Brain Res. Mol. Brain Res.* 70, 242–252.

Starbäck, P., Wraith, A., Eriksson, H., and Larhammar, D. (2000). Neuropeptide Y receptor gene y6: multiple deaths or resurrection? *Biochem. Biophys. Res. Commun.* 277, 264–269.

Sundstrom, G., Dreborg, S., and Larhammar, D. (2010). Concomitant duplications of opioid peptide and receptor genes before the origin of jawed vertebrates. *PLoS ONE* 5:e10512. doi:10.1371/journal.pone.0010512

Sundstrom, G., Larsson, T. A., Brenner, S., Venkatesh, B., and Larhammar, D. (2008). Evolution of the neuropeptide Y family: new genes by chromosome duplications in early vertebrates and in teleost fishes. *Gen. Comp. Endocrinol.* 155, 705–716.

Sundstrom, G., Xu, B., Larsson, T. A., Heldin, J., Bergqvist, C. A., Fredriksson, R., et al. (2012). Characterization of the neuropeptide Y system in the frog Silurana tropicalis (Pipidae): three peptides and six receptor subtypes. *Gen. Comp. Endocrinol.* 177, 322–331.

Tostivint, H., Lihrmann, I., and Vaudry, H. (2008). New insight into the molecular evolution of the somatostatin family. *Mol. Cell. Endocrinol.* 286, 5–17.

Wall, A., and Volkoff, H. (2013). Effects of fasting and feeding on the brain mRNA expressions of orexin, tyrosine hydroxylase (TH), PYY and CCK in the Mexican blind cavefish (Astyanax fasciatus mexicanus). *Gen. Comp. Endocrinol.* 183, 44–52.

Waterhouse, A. M., Procter, J. B., Martin, D. M., Clamp, M., and Barton, G. J. (2009). Jalview version 2: a multiple sequence alignment editor and analysis workbench. *Bioinformatics* 25, 1189–1191.

Wolak, M. L., Dejoseph, M. R., Cator, A. D., Mokashi, A. S., Brownfield, M. S., and Urban, J. H. (2003). Comparative distribution of neuropeptide Y Y1 and Y5 receptors in the rat brain by using immunohistochemistry. *J. Comp. Neurol.* 464, 285–311.

Wraith, A. (1999). *Molecular Evolution of the Neuropeptide Y Receptor Family. Insights from Mammals and Fish.* Uppsala: Uppsala University. [Comprehensive Summaries of Uppsala Dissertations from the Faculty of Medicine 893, ISBN 91-554-4611-6].

Wraith, A., Törnsten, A., Chardon, P., Harbitz, I., Chowdhary, B. P., Andersson, L., et al. (2000). Evolution of the neuropeptide Y receptor family: gene and chromosome duplications deduced from the cloning of the five receptor subtype genes in pig. *Genome Res.* 10, 302–310.

Xu, B., Sundstrom, G., Kuraku, S., Lundell, I., and Larhammar, D. (2012). Cloning and pharmacological characterization of the neuropeptide Y receptor Y5 in the sea lamprey, Petromyzon marinus. *Peptides* 39C, 64–70.

Yamaguchi, Y., Kaiya, H., Konno, N., Iwata, E., Miyazato, M., Uchiyama, M., et al. (2012). The fifth neurohypophysial hormone receptor is structurally related to the V2-type receptor but functionally similar to V1-type receptors. *Gen. Comp. Endocrinol.* 178, 519–528.

Zhang, L., Bijker, M. S., and Herzog, H. (2011). The neuropeptide Y system: pathophysiological and therapeutic implications in obesity and cancer. *Pharmacol. Ther.* 131, 91–113.

17

Isolation of the bioactive peptides CCHamide-1 and CCHamide-2 from *Drosophila* and their putative role in appetite regulation as ligands for G protein-coupled receptors

Takanori Ida[1]*, Tomoko Takahashi[2], Hatsumi Tominaga[1], Takahiro Sato[3], Hiroko Sano[3], Kazuhiko Kume[4], Mamiko Ozaki[5], Tetsutaro Hiraguchi[5], Hajime Shiotani[5], Saki Terajima[5], Yuki Nakamura[5], Kenji Mori[6], Morikatsu Yoshida[6], Johji Kato[7], Noboru Murakami[8], Mikiya Miyazato[6], Kenji Kangawa[6] and Masayasu Kojima[3]

[1] *Interdisciplinary Research Organization, University of Miyazaki, Miyazaki, Japan*
[2] *Department of Biology, School of Medicine, Kurume University, Fukuoka, Japan*
[3] *Molecular Genetics, Institute of Life Sciences, Kurume University, Fukuoka, Japan*
[4] *Department of Stem Cell Biology, Institute of Molecular Embryology and Genetics, Kumamoto University, Kumamoto, Japan*
[5] *Department of Biology, Graduate School of Science, Kobe University, Hyogo, Japan*
[6] *Department of Biochemistry, National Cerebral and Cardiovascular Center Research Institute, Osaka, Japan*
[7] *Frontier Science Research Center, University of Miyazaki, Miyazaki, Japan*
[8] *Department of Veterinary Physiology, Faculty of Agriculture, University of Miyazaki, Miyazaki, Japan*

Edited by:
Hubert Vaudry, University of Rouen, France

Reviewed by:
Young-Joon Kim, Gwangju Institute of Science and Technology, South Korea
Liliane Schoofs, Catholic University of Leuven, Belgium
Christian Wegener, Universität Würzburg, Germany

****Correspondence:***
Takanori Ida, Interdisciplinary Research Organization, University of Miyazaki, Miyazaki 889-1692, Japan
e-mail: a0d203u@cc.miyazaki-u.ac.jp

There are many orphan G protein-coupled receptors (GPCRs) for which ligands have not yet been identified. One such GPCR is the bombesin receptor subtype 3 (BRS-3). BRS-3 plays a role in the onset of diabetes and obesity. GPCRs in invertebrates are similar to those in vertebrates. Two *Drosophila* GPCRs (CG30106 and CG14593) belong to the BRS-3 phylogenetic subgroup. Here, we succeeded to biochemically purify the endogenous ligands of *Drosophila* CG30106 and CG14593 from whole *Drosophila* homogenates using functional assays with the reverse pharmacological technique, and identified their primary amino acid sequences. The purified ligands had been termed CCHamide-1 and CCHamide-2, although structurally identical to the peptides recently predicted from the genomic sequence searching. In addition, our biochemical characterization demonstrated two N-terminal extended forms of CCHamide-2. When administered to blowflies, CCHamide-2 increased their feeding motivation. Our results demonstrated these peptides actually present as the major components to activate these receptors in living *Drosophila*. Studies on the effects of CCHamides will facilitate the search for BRS-3 ligands.

Keywords: GPCR, novel bioactive peptide, *Drosophila*, CCHamide, bombesin receptor subtype 3

INTRODUCTION

G protein-coupled receptors (GPCRs) constitute a large protein superfamily that shares a 7-transmembrane motif as a common structure. Human genome sequencing has identified several hundred orphan GPCRs for which ligands have not yet been identified (Vassilatis et al., 2003). GPCRs play crucial roles in cell-to-cell communication involved in a variety of physiological phenomena and are the most common target of pharmaceutical drugs. Therefore, the identification of endogenous ligands for orphan GPCRs will lead to clarification of novel physiological regulatory mechanisms and potentially facilitate the development of new GPCR-targeted therapeutics. Many bioactive molecules have been discovered or identified as endogenous ligands of orphan GPCRs through reverse pharmacology to date (Civelli et al., 2012). These molecules include nociceptin, prolactin-releasing peptide, orexin, apelin, ghrelin, metastin, and neuromedin S. The discovery of novel endogenous ligands for orphan GPCRs in mammals is currently challenging, possibly because of the restricted timing of expression or distribution of GPCR ligands. One orphan receptor in mammals is the bombesin receptor subtype 3 (BRS-3). BRS-3 is primarily expressed in the hypothalamus and plays a role in the onset of diabetes and obesity (Ohki-Hamazaki et al., 1997). Although several small molecules that are agonists and antagonists for BRS-3 have been synthesized, the native ligand of BRS-3 has not yet been identified (Majumdar and Weber, 2012).

The recent sequencing of the *Drosophila melanogaster* genome has enabled the identification of at least 160 fly GPCRs (Brody and Cravchik, 2000). *Drosophila* is an excellent animal model for genetic analysis of developmental and behavioral processes, as it is a small, genetically modifiable organism with a relatively short lifecycle and can be bred easily under laboratory conditions. Structural or sequence comparison of newly discovered peptides in *Drosophila* with candidate molecules in mammals may lead to the discovery of new peptide signaling modules. We recently reported the discovery of dRYamide-1, dRYamide-2, and trissin as ligands

Abbreviations: BRS-3, bombesin receptor subtype 3; GPCR, G protein coupled receptors.

for *Drosophila* orphan GPCRs (Ida et al., 2011a,b). We consider it likely that additional novel bioactive peptides can be discovered for orphan GPCRs. Two *Drosophila* GPCRs (CG14593 and CG30106) belong to the BRS-3 phylogenetic subgroup (Hewes and Taghert, 2001).

Here, we report the identification of CCHamide-1 and CCHamide-2, which are ligands for GPCRs CG30106 and CG14593, respectively, in *D. melanogaster*. Injection of CCHamide-2 resulted in the stimulation of feeding motivation in blowflies. These bioactive peptides may provide new insights in the search for BRS-3 ligands and the elucidation of *D. melanogaster* feeding mechanisms.

MATERIALS AND METHODS

PURIFICATION OF *Drosophila* CCHamide-1 AND CCHamide-2

An assay system using CG30106- or CG14593-expressing cells was prepared as previously described (Ida et al., 2011a,b). The full-length cDNA of *Drosophila* CG30106 (GenBank accession number: NM_136355; residues −31 to 1700) and CG14593 (GenBank accession number: NM_136355; residues 656–2185) was obtained by RT-PCR using *Drosophila* cDNA as the template. The sense and antisense primers for CG30106 were 5′-aaatcgagcggactcagtacat-3′ and 5′-gtggcctgtaattcctgtaaactc-3′, respectively. The sense and antisense primers for CG14593 were 5′-tgagacatcttgcccaggag-3′ and 5′-gtgtttcggtacctccatttat-3′, respectively. The amplified cDNA was ligated into the pcDNA3.1 vector (Invitrogen). The expression vector, i.e., CG30106 or CG14593-pcDNA3.1, was transfected into Chinese hamster ovary (CHO) cells by using with Fugene6 transfection reagent (Roche), and stably expressing cells were selected using 1 mg/ml G418. The selected cell line, i.e., CHO-CG30106-line 2-4 or CHO-CG14593-line 10-1, showed the highest expression of CG3106 or CG14593 mRNA, respectively. Cells were cultured in a humidified environment of 95% air and 5% CO_2. Changes in intracellular Ca^{2+} concentrations ($[Ca^{2+}]_i$) were measured using the FlexStation 3 fluorometric imaging plate reader to conduct high-throughput measurements of intracellular Ca^{2+} concentration (Molecular Devices, CA, USA; Marshall et al., 2005). CHO-CG30106 or CHO-CG14593 cells (3×10^4 cells) were plated into 96-well black-wall microplates (Corning, NY, USA) 20 h before each assay. The cells were incubated with 100 μl of Calcium 4 assay kit reagent (Molecular Devices) for 1 h, and then 50 μl of each sample was added to the CHO-CG30106 or CHO-CG14593 cells to induce changes in fluorescence. The maximum $[Ca^{2+}]_i$ changes were recorded.

Drosophila melanogaster flies (Canton S.; 350 g) were collected on dry ice. The whole body of each fly was boiled for 10 min in 10 volumes of water to inactivate intrinsic proteases. The solution was adjusted to 1 M AcOH. Peptides were extracted by homogenization using a Polytron mixer. The supernatant of the extracts, obtained after 30 min of centrifugation at 11,000 rpm, was concentrated to approximately 1/10 by an evaporator. The residual concentrate was subjected to acetone precipitation using 66% acetone. After the precipitates were removed, the supernatant acetone was evaporated and loaded onto a 40-g cartridge of Sep-Pak C18 (Waters), which was pre-equilibrated with 0.1% trifluoroacetic acid (TFA). The Sep-Pak cartridge was washed with 10% CH_3CN/0.1% TFA, and then eluted with 60% CH_3CN/0.1% TFA. The eluate was evaporated and lyophilized. The residual materials were redissolved in 1 M AcOH and then adsorbed on a column of SP-Sephadex C-25 (H^+ form) that had been pre-equilibrated with 1 M AcOH. Successive elutions with 1 M AcOH, 2 M pyridine, and 2 M pyridine–AcOH (pH 5.0) provided three fractions of SP-I, SP-II, and SP-III. A basic peptide fraction (SP-III) was fractionated on a Sephadex G-50 gel filtration column (2.9 cm × 142 cm; GE Healthcare, Tokyo, Japan). A portion of each fraction, equivalent to 1.16 g of flies, was subjected to the assay using CHO-CG30106 or CHO-CG14593 cells. The active fraction was separated by carboxymethyl (CM)-ion-exchange high-performance liquid chromatography (HPLC) on a TSK CM-2SW column (4.6 mm × 250 mm; Tosoh, Tokyo, Japan) with an ammonium formate ($HCOONH_4$; pH 6.5) gradient of 10 mM to 1 M in the presence of 10% acetonitrile (ACN) at a flow rate of 1 ml/min for 160 min. The active fractions were separated by reverse-phase (RP)-HPLC with a μBondasphere C18 column (3.9 mm × 150 mm, Waters, MA, USA) by using a 10–60% ACN/0.1% TFA linear gradient at a flow rate of 1 ml/min for 80 min. The active fractions were further purified by RP-HPLC using a diphenyl column (2.1 mm × 150 mm, 219TP5125; Vydac, Hesperia, CA, USA) for 80 min by using a linear gradient of 10–60% ACN/0.1% TFA at a flow rate of 0.2 ml/min. Fractions corresponding to absorption peaks were collected, and an aliquot of each fraction (2 g tissue equivalent) was assayed by using the FLEX system. The active fractions were further purified by RP-HPLC by using a Chemcosorb 3ODSH column (2.1 mm × 75 mm; Chemco, Osaka, Japan) for 80 or 160 min by using a linear gradient of 10–60% ACN/0.1% TFA at a flow rate of 0.2 ml/min. Fractions corresponding to absorption peaks were collected, and an aliquot of each fraction (2 g tissue equivalent) was assayed by using the FLEX system. Approximately 20 pmol of the final purified peptides was analyzed using a protein sequencer (model 494; Applied Biosystems, CA, USA), and approximately 1 pmol of each active fraction was subjected to determination of molecular weight by matrix-assisted laser desorption–ionization time of flight (MALDI-TOF) mass spectrometry by using a Voyager-DE PRO instrument (Applied Biosystems).

CLONING OF *Drosophila* PREPRO-CCHamide-1 AND CCHamide-2 cDNA

A tBLASTn search of the *Drosophila* genome resources was performed by using sequence of the purified peptides, and we obtained *D. melanogaster* mRNA sequences [CG14358 (CCHamide-1), NM_001104314; and CG14375 (CCHamide-2), NM_142028] derived from an annotated genomic sequence. We searched for open reading frames upstream and downstream of the genome sequences of CCHamide-1 and CCHamide-2 by using specific primers 5′-cgtgcagcttgcgaaataata-3′ and 5′-cttctggcttagctagcgtgttatc-3′ for CCHamide-1 and 5′-caccagccaagtgcaagtatc-3′ and 5′-cggtttttaatgtacgttgtgg-3′ for CCHamide-2. The candidate PCR product was subcloned into the pCR-II TOPO vector and sequenced. The nucleotide sequence of the isolated cDNA fragment was determined by automated sequencing (DNA sequencer model 3100; Applied Biosystems) according to the protocol for the BigDye terminator cycle sequencing kit (Applied Biosystems).

PEPTIDES

CCHamide-1 (SCLEYGHSCWGAH-NH_2), CCHamide-2 (GCQAYGHVCYGGH-NH_2), CCHamide-1 C-terminal free (SCLEYGHSCWGAH), CCHamide-2 C-terminal free (GCQAYGHVCYGGH), long-form CCHamide-2 (AQQSQAKKGCQAYGHVCYGGH-NH_2), and long-form CCHamide-2 C-terminal free (AQQSQAKKGCQAYGHVCYGGH) were synthesized by Peptide Institute Inc. (Osaka, Japan).

PROBOSCIS EXTENSION REFLEX TEST FOR APPETITE MEASUREMENT

The proboscis extension reflex (PER) test and feeding test were performed for the blowfly *Phormia regina* as previously described (Nisimura et al., 2005; Ida et al., 2011a). CCHamide-2 was dissolved in blowfly linger solution at a concentration of 10 pμol/ml. Twenty flies were secured by their wings using washing pins, and the first PER test was performed by using 12 steps of sucrose concentrations that had been prepared by twofold serial dilutions in distilled water, beginning from a sucrose concentration of 1 M. We investigated the PER in three different groups of 20 flies each: no injection, fly linger injection, and fly linger plus peptide injection. The PER tests were performed 30 min after 1 μl of blowfly linger solution with or without peptide was injected into the shoulder of each fly. We repeated five sets of PER tests each, in which 20 flies were used in each batch.

STATISTICAL ANALYSIS

Results are presented as the mean ± SEM for each group. To compare the PER thresholds among the three groups, we used a non-parametric Steel–Dwass test. The criterion for statistical significance was $p < 0.05$ for all tests. The statistical software program GraphPad PRISM (GraphPad software, CA, USA) was used for analyses.

RESULTS

STRUCTURAL DETERMINATION OF CCHamide-1 FOR CG30106

$[Ca^{2+}]_i$ assays were performed by using the gel filtration samples to isolate the endogenous ligands of CG30106 (**Figure 1A**). The active fractions were observed in eight sequential fractions (numbers 48–55). The fractions (51–55) with particularly high activity were separated by CM-ion-exchange HPLC at pH 6.5. The active fractions were separated by RP-HPLC. The active fraction was purified as a single peak in the final RP-HPLC (**Figure 1B**, P1). The amino acid sequence of the purified peptide was determined as SXLEYGHSXWGAH (P1; where X is a position that was not identified) using a protein sequencer. To elucidate the complete amino acid sequence of this peptide, *Drosophila* cDNA encoding the purified peptides was isolated by RT-PCR. The cDNA encoded a 182-residue protein (CG14358; **Figure 1C**) that contained features characteristic of an N-terminal signal peptide immediately preceding the purified peptide sequence. Every X residue was a cysteine, and the rest of the sequence was identical to that determined by peptide sequencing (**Figure 1C**). Sequencing resulted in a very low yield of phenyl thiohydantoin (PTH) at the steps involving X, which suggests that two cysteines may form disulfide bonds (S–S bonds). The preproprotein contained a potential processing site at the C-terminal end of the purified peptide sequence. This peptide contained Gly residues that presumably serve as an amide donor for C-terminal amidation. We therefore deduced the primary structure of the peptide to be SCLEYGHSCWGAH-NH_2. This peptide had been named CCHamide-1 (Roller et al., 2008). Mass spectrometric analysis revealed that the observed monoisotopic *m/z* value of the purified peptide (1445.30) was very similar to the theoretically predicted value for this peptide (1445.55) when including an intrachain disulfide bond and C-terminal amidation. We generated the synthetic peptide SCLEYGHSCWGAH-NH_2 (CCHamide-1). The retention time of the P1 active fraction was identical to that of the synthetic SCLEYGHSCWGAH-NH_2 peptide (which has an intrachain disulfide bond) on RP-HPLC (**Figure 1D**). Thus, these data suggest that both natural peptides have an intrachain disulfide bond and C-terminal amidation. **Figure 1E** shows the active fractions of each chromatography and the amino acid sequence of CCHamide-1.

STRUCTURAL DETERMINATION OF CCHamide-2 FOR CG14593

The endogenous ligands of CG14593 were isolated in the same manner as those of CG30106 (**Figure 2A**). Three separate active fractions were revealed (**Figure 2G**, P2, P3, and P4), and each active fraction was purified as a single peak in the final RP-HPLC (**Figures 2B–D**). From the results obtained by using a protein sequencer and *Drosophila* cDNA encoding the purified peptides (**Figure 2E**), we deduced the primary structure of the peptide to be AQQSQAKKGCQAYGHVCYGGH-NH_2 (P2), GCQAYGHVCYGGH-NH_2 (P3), and KKGCQAYGHVCYGGH-NH_2 (P4; **Figure 2G**). All of these cysteines may form S–S bonds. The shortest peptide (P3) had been named CCHamide-2. The cDNA encoded a 136-residue protein (CG14375; **Figure 2E**) that contained features characteristic of an N-terminal signal peptide immediately preceding the purified longest peptide sequence (P2). All peptides were derived from the same precursor (CG14375), but the length of the N-terminal peptide was different. Mass spectrometric analysis revealed that the observed monoisotopic *m/z* values of the purified peptides (P2, 2216.80; P3, 1347.69; and P4, 1603.60) were similar to the theoretically predicted values (2216.99, 1347.52, and 1603.71, respectively) for a peptide that has an intrachain S–S bonds and C-terminal amidation. We generated the synthetic peptides AQQSQAKKGCQAYGHVCYGGH-NH_2 (long-form CCHamide-2) and GCQAYGHVCYGGH-NH_2 (CCHamide-2). The retention times of the P2 and P3 active fractions were identical to those of the synthetic AQQSQAKKGCQAYGHVCYGGH-NH_2 and GCQAYGHVCYGGH-NH_2 peptides (which have an intrachain disulfide bond) on RP-HPLC, respectively (**Figure 2F**). Thus, these data suggest that both natural peptides have an intrachain disulfide bond and C-terminal amidation.

PHARMACOLOGICAL CHARACTERIZATION

The interaction of CCHamide-1 and CCHamide-2 with CG30106 or CG14593 was examined using synthetic peptides. CCHamide-1 induced concentration-dependent, robust increases in $[Ca^{2+}]_i$ in CHO-CG30106 cells, with a half-maximal response concentration (EC_{50}) of 1.80×10^{-11} M (**Figure 3A**). CCHamide-2 potently activated CG30106 (EC_{50}; 4.86×10^{-9} M (**Figure 3A**). CCHamide-2 induced dose-dependent, robust increases in $[Ca^{2+}]_i$ in CHO-CG14593 cells, with an EC_{50} of 4.80×10^{-11} M (**Figure 3B**).

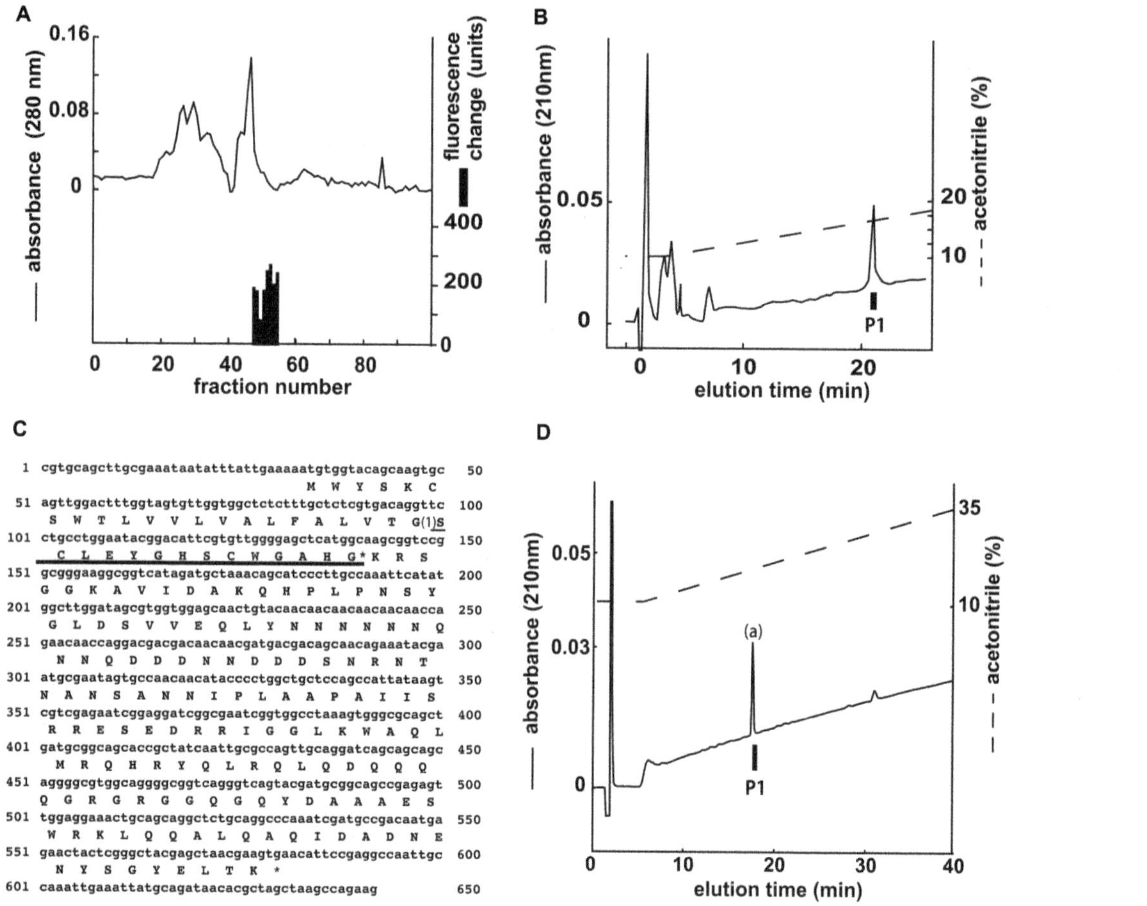

E

gel filtration	ion-exchange-HPLC (ammonium formate : mM)	reverse-phase-HPLC (acetonitrile : %)		sequence
fr51-55	fr23-24 (171-191 mM)	fr31-32 (19.4-20.0%)	P1	SCLEYGHSCWGAH-NH2

※ C C disulfide bond

FIGURE 1 | Purification of CCHamide-1 from fly extracts. *Black bars* indicate changes of $[Ca^{2+}]_i$ fluorescence signal in CHO-CG30106 cells. **(A)** G-50 gel filtration of the SP-III fraction of fly extracts. The active fraction was subjected to one step of CM-ion-exchange HPLC and three steps of RP-HPLC. **(B)** Final purification of the active fraction by RP-HPLC. **(C)** Nucleotide sequence and deduced amino acid sequence of CCHamide-1 cDNA. CCHamide-1 cDNA encode 182-residue peptides. The asterisk indicates a glycine residue that serves as an amide donor for C-terminal amidation. The CCHamide-1 sequence is underlined as (1). **(D)** Chromatographic comparison by RP-HPLC of natural CCHamide-1 and synthetic CCHamide-1. *Black bar* (P1) indicates the changes of $[Ca^{2+}]_i$ fluorescence signal in CHO-CG30106 cells. Each peptide was applied to a Symmetry C18 column (3.9 mm × 150 mm, Waters, MA, USA) with a 10–60% ACN/0.1% trifluoroacetic acid (TFA) linear gradient at a flow rate of 1 ml/min for 80 min. P1 represent active fraction containing natural CCHamide-1. (a) Synthetic CCHamide-1. **(E)** Active fractions of each chromatography and the amino acid sequence of CCHamide-1.

CCHamide-1 potently activated CG14593 (EC_{50}; 3.32×10^{-8} M (**Figure 3B**). Neither CCHamide-2 nor CCHamide-1 induced a response in CHO cells transfected with the vector alone (data not shown). In the investigation of the interaction between non-C-terminal amidated synthetic peptides or long-form CCHamide-2 and CG30106, the EC_{50} values were as follows: non-C-terminal amidated CCHamide-1, 1.66×10^{-10} M; non-C-terminal amidated long-form CCHamide-2, 8.93×10^{-8} M; long-form CCHamide-2, 6.45×10^{-8} M; and non-C-terminal amidated CCHamide-2, 1.22×10^{-7} M (**Figure 3C**). For CG14593, the EC_{50} values were as follows: long-form CCHamide-2, 1.49×10^{-10} M; non-C-terminal amidated long-form CCHamide-2, 1.18×10^{-9} M; non-C-terminal amidated CCHamide-2, 1.13×10^{-8} M; and non-C-terminal amidated CCHamide-1, 1.02×10^{-7} M (**Figure 3D**).

PER TEST FOR MEASURING FEEDING SENSITIVITY

As shown in **Figure 4**, a significant decrease was observed in the mean PER threshold, which was defined as the sucrose concentration at which 50% of flies show PER, after the injection of 10 pmol

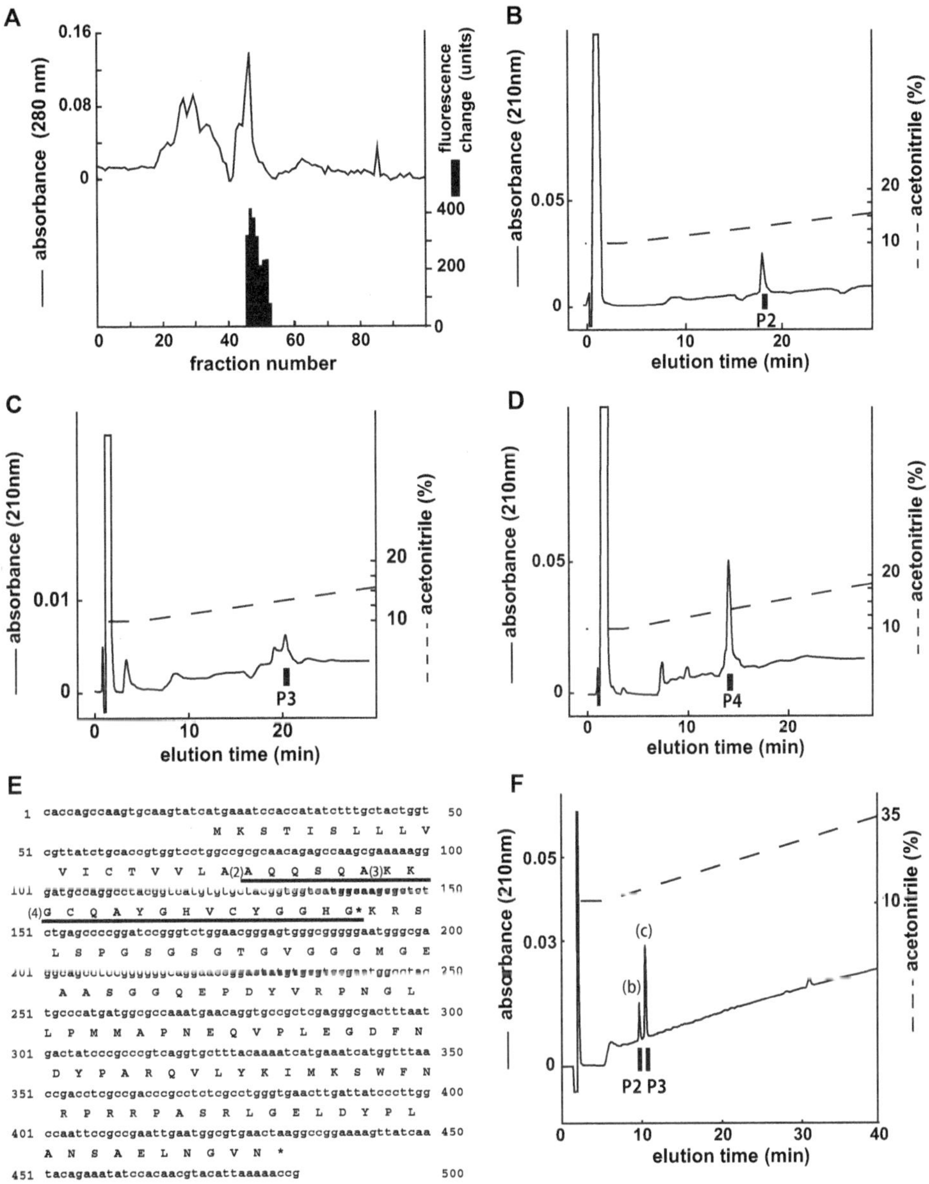

G

gel filtration	ion-exchange-HPLC (ammonium formate : mM)	reverse-phase-HPLC (acetonitrile : %)		sequence
fr47-50	fr38-41 (322-362 mM)	fr15-16 (14.4-15.0%)	P2	AQQSQAKKGCQAYGHVCYGGH-NH2
		fr17-18 (15.0-15.6%)	P3	GCQAYGHVCYGGH-NH2
	fr50-51 (443-463 mM)	fr15-16 (14.4-15.0%)	P4	KKGCQAYGHVCYGGH-NH2

※ C C disulfide bond

FIGURE 2 | Purification of CCHamide-2 from fly extracts. *Black bars* indicate changes of $[Ca^{2+}]_i$ fluorescent signal in CHO-CG14593 cells. **(A)** G-50 gel filtration of the SP-III fraction of fly extracts. The active fraction was subjected to one step of CM-ion-exchange HPLC and three steps of RP-HPLC. **(B–D)** Final purification of the active fraction by RP-HPLC. **(E)** Nucleotide sequence and deduced amino acid sequence of CCHamide-2 cDNA. CCHamide-2 cDNA encodes a 136-residue peptides. The asterisk indicates a glycine residue that serves as an amide donor for C-terminal amidation. The CCHamide-2 sequence is underlined as (4). The other long-form of CCHamide-2 is translated from (2) or (3). **(F)** Chromatographic comparison by RP-HPLC of natural CCHamide-2 and synthetic CCHamide-2. *Black bars* (P2, P3) indicate the changes of $[Ca^{2+}]_i$ fluorescence signal in CHO-CG14593 cells. Each peptide was applied to a Symmetry C18 column with a linear gradient elution for 80 min. P2 and P3 represent active fractions containing natural CCHamide-2. (b) Synthetic long-form of CCHamide-2. (c) Synthetic CCHamide-2. **(G)** Active fractions of each chromatography and the amino acid sequence of CCHamide-2.

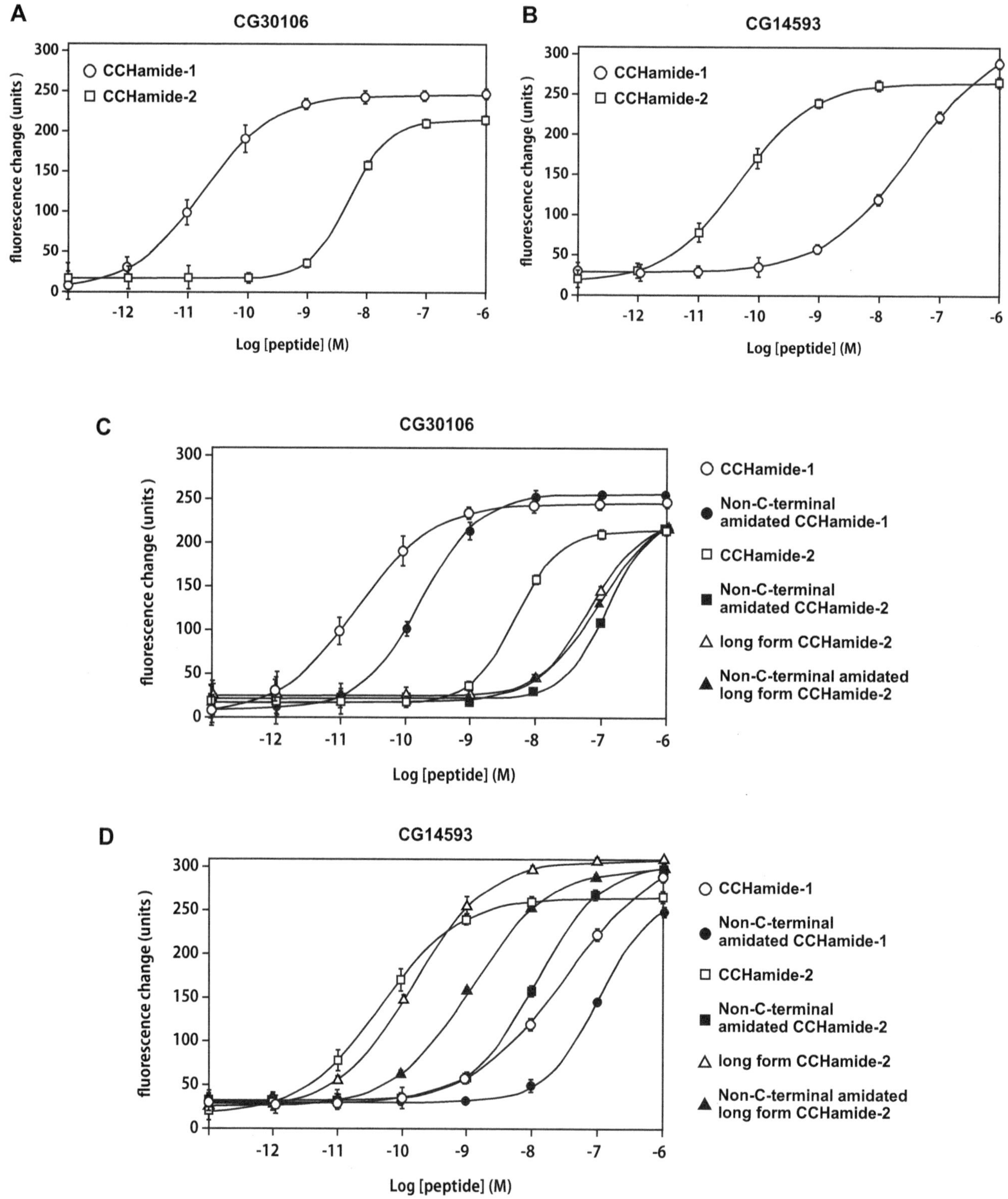

FIGURE 3 | Pharmacological characterization of synthetic peptides using CG30106 or CG14593 stably expressed in CHO cells. (A,B) Concentration–response relationships of changes in $[Ca^{2+}]_i$ for CCHamide-1 (open circle) and CCHamide-2 (open square), in CHO-CG30106 cells **(A)** or CHO-CG14593 cells **(B)**. **(C,D)** Concentration–response relationships of changes in $[Ca^{2+}]_i$ for various peptides, CCHamide-1 (open circle), and CCHamide-2 (open square) in CHO-CG30106 cells **(C)** or CHO-CG14593 cells **(D)**. Non-C-terminal amidated CCHamide-1 (filled circle), non-C-terminal amidated CCHamide-2 (filled square), long-form CCHamide-2 (open triangle), and non-C-terminal amidated long-form CCHamide-2 (filled triangle). Each symbol on the line graph represents the mean ± SEM of data from six replicates for each experiment.

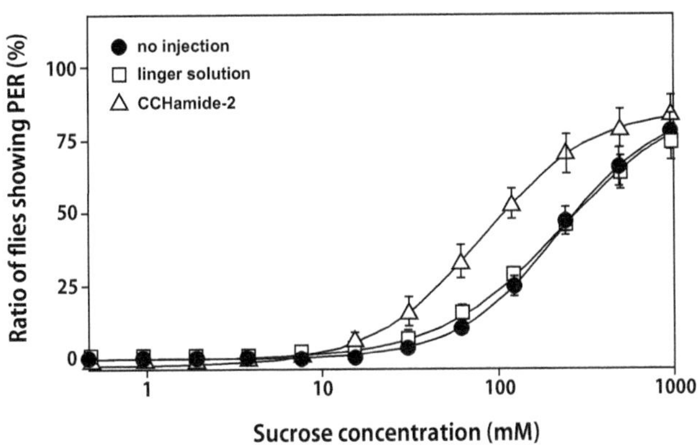

FIGURE 4 | Effect of CCHamide-2 on PER of the blowfly. Sigmoidal curves show the sucrose concentration–PER relationship for three fly groups: no injection (closed circle), injection with linger solution (open square), and injection of CCHamide-2 (open triangle). Each symbol on the line graph represents the mean ± SEM of data from five replicates for each experiment.

of CCHamide-2: the mean PER threshold decreased from 236 mM (30 min after linger solution injection) to 77.2 mM (30 min after CCHamide-2 injection; $p < 0.05$). In contrast, no difference was observed between the mean PER threshold without any injection and 30 min after linger solution injection (222 and 236 mM, respectively, $p > 0.05$).

DISCUSSION

In this study, we biochemically purified 2 *Drosophila* peptides (CCHamide-1 and CCHamide-2) as endogenous ligands for *Drosophila* GPCRs CG30106 and CG14593. Recently, Hansen et al. (2011) independently identified these peptides from genome database and reported that synthetic CCHamide-1 and CCHamide-2 potently activated CHO/G-16 cells expressing recombinant CG30106 and CG14593. Then, Reiher et al. (2011) characterized CCHamide-1 and CCHamide-2 from the *Drosophila* midgut by capillary offline RP-HPLC coupled with MALDI-TOF MS/MS. Our biochemical characterization, however, for the first time, demonstrated three forms of CCHamide-2. The CCHamide-2 preproprotein is 136 amino acid residues long and contains three forms of CCHamide-2. The CCHamide-1 preproprotein is 182 amino acid residues long and contains one form of CCHamide-1. Pharmacological characterization by using CHO cells expressing GPCRs indicated that CCHamide-1 had a high potency for activating recombinant CG30106, but CCHamide-2 rather potently activated CG30106. In contrast, CCHamide-2 had a high potency for activating recombinant CG14593, but CCHamide-1 rather potently activated CG14593. Long-form CCHamide-2 and CCHamide-2 shared a highly similar potency for activating recombinant CG14593. Although we did not generate synthetic KKGCQAYGHVCYGGH-NH_2, it is predicted to have a high potency similar to that of other forms of CCHamide-2 for activating CG14593 because of the relationship between the amount of purified peptide and the specific activity. KKGCQAYGHVCYGGH-NH_2 (P4) and AQQSQAKKGCQAYGHVCYGGH-NH_2 (P2) may be incomplete processing intermediates of GCQAYGHVCYGGH-NH_2 (P3), originating from two alternative signal peptide cleavage sites and incomplete KK prohormone convertase processing. The quantity of the purified peptide could not be accurately measured at the time of the experiments. Because the gel filtration fractions with particularly high activity were separated by CM-ion-exchange HPLC at pH 6.5, we did not purify all peptides for their receptors from the flies collected. However, we purified peptide KKGCQAYGHVCYGGH-NH_2 (P4) > AQQSQAKKGCQAYGHVCYGGH-NH_2 (P2) > GCQAYGHVCYGGH-NH_2 (P3) in amount. Therefore, in this study, we cannot conclude whether P4 and P2 are mature peptides or incomplete processing intermediates of P3. Because both CCHamide-1 and CCHamide-2 have a disulfide bond and a YGH motif, the disulfide bond is predicted to be an important structure for GPCR activation. Additionally, both peptides have a GXG-NH_2 motif at the C-terminus. Therefore, we synthesized non-C-terminal amidated peptides to determine whether the C-terminal amide was necessary for the activation of each receptor. These results show that these peptides are considered to require both disulfide bonds and C-terminal amides to activate their respective GPCRs. Because we biochemically purified these ligands for the receptors by using the reverse pharmacological technique, we propose that no further modified forms or unknown ligands exist for these receptors in the fruit fly. CCHamide-1 is a cognate ligand for CG30106 and the three forms of CCHamide-2 are cognate ligands for CG14593.

BRS-3 is a mammalian orphan receptor (Ohki-Hamazaki et al., 1997). *Drosophila* CG30106 and CG14593 belong to the BRS-3 phylogenetic subgroup (Hewes and Taghert, 2001). To provide new insights into the search for BRS-3 ligands, we examined whether CCHamides activate BRS-3, but we did not find any effect (data not shown).

CCHamide-1 and CCHamide-2 have been shown to be expressed predominantly in the brain and midgut (by FlyAtlas; http://www.flyatlas.org/; Chintapalli et al., 2007). In addition, CCHamide-1 and CCHamide-2 have been detected in the nervous system and midgut in a mass spectrometry study performed by Reiher et al. (2011). Therefore, CCHamides are suggested to be brain–gut peptides in insects. It is generally accepted that brain–gut peptides regulate feeding behavior in mammals (Williams et al., 2001). These peptides include neuropeptide Y, peptide YY, gastrin-releasing peptide, vasoactive intestinal peptide, adrenomedullin, cholecystokinin, galanin, glucagon-like peptide-1, and neuromedin U (Zimanyi et al., 1998; Beck, 2001). In addition, CCHamide-2 was distributed in the larval fat body (by FlyAtlas). The insect fat body is a functional counterpart of the mammalian adipose tissue and liver (Gutierrez et al., 2007). In mammal adipose tissue, leptin and adiponectin are important for feeding modulation. Therefore, we evaluated the effects of CCHamide on feeding by using the PER test in the blowfly *Phormia regina*. In flies and certain other insects, the PER test has long been used to investigate behavioral sensitivity to phagostimulative tastes (Nisimura et al., 2005). Flies extend their proboscis when the contact chemosensilla on their labella detects sweetness of sugar above a certain threshold concentration. Thus, we estimated the appetite or feeding motivation of the flies on the basis of the PER test for sucrose, in which the threshold concentration of sucrose was evaluated as an indicator of feeding sensitivity. The injection of CCHamide-2 decreased the threshold for feeding on a sucrose solution. These data suggest that CCHamide-2 stimulates the feeding motivation of flies. Indeed, administration of CCHamide-2 significantly increased the sucrose intake (Hiraguchi et al., paper in preparation). In the presence of amino acids in the diet, target-of-rapamycin complex 1 (TORC1) signaling in fat cells generates a positive messenger that is released into the hemolymph (Colombani et al., 2003). This signal reaches the brain insulin-producing cells (IPCs), where it remotely controls the secretion of *Drosophila* insulin-like peptides (Dilp). Insulin-like peptides couple growth, metabolism, longevity, and fertility with changes in nutritional availability (Géminard et al., 2009). If CCHamide is a humoral factor that is secreted from the fat body like unpaired 2, it may play an important role in the modulation of nutrient status and growth (Rajan and Perrimon, 2012). Mice lacking functional BRS-3 develop metabolic defects and obesity (Ohki-Hamazaki et al., 1997). Therefore, the natural ligand of BRS-3 is expected to be a prominent inhibitor of appetitive behavior. The difference between CCHamide and the unknown ligand for BRS-3 with regard to feeding behavior is not clear. Further studies should de-orphanize BRS-3 by considering CCHamide by using bioinformatics or antibodies for CCHamide or *Drosophila* GPCRs.

ACKNOWLEDGMENTS

We thank Kaori Shirouzu, Masako Naito, and Eri Iwamoto for their technical assistance. This work was financially supported in part by the Improvement of Research Environment for Young Researchers Program of the Ministry of Education, Culture, Sports, Science and Technology; a grant for Scientific Research on Priority Areas from the University of Miyazaki; grants-in-aid from the Ministry of Education, Culture, Sports, Science and Technology, Japan; the Program for Promotion of Basic Research Activities for Innovative Bioscience (PROBRAIN); Suzuken Memorial Foundation; Shimadzu Scientific Foundation; and Uehara Memorial Foundation.

REFERENCES

Beck, B. (2001). KO's and organisation of peptidergic feeding behavior mechanisms. *Neurosci. Biobehav. Rev.* 25, 143–158.

Brody, T., and Cravchik, A. (2000). *Drosophila melanogaster* G protein-coupled receptors. *J. Cell Biol.* 150, 83–88.

Chintapalli, V. R., Wang, J., and Dow, J. A. (2007). Using FlyAtlas to identify better *Drosophila melanogaster* models of human disease. *Nat. Genet.* 39, 715–720.

Civelli, O., Reinscheid, R. K., Zhang, Y., Wang, Z., Fredriksson, R., and Schiöth, H. B. (2012). G protein-coupled receptor deorphanizations. *Annu. Rev. Pharmacol. Toxicol.* doi: 10.1146/annurev-pharmtox-010611-134548 [Epub ahead of print].

Colombani, J., Raisin, S., Pantalacci, S., Radimerski, T., Montagne, J., and Leopold, P. (2003). A nutrient sensor mechanism controls *Drosophila* growth. *Cell* 114, 739–749.

Géminard, C., Rulifson, E. J., and Léopold, P. (2009). Remote control of insulin secretion by fat cells in *Drosophila*. *Cell Metab.* 10, 199–207.

Gutierrez, E., Wiggins, D., Fielding, B., and Gould, A. P. (2007). Specialized hepatocyte-like cells regulate *Drosophila* lipid metabolism. *Nature* 445, 275–280.

Hewes, R. S., and Taghert, P. H. (2001). Neuropeptides and neuropeptide receptors in the *Drosophila melanogaster* genome. *Genome Res.* 11, 1126–1142.

Hansen, K. K., Hauser, F., Williamson, M., Weber, S. B., and Grimmelikhuijzen, C. J. (2011). The *Drosophila* genes CG14593 and CG30106 code for G-protein-coupled receptors specifically activated by the neuropeptides CCHamide-1 and CCHamide-2. *Biochem. Biophys. Res. Commun.* 404, 184–189.

Ida, T., Takahashi, T., Tominaga, H., Sato, T., Kume, K., Ozaki, M., et al. (2011a). Identification of the novel bioactive peptides dRYamide-1 and dRYamide-2, ligands for a neuropeptide Y-like receptor in *Drosophila*. *Biochem. Biophys. Res. Commun.* 410, 872–77.

Ida, T., Takahashi, T., Tominaga, H., Sato, T., Kume, K., Yoshizawa-Kumagaye, K., et al. (2011b). Identification of the endogenous cysteine-rich peptide trissin, a ligand for an orphan G protein-coupled receptor in *Drosophila*. *Biochem. Biophys. Res. Commun.* 414, 44–48.

Majumdar, I. D., and Weber, H. C. (2012). Biology and pharmacology of bombesin receptor subtype-3. *Curr. Opin. Endocrinol. Diabetes Obes.* 19, 3–7.

Marshall, I. C., Boyfield, I., and McNulty, S. (2005). Ratiometric Ca^{2+} measurements using the FlexStation® Scanning Fluorometer. *Methods Mol. Biol.* 312, 119–124.

Nisimura, T., Seto, A., Nakamura, K., Miyama, M., Nagao, T., Tamotsu, S., et al. (2005). Experiential effects of appetitive and nonappetitive odors on feeding behavior in the blowfly, *Phormia regina*: a putative role for tyramine in appetite regulation. *J. Neurosci.* 25, 7507–7516.

Ohki-Hamazaki, H., Watase, K., Yamamoto, K., Ogura, H., Yamano, M., Yamada, K., et al. (1997). Mice lacking bombesin receptor subtype-3 develop metabolic defects and obesity. *Nature* 390, 165–169.

Rajan, A., and Perrimon, N. (2012). *Drosophila* cytokine unpaired 2 regulates physiological homeostasis by remotely controlling insulin secretion. *Cell* 151, 123–137.

Reiher, W., Shirras, C., Kahnt, J., Baumeister, S., Isaac, R. E., and Wegener, C. (2011). Peptidomics and peptide hormone processing in the *Drosophila* midgut. *J. Proteome Res.* 10, 1881–1892.

Roller, L., Yamanaka, N., Watanabe, K., Daubnerova, I., Zitnan, D., Kataoka, H., et al. (2008). The unique evolution of neuropeptide genes in the silkworm *Bombyx mori*. *Insect Biochem. Mol. Biol.* 38, 1147–1157.

Vassilatis, D. K., Hohmann, J. G., Zeng, H., Li, F., Ranchalis, J. E., Mortrud, M. T., et al. (2003). The G protein-coupled receptor repertories of human and mouse. *Proc. Natl. Acad. Sci. U.S.A.* 100, 4903–4908.

Williams, G., Bing, C., Cai, X. J., Harrold, J. A., King, P. J., and Liu, X. H. (2001). The hypothalamus and the control of energy homeostasis: different circuits, different purposes. *Physiol. Behav.* 74, 683–701.

Zimanyi, I. A., Fathi, Z., and Poindexter, G. S. (1998). Central control of feeding behavior by neuropeptide Y. *Curr. Pharm. Des.* 4, 349–366.

18

More than two decades of research on insect neuropeptide GPCRs

Jelle Caers, Heleen Verlinden, Sven Zels, Hans Peter Vandersmissen, Kristel Vuerinckx and Liliane Schoofs*

Animal Physiology and Neurobiology, Department of Biology, Zoological Institute, KU Leuven, Leuven, Belgium

Edited by:
Hubert Vaudry, University of Rouen, France

Reviewed by:
Dick R. Nässel, Stockholm University, Sweden
Hoffmann Klaus H., University of Bayreuth, Germany

****Correspondence:***
Liliane Schoofs, Department of Biology, Research Group of Functional Genomics and Proteomics, Naamsestraat 59, KU Leuven, 3000 Leuven, Belgium.
e-mail: liliane.schoofs@bio.kuleuven.be

This review focuses on the state of the art on neuropeptide receptors in insects. Most of these receptors are G protein-coupled receptors (GPCRs) and are involved in the regulation of virtually all physiological processes during an insect's life. More than 20 years ago a milestone in invertebrate endocrinology was achieved with the characterization of the first insect neuropeptide receptor, i.e., the *Drosophila* tachykinin-like receptor. However, it took until the release of the *Drosophila* genome in 2000 that research on neuropeptide receptors boosted. In the last decade a plethora of genomic information of other insect species also became available, leading to a better insight in the functions and evolution of the neuropeptide signaling systems and their intracellular pathways. It became clear that some of these systems are conserved among all insect species, indicating that they fulfill crucial roles in their physiological processes. Meanwhile, other signaling systems seem to be lost in several insect orders or species, suggesting that their actions were superfluous in those insects, or that other neuropeptides have taken over their functions. It is striking that the deorphanization of neuropeptide GPCRs gets much attention, but the subsequent unraveling of the intracellular pathways they elicit, or their physiological functions are often hardly examined. Especially in insects besides *Drosophila* this information is scarce if not absent. And although great progress made in characterizing neuropeptide signaling systems, even in *Drosophila* several predicted neuropeptide receptors remain orphan, awaiting for their endogenous ligand to be determined. The present review gives a précis of the insect neuropeptide receptor research of the last two decades. But it has to be emphasized that the work done so far is only the tip of the iceberg and our comprehensive understanding of these important signaling systems will still increase substantially in the coming years.

Keywords: insects, neuropeptides, G protein-coupled receptors, signal transduction, neurobiology

INTRODUCTION

The class of Insecta, which consists of more than 30 orders, forms the most diverse animal group on earth. With about one million documented species and presumably 10–30 million awaiting to be described, insects probably account for 50–70% of all existing animals (Scherkenbeck and Zdobinsky, 2009; Bellés, 2010; Van Hiel et al., 2010). Basically all the physiological processes during an insect's life cycle are regulated by neuropeptides, including developmental processes, behavioral functions, metabolic events and reproduction. As such, neuropeptides are the largest (very versatile) class of extracellular signaling molecules that are involved in communication between insect cells (Gäde and Goldsworthy, 2003; Meeusen et al., 2003; Claeys et al., 2005a). The insect neuropeptides and their actions have extensively been reviewed in the past (Nässel, 2002; Gäde and Auerswald, 2003; Gäde and Goldsworthy, 2003; Meeusen et al., 2003; Altstein, 2004; Gäde, 2004; Isaac et al., 2004; Simonet et al., 2004; Claeys et al., 2005a; Coast and Garside, 2005; Ewer, 2005; Predel and Wegener, 2006; Mertens et al., 2007; Stay and Tobe, 2007; De Loof, 2008; Audsley and Weaver, 2009; Scherkenbeck and Zdobinsky, 2009; Verleyen et al., 2009; Verlinden et al., 2009; Weaver and Audsley, 2009; Altstein and Nässel, 2010; Bendena, 2010; Nässel and Winther, 2010; Van Hiel et al., 2010; Van Loy et al., 2010; Nässel and Wegener, 2011; Herrero, 2012; Spit et al., 2012; Taghert and Nitabach, 2012).

Neuropeptides exert their physiological functions by interacting with specific signal-transducing membrane receptors, resulting in intracellular responses (Zupanc, 1996). Most of these neuropeptide receptors belong to the G protein-coupled receptors (GPCRs), the largest family of cell surface proteins. However, there are some exceptions like the prothoracicotropic hormone (PTTH), which executes its role in metamorphosis through the activation of a receptor tyrosine kinase (RTK) (Rewitz et al., 2009). Most of the insulin-like peptides (ILPs) also interact with RTKs (Fernandez et al., 1995; Graf et al., 1997; Brogiolo et al., 2001; Wheeler et al., 2006; Wen et al., 2010; Iga and Smagghe, 2011). The eclosion hormone (EH), involved in ecdysis, interacts with a membrane-bound guanylate cyclase receptor (Chang et al., 2009) as does the neuropeptide-like precursor peptide 1 (NPLP1) (Overend et al., 2012).

The functional characterization of the first insect neuropeptide receptor, the *Drosophila melanogaster* tachykinin-like receptor (DTKR) took place in 1991 (Li et al., 1991). Subsequently, another *Drosophila* tachykinin-like receptor (NKD) (Monnier et al., 1992) and a neuropeptide Y (NPY)-like receptor (Li et al., 1992) were identified. The latter has recently been deorphanized as the *Drosophila* RYamide receptor (Collin et al., 2011; Ida et al., 2011a). In the following years only a few more insect GPCRs were cloned, e.g., the diuretic hormone receptors of *Manduca sexta* and *Acheta domesticus* (Reagan, 1994, 1996), the *Drosophila* gonadotropin-releasing hormone receptor (Hauser et al., 1998), which later on was deorphanized as an adipokinetic hormone (AKH) receptor (Staubli et al., 2002) and the *Drosophila* allatostatin (AST) receptor (DAR-1) (Birgül et al., 1999).

The real breakthrough in the field of insect neuropeptide receptor research came with the publication of the *Drosophila* genome in 2000 (Adams et al., 2000). This opened the opportunity to predict receptors based on genomic data (Hewes and Taghert, 2001), which clearly boosted the receptor deorphanization rate. At present, 35 GPCRs are functionally characterized in *Drosophila*. One receptor (Dmel\SPR) is activated by seemingly different neuropeptides, the myoinhibitory peptide (MIP) and the sex peptide SP. The others mainly respond to one neuropeptide type, which underlines the specificity of the receptor/ligand couples. Another 14 GPCRs are predicted to be involved in neuropeptide signaling pathways, but their ligands are still unknown and therefore they are classified as "orphan" receptors (**Table 1**) (Meeusen et al., 2003; Hauser et al., 2006, 2008; Clynen et al., 2010a). In section "Methuselah (CG6936) and Methuselah-like Receptors" the methuselah receptor is also briefly discussed. In spite the fact that several studies have been performed on this receptor, it still is not clear if it is really a neuropeptide receptor and if the *stunted* gene really encodes for its endogenous ligands.

Despite the diversity in their endogenous ligands, GPCRs have been rather well conserved during evolution. This has facilitated the search for neuropeptide receptors in newly released genomes like those of *Apis mellifera* (Hauser et al., 2006), *Tribolium castaneum* (Hauser et al., 2008), and *Bombyx mori* (Yamanaka et al., 2008; Fan et al., 2010). Research in other insects also revealed a set of new neuropeptide signaling systems that are not present in *Drosophila*, e.g., AKH/corazonin-related peptide (ACP) discovered in *Anopheles gambiae* (Hansen et al., 2010), allatotropin (AT) discovered in *B. mori* (Yamanaka et al., 2008), and inotocin discoverd in *T. castaneum* (Stafflinger et al., 2008) (**Table 1**).

Hitherto, 149 insect genome projects are either completed or in progress (http://www.ncbi.nlm.nih.gov/sites/entrez?db=bioproject) and in 2011, the i5K project was initiated, which aims to sequence 5000 insect genomes in the next 5 years (Robinson et al., 2011). With this overload of genomic information coming up, we intend to give the reader a clear overview of what is currently known on insect neuropeptide receptors. First, we will discuss some general characteristics of GPCRs and the deorphanizing strategies. Next, we will highlight the area of peptidomics, which facilitated the prediction and detection of ligands enormously, followed by a genetics part to discuss some commonly used tools to unravel the physiological functions of the neuropeptide-receptor systems. Thereafter, the current status of the insect neuropeptide GPCRs will be reviewed. To conclude, a short discussion about the importance of neuropeptide research in insects will be given.

G PROTEIN-COUPLED RECEPTORS

Several GPCR-(sub)families originated prior to the divergence of protostomian and deuterostomian animals. This led to a great diversification in chemical specificity to external stimuli like neuropeptides, glycoproteins, nucleotides, biogenic amines, odorants, taste ligands, and photons. Although GPCRs do not share any overall sequence homology, they do expose a similar topographical structure which is remarkably well conserved during evolution. They are typically composed of seven transmembrane (7TM) α-helices, each consisting of 20–30 hydrophobic amino acids, and three extracellular and intracellular loops connecting the different helices. The N-terminus is located at the extracellular site and often possesses several glycosylation sites; the C-terminus, on the other hand, is orientated into the cytoplasm and offers some potential phosphorylation sites. The extracellular parts are involved in ligand-specific binding, while the intracellular areas interact with a member of the family of heterotrimeric GTP-binding proteins (G proteins), consisting of an α-, β-, and γ-subunit (Bockaert and Pin, 1999). Based on shared sequence motifs, the GPCRs are categorized into at least six subfamilies. The evolutionary relationship between the different families is still unclear because of the lack of significant sequence homology. They probably evolved independently of each other or have adopted the G protein signal transduction pathways through convergent evolution (Brody and Cravchik, 2000; Gether, 2000; Horn et al., 2000). All the neuropeptide GPCRs belong to the rhodopsin-like (family A) or the secretin-like (family B) subfamily.

When a GPCR becomes activated by its ligand, the extracellular signal will be transduced into intracellular physiological responses. An activated receptor will undergo a conformational change, which in turn leads to the activation of the associated G protein. This promotes the release of GDP from the α-subunit, followed by binding of GTP. Next, the GTP-bound α-subunit dissociates from the $\beta\gamma$-dimer and both will be released in the cytoplasm. Subsequently, they can interact with their specific effector proteins to elicit cellular signaling pathways. The effector proteins involved depend on the type of the α-subunit. The most common α-subunits are G_q, G_s, and $G_{i/o}$. The G_q subunits interact with phospholipase Cβ (PLCβ) in order to initiate the hydrolysis of the membrane-bound phosphoinositol-biphospholipid-bisphosphates resulting in diacylglycerol (DAG) and inositol triphosphate (IP_3). DAG activates protein kinase C (PKC) and IP_3 mobilizes Ca^{2+} from intracellular stores like the endoplasmic reticulum. The G_s and $G_{i/o}$ subunits, respectively, activate or inhibit adenylyl cyclase provoking a subsequent increase or decrease of the cyclic adenosine monophosphate (cAMP) concentration within the cell. The G_s proteins are also capable of activating Ca^{2+} channels, while the $G_{i/o}$ proteins are able to interact with K^+-channels. The intrinsic GTPase activity of Gα induces the hydrolysis of GTP to GDP, resulting in the reassociation of the subunits (Hepler and Gilman, 1992; Lustig et al., 1993; Vanden Broeck, 1996, 2001; Brody and Cravchik, 2000).

Table 1 | Characterized *Drosophila* neuropeptide receptors—Neuropeptide receptors not present in *Drosophila*—Orphan *Drosophila* neuropeptide receptors.

	Symbol	Receptor gene	Endogenous ligand	Ligand gene	Reference*
***Drosophila melanogaster* receptor**					
Adipokinetic hormone receptor	Dme\GRHR	CG11325	Adipokinetic hormone	CG1171	Staubli et al., 2002
Allatostatin A receptor 1	Dme\AlstR	CG2872	Allatostatin A	CG13633	Larsen et al., 2001
Allatostatin A receptor 2	Dme\AR-2	CG10001	Allatostatin A	CG13633	Larsen et al., 2001
Allatostatin C receptor 1	Dme\star1	CG7285	Allatostatin C	CG14919	Kreienkamp et al., 2002
Allatostatin C receptor 2	Dme\AICR2	CG13702	Allatostatin C	CG14919	Kreienkamp et al., 2002
Calcitonin-like diuretic hormone receptor	Dme\Dh31-R1	CG32843/CG17415/CG17043	Diuretic hormone 31	CG13094	Johnson et al., 2005
CAPA receptor	Dme\capaR	CG14575	Capa-1/Capa-2	CG15520	Iversen et al., 2002a
CCHamide-1 receptor	Dme\CCHa1r	CG30106/CG14484	CCHamide-1	CG14358	Hansen et al., 2011
CCHamide-2 receptor	Dme\CCHa2r	CG14593	CCHamide-2	CG14375	Hansen et al., 2011
Cholecystokinin (CCK)-like receptor	Dme\CCKLR-17D1	CG42301/CG6857	Drosulfakinin	CG18090	Chen et al., 2012
Corazonin receptor	Dme\GRHRII	CG10698	Corazonin	CG3302	Cazzamali et al., 2002
CRF-like diuretic hormone receptor 1	Dme\Dh44-R1	CG8422	Diuretic hormone 44	CG8348	Johnson et al., 2004
CRF-like diuretic hormone receptor 2	Dme\Dh44-R2	CG12370	Diuretic hormone 44	CG8348	Hector et al., 2009
Crustacean cardioactive peptide receptor	Dme\CcapR	CG33344/CG6111/CG14547	Cardioacceleratory peptide	CG4910	Cazzamali et al., 2003
Ecdysis triggering hormone receptor	Dme\ETHR	CG5911	Ecdysis triggering hormone	CG18105	Iversen et al., 2002b
FMRFamide receptor	Dme\FR	CG2114	FMRFamide	CG2346	Cazzamali and Grimmelikhuijzen, 2002
Glycoprotein A2/Glycoprotein B5 receptor	Dme\Lgr1	CG7665	GPA2/GPB5	CG17878/CG40041	Sudo et al., 2005
Kinin receptor	Dme\Lkr	CG10626	Leucokinin	CG13480	Radford et al., 2002
Myosuppressin receptor 1	Dme\DmsR-1	CG8985	Dromyosuppressin	CG6440	Egerod et al., 2003a
Myosuppressin receptor 2	Dme\DmsR-2	CG43745/CG13803	Dromyosuppressin	CG6440	Egerod et al., 2003a
Neuropeptide F receptor	Dme\NPFR1	CG1147	Neuropeptide F	CG10342	Garczynski et al., 2002
Pigment dispersing factor receptor	Dme\Pdfr	CG13758	Pigment-dispersing factor	CG6496	Hyun et al., 2005; Mertens et al., 2005
Proctolin receptor	Dme\Proc-R	CG6986	Proctolin	CG7105	Johnson et al., 2003a
Pyrokinin 1 receptor	Dme\Pk1r	CG9918	Drm-PK-1	CG15520	Cazzamali et al., 2005
Pyrokinin 2 receptor	Dme\CG8784	CG8784	Drm-PK-2	CG6371	Rosenkilde et al., 2003
Pyrokinin 2 receptor	Dme\CG8795	CG8795	Drm-PK-2	CG6371	Rosenkilde et al., 2003
Rickets	Dme\rk	CG8930	Bursicon/Partner of burs	CG13419/CG15284	Luo et al., 2005
RYamide receptor	Dme\NepYr	CG5811	RYamide	CG40733	Ida et al., 2011a
Sex peptide receptor	Dme\SPR	CG16752/CG12731	Sex peptides** and myoinhibiting peptide precursor	CG17673/CG33495 and CG6456	Yapici et al., 2008; Kim et al., 2010
Short neuropeptide F receptor	Dme\sNPF-R	CG7395/CG18639	Short neuropeptide F	CG13968	Mertens et al., 2002
SIFamide receptor	Dme\SIFR	CG10823	SIFamide	CG33527	Jørgensen et al., 2006
Sulfakinin receptor	Dme\CCKLR-17D3	CG32540/CG6894/CG6881	Drosulfakinin	CG18090	Kubiak et al., 2002
Tachykinin receptor	Dme\Takr86C	CG6515	Tachykinin	CG14734	Poels et al., 2009
Tachykinin receptor	Dme\Takr99D	CG7887	Tachykinin	CG14734	Birse et al., 2006
Trissin receptor	Dme\TrissinR	CG34381/CG14003	Trissin	CG14871	Ida et al., 2011b

(Continued)

Table 1 | Continued

	Symbol	Receptor gene	Endogenous ligand	Ligand gene	Reference*
Receptors not present in *Drosophila*					
AKH/corazonin-related peptide receptor	GPRGNR3	XP_321591	ACP	3290616	Hansen et al., 2010
Allatotropin receptor	NGR-A16	NP_001127714	Allatotropin	692738	Yamanaka et al., 2008
Inotocin receptor	ITR	NP_001078830	Inotocin	100038343	Stafflinger et al., 2008
Orphan *Drosophila* receptors					
Hector	Dme\hec	CG4395			
Lgr3	Dme\Lgr3	CG31096/CG5042			
Lgr4	Dme\CG34411	CG34411/CG4187			
Moody receptor	Dme\moody	CG4322			
Trapped in endoderm 1	Dme\Tre1	CG3171			
Orphan receptor	Dme\CG4313	CG4313			
Orphan receptor	Dme\CG12290	CG12290			
Orphan receptor	Dme\CG32547	CG32547/CG12610			
Orphan receptor	Dme\CG13229	CG13229			
Orphan receptor	Dme\CG13995	CG13995			
Orphan receptor	Dme\CG33696	CG33696/CG16726			
Orphan receptor	Dme\CG33639	CG33639/CG5936			
Orphan receptor	Dme\CG30340	CG30340			
Orphan receptor	Dme\CG13575	CG13575			

**The first published paper in which the full coding cDNA of the receptor was transfected and deorphanized using a reverse pharmacology approach resulting in a physiological relevant EC_{50} value.*

****Accessory gland peptide 70A (Acp70A)/Ductus ejaculatorius peptide 99B (Dup99B).*

DEORPHANIZING STRATEGIES

There is a clear distinction between the techniques used to deorphanize receptors before and after the genomic era. In the past, one started with a bioactive ligand, purified from tissue extracts, in order to identify its corresponding receptor (the classic approach). Nowadays, an orphan receptor is used to explore its activating ligand from a library of synthetic compounds consisting of predicted neuropeptides (reverse pharmacology) (Meeusen et al., 2003). This strategy makes use of appropriate cellular expression systems used to express orphan receptors of interest. These systems hold the opportunity to measure one of the many second messenger reporter molecules released after receptor activation. The most commonly used expression systems are mammalian cell lines (Chinese Hamster Ovary [CHO] cells or Human Embryonic Kidney [HEK] 293 cells) and *Xenopus* oocytes. These are used in the bioluminescence-based assay (CHO cells), the fluorescence-based assay (HEK293 cells), the luciferase-based assay (HEK293 cells) and the electrophysiological assay (*Xenopus* oocytes).

Because it is nearly impossible to predict which kind of G protein interacts with an orphan receptor, a universal tool was required to predict the signaling cascade. This problem was circumvented with the discovery of the promiscuous G protein α subunits $G\alpha_{16}$ (human) and $G\alpha_{15}$ (murine). These $G\alpha$ proteins regulate PLCβ, and possess the ability to interact with most GPCRs and, as such, their signaling pathways are redirected toward the release of Ca^{2+} (Offermanns and Simon, 1995). Both, the bioluminescence and the fluorescence assay are based on the measurement of the release of intracellular Ca^{2+} upon receptor activation. The bioluminescence assay makes use of bioluminescent proteins such as aequorine, purified from the jellyfish, *Aequoria victoria*, that interact with Ca^{2+} (Prasher et al., 1987; Stables et al., 1997). In the fluorescence assay usually HEK293 cells are charged with a Ca^{2+} sensitive fluorophore that serves as readout (Bender et al., 2002). The luciferase assay makes use of a reporter gene plasmid consisting of a cAMP response element (CRE) as readout for measuring intracellular cAMP levels (Janssen et al., 2008; Horodyski et al., 2011; Vuerinckx et al., 2011). For the electrophysiological assay, *Xenopus* oocytes are injected with a mix of the orphan receptor and the G protein gated inwardly rectifying K^+ (GIRK) channels that are activated upon ligand binding. This leads to subsequent inward K^+ currents that can be measured (Kofuji et al., 1995; Ho and Murrell-Lagnado, 1999; Ulens et al., 1999).

Besides the use of these heterologous expression systems, one can also make use of a homologous expression system in which the orphan receptor is expressed in *Drosophila* Schneider-2 (S2) cells (Vanden Broeck et al., 1998). The use of heterologous expression systems, however, prevents that compounds present in an insect extract, or predicted insect ligands would activate endogenous mammalian or amphibian receptors (for reviews, see: Meeusen et al., 2003; Mertens et al., 2004; Beets et al., 2011; Bendena et al., 2012).

NEUROPEPTIDES AND PEPTIDOMICS

An important feature of the currently used deorphanizing strategies is the ability to screen orphan receptors with compound libraries containing potential neuropeptides. The possibility to create such libraries coincided with the availability of the first whole genome databases. This also launched the era of peptidomics, which encloses the purpose to simultaneously identify and/or visualize all peptides present in a cell, tissue, body liquid, or organism. Peptidomics studies are based on two major elements, the *in silico* prediction of neuropeptides and the discovery and identification of neuropeptides using mass spectrometric devices (Baggerman et al., 2002; Predel et al., 2004; Wegener et al., 2006).

Endogenous neuropeptides are enclosed in larger preprohormones, mostly between 50 and 500 amino acids long (Baggerman et al., 2005a). They can code for multiple structurally related or unrelated neuropeptides, as well as for just one neuropeptide. The only common feature of preprohormones is the presence of an amino-terminal signal peptide, with exception of a predicted AST CC neuropeptide in *Drosophila* which has an amino-terminal peptide anchor (Veenstra, 2009a). This peptide is immediately cleaved off after arrival in the endoplasmic reticulum. The residual prohormone undergoes enzymatic cleavage at mono- or dibasic amino acid residues to release the neuropeptides (Hook et al., 2008; Rholam and Fahy, 2009). Most neuropeptides require post-translational modifications to become bioactive or to improve stability.

Because of the poor sequence conservation between preprohormones and the short length of the neuropeptides, the majority consists only of 4–20 amino acids, their prediction from genome databases is not straightforward. Nevertheless, classical BLAST analyses have revealed 36 neuropeptide genes in *D. melanogaster* (Hewes and Taghert, 2001; Vanden Broeck, 2001), and 35 in *A. gambiae* (Riehle et al., 2002). Later on, the combined use of different bioinformatic tools, to overcome the low sensitivity of a BLAST analysis alone, revealed a total of 119 potential neuropeptide-coding genes in *Drosophila* (Liu et al., 2006; Clynen et al., 2010a). All neuropeptides predicted by these methods can be synthesized to construct synthetic peptide libraries applied in the reverse pharmacology assays.

The bioinformatic predictions, though, do not reveal which neuropeptides are ultimately produced, and endogenous bioactive neuropeptides may be overlooked in the genomic data. The processing of a precursor can also differ during developmental stages or between tissues, and post-translational modifications are hard to predict based on sequence information. Therefore, a biochemical characterization of neuropeptides is necessary. There are several possible peptidomics methods available to provide in these needs, all based on mass spectrometry. The most common tool is a combination of liquid chromatography, tandem mass spectrometry and database mining, which allows the detection and sequencing of low concentrations of neuropeptides from complex mixtures (Clynen et al., 2010b). Mass spectrometry applications led to the discovery of hundreds of neuropeptides. As is often the case, *Drosophila* peptidomics (Baggerman et al., 2002; Baggermanet al., 2005b; Schoofs and Baggerman, 2003) paved the way for peptidomic studies in other insects, e.g., *A. mellifera* (Hummon et al., 2006; Boerjan et al., 2010a), *Nasonia vitripennis* (Hauser et al., 2010), *T. castaneum* (Li et al., 2008), and *Aedes aegypti* (Predel et al., 2010). Also in insects with no completely sequenced genome, peptidomics may prove useful, e.g., *Locusta migratoria* (Clynen et al., 2006; for reviews, see: Hummon et al., 2006; Boonen et al., 2008; Menschaert et al., 2010).

FUNCTIONAL GENOMICS

Upon the characterization of a neuropeptide receptor and its ligand, the question remains which function they possess in a specific organism. These functions can be determined with genetic tools. In the classic approach the phenotype of interest is chosen first and then attempts are made to identify the genes responsible for this phenotype (forward genetics). With the rise of the whole genome era, a tremendous number of genes with unknown functions were identified. This made it possible to start with a gene of interest and to study its function (reverse genetics). Currently, the most used techniques to perform reverse genetics are silencing of genes of interest by RNA interference (RNAi), generating knockouts, and overexpressing specific genes using the GAL4/UAS system.

The generation of loss-of-function phenotypes through the application of RNAi is a fairly new technique as it was described for the first time in 1998 in *Caenorhabditis elegans* (Fire et al., 1998), immediately followed by a report of RNAi usage in *D. melanogaster* (Kennerdell and Carthew, 1998). RNAi studies are widely used in the field of insect research and have proven to be appropriate to unravel functions of neuropeptides and their receptors in various species (Bellés, 2010; An et al., 2012). There is a genome-wide transgenic RNAi library available for *Drosophila*, consisting of short gene fragments cloned as inverted repeats and expressed using the binary GAL4/UAS system (Dietzl et al., 2007). The usage of the GAL4/UAS system to perform RNAi experiments becomes also more established in other insects like *B. mori* (Dai et al., 2008) and *T. castaneum* (Schinko et al., 2010).

RNAi can not entirely impede the expression of a gene of interest. To generate a complete knockout of a gene, mutagenic or homologous recombination tools are frequently used. Mutagenesis relies on the incorporation of mutations, which can be obtained by the application of chemical mutagenesis or by transposable element mutagenesis, followed by a thorough screen to detect the samples containing mutations in the gene of interest. Homologous recombination is based on the host DNA repair system for the alteration of a target sequence in the genome by a donor sequence. This donor sequence exhibits homology to the target sequence, but contains the desired genetic modifications. The alteration is preceded by the generation of a double strand break in the target or donor sequence, inducing the homologous recombination repair system (for reviews, see: Reumer et al., 2008; Wesolowska and Rong, 2010; An et al., 2012).

Besides studying the effects of a knockdown or a complete knockout of a certain gene, overexpressing a gene can also yield important information about its function. To obtain overexpression, the gene of interest can be coupled to a binary GAL4/UAS system as well.

The previous described techniques to identify, deorphanize and determine the functions of neuropeptide signaling systems are widely applied in insect research, yielding an enormous amount of information. **Table 2** summarizes the neuropeptide receptors that have been predicted and/or functionally characterized for a selection of model insects. In the next section we aim to give a brief summary of what is known so far relating to these insect neuropeptide receptors. For convenience all intertitles are accompanied with the corresponding computed gene (CG) numbers of the *Drosophila* receptors. These numbers were used for genes identified during the annotation of the whole *Drosophila* genome sequence. For those receptor genes not annotated in *Drosophila*, the accession number of the receptor gene for the insect in which it was first deorphanized is added.

DEORPHANIZED NEUROPEPTIDE RECEPTORS

ADIPOKINETIC HORMONE RECEPTORS (CG11325 ORTHOLOGS)

The first structural characterization of an AKH neuropeptide was achieved in 1976 (Stone et al., 1976). Currently, around 55 isoforms, derived from various insect species, have been described (Gäde, 2009; Caers et al., 2012; Gäde and Marco, 2012; Jedlička et al., 2012; Malik et al., 2012; Weaver et al., 2012). They consist of 8–10 amino acids, and are characterized by a blocked N-terminus (pyroglutamate) and C-terminus (amidation) (Gäde and Auerswald, 2003). The main function of AKH is the regulation of the energy metabolism. During energy requiring processes like flight, the AKH neuropeptides are released from the corpora cardiac (CC) and will interact with their receptors, present in the membrane of the fat body adipocytes. This will induce the release of energy rich substrates (lipids, trehalose, or proline) (Lorenz and Gäde, 2009). The kind of substrates released, depends on the coupled G protein. When AKH binds to a G_q protein-coupled receptor, glycogen phosphorylase will be activated and trehalose will be set free. If the signaling pathway acts by a G_s protein-coupled receptor, triacylglycerol lipase will be activated, resulting in the production of DAG or free fatty acids (Gäde and Auerswald, 2003). The last years it became clear that the function of AKH is not restricted to locomotory activity alone, but that it acts as a general regulator of homeostasis in insects, influencing all energy requiring processes (e.g., egg production, feeding behavior, larval growth, molting, and immune response) (Goldsworthy et al., 2002, 2003; Lorenz, 2003; Lee and Park, 2004; Isabel et al., 2005; Grönke et al., 2007; Bharucha et al., 2008; Lorenz and Gäde, 2009; Arrese and Soulages, 2010; Attardo et al., 2012; Konuma et al., 2012). AKH also serves as an anti-stress hormone in oxidative stress situations (Kodrík et al., 2007; Večeřa et al., 2007; Kodrík, 2008; Huang et al., 2011a).

The AKH receptors (AKHR) are closely related to the ACP receptors and constitute the invertebrate AKH/ACP receptor family. Together with the invertebrate corazonin/gonadotropin releasing hormone (GnRH) receptor family and the vertebrate/protochordate GnRH receptor family they compose the GnRH receptor superfamily (Lindemans et al., 2011; Roch et al., 2011). The first AKHR was determined in *M. sexta* by using fat body fractions to ascertain the optimal binding conditions for tritium-labeled *Manse*-AKH (Ziegler et al., 1995). The *Drosophila* AKHR was the first to be cloned and was deorphanized by making use of the electrophysiological assay (Park et al., 2002), and its characterization was confirmed by Staubli et al. (2002) using a bioluminescence assay. Later, AKHRs were also identified and characterized in other insect species: *Periplaneta americana* (Hansen et al., 2006; Wicher et al., 2006a), *A. gambiae* (Belmont

Table 2 | Characterized and predicted neuropeptide receptors in insect species of varying insect orders.

	Drosophila melanogaster	*Aedes aegypti*	*Anopheles gambiae*	*Apis mellifera*	*Nasonia vitripennis*	*Tribolium castaneum*	*Acyrthosiphon pisum*	*Bombyx mori*
	Diptera	**Diptera**	**Diptera**	**Hymenoptera**	**Hymenoptera**	**Coleoptera**	**Hemiptera**	**Lepidoptera**
Adipokinetic hormone receptor	CG11325	XP_001655248 XP_001655249	XP_001687839	NP_001035354	NP_001161243	NP_001076809	XP_001945436 XP_003245941	NP_001037049
AKH/corazonin-related peptide receptor	na	XP_001653920	XP_321591	na	XP_001605342	ABX52400	na	NP_001127726 NP_001127745
Allatostatin A receptor 1	CG2872	XP_001652590	XP_003435928	XP_397024	XP_001607985	na	XP_001952361	NP_001037035
Allatostatin A receptor 2	CG10001							
Allatostatin C receptor 1	CG7285	XP_001662510	XP_320274	XP_396335	XP_001600654	XP_971178	XP_001950448	NP_001127736
Allatostatin C receptor 2	CG13702	XP_001663106						
Allatotropin receptor	na	AEN03789	XP_318029	XP_001120335	XP_001604582	XP_973738	XP_003245221	NP_001127714 NP_001127740
Calcitonin-like diuretic hormone receptor	CG32843	XP_001660594	XP_318856	XP_396046	XP_001601649 XP_003424370	XP_969030	XP_001943752 XP_001945278	NP_001127732
CAPA receptor	CG14575	na	AAX84796 XP_312952 XP_312953	NP_001091702 NP_001073563	XP_001600587	XP_973937	XP_001950333	NP_001127723 NP_001127725
CCHamide-1 receptor	CG30106	XP_001656825	XP_317851	XP_395101	XP_001604352	XP_974772	XP_001948574	NP_001127712
CCHamide-2 receptor	CG14593	XP_001662526	XP_313395	XP_396992	XP_001604277	XP_974786	XP_001943863	NP_001127711
Corazonin receptor	CG10698	XP_001655399	AAQ67361 XP_321555	NP_001137393	na	na	na	NP_001127719
CRF-like diuretic hormone receptor 1	CG8422	ABX57919	XP_315468	XP_397268	XP_001606711 XP_003427176	NP_001167548	XP_001944842	na
CRF-like diuretic hormone receptor 2	CG12370	ABX57920				XP_975416	XP_003244979	na
Crustacean cardioactive peptide receptor	CG33344	XP_001659389	AAS77205	XP_001122652	XP_001602277	NP_001076796 NP_001076795	XP_003240503 XP_003245097	NP_001127724 NP_001127746
Ecdysis triggering hormone receptor	CG5911	ABI93273 ABI93274	XP_312031 XP_003436278	XP_001120367	XP_001606566	NP_001076792 NP_001076793	XP_001944756 XP_001944816	NP_001127741 NP_001165739
FMRFamide receptor	CG2114	na	AAQ73620	ACI90286	XP_001605409	XP_969392	XP_001947807	NP_001037007
Glycoprotein A2/Glycoprotein B5 receptor	CG7665	XP_001649032	XP_309589	na	na	XP_968907	XP_001945379	NP_001037033
Inotocin receptor	na	na	na	na	NP_001165745	NP_001078830	na	na
Kinin receptor	CG10626	AAT95982	EAU77489	XP_396025	na	na	XP_001944708	NP_001127721
Myosuppressin receptor 1	CG8985	XP_001651852	XP_314133	ACI90287	XP_001601584	XP_969504	XP_001949220	NP_001036929
Myosuppressin receptor 2	CG13803							NP_001127710

(Continued)

Table 2 | Continued

	Drosophila melanogaster	***Aedes aegypti***	***Anopheles gambiae***	***Apis mellifera***	***Nasonia vitripennis***	***Tribolium castaneum***	***Acyrthosiphon pisum***	***Bombyx mori***
	Diptera	**Diptera**	**Diptera**	**Hymenoptera**	**Hymenoptera**	**Coleoptera**	**Hemiptera**	**Lepidoptera**
Neuropeptide F receptor	CG1147	XP_001660966	AAT81602	na	na	XP_967689	na	NP_001127739
Pigment dispersing factor receptor	CG13758	na	XP_313426	XP_395896	XP_003427082	XP_971738	na	NP_001127733
Proctolin receptor	CG6986	na	na	na	na	EFA01332	XP_003247524	na
Pyrokinin 1 receptor	CG9918	XP_001662936	AAX84797	NP_001157480	XP_001606201	EEZ97715	XP_003241084	NP_001036913
Pyrokinin 2 receptor	CG8795 CG8784	XP_001657210	AAX84798	NP_001153387	NP_001153387	EEZ97729 EEZ97728	XP_001950091	NP_001036977
Rickets	CG8930	XP_001649742	XP_317111	XP_395206	XP_001605837	XP_975514	XP_001948776	NP_001037033
RYamide receptor	CG5811	AAY46405 XP_001653188 XP_001647749	XP_310762 XP_311031 XP_001237302	XP_395084	XP_003427563 XP_003427654	ADZ17181	XP_001946360 XP_001946314 XP_003241610	NP_001127717 NP_001127720
Sex peptide receptor	CG16752	ABW86944	ABW86945	na	na	NP_001106940	XP_001944453	NP_001108346
Short neuropeptide F receptor	CG7395	XP_001663694	ABD96049	XP_001123033	XP_001601972	XP_966794	XP_001952283	NP_001127707 NP_001127708 NP_001127742
SIFamide receptor	CG10823	EAT38404	XP_314231	NP_001106756	XP_001600098	XP_970225	XP_001947491	DAA35192
Sulfakinin receptor	CG6881	XP_001654357	XP_001237203	XP_003250082	na	XP_972750	na	NP_001127744
CCK-like receptor	CG42301		XP_309215			XP_975226		
Tachykinin receptor	CG6515	na	XP_312088	XP_395081	na	XP_971383	XP_001946954	NP_001127748 NP_001127749
Tachykinin receptor	CG7887	XP_001652376	CAD27763 XP_003435887 XP_321512	na	XP_001607956	XP_970102	XP_001946949	NP_001127722
Trissin receptor	CG34381	na	na	na	na	na	na	na

Black box: functionally characterized neuropeptide receptors.

Gray box: previously predicted neuropeptide receptors.

White box: predicted neuropeptide receptors based on our own blast analysis.

na: not annotated.

et al., 2006), *B. mori* (Staubli et al., 2002; Zhu et al., 2009; Huang et al., 2010), and *T. castaneum* (Li, unpublished data). Two putative AKHR variants have been predicted in *A. aegypti* (Kaufmann et al., 2009) and one AKHR is identified in the *Apis* genome (Hauser et al., 2006). However, it remains doubtful if this receptor is really functional in the honeybee, because mass spectrometric techniques have failed to detect the predicted *Apis* AKH neuropeptide (Veenstra et al., 2012). Besides expression in the fat body (Kaufmann and Brown, 2006; Ziegler et al., 2011), the AKHR is also expressed in various neurons of *P. americana*, including the abdominal dorsal unpaired medial (DUM) neurons, which are responsible for the release of octopamine. As such, octopamine may be the link between elevated AKH-titers and the increase in locomotion (Wicher et al., 2006b, 2007; Verlinden et al., 2010).

ADIPOKINETIC HORMONE/CORAZONIN-RELATED PEPTIDE RECEPTOR (XP_321591 ORTHOLOGS)

In 2006, an *A. gambiae* receptor was annotated and cloned that was closely related to the AKH and corazonin receptors, but could not be activated by these neuropeptides (Belmont et al., 2006). Hansen et al. (2010) detected a neuropeptide closely related to both AKH and corazonin and named it ACP. This neuropeptide was able to activate the receptor expressed in CHO/Gα_{16} cells in a dose-responsive manner (Hansen et al., 2010). Subsequently, the ACP receptor was also characterized in *T. castaneum* (Hansen et al., 2010). Recently, two predicted ACP receptors of *B. mori* (Yamanaka et al., 2008; Hansen et al., 2010) were also characterized, but were indicated as AKHR (Shi et al., 2011). The ACP neuropeptides were in fact already described in *L. migratoria* (Siegert, 1999) and in *A. gambiae* (Kaufmann and Brown, 2006), but were classified as AKH neuropeptides with unknown functions. ACP and its receptor are structurally intermediate between the AKH and corazonin neuropeptides and their receptors, which is a prominent example of receptor/ligand co-evolution. An ancestral receptor and ligand gene have probably duplicated several times followed by mutations and evolutionary selection, leading to three signaling systems. However, the ACP signaling system is absent in all investigated *Drosophila* species as well as in *A. mellifera*, *Acyrthosiphon pisum*, *Pediculus humanus*, and in the crustacean *Daphnia pulex*, suggesting that it may have been lost several times during arthropod evolution (Hansen et al., 2010). So far no functions are assigned to the ACP signaling system, but the high expression shortly before and after hatching of *T. castaneum* suggests a role in early larval development (Hansen et al., 2010).

ALLATOSTATIN A RECEPTORS (CG2872 AND CG10001 ORTHOLOGS)

The endogenous ligands of the AST A receptor are the A-type AST neuropeptides which belong to the group of allatoregulatory neuropeptides together with the B-, and C-type allatostins and the ATs (for a review, see: Weaver and Audsley, 2009) and the recently discovered AST CC neuropeptides (Veenstra, 2009a). Allatoregulatory peptides are named after their ability to either inhibit (ASTs) or stimulate (ATs) juvenile hormone (JH) synthesis (Audsley et al., 2008). The B-type ASTs are also known as myoinhibiting peptides and were found to activate the SP receptor [see section "Sex Peptide/Myoinhibiting Peptide Receptor (CG16752/CG12731 Orthologs)"].

The A-type AST-As, or FGLamides were first isolated of brain extracts of cockroaches (Woodhead et al., 1989; Pratt et al., 1991), and have since been found in every investigated insect species, except for *T. castaneum* (Li et al., 2008). They are characterized by a conserved (Y/F)XFG(L/I)-NH_2 sequence (Hayes et al., 1994; Audsley et al., 1998). AST-As regulate JH biosynthesis in cockroaches, crickets, and termites (Pratt et al., 1989, 1991; Woodhead et al., 1989, 1994; Bellés et al., 1994; Weaver et al., 1994; Lorenz et al., 1995, 1999; Yagi et al., 2005; for a review, see: Stay and Tobe, 2007). A property attributed to all AST-As is myoinhibition of visceral muscles (Hoffmann et al., 1999; Stay, 2000; Aguilar et al., 2003; Weaver and Audsley, 2009; Zandawala et al., 2012). Recently, *Drosophila* AST-A was linked to food intake and foraging behavior (Hergarden et al., 2012; Wang et al., 2012). In *Drosophila*, two A-type AST receptors are identified: DAR-1 and DAR-2 (Birgül et al., 1999; Larsen et al., 2001). DAR-1, when expressed in *Xenopus* oocytes was shown to couple to a G-protein of the $G_{i/o}$ family. When expressed in CHO cells, DAR-1 and -2 are activated by AST-A and mobilize intracellular Ca^{2+} (Larsen et al., 2001). AST-A receptors were also characterized in *P. americana* (Auerswald et al., 2001), *B. mori* (Secher et al., 2001), and *Diploptera punctata* (Lungchukiet et al., 2008). Northern blot experiments showed that the *B. mori* receptor is expressed in the midgut of fifth larval instars and to a much lesser extend in the brain (Secher et al., 2001).

ALLATOSTATIN C RECEPTORS (CG7285 AND CG13702 ORTHOLOGS)

The first C- or PISCF-type AST was characterized in the late pupae of *M. sexta*. AST-Cs contain a typical C-terminal PISCF-OH sequence, a blocked N-terminus and a disulfide bridge linking Cys-7 and Cys-14 (Kramer et al., 1991). Orthologs are found in other lepidopteran, dipteran and coleopteran species (Li et al., 2006). In several insects, C-type or C-type-like ASTs can have both allatostatic and allatotropic properties, depending on the age of the animal (Abdel-Latief et al., 2004; Clark et al., 2008; Griebler et al., 2008; Abdel-Latief and Hoffmann, 2010). In Diptera two AST-C receptors have been characterized for *Drosophila* using *Xenopus* oocytes (Kreienkamp et al., 2002) and for *Aedes* using HEK cells (Mayoral et al., 2010). Only one AST-C receptor was found to be present in *Bombyx* (Yamanaka et al., 2008) and in *Tribolium* (Audsley et al., 2012). Activation of the *Bombyx* AST-C receptor elicits an increase in intracellular cAMP levels (Yamanaka et al., 2008), while the *Tribolium* receptor was deorphanized in HEK cells, inducing a Ca^{2+} response (Audsley et al., 2012). In adult fruit flies, both *drostar* genes are expressed in the optic lobes and the pars intercerebralis, where the AST-C neuropeptide was also found to be present. This suggests a function in the modulation of visual information processing. In the last larval stage, receptor expression was found in the brain and corpora allata (CA) (Kreienkamp et al., 2002). In *Aedes* significant differences were observed in tissue distribution and expression levels for the two receptor paralogs (Mayoral et al., 2010). In *Tribolium* the highest transcript levels were noticed in the head and the gut, with variable amounts in the fat body and reproductive organs.

These transcript levels were also shown to be sex-dependent (Audsley et al., 2012).

The recently discovered AST CC neuropeptide (AST CC) (Veenstra, 2009a) was also identified in *Tribolium* and showed to be capable of activating the AST-C receptor in a dose-dependent manner (Audsley et al., 2012). A knock out of the *Drosophila Ast-CC* gene is embryonic lethal, suggesting that it is an essential gene (Veenstra, 2009a).

ALLATOTROPIN RECEPTORS (NP_001127714 ORTHOLOGS)

AT was named after its ability to stimulate JH biosynthesis in the CA but is also linked to other functions like myostimulation, cardio-acceleration, regulation of photic entrainment, ion exchange regulation, and the up-regulation of the secretion of digestive enzymes (Veenstra et al., 1994; Würden and Homberg, 1995; Lee et al., 1998; Koladich et al., 2002; Petri et al., 2002; Homberg et al., 2003; Hofer and Homberg, 2006; Lwalaba et al., 2010; Sterkel et al., 2010), of which the myotropic role of AT is probably the most ancestral (Elekonich and Horodyski, 2003). ATs are found in several invertebrate EST and genomic databases (for reviews, see: Clynen and Schoofs, 2009; Weaver and Audsley, 2009) and they all have a TARGF/Y motif at the C-terminus. In *Manduca* and *Bombyx*, also AT-like (ATL) neuropeptides were found, which arise by alternative splicing of the AT gene (Horodyski et al., 2001; Nagata et al., 2012a). In 2008, the AT receptor (ATR) was characterized in *B. mori* (Yamanaka et al., 2008). Remarkable, this receptor was mainly localized in the Short neuropeptide F (sNPF)-producing cells in the CC, but not in the JH producing CA. It was suggested that AT regulates the production and/or release of sNPFs from the CC and that these sNPFs are responsible for some of the allatotropic functions assigned to the ATs (Yamanaka et al., 2008). In 2011, the ATRs of *M. sexta*, *T. castaneum*, and *A. aegypti* were characterized (Horodyski et al., 2011; Vuerinckx et al., 2011; Nouzova et al., 2012) and show, unlike the ligand, remarkable similarity with the vertebrate orexin receptors (Yamanaka et al., 2008; Vuerinckx et al., 2011). Upon activation by AT or ATLs, *Manse*-ATR, and *Trica*-ATR elevate both intracellular Ca^{2+} and cAMP concentrations in cellular expression systems (Horodyski et al., 2011; Vuerinckx et al., 2011). Expression of ATs and ATRs in the different insect species is likely to be strongly regulated, since large differences were measured between developmental stages, sexes, feeding conditions, *etc.* (Elekonich and Horodyski, 2003; Horodyski et al., 2011; Vuerinckx et al., 2011; Nouzova et al., 2012). Possibly additional ATRs may be present in some insect species, since very similar additional receptors have been predicted from *Bombyx* and *Aedes* genomes (Yamanaka et al., 2008; Nouzova et al., 2012).

CALCITONIN-LIKE DIURETIC HORMONE RECEPTORS (CG32843/CG17415/CG17043 ORTHOLOGS)

The first calcitonin-like diuretic hormone (CT/DH), called *Dippu*-DH_{31} was identified in *D. punctata* (Furuya et al., 2000). More orthologs were discovered by phylogenetic analysis (Zandawala, 2012). CT/DH stimulates fluid secretion by Malpighian tubules and seems to work via a Ca^{2+}-dependent mechanism in *D. punctata* (Furuya et al., 2000). In *Drosophila*, CT/DH stimulates fluid secretion by activating the apical membrane V-ATPases via cAMP as second messenger (Coast et al., 2001) and in *Anopheles* the fluid excretion in Malpighian tubules is also cAMP driven (Coast et al., 2005). In *Rhodnius*, diuresis by CT/DH seems to be independent of cAMP (Te Brugge et al., 2011). CT/DH is also involved in contractions of the gut and associated glands (Te Brugge et al., 2009) and may play a role in ecdysis (Kim et al., 2006a,b). The *Drosophila* CT/DH receptor (DH31-R1) is activated by *Drome*-DH_{31} and is expressed in the Malpighian tubules. The signaling in HEK293 cells was dependent upon co-expression of the receptor component protein (RCP), which is critical for downstream signaling from the mammalian calcitonin-like receptor (Johnson et al., 2005). One CT/DH receptor has been predicted in *A. aegypti*, *A. gambiae*, *A. mellifera*, *N. vitripennis*, and *T. castaneum* and two CT/DH receptors were found in *A. pisum*, although it is not yet clear whether both paralogues encode a functional CT/DH receptor.

CAPA RECEPTORS (CG14575 ORTHOLOGS)

The insect capa neuropeptides, or periviscerokinin peptides, usually possess the C-terminal sequence FPRVamide. The insect *capability* gene encodes a preprohormone containing two capa neuropeptides (capa-1 and capa-2) and one or more pyrokinin-1 (Kean et al., 2002), but they do not activate each other's receptors (Iversen et al., 2002a; Rosenkilde et al., 2003; Cazzamali et al., 2005). Capa neuropeptides have a diuretic effect on the Malpighian tubules of *Drosophila* (Pollock et al., 2004), but in *R. prolixus* and other insects they act antidiuretic (Coast and Garside, 2005; Paluzzi and Orchard, 2006). Recently, it was shown that the *Aedes* capa neuropeptide can induce either diuretic or antidiuretic effects depending on the dose (Ionescu and Donini, 2012). In addition, capa neuropeptides have myotropic effects in a variety of insects (Wegener et al., 2002; Predel and Wegener, 2006). Capa receptors have been characterized in *Drosophila* and in *Anopheles* (Iversen et al., 2002a; Park et al., 2002; Olsen et al., 2007; Terhzaz et al., 2012). Both capa-1 and capa-2 elicited a dose-dependent response. The gene encoding the *Drosophila* capa receptor is highly expressed in larval and adult tubules (Terhzaz et al., 2012).

Capa receptors are found in different mosquito species, although not in *A. aegypti*. In other holometabolous insects, orthologs are found in representatives of the major orders, including Hymenoptera, Coleoptera, and Lepidoptera. The honey bee genome contains two paralogues, as does the *B. mori* and *M. sexta* genome. Also *N. vitripennis* contains a paralogue (XP_001600587.2), formerly suggested lacking this receptor (Hauser et al., 2006, 2010; Yamanaka et al., 2008). Also in Coleoptera, a capa receptor is found in *Tribolium* (Hauser et al., 2008).

CCHAMIDE-1 AND -2 RECEPTORS (CG30106/CG14484 AND CG14593 ORTHOLOGS)

The first CCHamide neuropeptide has only recently been identified in *B. mori* and it was found to be expressed in the central nervous system and the midgut (Roller et al., 2008). Subsequently, two CCHamide neuropeptides were detected in all insects with a sequenced genome (Hansen et al., 2011). In *D. melanogaster*, cognate receptors have been identified for both CCHamide neuropeptides. CG30106 expressed in CHO/Gα_{16} cells was activated by CCHamide-1 at nanomolar concentrations but also responded to high concentrations of CCHamide-2. CG14593 was activated by nanomolar concentrations of CCHamide-2 as well as by micromolar concentrations of CCHamide-1 (Hansen et al., 2011). Previously, CG30106 had been described as a receptor for myoinhibiting neuropeptides (Johnson et al., 2003b), but as several independent attempts to repeat this result were fruitless, this was likely an erroneous characterization.

CORAZONIN RECEPTORS (CG10698 ORTHOLOGS)

The first corazonin was isolated and identified from the CC of *P. americana* and was presented as a new cardioaccelerating neuropeptide (Veenstra, 1989). Corazonin is present in most insects (excluding beetles and aphids) (for reviews, see: Gäde et al., 2008; Li et al., 2008; Weaver and Audsley, 2008; Huybrechts et al., 2010) and the most common corazonin sequence among insects is pQT-FQYSRGWTNamide (Predel et al., 2007). The role of corazonin, however, is not restricted to cardio-excitatory actions. In locusts, corazonin is involved in cuticular melanization in the gregarious phase (Tawfik et al., 1999; Tanaka et al., 2002), in *M. sexta* a role in the initiation of ecdysis behavior is noticed (Kim et al., 2004; Žitňan et al., 2007) and it has been suggested that corazonin is involved in sex-dependent stress responses (Zhao et al., 2010) and in the regulation of insulin producing cells in *Drosophila* ((Kapan et al., 2012); for reviews, see: Veenstra, 2009b; Boerjan et al., 2010b).

The corazonin receptor was first characterized in *Drosophila* by making use of a bioluminescence assay (Cazzamali et al., 2002), which was confirmed using *Xenopus* oocytes (Park et al., 2002). Subsequently, the corazonin receptors for *M. sexta* (Kim et al., 2004), *A. gambiae* (Belmont et al., 2006) and *B. mori* (Shi et al., 2011) were characterized, and a putative corazonin receptor for *Musca domestica*, was cloned (Sha et al., 2012). Neither the corazonin neuropeptide nor its receptor could be identified in *Tribolium* (Hauser et al., 2008) or *Acyrthosiphon*. In *N. vitripennis*, despite the presence of a corazonin neuropeptide, so far no corazonin receptor could be predicted (Hauser et al., 2010). The invertebrate corazonin receptors are part of the GnRH receptor superfamily [see section "Adipokinetic Hormone Receptors (CG11325 Orthologs)"] (Lindemans et al., 2011; Roch et al., 2011). The *Drosophila* receptor is expressed in all developmental stages (Cazzamali et al., 2002). The *Manduca* corazonin receptor is present in endocrine Inka cells, the source of preecdysis- and ecdysis-triggering hormones, suggesting a role upstream of ecdysis triggering hormone (ETH) (Kim et al., 2004). In *Anopheles*, there are pronounced spikes of corazonin receptor expression in 2nd instar larvae and around the transition from pupa to adult (Hillyer et al., 2012). In *Musca*, a high level of corazonin receptor expression was noticed in the larval salivary glands and a moderate level in the central nervous system. In adults, the receptor was expressed both in the head and body (Sha et al., 2012).

CRF-LIKE DIURETIC HORMONE RECEPTORS (CG8422 AND CG12370 ORTHOLOGS)

The first corticotropin-releasing factor like diuretic hormone (CRF/DH) was identified in *M. sexta* as a diuretic peptide (DP) consisting of 41 amino acids that shows sequence similarity to corticotropin releasing factor, urotensin I and sauvagine (Kataoka et al., 1989). A second CRF/DH was also discovered in *M. sexta* (Blackburn et al., 1991). CRF/DHs are also referred to as DH_{44}, after the number of amino acids in the CRF/DH of *D. melanogaster* (Cabrero et al., 2002). CRF/DH increases fluid excretion *in vivo* (Kataoka et al., 1989) and *in vitro* (Kay et al., 1991, 1992; Lehmberg et al., 1991; Clottens et al., 1994) and increases cAMP levels in Malpighian tubules (Lehmberg et al., 1991; Kay et al., 1992; Clottens et al., 1994; Furuya et al., 1995). Besides its diuretic function, CRF/DH negatively influences feeding and reproduction (Keeley et al., 1992; Van Wielendaele et al., 2012) and stimulates gut contractions (Te Brugge et al., 2009). The *M. sexta* CRF/DH receptor was the first to be cloned and was activated by *Manse*-DH, making use of cAMP as second messenger (Reagan, 1995). Also the CRF/DH receptor in *A. domesticus* uses cAMP as secondary messenger (Reagan, 1996). The first *D. melanogaster* CRF/DH receptor (DH44-R1), encoded by CG8422, may couple to multiple second messengers as both cAMP and Ca^{2+} were stimulated upon binding of *Drome*-DH to the receptor (Johnson et al., 2004). The second *D. melanogaster* CRF/DH receptor (DH44-R2), encoded by CG12370, is also activated by *Drome*-DH resulting in an increase of intracellular cAMP and causes specific β-arrestin translocation to the plasma membrane. DH44-R2 is probably the receptor that modulates DH sensitivity at the level of the microtubules (Hector et al., 2009). A CRF/DH receptor was also cloned in *B. mori* and in *A. aegypti* (Ha et al., 2000). The *Aedes* DH-I receptor is by far the most abundant receptor in Malpighian tubules and its transcript levels increase after a blood meal (Jagge and Pietrantonio, 2008). More CRF/DH receptor orthologs were found in *T. castaneum* and *A. pisum*, but only one orthologue is found in *A. gambiae*, *A. mellifera*, and *N. vitripennis* up to date. Although the number of receptors seems to differ, CRF/DH signaling is likely to be conserved in all major insect orders.

CRUSTACEAN CARDIOACTIVE PEPTIDE RECEPTORS (CG33344/CG6111/CG14547 ORTHOLOGS)

Crustacean cardioactive peptide (CCAP) was originally identified in the shore crab *Carcinus maenas* and exhibited an acceleratory effect on semi-isolated heart tissue (Stangier et al., 1987). An identical neuropeptide was subsequently isolated from *L. migratoria* (Stangier et al., 1989). The structure of CCAP is identical in all examined insects and consists of the cyclic nonapeptide PFCNAFTGCamide. CCAP stimulates heart contractions (Cheung et al., 1992; Furuya et al., 1993; Li et al., 2011a) and contractions of visceral muscles (Stangier et al., 1989; Donini et al., 2001, 2002; Donini and Lange, 2002), and promotes the release of AKH (Veelaert et al., 1997) and digestive enzymes (Sakai et al., 2006). CCAP also plays a role in ecdysis in several insects (Gammie and Truman, 1997; Ewer et al., 1998; Kim et al., 2006a,b; Arakane et al., 2008). *Drosophila* and *Anopheles* CCAP receptors have been expressed in CHO/Gα_{16} cells and are activated by CCAP (Cazzamali et al., 2003; Belmont et al., 2006). In *T. castaneum*, two genes encode for CCAP receptors (Hauser et al., 2008) and both showed a dose-dependent response to CCAP (Li et al., 2011a). Functional analysis using RNAi revealed that only

TcCCAPR-2 is essential for cardioacceleratory activity (Li et al., 2011a). CCAP receptor orthologs have been found in *A. mellifera* (Hauser et al., 2006), *A. aegypti, A. pisum, B. mori,* and *N. vitripennis* and thus the CCAP receptor seems to be conserved in many insect orders.

ECDYSIS TRIGGERING HORMONE RECEPTORS (CG5911 ORTHOLOGS)

To be able to grow and undergo metamorphosis, insects need to shed their exoskeleton, the process known as ecdysis (Truman, 1996). This process is initiated and regulated by the ETH (for a review, see: Žitňan et al., 2007). The *eth* gene encodes for two active neuropeptides named pre-ETH and ETH in moths and ETH1 and ETH2 in other insects. The ETHs have a common PRX_1-amide (X_1 is I, V, L, or M) sequence at the C-terminus (Park et al., 2002). In *Drosophila, Manduca,* and *Bombyx*, the two ETHs differ in length. In *Drosophila* and *Manduca* the short form only can elicit a part of the ecdysis behaviors, whereas the long one can elicit whole ecdysis (Žitňan et al., 1999; Park et al., 2002). In *Bombyx* and *Aedes*, both neuropeptides seemed to be equally potent (Žitňan et al., 2002; Dai and Adams, 2009). In *Apis, Nasonia,* and *Acyrthosiphon* only one form is found, that in *Apis* is shown to be sufficient to elicit ecdysis (Žitňan et al., 1999; Park et al., 2002). These neuropeptides are released in the bloodstream and activate the ETH receptors (ETHRs) situated in the central nervous system. The *ethr* gene encodes for two splice variants of the receptor, ETRH-A and ETRH-B (Iversen et al., 2002b; Park et al., 2002; Dai and Adams, 2009; Roller et al., 2010), and the first ETHRs were identified in *Drosophila* (Iversen et al., 2002b; Park et al., 2002). The two forms are expressed in different central neurons (Kim et al., 2006a,b). ETHR-A is expressed in inhibitory and/or excitatory neuropeptide producing neurons, releasing the neuropeptides in response to ETH to regulate ecdysis (Kim et al., 2006a,b). In *B. mori* ETHR-B is highly expressed in the CA, pointing to a possible allatoregulatory function (Yamanaka et al., 2008). In *Drosophila, Manduca,* and *Aedes* activation of both receptors expressed in CHO cells could increase intracellular Ca^{2+} levels (Iversen et al., 2002b; Park et al., 2002; Kim et al., 2006a,b; Dai and Adams, 2009). In *Bombyx*, ETHR-B was expressed in HEK293 cells and was shown to be able to increase intracellular cAMP levels (Yamanaka et al., 2008). In *Tribolium*, the function of the ETRHs was confirmed through RNAi experiments (Arakane et al., 2008). ETRHs were also found in several holo- and hemimetabolous insects (Riehle et al., 2002; Žitňan et al., 2003; Clynen et al., 2006; Roller et al., 2010).

FMRFAMIDE RECEPTORS (CG2114 ORTHOLOGS)

The family of (N-terminally extended) FMRFamides is named after the tetrapeptide FMRFamide that was identified in the sunray venus clam *Macrocallista nimbosa* (Price and Greenberg, 1977), but not all extended FMRFamides retain the exact C-terminal motif. The first extended FMRFamide in insects was cloned and characterized in *D. melanogaster* (Nambu et al., 1988; Schneider and Taghert, 1988). More extended FMRFamides were detected by mass spectrometric analysis in various major insect orders (Verleyen et al., 2004a; Neupert and Predel, 2005; Li et al., 2008; Ons et al., 2009; Rahman et al., 2009; Huybrechts et al., 2010; Audsley et al., 2011; Zoephel et al., 2012). FMRFamides modulate heart and gut contractions in insects (Banner and Osborne, 1989; Robb and Evans, 1990; Duttlinger et al., 2002). The FMRFamide neurons become active at the early stages of pre-ecdysis in *D. melanogaster*, suggesting a role in the ecdysis process (Kim et al., 2006b). The *Drosophila* FMRFamide receptor is the only deorphanized insect FMRFamide receptor so far and was found to be activated by six of the seven endogenous *D. melanogaster* extended FMRFamides (Cazzamali and Grimmelikhuijzen, 2002; Meeusen et al., 2002). Orthologous FMRFamide receptors are found in *A. gambiae* (Duttlinger et al., 2003), *A. mellifera, N. vitripennis, T. castaneum, A. pisum,* and *B. mori* but have not been characterized up to date. FMRFamide receptors are conserved throughout insects, but our knowledge about these receptors is very limited.

INOTOCIN RECEPTOR (NP_001078830 ORTHOLOGS)

This neuropeptide was first discovered in the 1980s in *L. migratoria* and showed similarity to the oxytocin/vasopressin peptide family in Mammalia. The antiparallel dimer of the neuropeptide was described to have diuretic properties (Proux et al., 1987). Although the neuropeptide could not be identified in most insect species with sequenced genomes, it was recently found in *T. castaneum* and *N. vitripennis.* The mature neuropeptide shows C-terminal amidation. The *T. castaneum* inotocin receptor was characterized in $CHO/G\alpha_{16}$ cells displaying strong activation in the nanomolar range. For both the neuropeptide precursor and its receptor transcript levels have been reported throughout development of *T. castaneum*, but in larvae and the head of adult beetles high levels were detected (Aikins et al., 2008; Stafflinger et al., 2008). Inotocin was shown to act indirectly as a diuretic factor on *Tenebrio molitor* Malpighian tubules in the presence of central nervous system and CC-CA (Aikins et al., 2008).

KININ (MYOKININ) RECEPTORS (CG10626 ORTHOLOGS)

Insect kinins are small neuropeptides that function as myotropic, neuromodulatory, and diuretic hormones in the insect Malphigian tubules (Hayes et al., 1989; Terhzaz et al., 1999; Coast and Garside, 2005). These neuropeptides, which are characterized by the C-terminal sequence FX_1X_2WGamide (where X_1 is F, H, N, S or Y and X_2 is A, P, or S), were first isolated from *Leucophea maderae* (Holman et al., 1987; Hayes et al., 1989). The *Drosophila* kinin receptor was deorphanized in S2 cells using a bioluminescence assay (Radford et al., 2002). Antibodies raised against the receptor identified sites of myokinin action like stellate cells of the Malphigian tubules, two triplets of cells in the pars intercerebralis of the adult central nervous sytem and additional cells in the larval nervous system. Western blots and reverse transcription-PCR confirmed these locations, but also identified expression in male and female gonads. These tissues also displayed elevated Ca^{2+} in response to myokinin, demonstrating novel roles for these neuropeptides (Radford et al., 2002). In *A. aegypti* the myokinin receptor was shown to be critical for *in vivo* fluid excretion post blood feeding (Kersch and Pietrantonio, 2011). In *Drosophila* the receptor was shown to be involved in appetite, chemosensory responses, and metabolism (Al-Anzi et al., 2010; de Haro et al., 2010; Cognigni et al., 2011; López-Arias et al., 2011). Receptor orthologs are also present in *A. mellifera* (Hauser et al., 2006), *A. gambiae*, *Culex quinquefasciatus*, *A. pisum*, *P. humanus*, and *B. mori*, but seem to be absent in *N. vitripennis* and *T. castaneum*.

LEUCINE-RICH REPEATS CONTAINING GPCRs (LGRs)

These receptors, which belong to the rhodopsin-like GPCRs, can be considered "the odd ones out" within this receptor family as they display ectodomains that are much larger than is generally the case for rhodopsin-like GPCRs. Based on the structure of the ectodomain and the hinge region which links the ectodomain to the serpentine domain, three major types can be identified within the LGR family (Hsu et al., 2000; Van Hiel et al., 2012).

Type A LGRs (CG7665 orthologs)

Type A LGRs typically have 7–9 leucine-rich repeats (LRRs) in their ectodomain. Although little data are available on these receptors in insects, they are thought to be of significant importance as they are homologous to the three vertebrate receptors for the glycoprotein hormones (follicle stimulating hormone, thyroid stimulating hormone, luteinizing hormone, and choriogonadotropin). In contrast to the situation in vertebrates, invertebrate genomes encode only one type A LGR and the receptor is conserved in most sequenced insect genomes, but seems to be lost in Hymenoptera (Hauser et al., 2006, 2010; Fan et al., 2010). Another exception is the *T. castaneum* genome which encodes two type A LGRs (Hauser et al., 2008; Van Hiel et al., 2012).

LGR1 from *D. melanogaster* is activated by a heterodimer formed by GPA2 and GPB5 (Sudo et al., 2005) which are produced in neuroendocrine cells of the ventral nervous system (Sellami et al., 2011). As is the case for the vertebrate glycoprotein hormones, both of these subunits are cystine knot proteins with complex three dimensional structures (Vitt et al., 2001). Based on transcript studies, *dLgr1* gene expression has been detected throughout all developmental stages of the fruit fly (Hauser et al., 1997; Graveley et al., 2011). In wandering larvae and adults, high transcript abundance has been reported for the hindgut and the salivary glands (Chintapalli et al., 2007).

Type B LGRs (CG8930 orthologs)

LGRs from type B feature 16–18 LRRs, about twice the number found in the other two types (Van Hiel et al., 2012). In vertebrates, three type B LGRs can be identified, whereas in insect genomes only one type B has been found. The *D. melanogaster* member of the type B LGRs, LGR2 (*rk*) was cloned in 2000 (Eriksen et al., 2000) and was activated by bursicon (Luo et al., 2005; Mendive et al., 2005). Analogous to the known ligands of the LGR type A receptors, this hormone is a heterodimer of cystine knot glycoproteins. The bursicon hormone itself had already been described in the 1960s (Fraenkel et al., 1966), but it took until 2004 before its sequence was unraveled (Dewey et al., 2004; Honegger et al., 2004). Bursicon was found to induce the hardening and darkening of the cuticle of newly eclosed adult flies as well as the expansion of the wings (Luo et al., 2005; Mendive et al., 2005). More recently, bursicon has been shown to be responsible for the maturation of the wing, driving the epithelial-mesenchymal transition of the wing epithelial cells (Natzle et al., 2008), but the authors reported that apoptosis associated with wing maturation was not bursicon-regulated in contrast to previous results (Kimura et al., 2004). With regard to wing expansion, it has been proposed that the bursicon secreting neurons in the abdominal ganglion are responsible for neurohemal release, whereas the bursicon-positive neurons in the subesophageal ganglion would orchestrate wing expansion behavior (Peabody et al., 2008). Also, there are indications that bursicon is released preceding the initiation of larval ecdysis and that it is responsible for tanning the pupal case (Loveall and Deitcher, 2010). Additionally, recent data indicate that homodimers of the bursicon α- and β-subunits induced innate immunity genes in the fruit fly (An et al., 2012).

In addition to *D. melanogaster*, LGR2 homologues have been identified in representatives of most insect orders including in *A. mellifera*, *T. castaneum*, and *A. pisum* (Hauser et al., 2006, 2008, 2010; Van Hiel et al., 2012). Interestingly, in *A. mellifera* a single gene was found to encode bursicon. This protein features two cystine knot domains similar to the dimer of two cystine-knot proteins as is the case in the fruit fly and the silk moth (Mendive et al., 2005).

Type C LGRs (CG31096/CG6857 and CG34411/CG4187 orthologs)

In contrast to the vertebrate type C LGRs which are activated by members of the insulin-relaxin peptide family, in insects these receptors are largely uncharacterized. In *D. melanogaster*, two members of the type C LGRs can be identified, dLGR3 and dLGR4. In contrast, in *A. mellifera* and *T. castaneum*, only one receptor has been found which is, respectively, most closely related to dLGR3 and dLGR4 (Hauser et al., 2008). The ligands of these receptors are still unknown.

MYOSUPPRESSIN RECEPTORS (CG8985 AND CG43745/CG13803 ORTHOLOGS)

Myosuppressins have a conserved C-terminal FLRFamide. The first myosuppressin was isolated from *L. maderae* (Holman et al., 1986). Myosuppressins inhibit gut contractions and regulate heart contractions (Holman et al., 1986; Lange and Orchard, 1998; Wasielewski and Skonieczna, 2008; Maestro et al., 2011). They also contribute to the regulation of digestive processes by controlling the release of several digestive enzymes in the alimentary canal (Harshini et al., 2002; Hill and Orchard, 2005). Furthermore, myosuppressins inhibit food uptake and thus seem to classify as anorexic factors (Matthews et al., 2008; Vilaplana et al., 2008; Down et al., 2011; Nagata et al., 2011). The first putative myosuppressin receptor was characterized in *L. migratoria*. Cold competition binding studies and kinetic binding assays with a radiolabeled ligand were used to calculate the dissociation constant of the receptor (Kwok and Orchard, 2002). *D. melanogaster* possesses two myosuppressin receptors, DMSR-1 (CG8985) and DMSR-2 (CG43745/CG13803), and were activated by *D. melanogaster* myosuppressin in a dose-dependent manner. Another myosuppressin receptor was characterized in *A. gambiae* (Schöller et al., 2005). Additional myosuppressin receptors have been annotated in *A. aegypti*, *A. mellifera*, *N. vitripennis*, *T. castaneum*, *A. pisum*, and *B. mori*. DMSR-2 is expressed in the head and the body and possibly regulates the actions of myosuppressin on visceral muscles. DMSR-1 is only expressed in the head (Egerod et al., 2003a). Myosuppressin receptors are not evolutionary related to FMRFamide receptors and both represent two separately evolved signaling systems, despite the resemblance of their ligands (Schöller et al., 2005).

NEUROPEPTIDE F RECEPTORS (CG1147 ORTHOLOGS)

Invertebrate neuropeptide F (NPF) peptides are structural homologues of the vertebrate NPY family. The *Drosophila* NPF neuropeptide was the first full length member of the NPY/NPF family identified in insects (Brown et al., 1999). The insect NPF neuropeptides are characterized by the consensus sequence $x_nPxRx_nYLx_2Lx_2YYx_4$RPRFamide (Nässel and Wegener, 2011). NPF is involved in various processes in *Drosophila* like foraging, feeding, alcohol sensitivity, stress, aggression, reproduction, learning, and locomotion (Shen and Cai, 2001; Wu et al., 2003, 2005a,b; Wen et al., 2005; Lee et al., 2006; Dierick and Greenspan, 2007; Lingo et al., 2007; Chen et al., 2008; Krashes et al., 2009; Xu et al., 2010; Hermann et al., 2012; Shohat-Ophir et al., 2012, for a review, see: Nässel and Wegener, 2011). In several other insects NPF is also (predicted to be) involved in feeding behavior (Zhu et al., 1998; Stanek et al., 2002; Garczynski et al., 2005; Gonzalez and Orchard, 2008, 2009; Nuss et al., 2008, 2010; Ament et al., 2011; Huang et al., 2011b). NPF has also an effect on cardiac activity in the blowfly *Protophormia terraenovae* (Setzu et al., 2012). The *Drosophila* NPF receptor was characterized by means of a radioreceptor approach. The signaling pathway probably acts via Gi and adenylate cyclase as determined by NPF-induced inhibition of forskolin-stimulated cAMP production (Garczynski et al., 2002). The NPF receptor was also characterized in *Anopheles* (Garczynski et al., 2005) and has been predicted in several other insects like *Bombyx* and *Tribolium* (Hauser et al., 2008; Yamanaka et al., 2008; Fan et al., 2010). The proposed *Nasonia* NPF receptor (Hauser et al., 2010) is more likely to be a short NPF receptor; consequently there is probably no NPF receptor present in *Nasonia*. Expression of the *Drome*-NPF receptor was observed in cells of the midgut and numerous neurons in the brain and ventral nerve cord of the third instar larva (Garczynski et al., 2002). The NPF receptor was also located in the adult brain (Wen et al., 2005; Krashes et al., 2009). The *Anoga*-NPF receptor was detected in all life stages except for eggs (Garczynski et al., 2005).

PIGMENT DISPERSING FACTOR RECEPTORS (CG13758 ORTHOLOGS)

The first pigment dispersing factor (PDF) neuropeptide in insects was characterized in *Romalea microptera* (Rao et al., 1987). The best know function of PDF is its role in the circadian clock as a network coordinator, output factor and regulator of its plasticity similar to the vertebrate vasoactive intestinal peptide (VIP). Further processes that where associated with PDF are activity, reproduction, arousal, and geotaxis (for a review, see: Meelkop et al., 2011). Recently, also a role for PDF in the control of visceral physiology in *Drosophila* was described, thereby extending the similarities between fly PDF and VIP in mammals (Talsma et al., 2012). In 2005, three research groups simultaneously identified the PDF receptor in *Drosophila*. Mertens et al. (2005) found the receptor to be specifically responsive to PDF and to couple with Gs, leading to an elevated cAMP concentration upon receptor activation. Mutants showed an aberrant behavioral rhythmicity and a severe negative geotaxis. In a large-scale temperature preference behavior screen in *Drosophila*, Hyun et al. (2005) identified a mutant that preferred colder temperatures during the night and named it *han* (Korean for cold). *Han* seems to be a mutant of a P element controlling the CG13758 gene. But mutations in the latter gene did not cause temperature preference difference. Instead it shows arrhythmic circadian behavior in constant darkness as seen in *pdf* null mutants. PDF specifically binds to S2 cells expressing HAN and thereby elevates the cAMP level. The third research group also identified a mutant with the same disrupted circadian behavior as *pfd* mutants and named it *groom-of-PDF* (*gop*) (Lear et al., 2005). Later studies showed, however, that only the advanced evening activity is common with the *pdf* mutants. *pdfr* mutants, in contrast to *pdf* mutants, did have a morning peak (Im and Taghert, 2010). There are several indications that *pdfr* is regulated at steady-state level by the clock gene *period* (Lear et al., 2005; Mertens et al., 2005). Localization studies showed PDFR expression in the brain and visual system in close correspondence to PDF expression. PDFR expression shows also similarities to the clock pacemaker network of neurons. Furthermore expression is found dispersed in the anterior and posterior surfaces of the central brain and subesophageal ganglion (Shafer et al., 2008; Im and Taghert, 2010). In embryos no expression was noticed (Hyun et al., 2005). *Drosophila* is the only insect where the PDFR has been deorphanized so far. However, homologous sequences are found in many insects like several *Drosophila* species, *A. gambiae*, *A. mellifera*, *N. vitripennis*, *B. mori*, and *T. castaneum*.

PROCTOLIN RECEPTORS (CG6986 ORTHOLOGS)

Proctolin or RYLPT is a myo- and neurostimulatory neuropeptide of which the appearance seems to be restricted to arthropods (Starratt and Brown, 1975; Nässel, 2002). It stimulates or potentiates muscle contraction, is cardio-acceleratory and acts as a neurohormone (Orchard et al., 1989; Lange, 2002; Clark et al., 2006; Lange and Orchard, 2006; Nässel and Winther, 2010). The *Drosophila* gene for the proctolin receptor was identified and cloned (Egerod et al., 2003b; Johnson et al., 2003a,b; Taylor et al., 2004; Orchard et al., 2011). When the receptor was stably expressed in CHO/$G\alpha_{16}$ cells, a dose-dependent response was measured for proctolin (Egerod et al., 2003b). In competition-based studies, the proctolin receptor binds proctolin with high affinity (Johnson et al., 2003a). The proctolin and/or proctolin receptor gene was found in the genomes of only a few insect species, including *T. castaneum*, *T. molitor*, *P. humanus*, and *A. pisum* (Hauser et al., 2008; Li et al., 2008; Weaver and Audsley, 2008; Huybrechts et al., 2010). No proctolin gene has been identified in genomes of *A. aegypti*, *A. gambiae*, *A. mellifera*, *N. vitripennis*, *B. mori*, or *Acromyrmex echinatior* and three other ant species (Hauser et al., 2006, 2010; Roller et al., 2008; Predel et al., 2010; Nygaard et al., 2011), where proctolin and its receptor are now considered absent.

PYROKININ RECEPTORS (CG8784, CG8795 AND CG9918 ORTHOLOGS)

Pyrokinins are characterized by the C-terminal sequence FXPRLamide (X = S, T, K, A, or G) (Holman et al., 1986; Predel et al., 2001). They are involved in the stimulation of gut motility, the production and release of sex pheromones, diapause, and pupariation (Holman et al., 1986; Predel et al., 2001; Nässel, 2002; Altstein, 2004; Verleyen et al., 2004a; Homma et al., 2006). The pyrokinins can be subdivided into two groups, pyrokinin-1 (C-terminus WFGPRLamide) and pyrokinin-2 (C-terminus PFKPRLamide) (Cazzamali et al., 2005). The first identified insect pyrokinin receptors were those of *D. melanogaster*, where three pyrokinin receptors occur. CG9918 seems to be specific for pyrokinin-1 and CG8784 and CG8795 for pyrokinin-2 (Park et al., 2002; Rosenkilde et al., 2003; Cazzamali et al., 2005). Two pyrokinin receptors were cloned and pharmacologically characterized in *A. gambiae*, one being more specific for pyrokinin-1, the other for pyrokinin-2 (Olsen et al., 2007). The pyrokinin-2 receptor orthologue of *Helicoverpa zea* expressed in *Spodoptera frugiperda* (Sf) 9 cells also responded to pheromone biosynthesis-activating neuropeptide (PBAN) in the low nanomolar range (Choi et al., 2003).

A. mellifera has two pyrokinin receptor orthologs, but since they both have the same sequence identities (55–56%) to the *Drosophila* genes, it is difficult to classify them as pyrokinin-1 or -2 receptors (Hauser et al., 2006). The *T. castaneum* genome contains probably three pyrokinin receptors, which are currently classified according to their highest amino acid residue identities (Hauser et al., 2008). Pyrokinin receptors have been found in all insects so far, but it is difficult to classify them as pyrokinin-1 or -2 receptors (Jurenka and Nusawardani, 2011). This will remain problematic until *in vivo* studies using genetics will have solved this issue (Melcher et al., 2006).

RYAMIDE RECEPTORS (CG5811 ORTHOLOGS)

In 2010, a new class of neuropeptides was discovered from the genome of *N. vitripennis*. These RYamides are characterized by the C-terminal motif FFxxxRYamide (Hauser et al., 2010). Thereupon, RYamides were identified for all insects with a sequenced genome, except for some ant species (Hauser et al., 2010; Nygaard et al., 2011). Recently, the RYamide receptors for *D. melanogaster* and *T. castaneum* were characterized using CHO/Gα_{16} cells. Both *Drosophila* RYamides were capable of activating the receptor in the nanomolar range. For *T. castaneum* it was observed that *Trica*-RYamide-2 is somewhat more potent than *Trica*-RYamide-1 to activate the receptor (Collin et al., 2011; Ida et al., 2011a). Although the *Drosophila* receptor was also activated by high concentrations of mammalian NPY and NPYY (Li et al., 1992), a phylogenetic analysis seems to indicate that there is no significant structural relationship between NPY and RYamide receptors (Collin et al., 2011). A first study to unravel the function of the RYamides was performed in *Phormia regina*. Injections of *Drosophila* RYamide-1 attenuate the feeding motivation of these flies (Ida et al., 2011a). The receptor is mainly expressed in the hindgut, while it is not, or hardly present in other investigated tissues in *Drosophila* males and females. This strengthens the hypothesis that the signaling system has a role in digestion, or maybe water reabsorption (Collin et al., 2011; Ida et al., 2011a).

SEX PEPTIDE/MYOINHIBITING PEPTIDE RECEPTOR (CG16752/CG12731 ORTHOLOGS)

SP induces the post-mating effects that occur in female fruit flies (Kubli and Bopp, 2012). It is produced in the male accessory glands and transferred with the seminal fluid during copulation. It induces egg laying and loss of receptivity for additional mating (Chen et al., 1988), alters the female's sleep pattern (Isaac et al., 2010) and provokes antimicrobial peptide expression (Peng et al., 2005; Domanitskaya et al., 2007). Additionally, the food uptake and preference of females is altered after copulation (Carvalho et al., 2006; Barnes et al., 2007; Kubli, 2010; Ribeiro and Dickson, 2010; Vargas et al., 2010). The SP receptor (SPR) from *D. melanogaster* has been characterized and homologues of this receptor were identified in various insects with the exception of Hymenoptera (Yapici et al., 2008; Kim et al., 2010). Expression of this receptor is found in the female reproductive organs, especially the spermatheca, and the central nervous system of both males and females in very similar patterns (Yapici et al., 2008; Häsemeyer et al., 2009; Poels et al., 2010).

In addition to SP, the related ductus ejaculatorius peptide (DUP) 99B (Saudan et al., 2002) can activate SPR (Yapici et al., 2008). Although both SP and DUP99B have only been identified in *Drosophila* species, they can also elicit physiological responses in the lepidopteran *Helicoverpa armigera* (Fan et al., 1999). As SP and DUB99B so far have only been found in most—not all—*Drosophila* species, the receptor's evolutionary conservation was a puzzle that was only recently solved. SPR can be activated not only by SP, but also by myoinhibiting peptides (MIPs, also known as B-type ASTs) (Kim et al., 2010; Poels et al., 2010). These neuropeptides show the same evolutionary conservation as SPR and therefore likely correspond to the ancestral ligands of SPR. MIPs display a characteristic WX_6Wamide C-terminal motif and were first purified from *L. migratoria* (Schoofs et al., 1991), but members of the neuropeptide family were also identified in other species such as *Gryllus bimaculatus*, *D. melanogaster*, and *R. prolixus* (Lorenz et al., 1995; Williamson et al., 2001; Lange et al., 2012). MIPs display myoinhibiting activity in visceral muscle preparations *in vitro* (Schoofs et al., 1991; Blackburn et al., 1995, 2001; Predel et al., 2001). In *G. bimaculatus*, they inhibit JH biosynthesis (Lorenz et al., 1995), and in *D. melanogaster* and *M. sexta*, MIP may silence neurons that are not required during the ecdysis program (Kim et al., 2006a,b). Evidence from *B. mori* indicates that expression of the MIP receptor is strongly upregulated following a sudden decline of the 20-hydroxyecdysone titer. Therefore, MIP receptor signaling may be involved in the fine-tuning of ecdysteroid titers (Yamanaka et al., 2010).

SHORT NEUROPEPTIDE F RECEPTORS (CG7395/CG18639 ORTHOLOGS)

sNPF neuropeptides were first identified in *A. aegypti* and indicated as "*Aedes* head peptides" (Matsumoto et al., 1989). Nowadays, sNPFs are predicted in all insect with a sequenced genome and they are characterized by the C-terminal consensus sequence xPxLRLRFamide (Nässel and Wegener, 2011). The main functions of sNPF seem to be linked to the regulation of feeding behavior (Lee et al., 2004, 2008, 2009; Chen and Pietrantonio, 2006; Kahsai et al., 2010; Ament et al., 2011; Lu and Pietrantonio, 2011; Nagata et al., 2011, 2012b; Root et al., 2011; Hong et al., 2012; Mikani et al., 2012). Other processes in which sNPF is probably involved in are diapause, learning behavior, ovarian growth stimulation, metabolic stress, cardiac activity, the circadian rhythm, and the regulation of hormone production and hormonal release (Schoofs et al., 2001; Huybrechts et al., 2004; Johard et al., 2008; Nässel et al., 2008; Kahsai et al., 2010; Lu and Pietrantonio, 2011; Kapan et al., 2012; Setzu et al., 2012; for a review, see: Nässel and Wegener, 2011). As previously discussed in section "Allatotropin Receptors (NP_001127714 Orthologs)," sNPF peptides may also possess allatotropic activity (Yamanaka et al., 2008). The first sNPF receptor was identified in *Drosophila* and all four predicted *Drosophila* sNPF peptides activate the receptor in physiological concentrations (Mertens et al., 2002; Feng et al., 2003). Also in *Solenopsis invicta* (Chen and Pietrantonio, 2006), *A. gambiae* (Garczynski et al., 2007), and *B. mori* (Yamanaka et al., 2008) the sNPF receptor has been deorphaned. When co-expressed in *Xenopus* oocytes, the *Drosophila* sNPF receptor activates exogenously expressed inwardly rectifying K^+ channels (Reale et al., 2004). The sNPF receptor is present in a limited number of neurons in the nervous system of all developmental stages. Throughout development, the receptor is also expressed in peripheral tissues including the gut, Malpighian tubules, fat body, and ovaries as has been shown in various insects (Mertens et al., 2002; Feng et al., 2003; Chen and Pietrantonio, 2006; Garczynski et al., 2007; Yamanaka et al., 2008; Lu and Pietrantonio, 2011; Kahsai et al., 2012; Nagata et al., 2012b).

SIFAMIDE RECEPTORS (CG10823 ORTHOLOGS)

SIFamides are highly conserved during evolution and have been isolated from various insects (Verleyen et al., 2004b; Audsley and Weaver, 2006). SIFamide is present in four neurons in the insect pars intercerebralis and this specific pattern suggests a neuromodulatory role in combining visual, tactile and olfactory input. Targeted cell ablation and RNAi has revealed that SIFamide modulates sexual behavior in fruit flies (Terhzaz et al., 2007). The *Drosophila* SIFamide receptor is activated by the SIFamide (Jørgensen et al., 2006). The identification of well-conserved SIFamide receptor orthologs in all insects with a sequenced genome, suggests that SIFamide signaling regulates an essential function in arthropods (Hauser et al., 2006, 2008; Jørgensen et al., 2006; Verleyen et al., 2009).

SULFAKININ AND CHOLECYSTOKININ (CCK)-LIKE RECEPTORS (CG32540/CG6894/CG6881 AND CG42301/CG6857 ORTHOLOGS)

Sulfakinins (SKs) are the insect homologues of the vertebrate cholecystokinin (CCK) and gastrin neuropeptides (Nachman et al., 1986a,b; Staljanssens et al., 2011). They are named after the sulfated tyrosyl residue in their active core sequence YGHMRFamide that is usually required for biological activity. The first insect SKs were isolated from *L. maderae* and stimulated hindgut contractions (Nachman et al., 1986a,b). Peptidomic techniques elucidated SK peptides in all major insect orders (Verleyen et al., 2004a; Li et al., 2008; Ons et al., 2009; Hauser et al., 2010; Huybrechts et al., 2010; Audsley et al., 2011; Zoephel et al., 2012). SK regulates food uptake and works as a satiety factor that inhibits feeding in several insect species (Wei et al., 2000; Maestro et al., 2001; Downer et al., 2007; Meyering-Vos and Müller, 2007). Drosulfakinins are coreleased with ILPs and influence food choice in *D. Melanogaster* (Söderberg et al., 2012). It stimulates hindgut contractions (Nachman et al., 1986a,b; Marciniak et al., 2011), but inhibits contractions of the heart, oviduct and ejaculatory duct (Marciniak et al., 2011). Only one insect SK receptor, the *D. melanogaster* SK receptor 1 (*Drome*-SKR1) has been deorphanized so far. It is activated by [Leu^7]-*Drome*-SK-1 at nanomolar concentrations. [Leu^7]-*Drome*-SK-1 was tested instead of the endogenous [Met^7]-*Drome*-SK-1 for stability reasons. The sulphate residue is essential for high-affinity receptor binding in all tested cellular assays (Kubiak et al., 2002). SK receptors are widespread in insects: *T. castaneum* and *A. gambiae* have two SK receptors, while *A. aegypti*, *A. mellifera*, and *B. mori* contain at least one.

Drosophila contains a second, recently characterized, SK receptor, the CCK-like receptor (Chen et al., 2012). As both SK receptors probably arose through a gene duplication and because of the high homology between the two, it is likely that they also display similar ligand specificity (Hewes and Taghert, 2001; Kubiak et al., 2002). Both, CCKLR and DSK are strong positive growth regulators of the *D. melanogaster* larval neuromuscular junction (Chen and Ganetzky, 2012), by signaling via the cAMP-protein kinase A (PKA)-CRE binding protein (CREB) pathway, known for its role in structural synaptic plasticity in learning and memory (Chen and Ganetzky, 2012). A β-arrestin translocation assay in HEK cells was used to show that sulfated drosulfakinins are the endogenous ligands for CCKLR-17D1. Binding of DSK-1S or DSK-2S to the receptor promotes larval locomotion and evokes stress-induced larval escape behavior (Chen et al., 2012).

TACHYKININ RECEPTORS (CG6515 AND CG7887 ORTHOLOGS)

Insect tachykinins differ from mammalian tachykinins by their C-terminal consensus sequence, which is FX_1GX_2Ramide, rather than FXGLMamide as in mammals. There are many different tachykinin isoforms in each insect, which are all encoded by a single gene (Siviter et al., 2000). They play various roles in neuronal signaling and gut activity (Vanden Broeck, 2001; Nässel, 2002; Coast and Garside, 2005; Predel et al., 2005; Van Loy et al., 2010). The first insect GPCR capable of sensing tachykinin-related neuropeptides was cloned from *Drosophila* and is termed *Drosophila* tachykinin receptor (DTKR and CG7887) (Li et al., 1991). *Drosophila* tachykinin-related neuropeptides (*Drome*-TKs) are the endogenous ligands of DTKR and dose-dependently increased intracellular Ca^{2+} concentrations, as well as cyclic AMP levels, when applied on DTKR-expressing HEK293 or S2 cells (Birse et al., 2006; Poels et al., 2007). DTKR is involved in the regulation of insulin signaling and the olfactory sensory processing in the antennal lobe (Ignell et al., 2009; Birse et al., 2011).

A second tachykinin receptor in *Drosophila* is the neurokinin receptor (NKD and CG6515) (Monnier et al., 1992). *Drome*-TK-6 (with an Ala instead of Gly) is the only known fly neuropeptide with clear agonist activity on NKD-expressing cells (Poels et al., 2009), which suggests that NKD is able to discriminate between Ala- and Gly-containing isoforms of tachykinin ligands, a feature that does not apply to DTKR (Van Loy et al., 2010). A similar tachykinin receptor has been cloned from *Stomoxys calcitrans* (STKR) (Guerrero, 1997). Its endogenous ligand, *Stoca*-TK, which contains an Ala-residue instead of the highly conserved Gly-residue, behaves as a partial agonist (Poels et al., 2009; Van Loy et al., 2010).

A putative tachykinin receptor has been cloned from brain tissue of *L. maderae* (Johard et al., 2001). One or two tachykinin receptor orthologs have been identified in all insects with a sequenced genome (Hauser et al., 2006, 2008), pointing at an indispensable role of these proteins.

TRISSIN RECEPTOR (CG34381/CG14003 ORTHOLOGS)

Trissin is a recently identified neuropeptide that contains six Cys residues which form three intramolecular disulfide bridges. Trissin has been shown to activate the *D. melanogaster* GPCR CG34381 stably expressed in CHO/Gα_{16} cells at picomolar concentrations. Given the toxic and antimicrobial properties of many Cys containing neuropeptides, one hypothesis is that trissin may have an antimicrobial function. Transcript profiling data for trissin and its receptor on the other hand indicated that transcripts for both were present in the central nervous system of third instar larvae and adults, suggesting that trissin might be a neuropeptide (Ida et al., 2011b). Neuropeptides with high sequence similarity to trissin have been found in several *Drosophila* species and in three mosquitoes, *A. aegypti*, *A. gambiae*, and *C. quinquefasciatus* as well as in *B. mori* (Ida et al., 2011b). In *A. mellifera*, raalin displayed sequence similarity with trissin but this neuropeptide only features 5 Cys residues (Kaplan et al., 2007). Since currently no signal sequence or C-terminal processing sites have been identified for this neuropeptide, its sequence may still be incomplete.

REMAINING ORPHAN *DROSOPHILA* RECEPTORS

At least 14 GPCRs predicted to have a neuropeptide as cognate ligand are still orphan and include CG4313, CG12290, CG32547/CG12610, CG13229, CG13995, CG33696/CG16726, CG33639/CG5936, CG30340, and CG13575.

The orphan receptor *hector* (CG4395) is involved in the regulation of *Drosophila* male courtship behavior. It is expressed in numerous brain cells, mainly in the mushroom bodies, the central complex and, at lower levels, in a subset of glomeruli in the antennal lobes. However, only those cells that co-express *fruitless* (*fru*—one of the two main regulators of male courtship behavior besides *doublesex*) and *hector* are critical for male courtship (Li et al., 2011b).

The *moody* gene (CG4322) encodes two splice variants, Moody-α and Moody-β that differ in their long carboxy-terminal domains. Both receptors are coexpressed in glial cells that surround and insulate the nervous system, which is required for the formation and maintenance of the *Drosophila* blood-brain barrier (Bainton et al., 2005; Schwabe et al., 2005; Hatan et al., 2011). The moody receptors are also involved in drug sensitivity (Bainton et al., 2005; for a review, see: Daneman and Barres, 2005).

The receptor encoded by *trapped in endoderm 1* (*tre1*, CG3171) is a functional analog of the CXCR4 receptor of vertebrates, which is involved in tumor metastasis (Kamps et al., 2010). Tre1 is essential for the transepithelial migration of *Drosophila* germ cells from the posterior midgut toward the gonads (Kunwar et al., 2003). The receptor probably plays a role in three phases of early migration: polarization of germ cells, dispersal into individual cells, and transepithelial migration (Kunwar et al., 2008). Tre1 also regulates the relative orientation of cortical polarity in embryonic *Drosophila* neural stem cells (neuroblasts) (Yoshiura et al., 2012).

METHUSELAH (CG6936) AND METHUSELAH-LIKE RECEPTORS

The *methuselah* (*mth*) gene encodes a family B GPCR and is involved in stress response and biological ageing in *Drosophila* (Lin et al., 1998). Also 15 *methuselah-like* (*mthl*) relatives were identified in *Drosophila*, most of them characterized by a unique motif in the extracellular domain consisting of up to ten cysteine residues and several glycosylation sites (West et al., 2001; Patel et al., 2012). Two peptides were identified capable of activating the Mth receptor in a dose-dependent manner. These peptides correspond with the splice variants A and B of the *Drosophila* gene *stunted* (*sun*), which codes for the ε-subunit of mitochondrial ATP synthase (Cvejic et al., 2004; Kidd et al., 2005). The EC_{50} values for both polypeptides, however, were quite high with 4 μM for Sun A and 3.8 μM for Sun B. A second splice variant of the receptor was activated in somewhat lower doses with an EC_{50} value of 0.6 μM for Sun A and Sun B. The *stunted* gene was also shown to be involved in ageing and oxidative stress (Cvejic et al., 2004). Later on, the *Drosophila* SP and a non-physiological peptide with a randomly generated sequence, the serendipitous peptide activator of Mth (SPAM), were also identified as agonists of the Mth receptor. The peptides share almost no sequence homology with Sun A and B, indicating the promiscuity of Mth for activation (Ja et al., 2009). However, *mth* mutants do not affect behaviors controlled by SP, so it is doubtful that activation of the Mth receptor by these ligands is of any biological significance (Ja et al., 2009). An extensive developmental expression and sequence divergence study was performed by Patel et al. (2012). More studies are needed to affirm which are the cognate ligands of the Mth receptor and to unravel the physiological roles of the methuselah-like receptors.

REMAINING ORPHAN NEUROPEPTIDES

For several neuropeptides, including the ion transport peptides (ITPs), neuroparsins, orcokinins, and amnesiac, the cognate receptor is unknown at the moment. ITPs function as antidiuretic hormones in locusts (Audsley et al., 1992; Phillips et al., 2001). ITPs are found in the genomes of many insect orders including dipterans, lepidopterans, and coleopterans (Dircksen et al., 2008; Begum et al., 2009; Dircksen, 2009).

Neuroparsins are pleiotropic neuropeptides and are inter alia involved in reproduction and serve as molecular markers of the process of phase transition in locusts (Brown et al., 1998; Girardie et al., 1998; Claeys et al., 2005b, 2006; Badisco et al., 2007). It is noteworthy that in the genus *Drosophila*, the gene coding for the neuroparsins is absent from the *melanogaster* subgroup of the subgenus *Sophophora*, although present in other species of the genus (Veenstra, 2010).

Insect orcokinins were first identified in *B. germanica* and *S. gregaria* (Pascual et al., 2004; Hofer et al., 2005) and were subsequently detected in various other insects, excluding *Drosophila* and *Tribolium* (Roller et al., 2008). A study in *L. maderae* indicates that orcokinins are involved in circadian behavior (Hofer and Homberg, 2006). In *B. mori* it was demonstrated that orcokinins act as prothoracicotropic factors and as such are involved in ecdysteroidogenesis (Yamanaka et al., 2011). Recently, a new family of neuropeptides was discovered in *R. prolixus*, named Orcokinin B, because it arises due to alternative splicing of the *orcokinin* gene. Orcokinin B expression is observed in several insects, except *Drosophila* spp. and *A. pisum* (Sterkel et al., 2012).

The *amnesiac* (*amn*) gene, which encodes a putative neuropeptide precursor (Feany and Quinn, 1995; Moore et al., 1998), is important for stabilizing olfactory memory, and is involved in various aspects of other associative and non-associative learning (Quinn et al., 1979; Gong et al., 1998; DeZazzo et al., 1999; Keene et al., 2004, 2006; Yu et al., 2006; Motosaka et al., 2007). Additional studies have indicated that *amn* is also involved in ethanol sensitivity, sleep, temperature preference behavior and nociception (Moore et al., 1998; Hong et al., 2008; Liu et al., 2008; Aldrich et al., 2010). The *amn* gene was found to code for neuropeptides closely related to the vertebrate pituitary adenylate cyclase-activating polypeptide (PACAP) and submammalian glucagon/growth hormone-releasing hormone (GHRH) and were shown to possess phylogenetically conserved functions (Hashimoto et al., 2002).

DISCUSSION AND FUTURE PROSPECTS

This review clearly shows that during the last two decades a tremendous progress has been made on the field of insect neuropeptide signaling systems. This progress is mostly attributable to the increased availability of insect genomes and the advancing fields of genomics and peptidomics. It became clear that several of these systems are well conserved in all insect species, suggesting that they are indispensable in general insect physiological functions. Other neuropeptides and their receptors were apparantly lost during evolution in several insect species or orders, suggesting that they were otiose, or that their functions were taken over by other ligands. To gain more insight into the evolution of neuropeptide GPCRs across the Insecta, more insect genomes need to be sequenced, which may soon be accomplished due to the i5K project (Robinson et al., 2011). But despite the great progression made in insect endocrinology, the knowledge about the functions of many of the neuropeptides and their receptors involved is still scarce. Furthermore, even in *Drosophila*, the preeminent insect model organism, various receptors are still orphan and the physiological roles they play are still a mystery. It may be obvious that a lot of work has to be performed before the functions of the different signaling systems will be clearly understood and to unravel how these systems are intertwined with each other. This information is also necessary to get a better view on the evolutionary origin of the peptide-receptor couples and how they changed during evolution among species. It should be emphasized that sequence similarity between different insects does not necessarily implies functional similarity or *vice versa*. So, it remains a prerequisite to functionally characterize neuropeptide GPCRs in several insect model species. Reverse genetic tools including RNAi, or the application of the fairly new technique of genome editing using engineered zinc finger nucleases (Urnov et al., 2010) are only some of the methods being developed in several insects, which will likely boost GPCR functional research. Nevertheless, cross genome clustering of receptors based on sequence homology may be a good starting point to acquire a better view on their putative functions (Metpally and Sowdhamini, 2005).

The usefulness of research on insect neuropeptide signaling systems goes beyond the world of insects as several mammalian neuropeptides and/or their receptors have orthologs in insects. Well studied examples of such conserved signaling systems are the GnRH (Lindemans et al., 2011; Roch et al., 2011; De Loof et al., 2012), the tachykinin (Pennefather et al., 2004; Van Loy et al., 2010), the NPF/NPY (Nässel and Wegener, 2011), the capa-pyrokinin/neuromedin (Melcher et al., 2006; Terhzaz et al., 2012), the AST C/somatostatin (Birgül et al., 1999; Veenstra, 2009a), the myoinhibiting peptide/galanin (Blackburn et al., 1995), the PDF/VIP (Vosko et al., 2007; Talsma et al., 2012), the diuretic hormone/corticotropin releasing hormone (Lovejoy et al., 2009; De Loof et al., 2012), the diuretic hormone/calcitonin (Zandawala, 2012), and the SK/CCK (Staljanssens et al., 2011) orthologs, meaning that these signaling systems arose before the divergence of the Proto- and Deuterostomia (more than 700 million years ago). This strengthens the reasons to study insect endocrinology as these studies can help and learn vertebrate endocrinologists more about the current vertebrate receptors (Grimmelikhuijzen and Hauser, 2012a).

It should be clear that the importance of neuropeptides and their receptors in insect physiology can hardly be overestimated. The great variety among the neuropeptides and their receptors between different insect species makes them also potential targets for the development of a new generation of insecticides with high species specificity (Grimmelikhuijzen et al., 2007; Bendena, 2010; Grimmelikhuijzen and Hauser, 2012b). Such insecticides would ideally only be harmful for pest insects like insects acting as vectors for diseases or herbivorous insects detrimental for agriculture, while beneficial insects would be unharmed. The development of such new controlling agents is necessary because of the detrimental effects of the currently used insecticides on the environment and their toxicity to non-target organisms. The increasing resistance of pest insects against the used insecticides is also an expanding problem (Casida and Quistad, 1998; Van Hiel et al., 2010). As such, more and more research is performed on neuropeptides in order to develop synthetic ligands that can disturb the proper functioning of neuropeptide signaling systems, provoking detrimental effects on the insect's fitness. Once again we want to emphasize the importance of elucidating the biochemical pathways and the functions of the neuropeptides in order to be able to design these so called peptidomimetics. Hitherto, no neuropeptide-based insecticides are in use, but a lot of progress is made on a number of interesting neuropeptides (Teal et al., 1999; Gäde and Goldsworthy, 2003; Altstein, 2004; Scherkenbeck and Zdobinsky, 2009; Altstein and Nässel, 2010; Nachman and Pietrantonio, 2010).

ACKNOWLEDGMENTS

The authors acknowledge the Research Foundation Flanders (FWO-Vlaanderen, Belgium, G.0417.08) and the KU Leuven Research Foundation GOA/11/002. Heleen Verlinden is a postdoctoral research fellow of the FWO-Vlaanderen. Sven Zels is supported by the Flemish government agency for Innovation by Science and Technology (IWT-Vlaanderen, Belgium). Hans Peter Vandersmissen and Kristel Vuerinckx are supported by the KU Leuven.

REFERENCES

Abdel-Latief, M., Meyering-Vos, M., and Hoffmann, K. H. (2004). Characterization of a novel peptide with allatotropic activity in the fall armyworm *Spodoptera frugiperda*. *Regul. Pept.* 122, 69–78.

Abdel-Latief, M., and Hoffmann, K. H. (2010). Neuropeptide regulators of the juvenile hormone biosynthesis (*in vitro*) in the beetle, *Tenebrio molitor* (Coleoptera, Tenebrionidae). *Arch. Insect Biochem. Physiol.* 74, 135–146.

Adams, M. D., Celniker, S. E., Holt, R. A., Evans, C. A., Gocayne, J. D., Amanatides, P. G., et al. (2000). The genome sequence of *Drosophila melanogaster*. *Science* 287, 2185–2195.

Aguilar, R., Maestro, J. L., Vilaplana, L., Pascual, N., Piulachs, M.-D., and Bellés, X. (2003). Allatostatin gene expresión in brain and midgut, and activity of synthetic allatostatins on feeding-related processes in the cockroach *Blattella germanica*. *Regul. Pept.* 115, 171–177.

Aikins, M. J., Schooley, D. A., Begum, K., Detheux, M., Beeman, R. W., and Park, Y. (2008). Vasopressin-like peptide and its receptor function in an indirect diuretic signaling pathway in the red flour beetle. *Insect Biochem. Mol. Biol.* 38, 740–748

Al-Anzi, B., Armand, E., Nagamei, P., Olszewski, M., Sapin, V., Waters, C., et al. (2010). The leucokinin pathway and its neurons regulate meal size in *Drosophila*. *Curr. Biol.* 20, 969–978.

Aldrich, B. T., Kasuya, J., Faron, M., Ishimoto, H., and Kitamoto, T. (2010). The *amnesiac* gene is involved in the regulation of thermal nociception in *Drosophila melanogaster*. *J. Neurogenet.* 24, 33–41.

Altstein, M. (2004). Novel insect control agents based on neuropeptide antagonists: the PK/PBAN family as a case study. *J. Mol. Neurosci.* 22, 147–157.

Altstein, M., and Nässel, D. R. (2010). Neuropeptide signaling in insects. *Adv. Exp. Med. Biol.* 692, 155–165.

Ament, S. A., Velarde, R. A., Kolodkin, M. H., Moyse, D., and Robinson, G. E. (2011). Neuropeptide Y-like signalling and nutritionally mediated gene expression and behaviour in the honey bee. *Insect Mol. Biol.* 20, 335–345.

An, S., Dong, S., Wang, Q., Li, S., Gilbert, L. I., Stanley, D., et al. (2012). Insect neuropeptide bursicon homodimers induce innate immune and stress genes during molting by activating the NF-kappaB transcription factor relish. *PLoS ONE* 7:e34510. doi: 10.1371/journal.pone.0034510

Arakane, Y., Li, B., Muthukrishnan, S., Beeman, R. W., Kramer, K. J., and Park, Y. (2008). Functional analysis of four neuropeptides, EH, ETH, CCAP and bursicon, and their receptors in adult ecdysis behavior of the red flour beetle, *Tribolium castaneum*. *Mech. Dev.* 125, 984–995.

Arrese, E. L., and Soulages, J. L. (2010). Insect fat body: energy, metabolism, and regulation. *Annu. Rev. Entomol.* 55, 207–225.

Attardo, G. M., Benoit, J. B., Michalkova, V., Yang, G., Roller, L., Bohova, J., et al. (2012). Analysis of lipolysis underlying lactation in the tsetse fly, *Glossina morsitans*. *Insect Biochem. Mol. Biol.* 42, 360–370.

Audsley, N., Matthews, H. J., Down, R. E., and Weaver, R. J. (2011). Neuropeptides associated with the central nervous system of the cabbage root fly, *Delia radicum* (L). *Peptides* 32, 434–440.

Audsley, N., Matthews, H. J., Price, N. R., and Weaver, R. J. (2008). Allatoregulatory peptides in Lepidoptera, structures, distribution and functions. *J. Insect Physiol.* 54, 969–980.

Audsley, N., McIntosh, C., and Phillips, J. E. (1992). Isolation of a neuropeptide from locust corpus cardiacum which influences ileal transport. *J. Exp. Biol.* 173, 261–274.

Audsley, N., and Weaver, R. J. (2006). Analysis of peptides in the brain and corpora cardiaca-corpora allata of the honey bee, *Apis mellifera* using MALDI-TOF mass spectrometry. *Peptides* 27, 512–520.

Audsley, N., Weaver, R. J., and Edwards, J. P. (1998). Enzyme linked immunosorbent assay for *Manduca sexta* allatostatin (Mas-AS), isolation and measurement of Mas-AS immunoreactive peptide in *Lacanobia oleracea*. *Insect Biochem. Mol. Biol.* 28, 775–784.

Audsley, N., and Weaver, R. J. (2009). Neuropeptides associated with the regulation of feeding in insects. *Gen. Comp. Endocrinol.* 162, 93–104.

Audsley, N., Vandersmissen, H. P., Weaver, R., Dani, P., Matthews, J., Down, R., et al. (2012). Characterisation and tissue distribution of the PISCF allatostatin receptor in the red flour beetle, *Tribolium castaneum*. *Insect Biochem. Mol. Biol.* doi: 10.1016/j.ibmb.2012.09.007. [Epub ahead of print].

Auerswald, L., Birgül, N., Gäde, G., Kreienkamp, H. J., and Richter, D. (2001). Structural, functional, and evolutionary characterization of novel members of the allatostatin receptor family from insects. *Biochem. Biophys. Res. Commun.* 282, 904–909.

Badisco, L., Claeys, I., Van Loy, T., Van Hiel, M. B., Franssens, V., Simonet, G., et al. (2007). Neuroparsins, a family of conserved arthropod neuropeptides. *Gen. Comp. Endocrinol.* 153, 64–71.

Baggerman, G., Boonen, K., Verleyen, P., De Loof, A., and Schoofs, L. (2005b). Peptidomic analysis of the larval *Drosophila melanogaster* central nervous system by two-dimensional capillary liquid chromatography quadrupole time-of-flight mass spectrometry. *J. Mass Spectrom.* 40, 250–260.

Baggerman, G., Huybrechts, J., Clynen, E., Hens, K., Harthoorn, L., Van Der Horst, D., et al. (2002). New insights in Adipokinetic Hormone (AKH) precursor processing in *Locusta migratoria* obtained by capillary liquid chromatography tandem mass spectrometry. *Peptides* 23, 635–644.

Baggerman, G., Liu, F., Wets, G., and Schoofs, L. (2005a). Bioinformatic analysis of peptide precursor proteins. *Ann. N.Y. Acad. Sci.* 1040, 59–65.

Bainton, R. J., Tsai, L. T., Schwabe, T., DeSalvo, M., Gaul, U., and Heberlein, U. (2005). *moody* encodes two GPCRs that regulate cocaine behaviors and blood-brain barrier permeability in *Drosophila*. *Cell* 123, 145–156.

Banner, S. E., and Osborne, R. H. (1989). Modulation of 5-HT and proctolin receptors by FMRFamide in the foregut of the locust *Schistocerca gregaria*. *J. Insect Physiol.* 35, 887–892.

Barnes, A. I., Boone, J. M., Partridge, L., and Chapman, T. (2007). A functioning ovary is not required for sex peptide to reduce receptivity to mating in *D. melanogaster*. *J. Insect Physiol.* 53, 343–348.

Beets, I., Lindemans, M., Janssen, T., and Verleyen, P. (2011). Deorphanizing g protein-coupled receptors by a calcium mobilization assay. *Methods Mol. Biol.* 789, 377–391.

Begum, K., Li, B., Beeman, R. W., and Park, Y. (2009). Functions of ion transport peptide and ion transport peptide-like in the red flour beetle *Tribolium castaneum*. *Insect Biochem. Mol. Biol.* 39, 717–725.

Bellés, X. (2010). Beyond *Drosophila*: RNAi *in vivo* and functional genomics in insects. *Annu. Rev. Entomol.* 55, 111–128.

Bellés, X., Maestro, J.-L., Piulachs, M.-D., Johnsen, A. H., Duve, H., and Thorpe, A. (1994). Allatostatic neuropeptides from the cockroach *Blattella germanica* (L.) (Dictyoptera, Blattellidae). Identification, immunolocalization and activity. *Regul. Pept.* 53, 237–247.

Belmont, M., Cazzamali, G., Williamson, M., Hauser, F., and Grimmelikhuijzen, C. J. P. (2006). Identification of four evolutionarily related G protein-coupled receptors from the malaria mosquito *Anopheles gambiae*. *Biochem. Biophys. Res. Commun.* 344, 160–165.

Bendena, W. G. (2010). Neuropeptide physiology in insects. *Adv. Exp. Med. Biol.* 692, 166–191.

Bendena, W. G., Campbell, J., Zara, L., Tobe, S. S., and Chin-Sang, I. D. (2012). Select neuropeptides and their G-protein coupled receptors in *Caenorhabditis elegans* and *Drosophila melanogaster*. *Front. Endocrin.* 3:93. doi: 10.3389/fendo.2012.00093

Bender, E., Buist, A., Jurzak, M., Langlois, X., Baggerman, G., Verhasselt, P., et al. (2002). Characterization of an orphan G protein-coupled receptor localized in the dorsal root ganglia reveals adenine as a signaling molecule. *Proc. Natl. Acad. Sci. U.S.A.* 99, 8573–8578.

Bharucha, K. N., Tarr, P., and Zipursky, S. L. (2008). A glucagon-like endocrine pathway in *Drosophila* modulates both lipid and carbohydrate homeostasis. *J. Exp. Biol.* 211, 3103–3110.

Birgül, N., Weise, C., Kreienkamp, H. J., and Richter, D. (1999). Reverse physiology in *Drosophila*: identification of a novel allatostatin-like neuropeptide and its cognate receptor structurally related to the mammalian somatostatin/galanin/opioid receptor family. *EMBO J.* 18, 5892–5900.

Birse, R. T., Johnson, E. C., Taghert, P. H., and Nässel, D. R. (2006). Widely distributed *Drosophila* G-protein-coupled receptor (CG7887) is activated by endogenous tachykinin-related peptides. *J. Neurobiol.* 66, 33–46.

Birse, R. T., Söderberg, J. A. E., Luo, J., Winther, Å. M. E., and Nässel, D. R. (2011). Regulation of insulin-producing cells in the adult *Drosophila* brain *via* the tachykinin peptide receptor DTKR. *J. Exp. Biol.* 214(Pt 24), 4201–4208.

Blackburn, M. B., Jaffe, H., Kochansky, J., and Raina, A. K. (2001). Identification of four additional myoinhibitory peptides (MIPs) from the ventral nerve cord of *Manduca sexta*. *Arch. Insect Biochem. Physiol.* 48, 121–128.

Blackburn, M. B., Kingan, T. G., Bodnar, W., Shabanowitz, J., Hunt, D. F., Kempe, T., et al. (1991). Isolation and identification of a new diuretic peptide from the tobacco hornworm, *Manduca sexta*. *Biochem. Biophys. Res. Commun.* 181, 927–932.

Blackburn, M. B., Wagner, R. M., Kochansky, J. P., Harrison, D. J., Thomas-Laemont, P., and Raina, A. K. (1995). The identification of two myoinhibitory peptides, with sequence similarities to the galanins, isolated from the ventral nerve cord of *Manduca sexta*. *Regul. Pept.* 57, 213–219.

Bockaert, J., and Pin, J. P. (1999). Molecular tinkering of G protein-coupled receptors: an evolutionary success. *EMBO J.* 18, 1723–1729.

Boerjan, B., Cardoen, D., Bogaerts, A., Landuyt, B., Schoofs, L., and Verleyen, P. (2010a). Mass spectrometric profiling of (neuro)-peptides in the worker honeybee, *Apis mellifera*. *Neuropharmacology* 58, 248–258.

Boerjan, B., Verleyen, P., Huybrechts, J., Schoofs, L., and De Loof, A. (2010b). In search for a common denominator for the diverse functions of arthropod corazonin: a role in the physiology of stress? *Gen. Comp. Endocrinol.* 166, 222–233.

Boerjan, B., Cardoen, D., Verdonck, R., Caers, J., and Schoofs, L. (2012). Insect omics research coming of age. *Can. J. Zool.* 90, 440–455.

Boonen, K., Landuyt, B., Baggerman, G., Husson, S. J., Huybrechts, J., and Schoofs, L. (2008). Peptidomics: the integrated approach of MS, hyphenated techniques and bioinformatics for neuropeptide analysis. *J. Sep. Sci.* 31, 427–445.

Brody, T., and Cravchik, A. (2000). *Drosophila melanogaster* G protein-coupled receptors. *J. Cell Biol.* 150, F83–F88.

Brogiolo, W., Stocker, H., Ikeya, T., Rintelen, F., Fernandez, R., and Hafen, E. (2001). An evolutionarily conserved function of the *Drosophila* insulin receptor and insulin-like peptides in growth control. *Curr. Biol.* 11, 213–221.

Brown, M. R., Crim, J. W., Arata, R. C., Cai, H. N., Chun, C., and Shen, P. (1999). Identification of a *Drosophila* brain-gut peptide related to the neuropeptide Y family. *Peptides* 20, 1035–1042.

Brown, M. R., Graf, R., Swiderek, K. M., Fendley, D., Stracker, T. H., Champagne, D. E., et al. (1998). Identification of a steroidogenic neurohormone in female mosquitoes. *J. Biol. Chem.* 273, 3967–3971.

Cabrero, P., Radford, J. C., Broderick, K. E., Costes, L., Veenstra, J. A., Spana, E. P., et al. (2002). The Dh gene of *Drosophila melanogaster* encodes a diuretic peptide that acts through cyclic AMP. *J. Exp. Biol.* 205, 3799–3807.

Caers, J., Peeters, L., Janssen, T., De Haes, W., Gäde, G., and Schoofs, L. (2012). Structure-activity studies of *Drosophila* adipokinetic hormone (AKH) by a cellular expression system of dipteran AKH receptors. *Gen. Comp. Endocrinol.* 177, 332–337.

Carvalho, G. B., Kapahi, P., Anderson, D. J., and Benzer, S. (2006). Allocrine modulation of feeding behavior by the sex peptide of *Drosophila*. *Curr. Biol.* 16, 692–696.

Casida, J. E., and Quistad, G. B. (1998). Golden age of insecticide research: past, present, or future? *Annu. Rev. Entomol.* 43, 1–16.

Cazzamali, G., and Grimmelikhuijzen, C. J. P. (2002). Molecular cloning and functional expression of the first insect FMRFamide receptor. *Proc. Natl. Acad. Sci. U.S.A.* 99, 12073–12078.

Cazzamali, G., Hauser, F., Kobberup, S., Williamson, M., and Grimmelikhuijzen, C. J. P. (2003). Molecular identification of a *Drosophila* G protein-coupled receptor specific for crustacean cardioactive peptide. *Biochem. Biophys. Res. Commun.* 303, 146–152.

Cazzamali, G., Saxild, N., and Grimmelikhuijzen, C. J. P. (2002). Molecular cloning and functional expression of a Drosophila corazonin receptor. *Biochem. Biophys. Res. Commun.* 298, 31–36.

Cazzamali, G., Torp, M., Hauser, F., Williamson, M., and Grimmelikhuijzen, C. J. P. (2005). The Drosophila gene CG9918 codes for a pyrokinin-1 receptor. *Biochem. Biophys. Res. Commun.* 335, 14–19.

Chang, J. C., Yang, R. B., Adams, M. E., and Lu, K. H. (2009). Receptor guanylyl cyclases in Inka cells targeted by eclosion hormone. *Proc. Natl. Acad. Sci. U.S.A.* 106, 13371–13376.

Chen, J., Zhang, Y., and Shen, P. (2008). A protein kinase C activity localized to neuropeptide Y-like neurons mediates ethanol intoxication in *Drosophila melanogaster*. *Neuroscience* 156, 42–47.

Chen, M. E., and Pietrantonio, P. V. (2006). The short neuropeptide F-like receptor from the red imported fire ant, *Solenopsis invicta* Buren (Hymenoptera: Formicidae). *Arch. Insect Biochem. Physiol.* 61, 195–208.

Chen, P. S., Stumm-Zollinger, E., Aigaki, T., Balmer, J., Bienz, M., and Bohlen, P. (1988). A male accessory gland peptide that regulates reproductive behavior of female *D. melanogaster*. *Cell* 54, 291–298.

Chen, X., and Ganetzky, B. (2012). A neuropeptide signaling pathway regulates synaptic growth in *Drosophila*. *J. Cell Biol.* 196, 529–543.

Chen, X., Peterson, J., Nachman, R. J., and Ganetzky, B. (2012). Drosulfakinin activates CCKLR-17D1 and promotes larval locomotion and escape response in *Drosophila*. *Fly* 6, 1–8.

Cheung, C. C., Loi, P. K., Sylwester, A. W., Lee, T. D., and Tublitz, N. J. (1992). Primary structure of a cardioactive neuropeptide from the tobacco hawkmoth, *Manduca sexta*. *FEBS Lett.* 313, 165–168.

Chintapalli, V. R., Wang, J., and Dow, J. A. (2007). Using FlyAtlas to identify better *Drosophila melanogaster* models of human disease. *Nat. Genet.* 39, 715–720.

Choi, M. Y., Fuerst, E. J., Rafaeli, A., and Jurenka, R. (2003). Identification of a G protein-coupled receptor for pheromone biosynthesis activating neuropeptide from pheromone glands of the moth *Helicoverpa zea*. *Proc. Natl. Acad. Sci. U.S.A.* 100, 9721–9726.

Claeys, I., Poels, J., Simonet, G., Franssens, V., Van Loy, T., Van Hiel, M. B., et al. (2005a). Insect neuropeptide and peptide hormone receptors: current knowledge and future directions. *Vitam. Horm.* 73, 217–282.

Claeys, I., Simonet, G., Breugelmans, B., Van Soest, S., Franssens, V., Sas, F., et al. (2005b). Quantitative real-time RT-PCR analysis in desert locusts reveals phase dependent differences in neuroparsin transcript levels. *Insect Mol. Biol.* 14, 415–422.

Claeys, I., Breugelmans, B., Simonet, G., Van Soest, S., Sas, F., De Loof, A., et al. (2006). Neuroparsin transcripts as molecular markers in the process of desert locust (*Schistocerca gregaria*) phase transition. *Biochem. Biophys. Res. Commun.* 341, 599–606.

Clark, L., Lange, A. B., Zhang, J. R., and Tobe, S. S. (2008). The roles of *Dippu*-allatostatin in the modulation of hormone release in *Locusta migratoria*. *J. Insect Physiol.* 54, 949–958.

Clark, L., Zhang, J. R., Tobe, S. S., and Lange, A. B. (2006). Proctolin: a possible releasing factor in the corpus cardiacum/corpus allatum of the locust. *Peptides* 27, 559–566.

Clottens, F. L., Holman, G. M., Coast, G. M., Totty, N. F., Hayes, T. K., Kay, I., et al. (1994). Isolation and characterization of a diuretic peptide common to the house fly and stable fly. *Peptides* 15, 971–979.

Clynen, E., Huybrechts, J., Verleyen, P., De Loof, A., and Schoofs, L. (2006). Annotation of novel neuropeptide precursors in the migratory locust based on transcript screening of a public EST database and mass spectrometry. *BMC Genomics* 7:201. doi: 10.1186/1471-2164-7-201

Clynen, E., and Schoofs, L. (2009). Peptidomic survey of the locust neuroendocrine system. *Insect Biochem. Mol. Biol.* 39, 491–507.

Clynen, E., Liu, F., Husson, S. J., Landuyt, B., Hayakawa, E., Baggerman, G., et al. (2010b). Bioinformatic approaches to the identification of novel neuropeptide precursors. *Methods Mol. Biol.* 615, 357–374.

Clynen, E., Reumer, A., Baggerman, G., Mertens, I., and Schoofs, L. (2010a). Neuropeptide biology in *Drosophila*. *Adv. Exp. Med. Biol.* 692, 192–210.

Coast, G. M., and Garside, C. S. (2005). Neuropeptide control of fluid balance in insects. *Ann. N.Y. Acad. Sci.* 1040, 1–8.

Coast, G. M., Garside, C. S., Webster, S. G., Schegg, K. M., and Schooley, D. A. (2005). Mosquito natriuretic peptide identified as a calcitonin-like diuretic hormone in *Anopheles gambiae* (Giles). *J. Exp. Biol.* 208, 3281–3291.

Coast, G. M., Webster, S. G., Schegg, K. M., Tobe, S. S., and Schooley, D. A. (2001). The *Drosophila melanogaster* homologue of an insect calcitonin-like diuretic peptide stimulates V-ATPase activity in fruit fly Malpighian tubules. *J. Exp. Biol.* 204, 1795–1804.

Cognigni, P., Bailey, A. P., and Miguel-Aliaga, I. (2011). Enteric neurons and systemic signals couple nutritional and reproductive status with intestinal homeostasis. *Cell Metab.* 13, 92–104.

Collin, C., Hauser, F., Krogh-Meyer, P., Hansen, K. K., de Gonzalez, V., Williamson, M., et al. (2011). Identification of the Drosophila and Tribolium receptors for the recently discovered insect RYamide neuropeptides. *Biochem. Biophys. Res. Commun.* 412, 578–583.

Cvejic, S., Zhu, Z., Felice, S. J., Berman, Y., and Huang, X.-Y. (2004). The endogenous ligand stunted of the GPCR methuselah extends lifespan in *Drosophila*. *Nat. Cell Biol.* 6, 540–546.

Dai, H., Ma, L., Wang, J., Jiang, R., Wang, Z., and Fei, J. (2008). Knockdown of ecdysis-triggering hormone gene with a binary UAS/GAL4 RNA interference system leads to lethal ecdysis deficiency in silkworm. *Acta Biochim. Biophys. Sin. (Shanghai)* 40, 790–795.

Dai, L., and Adams, M. E. (2009). Ecdysis triggering hormone signaling in the yellow fever mosquito *Aedes aegypti*. *Gen. Comp. Endocrinol.* 162, 43–51.

Daneman, R., and Barres, B. A. (2005). The blood-brain barrier–lessons from moody flies. *Cell* 123, 9–12.

de Haro, M., Al-Ramahi, I., Benito-Sipos, J., López-Arias, B., Dorado, B., Veenstra, J. A., et al. (2010). Detailed análisis of leucokinin-expressing neurons and their candidate functions in the *Drosophila* nervous system. *Cell Tissue Res.* 339, 321–336.

De Loof, A. (2008). Ecdysteroids, juvenile hormone and insect neuropeptides: recent successes and remaining major challenges. *Gen. Comp. Endocrinol.* 155, 3–13.

De Loof, A., Lindemans, M., Liu, F., De Groef, B., and Schoofs, L. (2012). Endocrine archeology: do insects retain ancestrally inherited counterparts of the vertebrate releasing hormones GnRH, GHRH, TRH, and CRF? *Gen. Comp. Endocrinol.* 177, 18–27.

Dewey, E. M., McNabb, S. L., Ewer, J., Kuo, G. R., Takanishi, C. L., Truman, J. W., et al. (2004). Identification of the gene encoding bursicon, an insect neuropeptide responsible for cuticle sclerotization and wing spreading. *Curr. Biol.* 14, 1208–1213.

DeZazzo, J., Xia, S., Christensen, J., Velinzon, K., and Tully, T. (1999). Developmental expression of an amn^{+} transgene rescues the mutant memory defect of *amnesiac* adults. *J. Neurosci.* 19, 8740–8746.

Dierick, H. A., and Greenspan, R. J. (2007). Serotonin and neuropeptide F have opposite modulatory effects on fly aggression. *Nat. Genet.* 39, 678–682.

Dietzl, G., Chen, D., Schnorrer, F., Su, K. C., Barinova, Y., Fellner, M., et al. (2007). A genome-wide transgenic RNAi library for conditional gene inactivation in *Drosophila*. *Nature* 448, 151–156.

Dircksen, H. (2009). Insect ion transport peptides are derived from alternatively spliced genes and differentially expressed in the central and peripheral nervous system. *J. Exp. Biol.* 212, 401–412.

Dircksen, H., Tesfai, L. K., Albus, C., and Nassel, D. R. (2008). Ion transport peptide splice forms in central and peripheral neurons throughout postembryogenesis of *Drosophila melanogaster*. *J. Comp. Neurol.* 509, 23–41.

Domanitskaya, E. V., Liu, H., Chen, S., and Kubli, E. (2007). The hydroxyproline motif of male sex peptide elicits the innate immune response in *Drosophila* females. *FEBS J.* 274, 5659–5668.

Donini, A., Agricola, H., and Lange, A. B. (2001). Crustacean cardioactive peptide is a modulator of oviduct contractions in *Locusta migratoria*. *J. Insect Physiol.* 47, 277–285.

Donini, A., and Lange, A. B. (2002). The effects of crustacean cardioactive peptide on locust oviducts are calcium-dependent. *Peptides* 23, 683–691.

Donini, A., Ngo, C., and Lange, A. B. (2002). Evidence for crustacean cardioactive peptide-like innervation of the gut in *Locusta migratoria*. *Peptides* 23, 1915–1923.

Down, R. E., Matthews, H. J., and Audsley, N. (2011). Oral activity of FMRFamide-related peptides on the pea aphid *Acyrthosiphon pisum* (Hemiptera: Aphididae) and degradation by enzymes from the aphid gut. *Regul. Pept.* 171, 11–18.

Downer, K. E., Haselton, A. T., Nachman, R. J., and Stoffolano, J. G. Jr. (2007). Insect satiety: sulfakinin localization and the effect of drosulfakinin on protein and carbohydrate ingestion in the blow fly, *Phormia regina* (Diptera: Calliphoridae). *J. Insect Physiol.* 53, 106–112.

Duttlinger, A., Berry, K., and Nichols, R. (2002). The different effects of three *Drosophila melanogaster* dFMRFamide-containing peptides on crop contractions suggest these structurally related peptides do not play redundant functions in gut. *Peptides* 23, 1953–1957.

Duttlinger, A., Mispelon, M., and Nichols, R. (2003). The structure of the FMRFamide receptor and activity of the cardioexcitatory neuropeptide are conserved in mosquito. *Neuropeptides* 37, 120–126.

Egerod, K., Reynisson, E., Hauser, F., Cazzamali, G., Williamson, M., and Grimmelikhuijzen, C. J. P. (2003a). Molecular cloning and functional expression of the first two specific insect myosuppressin receptors. *Proc. Natl. Acad. Sci. U.S.A.* 100, 9808–9813.

Egerod, K., Reynisson, E., Hauser, F., Williamson, M., Cazzamali, G., and Grimmelikhuijzen, C. J. P. (2003b). Molecular identification of the first insect proctolin receptor. *Biochem. Biophys. Res. Commun.* 306, 437–442.

Elekonich, M. M., and Horodyski, F. M. (2003). Insect allatotropins belong to a family of structurally-related myoactive peptides present in several invertebrate phyla. *Peptides* 24, 1623 1632.

Eriksen, K. K., Hauser, F., Schiøtt, M., Pedersen, K.-M., Søndergaard, L., and Grimmelikhuijzen, C. J. P. (2000). Molecular cloning, genomic organization, developmental regulation, and a knock-out mutant of a novel leu-rich repeats-containing G protein-coupled receptor (DLGR-2) from *Drosophila melanogaster*. *Genome Res.* 10, 924–938.

Ewer, J. (2005). Behavioral actions of neuropeptides in invertebrates: insights from *Drosophila*. *Horm. Behav.* 48, 418–429.

Ewer, J., Wang, C. M., Klukas, K. A., Mesce, K. A., Truman, J. W., and Fahrbach, S. E. (1998). Programmed cell death of identified peptidergic neurons involved in ecdysis behavior in the Moth, *Manduca sexta*. *J. Neurobiol.* 37, 265–280.

Fan, Y., Rafaeli, A., Gileadi, C., Kubli, E., and Applebaum, S. W. (1999). *Drosophila melanogaster* sex peptide stimulates juvenile hormone synthesis and depresses sex pheromone production in *Helicoverpa armigera*. *J. Insect Physiol.* 45, 127–133.

Fan, Y., Sun, P., Wang, Y., He, X., Deng, X., Chen, X., et al. (2010). The G protein-coupled receptors in the silkworm, *Bombyx mori*. *Insect Biochem. Mol. Biol.* 40, 581–591.

Feany, M. B., and Quinn, W. G. (1995). A neuropeptide gene defined by the *Drosophila* memory mutant *amnesiac*. *Science* 268, 869–873.

Feng, G. P., Reale, V., Chatwin, H. M., Kennedy, K., Venard, R., Ericsson, C., et al. (2003). Functional characterization of a neuropeptide F-like receptor from *Drosophila melanogaster*. *Eur. J. Neurosci.* 18, 227–238.

Fernandez, R., Tabarini, D., Azpiazu, N., Frasch, M., and Schlessinger, J. (1995). The *Drosophila* insulin receptor homolog: a gene essential for embryonic development encodes two receptor isoforms with different signaling potential. *EMBO J.* 14, 3373–3384.

Fire, A., Xu, S., Montgomery, M. K., Kostas, S. A., Driver, S. E., and Mello, C. C. (1998). Potent and specific genetic interference by double-stranded RNA in *Caenorhabditis elegans*. *Nature* 391, 806–811.

Fraenkel, G., Hsiao, C., and Seligman, M. (1966). Properties of bursicon: an insect protein hormone that controls cuticular tanning. *Science* 151, 91–93.

Furuya, K., Liao, S., Reynolds, S. E., Ota, R. B., Hackett, M., and Schooley, D. A. (1993). Isolation and identification of a cardioactive peptide from *Tenebrio molitor* and *Spodoptera eridania*. *Biol. Chem. Hoppe Seyler* 374, 1065–1074.

Furuya, K., Milchak, R. J., Schegg, K. M., Zhang, J., Tobe, S. S., Coast, G. M., et al. (2000). Cockroach diuretic hormones: characterization of a calcitonin-like peptide in insects. *Proc. Natl. Acad. Sci. U.S.A.* 97, 6469–6474.

Furuya, K., Schegg, K. M., Wang, H., King, D. S., and Schooley, D. A. (1995). Isolation and identification of a diuretic hormone from the mealworm *Tenebrio molitor*. *Proc. Natl. Acad. Sci. U.S.A.* 92, 12323–12327.

Gammie, S. C., and Truman, J. W. (1997). Neuropeptide hierarchies and the activation of sequential motor behaviors in the hawkmoth, *Manduca sexta*. *J. Neurosci.* 17, 4389–4397.

Garczynski, S. F., Brown, M. R., Shen, P., Murray, T. F., and Crim, J. W. (2002). Characterization of a functional neuropeptide F receptor from *Drosophila melanogaster*. *Peptides* 23, 773–780.

Garczynski, S. F., Crim, J. W., and Brown, M. R. (2005). Characterization of neuropeptide F and its receptor from the African malaria mosquito, *Anopheles gambiae*. *Peptides* 26, 99–107.

Garczynski, S. F., Crim, J. W., and Brown, M. R. (2007). Characterization and expression of the short neuropeptide F receptor in the African malaria mosquito, *Anopheles gambiae*. *Peptides* 28, 109–118.

Gäde, G., and Auerswald, L. (2003). Mode of action of neuropeptides from the adipokinetic hormone family. *Gen. Comp. Endocrinol.* 132, 10–20.

Gäde, G., and Goldsworthy, G. (2003). Insect peptide hormones: a selective review of their physiology and potential application for pest control. *Pest Manag. Sci.* 59, 1063–1075.

Gäde, G. (2004). Regulation of intermediary metabolism and water balance of insects by neuropeptides. *Annu. Rev. Entomol.* 49, 93–113.

Gäde, G. (2009). Peptides of the adipokinetic hormone/red pigment-concentrating hormone family: a new take on biodiversity. *Ann. N.Y. Acad. Sci.* 1163, 125–136.

Gäde, G., and Marco, H. G. (2012). The adipokinetic hormone (AKH) of one of the most basal orders of Pterygota: structure and function of Ephemeroptera AKH. *J. Insect Physiol.* 58, 1390–1396.

Gäde, G., Marco, H. G., Simek, P., Audsley, N., Clark, K. D., and Weaver, R. J. (2008). Predicted versus expressed adipokinetic hormones, and other small peptides from the corpus cardiacum-corpus allatum: a case study with beetles and moths. *Peptides* 29, 1124–1139.

Gether, U. (2000). Uncovering molecular mechanisms involved in activation of G protein-coupled receptors. *Endocr. Rev.* 21, 90–113.

Girardie, J., Huet, J. C., tay-Kadiri, Z., Ettaouil, S., Delbecque, J. P., Fournier, B., et al. (1998). Isolation, sequence determination, physical and physiological characterization of the neuroparsins and ovary maturing parsins of *Schistocerca gregaria*. *Insect Biochem. Mol. Biol.* 28, 641–650.

Goldsworthy, G., Chandrakant, S., and Opoku-Ware, K. (2003). Adipokinetic hormone enhances nodule formation and phenoloxidase activation in adult locusts injected with bacterial lipopolysaccharide. *J. Insect Physiol.* 49, 795–803.

Goldsworthy, G., Opoku-Ware, K., and Mullen, L. (2002). Adipokinetic hormone enhances laminarin and bacterial lipopolysaccharide-induced activation of the prophenoloxidase cascade in the African migratory locust, *Locusta migratoria*. *J. Insect Physiol.* 48, 601–608.

Gong, Z.-F., Xia, S.-Z., Liu, L., Feng, C.-H., and Guo, A.-K. (1998). Operant visual learning and memory in *Drosophila* mutants *dunce*, *amnesiac* and *radish*. *J. Insect Physiol.* 44, 1149–1158.

Gonzalez, R., and Orchard, I. (2008). Characterization of neuropeptide F-like immunoreactivity in the blood-feeding hemipteran, *Rhodnius prolixus*. *Peptides* 29, 545–558.

Gonzalez, R., and Orchard, I. (2009). Physiological activity of neuropeptide f on the hindgut of the blood-feeding hemipteran, *Rhodnius prolixus*. *J. Insect Sci.* 9, 1–14.

Graf, R., Neuenschwander, S., Brown, M. R., and Ackermann, U. (1997). Insulin-mediated secretion of ecdysteroids from mosquito ovaries and molecular cloning of the insulin receptor homologue from ovaries of bloodfed *Aedes aegypti*. *Insect Mol. Biol.* 6, 151–163.

Graveley, B. R., Brooks, A. N., Carlson, J. W., Duff, M. O., Landolin, J. M., Yang, L., et al. (2011). The developmental transcriptome of *Drosophila melanogaster*. *Nature* 471, 473–479.

Griebler, M., Westerlund, S. A., Hoffmann, K. H., and Meyering-Vos, M. (2008). RNA interference with the allatoregulating neuropeptide genes from the fall armyworm *Spodoptera frugiperda* and its effects on the JH titer in the hemolymph. *J. Insect Physiol.* 54, 997–1007.

Grimmelikhuijzen, C. J. P., Cazzamali, G., Williamson, M., and Hauser, F. (2007). The promise of insect genomics. *Pest Manag. Sci.* 63, 413–416.

Grimmelikhuijzen, C. J. P., and Hauser, F. (2012a). Mini-review: the evolution of neuropeptide signaling. *Regul. Pept.* 177, S6–S9.

Grimmelikhuijzen, C. J. P., and Hauser, F. (2012b). "Arthropod genomics and pest management targeting GPCRs," in *Advanced Technologies for Managing Insect Pests*, eds I. Ishaaya, S. R. Palli, and A. R. Horowitz (Heidelberg: Springer Verlag), 165–177.

Grönke, S., Muller, G., Hirsch, J., Fellert, S., Andreou, A., Haase, T., et al. (2007). Dual lipolytic control of body fat storage and mobilization in *Drosophila*. *PLoS Biol.* 5:e137. doi: 10.1371/journal.pbio.0050137

Guerrero, F. D. (1997). Transcriptional expression of a putative tachykinin-like peptide receptor gene from stable fly. *Peptides* 18, 1–5.

Ha, S. D., Kataoka, H., Suzuki, A., Kim, B. J., Kim, H. J., Hwang, S. H., et al. (2000). Cloning and sequence analysis of cDNA for diuretic hormone receptor from the *Bombyx mori*. *Mol. Cells* 10, 13–17.

Hansen, K. K., Hauser, F., Cazzamali, G., Williamson, M., and Grimmelikhuijzen, C. J. P. (2006). Cloning and characterization of the adipokinetic hormone receptor from the cockroach *Periplaneta americana*. *Biochem. Biophys. Res. Commun.* 343, 638–643.

Hansen, K. K., Hauser, F., Williamson, M., Weber, S. B., and Grimmelikhuijzen, C. J. P. (2011). The *Drosophila* genes CG14593 and CG30106 code for G-protein-coupled receptors specifically activated by the neuropeptides CCHamide-1 and CCHamide-2. *Biochem. Biophys. Res. Commun.* 404, 184–189.

Hansen, K. K., Stafflinger, E., Schneider, M., Hauser, F., Cazzamali, G., Williamson, M., et al. (2010). Discovery of a novel insect neuropeptide signaling system closely related to the insect adipokinetic hormone and corazonin hormonal systems. *J. Biol. Chem.* 285, 10736–10747.

Harshini, S., Nachman, R. J., and Sreekumar, S. (2002). *In vitro* release of digestive enzymes by FMRF amide related neuropeptides and analogues in the lepidopteran insect *Opisina arenosella* (Walk.). *Peptides* 23, 1759–1763.

Häsemeyer, M., Yapici, N., Heberlein, U., and Dickson, B. J. (2009). Sensory neurons in the *Drosophila* genital tract regulate female reproductive behavior. *Neuron* 61, 511–518.

Hashimoto, H., Shintani, N., and Baba, A. (2002). Higher brain functions of PACAP and a homologous *Drosophila* memory gene *amnesiac*: insights from knockouts and mutants. *Biochem. Biophys. Res. Commun.* 297, 427–431.

Hatan, M., Shinder, V., Israeli, D., Schnorrer, F., and Volk, T. (2011). The *Drosophila* blood brain barrier is maintained by GPCR-dependent dynamic actin structures. *J. Cell Biol.* 192, 307–319.

Hauser, F., Cazzamali, G., Williamson, M., Blenau, W., and Grimmelikhuijzen, C. J. P. (2006). A review of neurohormone GPCRs present in the fruitfly *Drosophila melanogaster* and the honey bee *Apis mellifera*. *Prog. Neurobiol.* 80, 1–19.

Hauser, F., Cazzamali, G., Williamson, M., Park, Y., Li, B., Tanaka, Y., et al. (2008). A genome-wide inventory of neurohormone GPCRs in the red flour beetle *Tribolium castaneum*. *Front. Neuroendocrinol.* 29:3. doi: 10.1016/j.yfrne.2007.10.003

Hauser, F., Neupert, S., Williamson, M., Predel, R., Tanaka, Y., and Grimmelikhuijzen, C. J. P. (2010). Genomics and peptidomics of neuropeptides and protein hormones present in the parasitic wasp *Nasonia vitripennis*. *J. Proteome Res.* 9, 5296–5310.

Hauser, F., Nothacker, H. P., and Grimmelikhuijzen, C. J. P. (1997). Molecular cloning, genomic organization, and developmental regulation of a novel receptor from *Drosophila melanogaster* structurally related to members of the thyroid-stimulating hormone, follicle-stimulating hormone, luteinizing hormone/choriogonadotropin receptor family from mammals. *J. Biol. Chem.* 272, 1002–1010.

Hauser, F., Søndergaard, L., and Grimmelikhuijzen, C. J. P. (1998). Molecular cloning, genomic organization and developmental regulation of a novel receptor from *Drosophila melanogaster* structurally related to gonadotropin-releasing hormone receptors for vertebrates. *Biochem. Biophys. Res. Commun.* 249, 822–828.

Hayes, T. K., Guan, X. C., Johnson, V., Strey, A., and Tobe, S. S. (1994). Structure-activity studies of allatostatin 4 on the inhibition of juvenile hormone biosynthesis by corpora allata: the importance of individual side chains and stereochemistry. *Peptides* 15, 1165–1171.

Hayes, T. K., Pannabecker, T. L., Hinckley, D. J., Holman, G. M., Nachman, R. J., Petzel, D. H., et al. (1989). Leucokinins, a new family of ion transport stimulators and inhibitors in insect Malpighian tubules. *Life Sci.* 44, 1259–1266.

Hector, C. E., Bretz, C. A., Zhao, Y., and Johnson, E. C. (2009). Functional differences between two CRF-related diuretic hormone receptors in *Drosophila*. *J. Exp. Biol.* 212, 3142–3147.

Hepler, J. R., and Gilman, A. G. (1992). G proteins. *Trends Biochem. Sci.* 17, 383–387.

Hergarden, A. C., Tayler, T. D., and Anderson, D. J. (2012). Allatostatin-A neurons inhibit feeding behavior in adult *Drosophila*. *Proc. Natl. Acad. Sci. U.S.A.* 109, 3967–3972.

Hermann, C., Saccon, R., Senthilan, P. R., Domnik, L., Dircksen, H., Yoshii, T., et al. (2012). The circadian clock network in the brain of different *Drosophila* species. *J. Comp. Neurol.* doi: 10.1002/cne.23178. [Epub ahead of print].

Herrero, P. (2012). Fruit fly behavior in response to chemosensory signals. *Peptides.* 38, 228–237.

Hewes, R. S., and Taghert, P. H. (2001). Neuropeptides and neuropeptide receptors in the *Drosophila melanogaster* genome. *Genome Res.* 11, 1126–1142.

Hill, S. R., and Orchard, I. (2005). *In vitro* analysis of the digestive enzymes amylase and alpha-glucosidase in the midguts of *Locusta migratoria* L. in response to the myosuppressin,

*Schisto*FLRFamide. *J. Insect Physiol.* 51, 1–9.

Hillyer, J. F., Estevez-Lao, T. Y., Funkhouser, L. J., and Aluoch, V. A. (2012). *Anopheles gambiae* corazonin: gene structure, expression and effect on mosquito heart physiology. *Insect Mol. Biol.* 21, 343–355.

Ho, I. H. M., and Murrell-Lagnado, R. D. (1999). Molecular mechanism for sodium-dependent activation of G protein-gated K^+ channels. *J. Physiol.* 520(Pt 3), 645–651.

Hofer, S., Dircksen, H., Tollbäck, P., and Homberg, U. (2005). Novel insect orcokinins: characterization and neural distribution in the brains of selected dicondylian insects. *J. Comp. Neurol.* 490, 57–71.

Hofer, S., and Homberg, U. (2006). Evidence for a role of orcokinin-related peptides in the circadian clock controlling locomotor activity of the cockroach *Leucophaea maderae*. *J. Exp. Biol.* 209, 2794–2803.

Hoffmann, K. H., Meyering-Vos, M., and Lorenz, M. W. (1999). Allatostatins and allatotropins: is the regulation of corpora allata activity their primary function? *Eur. J. Entomol.* 96, 266.

Holman, G. M., Cook, B. J., and Nachman, R. J. (1986). Primary structure and synthesis of two additional neuropeptides from *Leucophaea maderae*: members of a new family of cephalomyotropins. *Comp. Biochem. Physiol. C* 84, 271–276.

Holman, G. M., Cook, B. J., and Nachman, R. J. (1987). Isolation, primary structure and synthesis of leucomyosuppressin, an insect neuropeptide that inhibits the spontaneous contractions of the cockroach hindgut. *Comp. Biochem. Physiol. B* 88, 27–30.

Homberg, U., Reischig, T., and Stengl, M. (2003). Neural organization of the circadian system of the cockroach *Leucophaea maderae*. *Chronobiol. Int.* 20, 577–591.

Homma, T., Watanabe, K., Tsurumaru, S., Kataoka, H., Imai, K., Kamba, M., et al. (2006). G protein-coupled receptor for diapause hormone, an inducer of *Bombyx* embryonic diapause. *Biochem. Biophys. Res. Commun.* 344, 386–393.

Honegger, H.-W., Dewey, E. M., and Kostron, B. (2004). From bioassays to *Drosophila* genetics: strategies for characterizing an essential insect neurohormone, bursicon. *Acta Biol. Hung.* 55, 91–102.

Hong, S.-T., Bang, S., Hyun, S., Kang, J., Jeong, K., Paik, D., et al. (2008). cAMP signaling in mushroom bodies modulates temperature preference behaviour in *Drosophila*. *Nature* 454, 771–775.

Hong, S. H., Lee, K. S., Kwak, S. J., Kim, A. K., Bai, H., Jung, M. S., et al. (2012). Minibrain/Dyrk1a regulates food intake through the Sir2-FOXO-sNPF/NPY pathway in *Drosophila* and mammals. *PLoS Genet.* 8:e1002857. doi: 10.1371/journal.pgen.1002857

Hook, V., Funkelstein, L., Lu, D., Bark, S., Wegrzyn, J., and Hwang, S. R. (2008). Proteases for processing proneuropeptides into peptide neurotransmitters and hormones. *Annu. Rev. Pharmacol. Toxicol.* 48, 393–423.

Horn, F., van der Wenden, E. M., Oliveira, L., IJzerman, A. P., and Vriend, G. (2000). Receptors coupling to G proteins: is there a signal behind the sequence? *Proteins* 41, 448–459.

Horodyski, F. M., Bhatt, S. R., and Lee, K. Y. (2001). Alternative splicing of transcripts expressed by the *Manduca sexta* allatotropin (Mas-AT) gene is regulated in a tissue-specific manner. *Peptides* 22, 263–269.

Horodyski, F. M., Verlinden, H., Filkin, N., Vandersmissen, H. P., Fleury, C., Reynolds, S. E., et al. (2011). Isolation and functional characterization of an allatotropin receptor from *Manduca sexta*. *Insect Biochem. Mol. Biol.* 41, 804–814.

Hsu, S. Y., Kudo, M., Chen, T., Nakabayashi, K., Bhalla, A., van der Spek, P. J., et al. (2000). The three subfamilies of leucine-rich repeat-containing G protein-coupled receptors (LGR): identification of LGR6 and LGR7 and the signaling mechanism for LGR7. *Mol. Endocrinol.* 14, 1257–1271.

Huang, H., He, X., Deng, X., Li, G., Ying, G., Sun, Y., et al. (2010). *Bombyx* adipokinetic hormone receptor activates extracellular signal-regulated kinase 1 and 2 via G protein-dependent PKA and PKC but beta-arrestin-independent pathways. *Biochemistry* 49, 10862–10872.

Huang, J. H., Bellés, X., and Lee, H. J. (2011a). Functional characterization of hypertrehalosemic hormone receptor in relation to hemolymph trehalose and to oxidative stress in the cockroach *Blattella germanica*. *Front. Endocrin. (Lausanne)* 2:114. doi: 10.3389/fendo.2011.00114

Huang, Y., Crim, J. W., Nuss, A. B., and Brown, M. R. (2011b). Neuropeptide F and the corn earworm, *Helicoverpa zea*: a midgut peptide revisited. *Peptides* 32, 483–492.

Hummon, A. B., Richmond, T. A., Verleyen, P., Baggerman, G., Huybrechts, J., Ewing, M. A., et al. (2006). From the genome to the proteome: uncovering peptides in the *Apis* brain. *Science* 314, 647–649.

Huybrechts, J., Bonhomme, J., Minoli, S., Prunier-Leterme, N., Dombrovsky, A., Abdel-Latief, M., et al. (2010). Neuropeptide and neurohormone precursors in the pea aphid, *Acyrthosiphon pisum*. *Insect Mol. Biol.* 19(Suppl. 2), 87–95.

Huybrechts, J., De Loof, A., and Schoofs, L. (2004). Diapausing colorado potato beetles are devoid of short neuropeptide F I and II. *Biochem. Biophys. Res. Commun.* 317, 909–916.

Hyun, S., Lee, Y., Hong, S. T., Bang, S., Paik, D., Kang, J., et al. (2005). *Drosophila* GPCR han is a receptor for the circadian clock neuropeptide, P. D. F. *Neuron* 48, 267–278.

Ida, T., Takahashi, T., Tominaga, H., Sato, T., Kume, K., Ozaki, M., et al. (2011a). Identification of the novel bioactive peptides dRYamide-1 and dRYamide-2, ligands for a neuropeptide Y-like receptor in *Drosophila*. *Biochem. Biophys. Res. Commun.* 410, 872–877.

Ida, T., Takahashi, T., Tominaga, H., Sato, T., Kume, K., Yoshizawa-Kumagaye, K., et al. (2011b). Identification of the endogenous cysteine-rich peptide trissin, a ligand for an orphan G protein-coupled receptor in *Drosophila*. *Biochem. Biophys. Res. Commun.* 414, 44–48.

Iga, M., and Smagghe, G. (2011). Relationship between larval-pupal metamorphosis and transcript expression of insulin-like peptide and insulin receptor in *Spodoptera littoralis*. *Peptides* 32, 531–538.

Ignell, R., Root, C. M., Birse, R. T., Wang, J. W., Nässel, D. R., and Winther, Å. M. E. (2009). Presynaptic peptidergic modulation of olfactory receptor neurons in *Drosophila*. *Proc. Natl. Acad. Sci. U.S.A.* 106, 13070–13075.

Im, S. H., and Taghert, P. H. (2010). PDF receptor expression reveals direct interactions between circadian oscillators in *Drosophila*. *J. Comp. Neurol.* 518, 1925–1945.

Ionescu, A., and Donini, A. (2012). *Aedes*CAPA-PVK-1 displays diuretic and dose dependent antidiuretic potential in the larval mosquito *Aedes aegypti* (Liverpool). *J. Insect Physiol.* 58, 1299–1306.

Isaac, R. E., Li, C., Leedale, A. E., and Shirras, A. D. (2010). *Drosophila* male sex peptide inhibits siesta sleep and promotes locomotor activity in the post-mated female. *Proc. Biol. Sci.* 277, 65–70.

Isaac, R. E., Taylor, C. A., Hamasaka, Y., Nässel, D. R., and Shirras, A. D. (2004). Proctolin in the post-genomic era: new insights and challenges. *Invert. Neurosci.* 5, 51–64.

Isabel, G., Martin, J. R., Chidami, S., Veenstra, J. A., and Rosay, P. (2005). AKH-producing neuroendocrine cell ablation decreases trehalose and induces behavioral changes in *Drosophila*. *Am. J. Physiol. Regul. Integr. Comp. Physiol.* 288, R531–R538.

Iversen, A., Cazzamali, G., Williamson, M., Hauser, F., and Grimmelikhuijzen, C. J. P. (2002a). Molecular cloning and functional expression of a *Drosophila* receptor for the neuropeptides capa-1 and -2. *Biochem. Biophys. Res. Commun.* 299, 628–633.

Iversen, A., Cazzamali, G., Williamson, M., Hauser, F., and Grimmelikhuijzen, C. J. P. (2002b). Molecular identification of the first insect ecdysis triggering hormone receptors. *Biochem. Biophys. Res. Commun.* 299, 924–931.

Ja, W. W., Carvalho, G. B., Madrigal, M., Roberts, R. W., and Benzer, S. (2009). The *Drosophila* G protein-coupled receptor, methuselah, exhibits a promiscuous response to peptides. *Protein Sci.* 18, 2203–2208.

Jagge, C. L., and Pietrantonio, P. V. (2008). Diuretic hormone 44 receptor in malpighian tubules of the mosquito *Aedes aegypti*: evidence for transcriptional regulation paralleling urination. *Insect Mol. Biol.* 17, 413–426.

Janssen, T., Husson, S. J., Lindemans, M., Mertens, I., Rademakers, S., Ver Donck, K., et al. (2008). Functional characterization of three G protein-coupled receptors for pigment dispersing factors in *Caenorhabditis elegans*. *J. Biol. Chem.* 283, 15241–15249.

Jedlička, P., Steinbauerová, V., Šimek, P., and Zahradníčková, H. (2012). Functional characterization of the adipokinetic hormone in the pea aphid, *Acyrthosiphon pisum*. *Comp. Biochem. Physiol. A* 162, 51–58.

Johard, H. A., Muren, J. E., Nichols, R., Larhammar, D. S., and Nässel, D. R. (2001). A putative tachykinin receptor in the cockroach brain: molecular cloning and analysis of expression by means of antisera to portions of the receptor protein. *Brain Res.* 919, 94–105.

Johard, H. A., Enell, L. E., Gustafsson, E., Trifilieff, P., Veenstra, J. A., and Nässel, D. R. (2008). Intrinsic neurons of *Drosophila* mushroom bodies express short neuropeptide F: relations to extrinsic neurons expressing different neurotransmitters. *J. Comp. Neurol.* 507, 1479–1496.

Johnson, E. C., Garczynski, S. F., Park, D., Crim, J. W., Nässel, D. R., and Taghert, P. H. (2003a). Identification and characterization of a G protein-coupled receptor for the neuropeptide proctolin in *Drosophila melanogaster*. *Proc. Natl. Acad. Sci. U.S.A.* 100, 6198–6203.

Johnson, E. C., Bohn, L. M., Barak, L. S., Birse, R. T., Nässel, D. R., Caron, M. G., et al. (2003b). Identification of *Drosophila* neuropeptide receptors by G protein-coupled receptors-beta-arrestin2 interactions. *J. Biol. Chem.* 278, 52172–52178.

Johnson, E. C., Bohn, L. M., and Taghert, P. H. (2004). *Drosophila* CG8422 encodes a functional diuretic hormone receptor. *J. Exp. Biol.* 207, 743–748.

Johnson, E. C., Shafer, O. T., Trigg, J. S., Park, J., Schooley, D. A., Dow, J. A., et al. (2005). A novel diuretic hormone receptor in *Drosophila*: evidence for conservation of CGRP signaling. *J. Exp. Biol.* 208, 1239–1246.

Jørgensen, L. M., Hauser, F., Cazzamali, G., Williamson, M., and Grimmelikhuijzen, C. J. P. (2006). Molecular identification of the first SIFamide receptor. *Biochem. Biophys. Res. Commun.* 340, 696–701.

Jurenka, R., and Nusawardani, T. (2011). The pyrokinin/ pheromone biosynthesis-activating neuropeptide (PBAN) family of peptides and their receptors in Insecta: evolutionary trace indicates potential receptor ligand-binding domains. *Insect Mol. Biol.* 20, 323–334.

Kahsai, L., Carlsson, M. A., Winther, A. M., and Nässel, D. R. (2012). Distribution of metabotropic receptors of serotonin, dopamine, GABA, glutamate, and short neuropeptide F in the central complex of *Drosophila*. *Neuroscience* 208, 11–26.

Kahsai, L., Kapan, N., Dircksen, H., Winther, A. M., and Nässel, D. R. (2010). Metabolic stress responses in *Drosophila* are modulated by brain neurosecretory cells that produce multiple neuropeptides. *PLoS ONE* 5:e11480. doi: 10.1371/journal.pone.0011480

Kamps, A. R., Pruitt, M. M., Herriges, J. C., and Coffman, C. R. (2010). An evolutionarily conserved arginine is essential for Tre1 G protein-coupled receptor function during germ cell migration in *Drosophila melanogaster*. *PLoS ONE* 5:e11839. doi: 10.1371/journal.pone.0011839

Kapan, N., Lushchak, O. V., Luo, J., and Nässel, D. R. (2012). Identified peptidergic neurons in the *Drosophila* brain regulate insulin-producing cells, stress responses and metabolism by coexpressed short neuropeptide F and corazonin. *Cell. Mol. Life Sci.* 69, 4051–4066.

Kaplan, N., Morpurgo, N., and Linial, M. (2007). Novel families of toxin-like peptides in insects and mammals: a computational approach. *J. Mol. Biol.* 369, 553–566.

Kataoka, H., Troetschler, R. G., Li, J. P., Kramer, S. J., Carney, R. L., and Schooley, D. A. (1989). Isolation and identification of a diuretic hormone from the tobacco hornworm, *Manduca sexta*. *Proc. Natl. Acad. Sci. U.S.A.* 86, 2976–2980.

Kaufmann, C., and Brown, M. R. (2006). Adipokinetic hormones in the African malaria mosquito, *Anopheles gambiae*: identification and expression of genes for two peptides and a putative receptor. *Insect Biochem. Mol. Biol.* 36, 466–481.

Kaufmann, C., Merzendorfer, H., and Gäde, G. (2009). The adipokinetic hormone system in Culicinae (Diptera: Culicidae): molecular identification and characterization of two adipokinetic hormone (AKH) precursors from *Aedes aegypti* and *Culex pipiens* and two putative AKH receptor variants from *A. aegypti*. *Insect Biochem. Mol. Biol.* 39, 770–781.

Kay, I., Coast, G. M., Cusinato, O., Wheeler, C. H., Totty, N. F., and Goldsworthy, G. (1991). Isolation and characterization of a diuretic peptide from *Acheta domesticus*. Evidence for a family of insect diuretic peptides. *Biol. Chem. Hoppe Seyler* 372, 505–512.

Kay, I., Patel, M., Coast, G. M., Totty, N. F., Mallet, A. I., and Goldsworthy, G. (1992). Isolation, characterization and biological activity of a CRF-related diuretic peptide from *Periplaneta americana L. Regul. Pept.* 42, 111–122.

Kean, L., Cazenave, W., Costes, L., Broderick, K. E., Graham, S., Pollock, V. P., et al. (2002). Two nitridergic peptides are encoded by the gene capability in *Drosophila melanogaster*. *Am. J. Physiol. Regul. Integr. Comp. Physiol.* 282, R1297–R1307.

Keeley, L. L., Chung, J. S., and Hayes, T. K. (1992). Diuretic and antifeedant actions by *Manduca sexta* diuretic hormone in lepidopteran larvae. *Cell. Mol. Life Sci.* 48, 1145–1148.

Keene, A. C., Krashes, M. J., Leung, B., Bernard, J. A., and Waddell, S. (2006). *Drosophila* dorsal paired medial neurons provide a general mechanism for memory consolidation. *Curr. Biol.* 16, 1524–1530.

Keene, A. C., Stratmann, M., Keller, A., Perrat, P. N., Vosshall, L. B., and Waddell, S. (2004). Diverse odor-conditioned memories require uniquely timed dorsal paired medial neuron output. *Neuron* 44, 521–533.

Kennerdell, J. R., and Carthew, R. W. (1998). Use of dsRNA-mediated genetic interference to demonstrate that frizzled and frizzled 2 act in the wingless pathway. *Cell* 95, 1017–1026.

Kersch, C. N., and Pietrantonio, P. V. (2011). Mosquito *Aedes aegypti* (L.) leucokinin receptor is critical for *in vivo* fluid excretion post blood feeding. *FEBS Lett.* 585, 3507–3512.

Kidd, T., Abu-Shumays, R., Katzen, A., Sisson, J. C., Jiménez, G., Pinchin, S., et al. (2005). The ε-subunit of mitochondrial ATP synthase is required for normal spindle orientation during the drosophila embryonic divisions. *Genetics* 170, 697–708.

Kim, Y. J., Bartalska, K., Audsley, N., Yamanaka, N., Yapici, N., Lee, J. Y., et al. (2010). MIPs are ancestral ligands for the sex peptide receptor. *Proc. Natl. Acad. Sci. U.S.A.* 107, 6520–6525.

Kim, Y. J., Žitňan, D., Cho, K. H., Schooley, D. A., Mizoguchi, A., and Adams, M. E. (2006a). Central peptidergic ensembles associated with organization of an innate behavior. *Proc. Natl. Acad. Sci. U.S.A.* 103, 14211–14216.

Kim, Y. J., Žitňan, D., Galizia, C. G., Cho, K. H., and Adams, M. E. (2006b). A command chemical triggers an innate behavior by sequential activation of multiple peptidergic ensembles. *Curr. Biol.* 16, 1395–1407.

Kim, Y. J., Spalovska-Valachova, I., Cho, K. H., Zitnanova, I., Park, Y., Adams, M. E., et al. (2004). Corazonin receptor signaling in ecdysis initiation. *Proc. Natl. Acad. Sci. U.S.A.* 101, 6704–6709.

Kimura, K., Kodama, A., Hayasaka, Y., and Ohta, T. (2004). Activation of the cAMP/PKA signaling pathway is required for post-ecdysial cell death in wing epidermal cells of *Drosophila melanogaster*. *Development* 131, 1597–1606.

Kodrík, D. (2008). Adipokinetic hormone functions that are not associated with insect flight. *Physiol. Entomol.* 33, 171–180.

Kodrík, D., Krishnan, N., and Habustova, O. (2007). Is the titer of adipokinetic peptides in *Leptinotarsa decemlineata* fed on genetically modified potatoes increased by oxidative stress? *Peptides* 28, 974–980.

Kofuji, P., Davidson, N., and Lester, H. A. (1995). Evidence that neuronal G-protein-gated inwardly rectifying K+ channels are activated by G beta gama subunits and function as heteromultimers. *Proc. Natl. Acad. Sci. U.S.A.* 92, 6542–6546.

Koladich, P. M., Cusson, M., Bendena, W. G., Tobe, S. S., and McNeil, J. N. (2002). Cardioacceleratory effects of *Manduca sexta* allatotropin in the true armyworm moth, *Pseudaletia unipuncta*. *Peptides* 23, 645–651.

Konuma, T., Morooka, N., Nagasawa, H., and Nagata, S. (2012). Knockdown of the adipokinetic hormone receptor increases feeding frequency in the two-spotted cricket *Gryllus bimaculatus*. *Endocrinology* 153, 3111–3122.

Kramer, S. J., Toschi, A., Miller, C. A., Kataoka, H., Quistad, G. B., Li, J. P., et al. (1991). Identification of an allatostatin from the tobacco hornworm *Manduca sexta*. *Proc. Natl. Acad. Sci. U.S.A.* 88, 9458–9462.

Krashes, M. J., DasGupta, S., Vreede, A., White, B., Armstrong, J. D., and Waddell, S. (2009). A neural circuit mechanism integrating motivational state with memory expression in *Drosophila*. *Cell* 139, 416–427.

Kreienkamp, H. J., Larusson, H. J., Witte, I., Roeder, T., Birgül, N., Hönck, H. H., et al. (2002). Functional annotation of two orphan G-protein-coupled receptors, Drostar1 and -2, from *Drosophila melanogaster* and their ligands by reverse pharmacology. *J. Biol. Chem.* 277, 39937–39943.

Kubiak, T. M., Larsen, M. J., Burton, K. J., Bannow, C. A., Martin, R. A., Zantello, M. R., et al. (2002). Cloning and functional expression of the first *Drosophila melanogaster* sulfakinin receptor DSK-R1. *Biochem. Biophys. Res. Commun.* 291, 313–320.

Kubli, E. (2010). Sexual behavior: dietary food switch induced by sex. *Curr. Biol.* 20, 474–476.

Kubli, E., and Bopp, D. (2012). Sexual behavior: how sex peptide flips the postmating switch of female flies. *Curr. Biol.* 22, 520–522.

Kunwar, P. S., Sano, H., Renault, A. D., Barbosa, V., Fuse, N., and

Lehmann, R. (2008). Tre1 GPCR initiates germ cell transepithelial migration by regulating *Drosophila melanogaster* E-cadherin. *J. Cell Biol.* 183, 157–168.

Kunwar, P. S., Starz-Gaiano, M., Bainton, R. J., Heberlein, U., and Lehmann, R. (2003). Tre1, a G protein-coupled receptor, directs transepithelial migration of *Drosophila* germ cells. *PLoS Biol.* 1:E80. doi: 10.1371/journal.pbio.0000080

Kwok, R., and Orchard, I. (2002). Characterization of a putative *Schisto*FLRFamide receptor in the CNS of *Locusta migratoria. Peptides* 23, 765–772.

Lange, A. B. (2002). A review of the involvement of proctolin as a cotransmitter and local neurohormone in the oviduct of the locust, *Locusta migratoria. Peptides* 23, 2063–2070.

Lange, A. B., Alim, U., Vandersmissen, H. P., Mizoguchi, A., Vanden Broeck, J., and Orchard, I. (2012). The distribution and physiological effects of the myoinhibiting peptides in the kissing bug, *Rhodnius Prolixus. Front Neurosci.* 6:98. doi: 10.3389/fnins.2012.00098

Lange, A. B., and Orchard, I. (1998). The effects of *Schisto*FLRFamide on contractions of locust midgut. *Peptides* 19, 459–467.

Lange, A. B., and Orchard, I. (2006). "Proctolin in insects," in *Handbook of Biologically Active Peptides*, ed A. J. Kastin (New York, NY: Academic Press, Elsevier), 177–180.

Larsen, M. J., Burton, K. J., Zantello, M. R., Smith, V. G., Lowery, D. L., and Kubiak, T. M. (2001). Type A allatostatins from *Drosophila melanogaster* and *Diplotera puncata* activate two *Drosophila* allatostatin receptors, DAR-1 and DAR-2, expressed in CHO cells. *Biochem. Biophys. Res. Commun.* 286, 895–901.

Lear, B. C., Merrill, C. E., Lin, J. M., Schroeder, A., Zhang, L., and Allada, R. (2005). A G protein-coupled receptor, groom-of-PDF, is required for PDF neuron action in circadian behavior. *Neuron* 48, 221–227.

Lee, G., and Park, J. H. (2004). Hemolymph sugar homeostasis and starvation-induced hyperactivity affected by genetic manipulations of the adipokinetic hormone-encoding gene in *Drosophila melanogaster. Genetics* 167, 311–323.

Lee, G. H., Bahn, J. H., and Park, J. H. (2006). Sex- and clock-controlled expression of the neuropeptide F gene in *Drosophila. Proc. Natl. Acad. Sci. U.S.A.* 103, 12580–12585.

Lee, K. S., Hong, S. H., Kim, A. K., Ju, S. K., Kwon, O. Y., and Yu, K. (2009). Processed short neuropeptide F peptides regulate growth through the ERK-insulin pathway in *Drosophila melanogaster. FEBS Lett.* 583, 2573–2577.

Lee, K. S., Kwon, O. Y., Lee, J. H., Kwon, K., Min, K. J., Jung, S. A., et al. (2008). *Drosophila* short neuropeptide F signalling regulates growth by ERK-mediated insulin signalling. *Nat. Cell Biol.* 10, 468–475.

Lee, K. S., You, K. H., Choo, J. K., Han, Y. M., and Yu, K. (2004). *Drosophila* short neuropeptide F regulates food intake and body size. *J. Biol. Chem.* 279, 50781–50789.

Lee, K. Y., Horodyski, F. M., and Chamberlin, M. E. (1998). Inhibition of midgut ion transport by allatotropin (Mas-AT) and *Manduca* FLRFamides in the tobacco hornworm *Manduca sexta. J. Exp. Biol.* 201, 3067–3074.

Lehmberg, E., Ota, R. B., Furuya, K., King, D. S., Applebaum, S. W., Ferenz, H. J., et al. (1991). Identification of a diuretic hormone of *Locusta migratoria. Biochem. Biophys. Res. Commun.* 179, 1036–1041.

Li, B., Beeman, R. W., and Park, Y. (2011a). Functions of duplicated genes encoding CCAP receptors in the red flour beetle, *Tribolium castaneum. J. Insect Physiol.* 57, 1190–1197.

Li, B., Predel, R., Neupert, S., Hauser, F., Tanaka, Y., Cazzamali, G., et al. (2008). Genomics, transcriptomics, and peptidomics of neuropeptides and protein hormones in the red flour beetle *Tribolium castaneum. Genome Res.* 18, 113–122.

Li, X. J., Wolfgang, W., Wu, Y. N., North, R. A., and Forte, M. (1991). Cloning, heterologous expression and developmental regulation of a *Drosophila* receptor for tachykinin-like peptides. *EMBO J.* 10, 3221–3229.

Li, X. J., Wu, Y. N., North, R. A., and Forte, M. (1992). Cloning, functional expression, and developmental regulation of a neuropeptide-Y receptor from *Drosophila melanogaster. J. Biol. Chem.* 267, 9–12.

Li, Y., Hernandez-Martinez, S., Fernandez, F., Mayoral, J. G., Topalis, P., Priestap, H., et al. (2006). Biochemical, molecular, and functional characterization of PISCF-allatostatin, a regulator of juvenile hormone biosynthesis in the mosquito *Aedes aegypti. J. Biol. Chem.* 281, 34048–34055.

Li., Y., Hoxha, V., Lama, C., Dinh, B. H., Vo, C. N., and Dauwalder, B. (2011b). The *hector* G-protein coupled receptor is required in a subset of *fruitless* neurons for male courtship behavior. *PLoS ONE* 6:e28269. doi: 10.1371/journal.pone.0028269

Lin, Y.-J., Seroude, L., and Benzer, S. (1998). Extended life-span and stress resistance in the *Drosophila* Mutant *methuselah. Science* 282, 943–946.

Lindemans, M., Janssen, T., Beets, I., Temmerman, L., Meelkop, E., and Schoofs, L. (2011). Gonadotropin-releasing hormone and adipokinetic hormone signaling systems share a common evolutionary origin. *Front. Endocrinol.* 2:16. doi: 10.3389/fendo.2011.00016

Lingo, P. R., Zhao, Z., and Shen, P. (2007). Co-regulation of cold-resistant food acquisition by insulin- and neuropeptide Y-like systems in *Drosophila melanogaster. Neuroscience* 148, 371–374.

Liu, F., Baggerman, G., D'Hertog, W., Verleyen, P., Schoofs, L., and Wets, G. (2006). *In silico* identification of new secretory peptide genes in *Drosophila melanogaster. Mol. Cell. Proteomics* 5, 510–522.

Liu, W., Guo, F., Lu, B., and Guo, A. (2008). *amnesiac* regulates sleep onset and maintenance in *Drosophila melanogaster. Biochem. Biophys. Res. Commun.* 372, 798–803.

López-Arias, B., Dorado, B., and Herrero, P. (2011). Blockade of the release of the neuropeptide leucokinin to determine its possible functions in fly behavior: chemoreception assays. *Peptides* 32, 545–552.

Lorenz, M. W., Kellner, R., and Hoffmann, K. H. (1995). Identification of two allatostatins from the cricket, *Gryllus bimaculatus* de Geer (Ensifera, Gryllidae): additional members of a family of neuropeptides inhibiting juvenile hormone biosynthesis. *Regul. Pept.* 57, 227–236.

Lorenz, M. W., Kellner, R., and Hoffmann, K. H. (1999). Allatostatins in *Gryllus bimaculatus* (Ensifera: Gryllidae): new structures and physiological properties. *Eur. J. Entomol.* 96, 267–274.

Lorenz, M. W. (2003). Adipokinetic hormone inhibits the formation of energy stores and egg production in the cricket *Gryllus bimaculatus. Comp. Biochem. Physiol. B Biochem Mol. Biol.* 136, 197–206.

Lorenz, M. W., and Gäde, G. (2009). Hormonal regulation of energy metabolism in insects as a driving force for performance. *Integr. Comp. Biol.* 49, 380–392.

Loveall, B. J., and Deitcher, D. L. (2010). The essential role of bursicon during *Drosophila* development. *BMC Dev. Biol.* 10:92. doi: 10.1186/1471-213X-10-92

Lovejoy, D. A., Rotzinger, S., and Barsyste-Lovejoy, D. (2009). Evolution of complementary peptide systems: teneurin C-terminal-associated peptides and corticotropin-releasing factor superfamilies. *Ann. N.Y. Acad. Sci.* 1163, 215–220.

Lu, H. L., and Pietrantonio, P. V. (2011). Immunolocalization of the short neuropeptide F receptor in queen brains and ovaries of the red imported fire ant (*Solenopsis invicta* Buren). *BMC Neurosci.* 12:57. doi: 10.1186/1471-2202-12-57

Lungchukiet, P., Donly, B. C., Zhang, J., Tobe, S. S., and Bendena, W. G. (2008). Molecular cloning and characterization of an allatostatin-like receptor in the cockroach *Diploptera punctata. Peptides* 29, 276–285.

Luo, C. W., Dewey, E. M., Sudo, S., Ewer, J., Hsu, S. Y., Honegger, H. W., et al. (2005). Bursicon, the insect cuticle-hardening hormone, is a heterodimeric cystine knot protein that activates G protein-coupled receptor LGR2. *Proc. Natl. Acad. Sci. U.S.A.* 102, 2820–2825.

Lustig, K. D., Conklin, B. R., Herzmark, P., Taussig, R., and Bourne, H. R. (1993). Type II adenylylcyclase integrates coincident signals from Gs, Gi, and Gq. *J. Biol. Chem.* 268, 13900–13905.

Lwalaba, D., Hoffmann, K. H., and Woodring, J. (2010). Control of the release of digestive enzymes in the larvae of the fall armyworm, *Spodoptera frugiperda. Arch. Insect Biochem. Physiol.* 73, 14–29.

Maestro, J. L., Aguilar, R., Pascual, N., Valero, M. L., Piulachs, M. D., Andreu, D., et al. (2001). Screening of antifeedant activity in brain extracts led to the identification of sulfakinin as a satiety promoter in the German cockroach. Are arthropod sulfakinins homologous to vertebrate gastrins-cholecystokinins? *Eur. J. Biochem.* 268, 5824–5830.

Maestro, J. L., Tobe, S. S., and Bellés, X. (2011). Leucomyosuppressin modulates cardiac rhythm in the cockroach *Blattella germanica. J. Insect Physiol.* 57, 1677–1681.

Malik, A., Gäde, G., and Lange, A. B. (2012). Sequencing and biological effects of an adipokinetic/hypertrehalosemic peptide in the stick insect, *Baculum extradentatum*. *Peptides* 34, 51–56.

Marciniak, P., Kuczer, M., and Rosinski, G. (2011). New physiological activities of myosuppressin, sulfakinin and NVP-like peptide in *Zophobas atratus* beetle. *J. Comp. Physiol. B* 181, 721–730.

Matsumoto, S., Brown, M. R., Crim, J. W., Vigna, S. R., and Lea, A. O. (1989). Isolation and primary structure ofneuropeptides from the mosquito, Aedes aegypti, immunoreactive to FMRFamide antiserum. *Insect Biochem. Mol. Biol.* 19, 277–283.

Matthews, H. J., Audsley, N., and Weaver, R. J. (2008). *In vitro* and *in vivo* effects of myo-active peptides on larvae of the tomato moth *Lacanobia oleracea* and the cotton leaf worm *Spodoptera littoralis* (Lepidoptera; Noctuidae). *Arch. Insect Biochem. Physiol.* 69, 60–69.

Mayoral, J. G., Nouzova, M., Brockhoff, A., Goodwin, M., Hernandez-Martinez, S., Richter, D., et al. (2010). Allatostatin-C receptors in mosquitoes. *Peptides* 31, 442–450.

Meelkop, E., Temmerman, L., Schoofs, L., and Janssen, T. (2011). Signalling through pigment dispersing hormone-like peptides in invertebrates. *Prog. Neurobiol.* 93, 125–147.

Meeusen, T., Mertens, I., Clynen, E., Baggerman, G., Nichols, R., Nachman, R. J., et al. (2002). Identification in *Drosophila melanogaster* of the invertebrate G protein-coupled FMRFamide receptor. *Proc. Natl. Acad. Sci. U.S.A.* 99, 15363–15368.

Meeusen, T., Mertens, I., De Loof, A., and Schoofs, L. (2003). G protein-coupled receptors in invertebrates: a state of the art. *Int. Rev. Cytol.* 230, 189–261.

Melcher, C., Bader, R., Walther, S., Simakov, O., and Pankratz, M. J. (2006). Neuromedin U and its putative *Drosophila* homolog hugin. *PLoS Biol.* 4:e68. doi: 10.1371/journal.pbio.0040068

Mendive, F. M., Van Loy, T., Claeysen, S., Poels, J., Williamson, M., Hauser, F., et al. (2005). *Drosophila* molting neurohormone bursicon is a heterodimer and the natural agonist of the orphan receptor DLGR2. *FEBS Lett.* 579, 2171–2176.

Menschaert, G., Vandekerckhove, T. T., Baggerman, G., Schoofs, L., Luyten, W., and Van Criekinge, W. (2010). Peptidomics coming of age: a review of contributions from a bioinformatics angle. *J. Proteome Res.* 9, 2051–2061.

Mertens, I., Meeusen, T., Huybrechts, R., De Loof, A., and Schoofs, L. (2002). Characterization of the short neuropeptide F receptor from *Drosophila melanogaster*. *Biochem. Biophys. Res. Commun.* 297, 1140–1148.

Mertens, I., Vandingenen, A., Meeusen, T., De Loof, A., and Schoofs, L. (2004). Postgenomic characterization of G-protein-coupled receptors. *Pharmacogenomics* 5, 657–672.

Mertens, I., Vandingenen, A., Johnson, E. C., Shafer, O. T., Li, W., Trigg, J. S., et al. (2005). PDF receptor signaling in *Drosophila* contributes to both circadian and geotactic behaviors. *Neuron* 48, 213–219.

Mertens, I., Husson, S. J., Janssen, T., Lindemans, M., and Schoofs, L. (2007). PACAP and PDF signaling in the regulation of mammalian and insect circadian rhythms. *Peptides* 28, 1775–1783.

Metpally, R. P. R., and Sowdhamini, R. (2005). Cross genome phylogenetic analysis of human and *Drosophila* G protein-coupled receptors: application to functional annotation of orphan receptors. *BMC Genomics* 6:106. doi: 10.1186/1471-2164-6-106

Meyering-Vos, M., and Müller, A. (2007). Structure of the sulfakinin cDNA and gene expression from the Mediterranean field cricket *Gryllus bimaculatus*. *Insect Mol. Biol.* 16, 445–454.

Mikani, A., Wang, Q. S., and Takeda, M. (2012). Brain-midgut short neuropeptide F mechanism that inhibits digestive activity of the American cockroach, *Periplaneta americana* upon starvation. *Peptides* 34, 135–144.

Monnier, D., Colas, J. F., Rosay, P., Hen, R., Borrelli, E., and Maroteaux, L. (1992). NKD, a developmentally regulated tachykinin receptor in *Drosophila*. *J. Biol. Chem.* 267, 1298–1302.

Moore, M. S., DeZazzo, J., Luk, A. Y., Tully, T., Singh, C. M., and Heberlein, U. (1998). Ethanol intoxication in *Drosophila*: genetic and pharmacological evidence for regulation by the cAMP signaling pathway. *Cell* 93, 997–1007.

Motosaka, K., Koganezawa, M., Narikawa, S., Furuyama, A., Shinozaki, K., Isono, K., et al. (2007). Cyclic AMP-dependent memory mutants are defective in the food choice behavior of *Drosophila*. *J. Comp. Physiol. A Neuroethol. Sens. Neural Behav. Physiol.* 193, 279–283.

Nachman, R. J., Holman, G. M., Cook, B. J., Haddon, W. F., and Ling, N. (1986a). Leucosulfakinin-II, a blocked sulfated insect neuropeptide with homology to cholecystokinin and gastrin. *Biochem. Biophys. Res. Commun.* 140, 357–364.

Nachman, R. J., Holman, G. M., Haddon, W. F., and Ling, N. (1986b). Leucosulfakinin, a sulfated insect neuropeptide with homology to gastrin and cholecystokinin. *Science* 234, 71–73.

Nachman, R. J., and Pietrantonio, P. V. (2010). Interaction of mimetic analogs of insect kinin neuropeptides with arthropod receptors. *Adv. Exp. Med. Biol.* 692, 27–48.

Nagata, S., Matsumoto, S., Mizoguchi, A., and Nagasawa, H. (2012a). Identification of cDNAs encoding allatotropin and allatotropin-like peptides from the silkworm, *Bombyx mori*. *Peptides* 34, 98–105.

Nagata, S., Matsumoto, S., Nakane, T., Ohara, A., Morooka, N., Konuma, T., et al. (2012b). Effects of starvation on brain short neuropeptide F-1, -2, and -3 levels and short neuropeptide F receptor expression levels of the silkworm, *Bombyx mori*. *Front. Endocrinol. (Lausanne)* 3:3. doi: 10.3389/fendo.2012.00003

Nagata, S., Morooka, N., Matsumoto, S., Kawai, T., and Nagasawa, H. (2011). Effects of neuropeptides on feeding initiation in larvae of the silkworm, *Bombyx mori*. *Gen. Comp. Endocrinol.* 172, 90–95.

Nambu, J. R., Murphy-Erdosh, C., Andrews, P. C., Feistner, G. J., and Scheller, R. H. (1988). Isolation and characterization of a *Drosophila* neuropeptide gene. *Neuron* 1, 55–61.

Natzle, J. E., Kiger, J. A. Jr., and Green, M. M. (2008). Bursicon signaling mutations separate the epithelial-mesenchymal transition from programmed cell death during *Drosophila melanogaster* wing maturation. *Genetics* 180, 885–893.

Nässel, D. R. (2002). Neuropeptides in the nervous system of *Drosophila* and other insects: multiple roles as neuromodulators and neurohormones. *Prog. Neurobiol.* 68, 1–84.

Nässel, D. R., Enell, L. E., Santos, J. G., Wegener, C., and Johard, H. A. (2008). A large population of diverse neurons in the *Drosophila* central nervous system expresses short neuropeptide F, suggesting multiple distributed peptide functions. *BMC Neurosci.* 9:90. doi: 10.1186/1471-2202-9-90

Nässel, D. R., and Winther, A. M. (2010). *Drosophila* neuropeptides in regulation of physiology and behavior. *Prog. Neurobiol.* 92, 42–104.

Nässel, D. R., and Wegener, C. (2011). A comparative review of short and long neuropeptide F signaling in invertebrates: any similarities to vertebrate neuropeptide Y signaling? *Peptides* 32, 1335–1355.

Neupert, S., and Predel, R. (2005). Mass spectrometric analysis of single identified neurons of an insect. *Biochem. Biophys. Res. Commun.* 327, 640–645.

Nouzova, M., Brockhoff, A., Mayoral, J. G., Goodwin, M., Meyerhof, W., and Noriega, F. G. (2012). Functional characterization of an allatotropin receptor expressed in the corpora allata of mosquitoes. *Peptides* 34, 201–208.

Nuss, A. B., Forschler, B. T., Crim, J. W., and Brown, M. R. (2008). Distribution of neuropeptide F-like immunoreactivity in the Eastern Subterranean termite, *Reticulitermes flavipes*. *J. Insect Sci.* 8, 1–18.

Nuss, A. B., Forschler, B. T., Crim, J. W., Te Brugge, V., Pohl, J., and Brown, M. R. (2010). Molecular characterization of neuropeptide F from the eastern subterranean termite *Reticulitermes flavipes* (Kollar) (Isoptera: Rhinotermitidae). *Peptides* 31, 419–428.

Nygaard, S., Zhang, G., Schiott, M., Li, C., Wurm, Y., Hu, H., et al. (2011). The genome of the leaf-cutting ant *Acromyrmex echinatior* suggests key adaptations to advanced social life and fungus farming. *Genome Res.* 21, 1339–1348.

Offermanns, S., and Simon, M. I. (1995). G alpha 15 and G alpha 16 couple a wide variety of receptors to phospholipase C. *J. Biol. Chem.* 270, 15175–15180.

Olsen, S. S., Cazzamali, G., Williamson, M., Grimmelikhuijzen, C. J. P., and Hauser, F. (2007). Identification of one capa and two pyrokinin receptors from the malaria mosquito *Anopheles gambiae*. *Biochem. Biophys. Res. Commun.* 362, 245–251.

Ons, S., Richter, F., Urlaub, H., and Pomar, R. R. (2009). The neuropeptidome of *Rhodnius prolixus* brain. *Proteomics* 9, 788–792.

Orchard, I., Belanger, J. H., and Lange, A. B. (1989). Proctolin: a review with emphasis on insects. *J. Neurobiol.* 20, 470–496.

Orchard, I., Lee, d. H., da, S. R., and Lange, A. B. (2011). The proctolin gene and biological effects of proctolin in the blood-feeding bug, *Rhodnius prolixus*. *Front.*

Endocrinol. (Lausanne) 2:59. doi: 10.3389/fendo.2011.00059

Overend, G., Cabrero, P., Guo, A. X., Sebastian, S., Cundall, M., Armstrong, H., et al. (2012). The receptor guanylate cyclase Gyc76C and a peptide ligand, NPLP1-VQQ, modulate the innate immune IMD pathway in response to salt stress. *Peptides* 34, 209–218.

Paluzzi, J. P., and Orchard, I. (2006). Distribution, activity and evidence for the release of an anti-diuretic peptide in the kissing bug *Rhodnius prolixus*. *J. Exp. Biol.* 209, 907–915.

Park, Y., Kim, Y. J., and Adams, M. E. (2002). Identification of G protein-coupled receptors for *Drosophila* PRXamide peptides, CCAP, corazonin, and AKH supports a theory of ligand-receptor coevolution. *Proc. Natl. Acad. Sci. U.S.A.* 99, 11423–11428.

Pascual, N., Castresana, J., Valero, M. L., Andreu, D., and Bellés, X. (2004). Orcokinins in insects and other invertebrates. *Insect Biochem. Mol. Biol.* 34, 1141–1146.

Patel, M. V., Hallal, D. A., Jones, J. W., Bronner, D. N., Zein, R., Caravas, J., et al. (2012). Dramatic expansion and developmental expression diversification of the *Methuselah* gene family during recent *Drosophila* evolution. *J. Exp. Zool. B Mol. Dev. Evol.* 318, 368–387.

Peabody, N. C., Diao, F., Luan, H., Wang, H., Dewey, E. M., Honegger, H. W., et al. (2008). Bursicon functions within the *Drosophila* CNS to modulate wing expansion behavior, hormone secretion, and cell death. *J. Neurosci.* 28, 14379–14391.

Peng, J., Zipperlen, P., and Kubli, E. (2005). *Drosophila* sex-peptide stimulates female innate immune system after mating via the Toll and Imd pathways. *Curr. Biol.* 15, 1690–1694.

Pennefather, J. N., Lecci, A., Candenas, M. L., Patak, E., Pinto, F. M., and Maggi, C. A. (2004). Tachykinins and tachykinin receptors: a growing family. *Life Sci.* 74, 1445–1463.

Petri, B., Homberg, U., Loesel, R., and Stengl, M. (2002). Evidence for a role of GABA and Mass-allatotropin in photic entranement of the circadian clock of the cockroach *Leucophaea maderae*. *J. Exp. Biol.* 205, 1459–1469.

Phillips, J. E., Meredith, J., Wang, Y., Zhao, Y., and Brock, H. (2001). "Ion transport peptide (ITP): structure, function, evolution," in *Perspectives in Comparative Endocrinology: Unity and Diversity*, eds H. J. Goos, R. K. Rastogi, H. Vaudry, and R. Pierantoni (Bologna: Medimond), 745–752.

Poels, J., Birse, R. T., Nachman, R. J., Fichna, J., Janecka, A., Vanden Broeck, J., et al. (2009). Characterization and distribution of NKD, a receptor for *Drosophila* tachykinin-related peptide 6. *Peptides* 30, 545–556.

Poels, J., Van Loy, T., Vandersmissen, H. P., Van Hiel, M. B., Van Soest, S., Nachman, R. J., et al. (2010). Myoinhibiting peptides are the ancestral ligands of the promiscuous *Drosophila* sex peptide receptor. *Cell. Mol. Life Sci.* 67, 3511–3522.

Poels, J., Verlinden, H., Fichna, J., Van Loy, T., Franssens, V., Studzian, K., et al. (2007). Functional comparison of two evolutionary conserved insect neurokinin-like receptors. *Peptides* 28, 103–108.

Pollock, V. P., McGettigan, J., Cabrero, P., Maudlin, I. M., Dow, J. A., and Davies, S. A. (2004). Conservation of capa peptide-induced nitric oxide signalling in Diptera. *J. Exp. Biol.* 207, 4135–4145.

Prasher, D. C., McCann, R. O., Longiaru, M., and Cormier, M. J. (1987). Sequence comparisons of complementary DNAs encoding aequorin isotypes. *Biochemistry* 26, 1326–1332.

Pratt, G. E., Farnsworth, D. E., Fok, K. F., Siegel, N. R., McCormack, A. L., Shabanowitz, J., et al. (1991). Identity of a second type of allatostatin from cockroach brains: an octadecapeptide amide with a tyrosine-rich address sequence. *Proc. Natl. Acad. Sci. U.S.A.* 88, 2412–2416.

Pratt, G. E., Farnsworth, D. E., Siegel, N. R., Fok, K. F., and Feyereisen, R. (1989). Identification of an allatostatin from adult *Diploptera punctata*. *Biochem. Biophys. Res. Commun.* 163, 1243–1247.

Predel, R., Nachman, R. J., and Gäde, G. (2001). Myostimulatory neuropeptides in cockroaches: structures, distribution, pharmacological activities, and mimetic analogs. *J. Insect Physiol.* 47, 311–324.

Predel, R., Neupert, S., Roth, S., Derst, C., and Nässel, D. R. (2005). Tachykinin-related peptide precursors in two cockroach species. *FEBS J.* 272, 3365–3375.

Predel, R., Neupert, S., Russell, W. K., Scheibner, O., and Nachman, R. J. (2007). Corazonin in insects. *Peptides* 28, 3–10.

Predel, R., Neupert, S., Garczynski, S. F., Crim, J. W., Brown, M. R., Russell, W. K., et al. (2010). Neuropeptidomics of the mosquito *Aedes aegypti*. *J. Proteome Res.* 9, 2006–2015.

Predel, R., Wegener, C., Russell, W. K., Tichy, S. E., Russell, D. H., and Nachman, R. J. (2004). Peptidomics of CNS-associated neurohemal systems of adult *Drosophila melanogaster*: a mass spectrometric survey of peptides from individual flies. *J. Comp. Neurol.* 474, 379–392.

Predel, R., and Wegener, C. (2006). Biology of the CAPA peptides in insects. *Cell. Mol. Life Sci.* 63, 2477–2490.

Price, D. A., and Greenberg, M. J. (1977). Purification and characterization of a cardioexcitatory neuropeptide from the central ganglia of a bivalve mollusc. *Prep. Biochem.* 7, 261–281.

Proux, J. P., Miller, C. A., Li, J. P., Carney, R. L., Girardie, A., Delaage, M., et al. (1987). Identification of an arginine vasopressin-like diuretic hormone from *Locusta migratoria*. *Biochem. Biophys. Res. Commun.* 149, 180–186.

Quinn, W. G., Sziber, P. P., and Booker, R. (1979). The *Drosophila* memory mutant *amnesiac*. *Nature* 277, 212–214.

Radford, J. C., Davies, S. A., and Dow, J. A. (2002). Systematic G-protein-coupled receptor analysis in *Drosophila melanogaster* identifies a leucokinin receptor with novel roles. *J. Biol. Chem.* 277, 38810–38817.

Rahman, M. M., Fromm, B., Neupert, S., Kreusch, S., and Predel, R. (2009). Extended FMRFamides in dipteran insects: conservative expression in the neuroendocrine system is accompanied by rapid sequence evolution. *Gen. Comp. Endocrinol.* 162, 52–58.

Rao, K. R., Mohrherr, C. J., Riehm, J. P., Zahnow, C. A., Norton, S., Johnson, L., et al. (1987). Primary structure of an analog of crustacean pigment-dispersing hormone from the lubber grasshopper *Romalea microptera*. *J. Biol. Chem.* 262, 2672–2675.

Reagan, J. D. (1994). Expression cloning of an insect diuretic hormone receptor. A member of the calcitonin/secretin receptor family. *J. Biol. Chem.* 269, 9–12.

Reagan, J. D. (1995). Functional expression of a diuretic hormone receptor in baculovirus-infected insect cells: evidence suggesting that the N-terminal region of diuretic hormone is associated with receptor activation. *Insect Biochem. Mol. Biol.* 25, 535–539.

Reagan, J. D. (1996) Molecular cloning and function expression of a diuretic hormone receptor from the house cricket, *Acheta domesticus*. *Insect Biochem. Mol. Biol.* 26, 1–6.

Reale, V., Chatwin, H. M., and Evans, P. D. (2004). The activation of G-protein gated inwardly rectifying K+ channels by a cloned *Drosophila melanogaster* neuropeptide F-like receptor. *Eur. J. Neurosci.* 19, 570–576.

Reumer, A., Van Loy, T., Clynen, E., and Schoofs, L. (2008). How functional genomics and genetics complements insect endocrinology. *Gen. Comp. Endocrinol.* 155, 22–30.

Rewitz, K. F., Yamanaka, N., Gilbert, L. I., and O'Connor, M. B. (2009). The insect neuropeptide PTTH activates receptor tyrosine kinase torso to initiate metamorphosis. *Science* 326, 1403–1405.

Rholam, M., and Fahy, C. (2009). Processing of peptide and hormone precursors at the dibasic cleavage sites. *Cell. Mol. Life Sci.* 66, 2075–2091.

Ribeiro, C., and Dickson, B. J. (2010). Sex peptide receptor and neuronal TOR/S6K signaling modulate nutrient balancing in *Drosophila*. *Curr. Biol.* 20, 1000–1005.

Riehle, M. A., Garczynski, S. F., Crim, J. W., Hill, C. A., and Brown, M. R. (2002). Neuropeptides and peptide hormones in *Anopheles gambiae*. *Science* 298, 172–175.

Robb, S., and Evans, P. D. (1990). FMRFamide-like peptides in the locust: distribution, partial characterization and bioactivity. *J. Exp. Biol.* 149, 335–360.

Robinson, G. E., Hackett, K. J., Purcell-Miramontes, M., Brown, S. J., Evans, J. D., Goldsmith, M. R., et al. (2011). Creating a buzz about insect genomes. *Science* 331, 1386.

Roch, G. J., Busby, E. R., and Sherwood, N. M. (2011). Evolution of GnRH: diving deeper. *Gen. Comp. Endocrinol.* 171, 1–16.

Roller, L., Yamanaka, N., Watanabe, K., Daubnerova, I., Žitňan, D., Kataoka, H., et al. (2008). The unique evolution of neuropeptide genes in the silkworm *Bombyx mori*. *Insect Biochem. Mol. Biol.* 38, 1147–1157.

Roller, L., Žitňanová, I., Dai, L., Šimo, L., Park, Y., Satake, H., et al. (2010). Ecdysis triggering hormone signaling in arthropods. *Peptides* 31, 429–441.

Root, C. M., Ko, K. I., Jafari, A., and Wang, J. W. (2011). Presynaptic facilitation by neuropeptide signaling mediates odor-driven food search. *Cell* 145, 133–144.

Rosenkilde, C., Cazzamali, G., Williamson, M., Hauser, F., Søndergaard, L., DeLotto, R., et al. (2003). Molecular cloning, functional expression, and gene silencing of two *Drosophila* receptors for the *Drosophila* neuropeptide pyrokinin-2. *Biochem. Biophys. Res. Commun.* 309, 485–494.

Sakai, T., Satake, H., and Takeda, M. (2006). Nutrient-induced alpha-amylase and protease activity is regulated by crustacean cardioactive peptide (CCAP) in the cockroach midgut. *Peptides* 27, 2157–2164.

Saudan, P., Hauck, K., Soller, M., Choffat, Y., Ottiger, M., Sporri, M., et al. (2002). Ductus ejaculatorius peptide 99B (DUP99B), a novel *Drosophila melanogaster* sex-peptide pheromone. *Eur. J. Biochem.* 269, 989–997.

Scherkenbeck, J., and Zdobinsky, T. (2009). Insect neuropeptides: structures, chemical modifications and potential for insect control. *Bioorg. Med. Chem.* 17, 4071–4084.

Schinko, J. B., Weber, M., Viktorinova, I., Kiupakis, A., Averof, M., Klingler, M., et al. (2010). Functionality of the GAL4/UAS system in *Tribolium* requires the use of endogenous core promoters. *BMC Dev. Biol.* 10:53. doi: 10.1186/1471-213X-10-53

Schneider, L. E., and Taghert, P. H. (1988). Isolation and characterization of a *Drosophila* gene that encodes multiple neuropeptides related to Phe-Met-Arg-Phe-NH2 (FMRFamide). *Proc. Natl. Acad. Sci. U.S.A.* 85, 1993–1997.

Schöller, S., Belmont, M., Cazzamali, G., Hauser, F., Williamson, M., and Grimmelikhuijzen, C. J. P. (2005). Molecular identification of a myosuppressin receptor from the malaria mosquito *Anopheles gambiae*. *Biochem. Biophys. Res. Commun.* 327, 29–34.

Schoofs, L., and Baggerman, G. (2003). Peptidomics in *Drosophila melanogaster*. *Brief. Funct. Genomic. Proteomic.* 2, 114–120.

Schoofs, L., Clynen, E., Cerstiaens, A., Baggerman, G., Wei, Z., Vercammen, T., et al. (2001). Newly discovered functions for some myotropic neuropeptides in locusts. *Peptides* 22, 219–227.

Schoofs, L., Holman, G. M., Hayes, T. K., Nachman, R. J., and De Loof, A. (1991). Isolation, primary structure, and synthesis of locustapyrokinin - a myotropic peptide of *Locusta migratoria*. *Gen. Comp. Endocrinol.* 81, 97–104.

Schwabe, T., Bainton, R. J., Fetter, R. D., Heberlein, U., and Gaul, U. (2005). GPCR signaling is required for blood-brain barrier formation in *Drosophila*. *Cell* 123, 133–144.

Secher, T., Lenz, C., Cazzamali, G., Sorensen, G., Williamson, M., Hansen, G. N., et al. (2001). Molecular cloning of a functional allatostatin gut/brain receptor and an allatostatin preprohormone from the silkworm *Bombyx mori*. *J. Biol. Chem.* 276, 47052–47060.

Sellami, A., Agricola, H., and Veenstra, J. A. (2011). Neuroendocrine cells in *Drosophila melanogaster* producing GPA2/GPB5, a hormone with homology to LH, FSH and TSH. *Gen. Comp. Endocrinol.* 170, 582–588.

Setzu, M., Biolchini, M., Lilliu, A., Manca, M., Muroni, P., Poddighe, S., et al. (2012). Neuropeptide F peptides act through unique signaling pathways to affect cardiac activity. *Peptides* 33, 230–239.

Sha, K., Conner, W. C., Choi, D. Y., and Park, J. H. (2012). Characterization, expression, and evolutionary aspects of Corazonin neuropeptide and its receptor from the House Fly, *Musca domestica* (Diptera: Muscidae). *Gene* 497, 191–199.

Shafer, O. T., Kim, D. J., Dunbar-Yaffe, R., Nikolaev, V. O., Lohse, M. J., and Taghert, P. H. (2008). Widespread receptivity to neuropeptide PDF throughout the neuronal circadian clock network of *Drosophila* revealed by real-time cyclic AMP imaging. *Neuron* 58, 223–237.

Shen, P., and Cai, H. N. (2001). *Drosophila* neuropeptide F mediates integration of chemosensory stimulation and conditioning of the nervous system by food. *J. Neurobiol.* 47, 16–25.

Shi, Y., Huang, H., Deng, X., He, X., Yang, J., Yang, H., et al. (2011). Identification and functional characterization of two orphan G-protein-coupled receptors for adipokinetic hormones from silkworm *Bombyx mori*. *J. Biol. Chem.* 286, 42390–42402.

Shohat-Ophir, G., Kaun, K. R., Azanchi, R., Mohammed, H., and Heberlein, U. (2012). Sexual deprivation increases ethanol intake in *Drosophila*. *Science* 335, 1351–1355.

Siegert, K. J. (1999). Locust corpora cardiaca contain an inactive adipokinetic hormone. *FEBS Lett.* 447, 237–240.

Simonet, G., Poels, J., Claeys, I., Van Loy, T., Franssens, V., De Loof, A., et al. (2004). Neuroendocrinological and molecular aspects of insect reproduction. *J. Neuroendocrinol.* 16, 649–659.

Siviter, R. J., Coast, G. M., Winther, A. M., Nachman, R. J., Taylor, C. A., Shirras, A. D., et al. (2000). Expression and functional characterization of a *Drosophila* neuropeptide precursor with homology to mammalian preprotachykinin A. *J. Biol. Chem.* 275, 23273–23280.

Söderberg, J. A. E., Carlsson, M. A., and Nässel, D. R. (2012). Insulin-producing cells in the *Drosophila* brain also express satiety-inducing cholecystokinin-like peptide, drosulfakinin. *Front. Endocrinol. (Lausanne)* 3:109. doi: 10.3389/fendo.2012.00109

Spit, J., Badisco, L., Verlinden, H., Van Wielendaele, P., Zels, S., Dillen, S., et al. (2012). Peptidergic control of food intake and digestion in insects. *Can. J. Zool.* 90, 489–506.

Stables, J., Green, A., Marshall, F., Fraser, N., Knight, E., Sautel, M., et al. (1997). A bioluminescent assay for agonist activity at potentially any G-protein-coupled receptor. *Anal. Biochem.* 252, 115–126.

Stafflinger, E., Hansen, K. K., Hauser, F., Schneider, M., Cazzamali, G., Williamson, M., et al. (2008). Cloning and identification of an oxytocin/vasopressin-like receptor and its ligand from insects. *Proc. Natl. Acad. Sci. U.S.A.* 105, 3262–3267.

Staljanssens, D., Azari, E. K., Christiaens, O., Beaufays, J., Lins, L., Van Camp, J., et al. (2011). The CCK(-like) receptor in the animal kingdom: functions, evolution and structures. *Peptides* 32, 607–619.

Stanek, D. M., Pohl, J., Crim, J. W., and Brown, M. R. (2002). Neuropeptide F and its expression in the yellow fever mosquito, *Aedes aegypti*. *Peptides* 23, 1367–1378.

Stangier, J., Hilbich, C., Beyreuther, K., and Keller, R. (1987). Unusual cardioactive peptide (CCAP) from pericardial organs of the shore crab *Carcinus maenas*. *Proc. Natl. Acad. Sci. U.S.A.* 84, 575–579.

Stangier, J., Hilbich, C., and Keller, R. (1989). Occurrence of crustacean cardioactive peptide (CCAP) in the nervous system of an insect, *Locusta migratoria*. *J. Comp. Physiol. B* 159, 5–11.

Starratt, A. N., and Brown, B. E. (1975). Structure of the pentapeptide proctolin, a proposed neurotransmitter in insects. *Life Sci.* 17, 1253–1256.

Staubli, F., Jørgensen, T. J. D., Cazzamali, G., Williamson, M., Lenz, C., Søndergaard, L., et al. (2002). Molecular identification of the insect adipokinetic hormone receptors. *Proc. Natl. Acad. Sci. U.S.A.* 99, 3446–3451.

Stay, B. (2000). A review of the role of neurosecretion in the control of juvenile hormone synthesis: a tribute to Berta Scharrer. *Insect Biochem. Mol. Biol.* 30, 653–662.

Stay, B., and Tobe, S. S. (2007). The role of allatostatins in juvenile hormone synthesis in insects and crustaceans. *Annu. Rev. Entomol.* 52, 277–299.

Sterkel, M., Riccillo, F. L., and Ronderos, J. R. (2010). Cardioacceleratory and myostimulatory activity of allatotropin in *Triatoma infestans*. *Comp. Biochem. Physiol. A Mol. Integr. Physiol.* 155, 371–377.

Sterkel, M., Oliveira, P. L., Urlaub, H., Hernandez-Martinez, S., Rivera-Pomar, R., and Ons, S. (2012). OKB, a novel family of brain-gut neuropeptides from insects. *Insect Biochem. Mol. Biol.* 42, 466–473.

Stone, J. V., Mordue, W., Batley, K. E., and Morris, H. R. (1976). Structure of locust adipokinetic hormone, a neurohormone that regulates lipid utilization during flight. *Nature* 263, 207–211.

Sudo, S., Kuwabara, Y., Park, J. I., Hsu, S. Y., and Hsueh, A. J. (2005). Heterodimeric fly glycoprotein hormone-alpha2 (GPA2) and glycoprotein hormone-beta5 (GPB5) activate fly leucine-rich repeat-containing G protein-coupled receptor-1 (DLGR1) and stimulation of human thyrotropin receptors by chimeric fly GPA2 and human GPB5. *Endocrinology* 146, 3596–3604.

Taghert, P. H., and Nitabach, M. N. (2012). Peptide neuromodulation in invertebrate model systems. *Neuron* 76, 82–97.

Talsma, A. D., Christov, C. P., Terriente-Felix, A., Linneweber, G. A., Perea, D., Wayland, M., et al. (2012). Remote control of renal physiology by the intestinal neuropeptide pigment-dispersing factor in *Drosophila*. *Proc. Natl. Acad. Sci. U.S.A.* 109, 12177–12182.

Tanaka, Y., Hua, Y., Roller, L., and Tanaka, S. (2002). Corazonin reduces the spinning rate in the silkworm, *Bombyx mori*. *J. Insect Physiol.* 48, 707–714.

Tawfik, A. I., Tanaka, S., De Loof, A., Schoofs, L., Baggerman, G., Waelkens, E., et al. (1999). Identification of the gregarization-associated dark-pigmentotropin in locusts through an albino mutant. *Proc. Natl. Acad. Sci. U.S.A.* 96, 7083–7087.

Taylor, C. A., Winther, A. M., Siviter, R. J., Shirras, A. D., Isaac, R. E., and Nässel, D. R. (2004). Identification of a proctolin preprohormone gene (Proct) of *Drosophila melanogaster*: expression and predicted prohormone processing. *J. Neurobiol.* 58, 379–391.

Teal, P. E., Meredith, J. A., and Nachman, R. J. (1999). Development of amphiphylic mimics of insect neuropeptides for pest control. *Ann. N.Y. Acad. Sci.* 897, 348–360.

Te Brugge, V., Ianowski, J. P., and Orchard, I. (2009). Biological activity of diuretic factors on the anterior midgut of the blood-feeding bug, *Rhodnius prolixus*. *Gen. Comp. Endocrinol.* 162, 105–112.

Te Brugge, V., Paluzzi, J. P., Schooley, D. A., and Orchard, I. (2011). Identification of the elusive peptidergic diuretic hormone in the blood-feeding bug *Rhodnius prolixus*: a CRF-related peptide. *J. Exp. Biol.* 214, 371–381.

Terhzaz, S., O'Connell, F. C., Pollock, V. P., Kean, L., Davies, S. A., Veenstra, J. A., et al. (1999). Isolation and characterization of a leucokinin-like peptide of *Drosophila melanogaster*. *J. Exp. Biol.* 202(Pt 24), 3667–3676.

Terhzaz, S., Rosay, P., Goodwin, S. F., and Veenstra, J. A. (2007). The neuropeptide SIFamide modulates sexual behavior in *Drosophila*. *Biochem. Biophys. Res. Commun.* 352, 305–310.

Terhzaz, S., Cabrero, P., Robben, J. H., Radford, J. C., Hudson, B. D., Milligan, G., et al. (2012). Mechanism and function of *Drosophila capa* GPCR: a desiccation stress-responsive receptor with functional homology to human neuromedinU receptor. *PLoS ONE* 7:e29897. doi: 10.1371/journal.pone.0029897

Truman, J. W. (1996). Ecdysis control sheds another layer. *Science* 271, 40–41.

Ulens, C., Daenens, P., and Tytgat, J. (1999). The dual modulation of GIRK1/GIRK2 channels by opioid receptor ligands. *Eur. J. Pharmacol.* 385, 239–245.

Urnov, F. D., Rebar, E. J., Holmes, M. C., Zhang, H. S., and Gregory, P. D. (2010). Genome editing with engineered zinc finger nucleases. *Nat. Rev. Genet.* 11, 636–646.

Van Hiel, M. B., Van Loy, T., Poels, J., Vandersmissen, H. P., Verlinden, H., Badisco, L., et al. (2010). Neuropeptide receptors as possible targets for development of insect pest control agents. *Adv. Exp. Med. Biol.* 692, 211–226.

Van Hiel, M. B., Vandersmissen, H. P., Van Loy, T., and Vanden Broeck, J. (2012). An evolutionary comparison of leucine-rich repeat containing G protein-coupled receptors reveals a novel LGR subtype. *Peptides* 34, 193–200.

Van Loy, T., Vandersmissen, H. P., Poels, J., Van Hiel, M. B., Verlinden, H., and Vanden Broeck, J. (2010). Tachykinin-related peptides and their receptors in invertebrates: a current view. *Peptides* 31, 520–524.

Van Wielendaele, P., Dillen, S., Marchal, E., Badisco, L., and Vanden Broeck, J. (2012). CRF-like diuretic hormone negatively affects both feeding and reproduction in the desert locust, *Schistocerca gregaria*. *PLoS ONE* 7:e31425. doi: 10.1371/journal.pone.0031425

Vanden Broeck, J. (1996). G-protein-coupled receptors in insect cells. *Int. Rev. Cytol.* 164, 189–268.

Vanden Broeck, J. (2001). Insect G protein-coupled receptors and signal transduction. *Arch. Insect Biochem. Physiol.* 48, 1–12.

Vanden Broeck, J., Poels, J., Simonet, G., Dicksens, L., and De Loof, A. (1998). Identification of G protein-coupled receptors in insect cells. *Ann. N.Y. Acad. Sci.* 839, 123–128.

Vargas, M. A., Luo, N., Yamaguchi, A., and Kapahi, P. (2010). A role for S6 kinase and serotonin in postmating dietary switch and balance of nutrients in *D. melanogaster*. *Curr. Biol.* 20, 1006–1011.

Večeřa, J., Krishnan, N., Alquicer, G., Kodrík, D., and Socha, R. (2007). Adipokinetic hormone-induced enhancement of antioxidant capacity of *Pyrrhocoris apterus* hemolymph in response to oxidative stress. *Comp. Biochem. Physiol. C Toxicol. Pharmacol.* 146, 336–342.

Veelaert, D., Schoofs, L., Verhaert, P., and De Loof, A. (1997). Identification of two novel peptides from the central nervous system of the desert locust, *Schistocerca gregaria*. *Biochem. Biophys. Res. Commun.* 241, 530–534.

Veenstra, J. A. (1989). Isolation and structure of corazonin, a cardioactive peptide from the American cockroach. *FEBS Lett.* 250, 231–234.

Veenstra, J. A. (2009a). Allatostatin C and its paralog allatostatin double C: the arthropod somatostatins. *Insect Biochem. Mol. Biol.* 39, 161–170.

Veenstra, J. A. (2009b). Does corazonin signal nutritional stress in insects? *Insect Biochem. Mol. Biol.* 39, 755–762.

Veenstra, J. A. (2010). What the loss of the hormone neuroparsin in the *melanogaster* subgroup of *Drosophila* can tell us about its function. *Insect Biochem. Mol. Biol.* 40, 354–361.

Veenstra, J. A., Lehman, H. K., and Davis, N. T. (1994). Allatotropin is a cardioacceleratory peptide in *Manduca sexta*. *J. Exp. Biol.* 188, 347–354.

Veenstra, J. A., Rodriguez, L., and Weaver, R. J. (2012). Allatotropin, leucokinin and AKH in honey bees and other Hymenoptera. *Peptides* 35, 122–130.

Verleyen, P., Huybrechts, J., Sas, F., Clynen, E., Baggerman, G., De Loof, A., et al. (2004a). Neuropeptidomics of the grey flesh fly, *Neobellieria bullata*. *Biochem. Biophys. Res. Commun.* 316, 763–770.

Verleyen, P., Huybrechts, J., Baggerman, G., Van Lommel, A., De Loof, A., and Schoofs, L. (2004b). SIFamide is a highly conserved neuropeptide: a comparative study in different insect species. *Biochem. Biophys. Res. Commun.* 320, 334–341.

Verleyen, P., Huybrechts, J., and Schoofs, L. (2009). SIFamide illustrates the rapid evolution in Arthropod neuropeptide research. *Gen. Comp. Endocrinol.* 162, 27–35.

Verlinden, H., Badisco, L., Marchal, E., Van Wielendaele, P., and Vanden Broeck, J. (2009). Endocrinology of reproduction and phase transition in locusts. *Gen. Comp. Endocrinol.* 162, 79–92.

Verlinden, H., Vleugels, R., Marchal, E., Badisco, L., Pfluger, H. J., Blenau, W., et al. (2010). The role of octopamine in locusts and other arthropods. *J. Insect Physiol.* 56, 854–867.

Vilaplana, L., Pascual, N., Perera, N., Leira, D., and Bellés, X. (2008). Antifeeding properties of myosuppressin in a generalist phytophagous leafworm, *Spodoptera littoralis* (Boisduval). *Regul. Pept.* 148, 68–75.

Vitt, U. A., Hsu, S. Y., and Hsueh, A. J. (2001). Evolution and classification of cystine knot-containing hormones and related extracellular signaling molecules. *Mol. Endocrinol.* 15, 681–694.

Vosko, A. M., Schroeder, A., Loh, D. H., and Colwell, C. S. (2007). Vasoactive intestinal peptide and the mammalian circadian system. *Gen. Comp. Endocrinol.* 152, 165–175.

Vuerinckx, K., Verlinden, H., Lindemans, M., Broeck, J. V., and Huybrechts, R. (2011). Characterization of an allatotropin-like peptide receptor in the red flour beetle, *Tribolium castaneum*. *Insect Biochem. Mol. Biol.* 41, 815–822.

Wang, C., Chin-Sang, I., and Bendena, W. G. (2012). The FGLamide-allatostatins influence foraging behavior in *Drosophila melanogaster*. *PLoS ONE* 7:e36059. doi: 10.1371/journal.pone.0036059

Wasielewski, O., and Skonieczna, M. (2008). Pleiotropic effects of the neuropeptides CCAP and myosuppressin in the beetle, *Tenebrio molitor L. J. Comp. Physiol. B* 178, 877–885.

Weaver, R. J., and Audsley, N. (2008). Neuropeptides of the beetle, *Tenebrio molitor* identified using MALDI-TOF mass spectrometry and deduced sequences from the *Tribolium castaneum* genome. *Peptides* 29, 168–178.

Weaver, R. J., and Audsley, N. (2009). Neuropeptide regulators of juvenile hormone synthesis: structures, functions, distribution, and unanswered questions. *Ann. N.Y. Acad. Sci.* 1163, 316–329.

Weaver, R. J., Freeman, Z. A., Pickering, M. G., and Edwards, J. P. (1994). Identification of two allatostatins from the CNS of the cockroach *Periplaneta americana*: Novel members of a family of neuropeptide inhibitors of insect juvenile hormone biosynthesis. *Comp. Biochem. Physiol. C Pharmacol. Toxicol. Endocrinol.* 107, 119–127.

Weaver, R. J., Marco, H. G., Simek, P., Audsley, N., Clark, K. D., and Gäde, G. (2012). Adipokinetic hormones (AKHs) of sphingid Lepidoptera, including the identification of a second *M. sexta* AKH. *Peptides* 34, 44–50.

Wegener, C., Herbert, Z., Eckert, M., and Predel, R. (2002). The periviscerokinin (PVK) peptide family in insects: evidence for the inclusion of CAP(2b) as a PVK family member. *Peptides* 23, 605–611.

Wegener, C., Reinl, T., Jänsch, L., and Predel, R. (2006). Direct mass spectrometric peptide profiling and fragmentation of larval peptide hormone release sites in *Drosophila melanogaster* reveals tagma-specific peptide expression and differential processing. *J. Neurochem.* 96, 1362–1374.

Wei, Z., Baggerman, G., Nachman, J., Goldsworthy, G., Verhaert, P., De Loof, A., et al. (2000). Sulfakinins reduce food intake in the desert locust, *Schistocerca gregaria*. *J. Insect Physiol.* 46, 1259–1265.

Wen, T., Parrish, C. A., Xu, D., Wu, Q., and Shen, P. (2005). Drosophila neuropeptide F and its receptor, NPFR1, define a signaling pathway that acutely modulates alcohol sensitivity. *Proc. Natl. Acad. Sci. U.S.A.* 102, 2141–2146.

Wen, Z., Gulia, M., Clark, K. D., Dhara, A., Crim, J. W., Strand, M. R., et al. (2010). Two insulin-like peptide family members from the mosquito *Aedes aegypti* exhibit differential biological and receptor binding activities. *Mol. Cell. Endocrinol.* 328, 47–55.

Wesolowska, N., and Rong, Y. S. (2010). The past, present and future of gene targeting in *Drosophila. Fly (Austin)* 4, 53–59.

West, A. P., Llamas, L. L., Snow, P. M., Benzer, S., and Bjorkman, P. J. (2001). Crystal structure of the ectodomain of Methuselah, a *Drosophila* G protein-coupled receptor associated with extended lifespan. *Proc. Natl. Acad. Sci. U.S.A.* 98, 3744–3749.

Wheeler, D. E., Buck, N., and Evans, J. D. (2006). Expression of insulin pathway genes during the period of caste determination in the honey bee, *Apis mellifera. Insect Mol. Biol.* 15, 597–602.

Wicher, D., Agricola, H., Sohler, S., Gundel, M., Heinemann, S. H., Wollweber, L., et al. (2006a). Differential receptor activation by cockroach adipokinetic hormones produces differential effects on ion currents, neuronal activity, and locomotion. *J. Neurophysiol.* 95, 2314–2325.

Wicher, D., Agricola, H., Schonherr, R., Heinemann, S. H., and Derst, C. (2006b). TRPgamma channels are inhibited by cAMP and contribute to pacemaking in neurosecretory insect neurons. *J. Biol. Chem.* 281, 3227–3236.

Wicher, D., Derst, C., Gautier, H., Lapied, B., Heinemann, S. H., and Agricola, H. (2007). The satiety signaling neuropeptide perisulfakinin inhibits the activity of central neurons promoting general activity. *Front. Cell. Neurosci.* 1:3. doi: 10.3389/neuro.03.003.2007

Williamson, M., Lenz, C., Winther, A. M., Nässel, D. R., and Grimmelikhuijzen, C. J. P. (2001). Molecular cloning, genomic organization, and expression of a C-type (Manduca sexta-type) allatostatin preprohormone from *Drosophila melanogaster. Biochem. Biophys. Res. Commun.* 282, 124–130.

Woodhead, A. P., Stay, B., Seidel, S. L., Khan, M. A., and Tobe, S. S. (1989). Primary structure of four allatostatins: neuropeptide inhibitors of juvenile hormone synthesis. *Proc. Natl. Acad. Sci. U.S.A.* 86, 5997–6001.

Woodhead, A. P., Khan, M. A., Stay, B., and Tobe, S. S. (1994). Two new allatostatins from the brains of *Diploptera punctata. Insect Biochem. Mol. Biol.* 24, 257–263.

Wu, Q., Wen, T., Lee, G., Park, J. H., Cai, H. N., and Shen, P. (2003). Developmental control of foraging and social behavior by the *Drosophila* neuropeptide Y-like system. *Neuron* 39, 147–161.

Wu, Q., Zhao, Z., and Shen, P. (2005a). Regulation of aversion to noxious food by *Drosophila* neuropeptide Y- and insulin-like systems. *Nat. Neurosci.* 8, 1350–1355.

Wu, Q., Zhang, Y., Xu, J., and Shen, P. (2005b). Regulation of hunger-driven behaviors by neural ribosomal S6 kinase in *Drosophila. Proc. Natl. Acad. Sci. U.S.A.* 102, 13289–13294.

Würden, S., and Homberg, U. (1995). Immunocytochemical mapping of serotonin and neuropeptides in the accessory medulla of the locust, *Schistocerca gregaria. J. Comp. Neurol.* 362, 305–319.

Xu, J., Li, M., and Shen, P. (2010). A G-protein-coupled neuropeptide Y-like receptor suppresses behavioral and sensory response to multiple stressful stimuli in *Drosophila. J. Neurosci.* 30, 2504–2512.

Yagi, K. J., Kwok, R., Chan, K. K., Setter, R. R., Myles, T. G., Tobe, S. S., et al. (2005). Phe-Gly-Leu-amide allatostatin in the termite *Reticulitermes flavipes*: Content in brain and corpus allatum and effect on juvenile hormone synthesis. *J. Insect Physiol.* 51, 357–365.

Yamanaka, N., Yamamoto, S., Žitňan, D., Watanabe, K., Kawada, T., Satake, H., et al. (2008). Neuropeptide receptor transcriptome reveals unidentified neuroendocrine pathways. *PLoS ONE* 3:e3048. doi: 10.1371/journal.pone.0003048

Yamanaka, N., Hua, Y. J., Roller, L., Spalovska-Valachova, I., Mizoguchi, A., Kataoka, H., et al. (2010). *Bombyx* prothoracicostatic peptides activate the sex peptide receptor to regulate ecdysteroid biosynthesis. *Proc. Natl. Acad. Sci. U.S.A.* 107, 2060–2065.

Yamanaka, N., Roller, L., Žitňan, D., Satake, H., Mizoguchi, A., Kataoka, H., et al. (2011). *Bombyx* orcokinins are brain-gut peptides involved in the neuronal regulation of ecdysteroidogenesis. *J. Comp. Neurol.* 519, 238–246.

Yapici, N., Kim, Y. J., Ribeiro, C., and Dickson, B. J. (2008). A receptor that mediates the post-mating switch in *Drosophila* reproductive behaviour. *Nature* 451, 33–37.

Yoshiura, S., Ohta, N., and Matsuzaki, F. (2012). Tre1 GPCR signaling orients stem cell divisions in the *Drosophila* central nervous system. *Dev. Cell* 22, 79–91.

Yu, D., Akalal, D.-B. G., and Davis, R. L. (2006). *Drosophila* α/β mushroom body neurons form a branch-specific, long-term cellular memory trace after spaced olfactory conditioning. *Neuron* 52, 845–855.

Zandawala, M. (2012). Calcitonin-like diuretic hormones in insects. *Insect Biochem. Mol. Biol.* 42, 816–825.

Zandawala, M., Lytvyn, Y., Taiakina, D., and Orchard, I. (2012). Cloning of the cDNA, localization, and physiological effects of FGLamide-related allatostatins in the blood-gorging bug, *Rhodnius prolixus. Insect Biochem. Mol. Biol.* 42, 10–21.

Zhao, Y., Bretz, C. A., Hawksworth, S. A., Hirsh, J., and Johnson, E. C. (2010). Corazonin neurons function in sexually dimorphic circuitry that shape behavioral responses to stress in *Drosophila. PLoS ONE* 5:e9141. doi: 10.1371/journal.pone.0009141

Zhu, C., Huang, H., Hua, R., Li, G., Yang, D., Luo, J., et al. (2009). Molecular and functional characterization of adipokinetic hormone receptor and its peptide ligands in *Bombyx mori. FEBS Lett.* 583, 1463–1468.

Zhu, W., Verhaert, P., Shaw, C., Maule, A., De Loof, A., and Vaudry, H. (1998). NPF immunolocalization in cockroaches and locusts: Comparison of antisera to beetle, tapeworm, and pig NPY/NPF-type peptides. *Ann. N.Y. Acad. Sci.* 839, 625–627.

Ziegler, R., Jasensky, R. D., and Morimoto, H. (1995). Characterization of the adipokinetic hormone receptor form the fat body of *Manduca sexta. Regul. Pept.* 57, 329–338.

Ziegler, R., Isoe, J., Moore, W., Riehle, M. A., and Wells, M. A. (2011). The putative AKH receptor of the tobacco hornworm, *Manduca sexta*, and its expression. *J. Insect Sci.* 11, 40.

Zoephel, J., Reiher, W., Rexer, K. H., Kahnt, J., and Wegener, C. (2012). Peptidomics of the agriculturally damaging larval stage of the cabbage root fly *Delia radicum* (Diptera: Anthomyiidae). *PLoS ONE* 7:e41543. doi: 10.1371/journal.pone.0041543

Zupanc, G. K. (1996). Peptidergic transmission: from morphological correlates to functional implications. *Micron* 27, 35–91.

Žitňan, D., Hollar, L., Spalovská, I., Takáč, P., Žitňanová, I., Gill, S. S., et al. (2002). Molecular cloning and function of ecdysis-triggering hormones in the silkworm *Bombyx mori. J. Exp. Biol.* 205, 3459–3473.

Žitňan, D., Ross, L. S., Žitňanová, I., Hermesman, J. L., Gill, S. S., and Adams, M. E. (1999). Steroid induction of a peptide hormone gene leads to orchestration of a defined behavioral sequence. *Neuron* 23, 523–535.

Žitňan, D., Kim, Y. J., Žitňanová, I., Roller, L., and Adams, M. E. (2007). Complex steroid-peptide-receptor cascade controls insect ecdysis. *Gen. Comp. Endocrinol.* 153, 88–96.

Žitňan, D., Žitňanová, I., Spalovská, I., Takáè, P., Park, Y., and Adams, M. E. (2003). Conservation of ecdysis-triggering hormone signalling in insects. *J. Exp. Biol.* 206, 1275–1289.

19

Neuropeptide GPCRs in *C. elegans*

Lotte Frooninckx†, Liesbeth Van Rompay†, Liesbet Temmerman, Elien Van Sinay, Isabel Beets, Tom Janssen, Steven J. Husson and Liliane Schoofs*

Laboratory of Functional Genomics and Proteomics, Department of Biology, Katholieke Universiteit Leuven, Leuven, Belgium

Edited by:
Hubert Vaudry, University of Rouen, France

Reviewed by:
Pascal Favrel, University of Caen Lower Normandy, France
William Bendena, Queen's University, Canada

***Correspondence:**
Liliane Schoofs, Laboratory of Functional Genomics and Proteomics, Zoological Institute, Naamsestraat 59, 3000 Leuven, Belgium.
e-mail: liliane.schoofs@bio.kuleuven.be

† Lotte Frooninckx and Liesbeth Van Rompay have contributed equally to this work.

Like most organisms, the nematode *Caenorhabditis elegans* relies heavily on neuropeptidergic signaling. This tiny animal represents a suitable model system to study neuropeptidergic signaling networks with single cell resolution due to the availability of powerful molecular and genetic tools. The availability of the worm's complete genome sequence allows researchers to browse through it, uncovering putative neuropeptides and their cognate G protein-coupled receptors (GPCRs). Many predictions have been made about the number of *C. elegans* neuropeptide GPCRs. In this review, we report the state of the art of both verified as well as predicted *C. elegans* neuropeptide GPCRs. The predicted neuropeptide GPCRs are incorporated into the receptor classification system based on their resemblance to orthologous GPCRs in insects and vertebrates. Appointing the natural ligand(s) to each predicted neuropeptide GPCR (receptor deorphanization) is a crucial step during characterization. The development of deorphanization strategies resulted in a significant increase in the knowledge of neuropeptidergic signaling in *C. elegans*. Complementary localization and functional studies demonstrate that neuropeptides and their GPCRs represent a rich potential source of behavioral variability in *C. elegans*. Here, we review all neuropeptidergic signaling pathways that so far have been functionally characterized in *C. elegans*.

Keywords: nematoda, *Caenorhabditis elegans*, G protein-coupled receptor, neuropeptidergic signaling, GPCR deorphanization

INTRODUCTION

Caenorhabditis elegans is a free-living, microscopic soil nematode. Since its isolation in 1963, this bacterivorous animal acquired the status of model organism in neurobiology (Brenner, 1974). *C. elegans* is easy to cultivate and has a short life cycle of about 3 days at 20°C. Before reaching its adult form, it goes through four larval stages (L1–L4). Hermaphrodites can either self-fertilize or mate with males, a feature that is commonly exploited during high-throughput genetic studies. The publication of its approximately 100 Mb genome in 1998 made *C. elegans* the first multicellular organism to have its entire genome sequenced (The *C. elegans* Sequencing Consortium, 1998). Genome-wide comparison of the predicted *C. elegans* genes and their vertebrate equivalents revealed an unexpected but notable resemblance between their nervous systems (Bargmann, 1998). The *C. elegans* nervous system comprises only 302 small neurons in adult hermaphrodites. It might seem simple at first sight, but appears to be chemically complex, equivalent to most vertebrate nervous systems. Chemical signaling in *C. elegans* occurs through a group of classical neurotransmitters which are important for synaptic communication and includes acetylcholine (ACh), γ-aminobutyric acid (GABA), glutamate, nitric oxide, serotonin, and other monoamines (Brownlee and Fairweather, 1999). These small-molecule neurotransmitters are packed into synaptic vesicles and subsequently released by exocytosis (Gasnier, 2000; Weimer and Jorgensen, 2003; Scalettar, 2006). In addition to classical neurotransmitters, cell-to-cell communication via chemical signaling in *C. elegans* also occurs through neuropeptides. Both bioinformatic predictions and peptidomic analyses demonstrated that the *C. elegans* genome comprises a rich diversity of small neuropeptide bioregulators (Li et al., 1999; Nathoo et al., 2001; Pierce et al., 2001; Husson et al., 2005, 2007a; Li and Kim, 2010). This abundant group of over 250 signaling molecules is derived from neuropeptide precursor genes and outnumbers the classical neurotransmitters. As observed in other animal species, one or multiple mature bioactive neuropeptides are generated out of each preproprotein precursor by proteolytic processing and extensive post-translational modifications (Husson et al., 2005, 2006, 2007b; Husson and Schoofs, 2007). Besides their role in key physiological processes, it seems that *C. elegans* neuropeptides are implicated in the modulation of essentially all behaviors including locomotion, reproduction, social behavior, mechano- and chemosensation, learning and memory (Li and Kim, 2008); and may be important for behavioral adaptation throughout evolution (Avery, 2010). Neuropeptides are primarily thought to act as neuromodulators but can also act as fast neurotransmitters. Despite the lack of a circulatory system in *C. elegans*, a neurohormonal role is also ascribed to neuropeptides, and its nervous system harbors a significant number of peptidergic neurosecretory cells (Hartenstein, 2006). It is assumed that possibly all *C. elegans* neurons synthesize and secrete neuropeptides (Holden-Dye and Walker, 2012). Currently, 119 neuropeptide precursor genes are known which can be subdivided into three major families according to the sequence and structural similarities of their derived peptides. Thirty-one neuropeptide-encoding genes are assigned to the FMRFamide (Phe-Met-Arg-Phe-amide)-like peptide (*flp*) gene family, while 40 genes belong to the family of insulin-like peptide (*ins*) genes. Peptides that bear no resemblance to FMRFamide- or insulin-like peptides are encoded by the family of neuropeptide-like protein (*nlp*) genes. So far, 48 *nlp* precursor genes are known. G protein-coupled receptors (GPCRs) are the principal neuropeptide targets through which intracellular signaling transduction pathways are triggered. GPCRs are defined as seven transmembrane receptors that signal through G proteins. They are found in almost any eukaryotic organism indicating they have an early evolutionary origin (Krishnan et al., 2012). GPCRs have a diverse array of ligands ranging from light, Ca^{2+} and odorants to small molecules such as amino acid residues, nucleotides, peptides, and proteins (Pin, 2000). About 7% of all predicted protein-coding genes in *C. elegans* are GPCRs (Bargmann, 1998; Fredriksson and Schiöth, 2005). Most of them (~1300) encode nematode-specific chemoreceptors, which are thought to compensate for the absence of visual and auditory systems in *C. elegans* (Thomas and Robertson, 2008). The remaining GPCRs can be classified according to the GRAFS classification system and comprise the Glutamate, Rhodopsin, Adhesion, Frizzled, and Secretin families (Schiöth and Fredriksson, 2005). In this review we will focus on the *C. elegans* neuropeptide GPCRs, which belong to the rhodopsin and secretin families. To date, only a limited number of nematode neuropeptide GPCRs of these families have been deorphanized and functionally characterized.

UNRAVELING NEUROPEPTIDERGIC SIGNALING IN THE MODEL ORGANISM *C. ELEGANS*

The flexible genetic tool box that comes with the use of *C. elegans* as a model has greatly expedited the functional characterization of neuropeptide GPCRs in this organism. Genome-wide RNA interference (RNAi) and mutant analyses have been used to shed light on the behavioral output of neuropeptidergic signaling (Keating et al., 2003; Rual et al., 2004; Ceron et al., 2007). With these techniques, it has become clear that neuropeptides and their receptors influence many if not all of the worm's behaviors. This conclusion is further supported by results from genetic studies on orphan *C. elegans* GPCRs. Recently, Jee et al. (2012) generated mutants for the SEB-3 receptor, an orphan corticotropin-releasing factor (CRF)-related GPCR, and showed that it is strongly implicated in the worm's stress response and ethanol tolerance. This is a perfect example of an earlier finding that several neuropeptide pathways are involved in *C. elegans* responses to ethanol (Mitchell et al., 2010). A genome-wide RNAi study of predicted *C. elegans* GPCRs was performed by Keating et al. (2003) amongst others, which were able to identify a number of neuropeptide receptors involved in reproduction and locomotion. *In vivo* localization of neuropeptide signaling components is facilitated by the worm's transparency and its simple but well-defined anatomy. The adult hermaphrodite has exactly 959 somatic nuclei ordered in fully differentiated tissues (Sulston et al., 1983; WormAtlas et al., 2002–2012). The developmental origin of every *C. elegans* neuron and the wiring diagram of its roughly 7000 synapses have been completely mapped (White et al., 1986; Jarrell et al., 2012). Using selective promoters that target gene expression to a cell or tissue of interest, combined with laser ablation and cell imaging techniques, gene function and neural activity can be studied at the level of individual neurons, of which several examples are described below. Together, these powerful molecular and genetics tools enable the dissection of neural networks underlying the neuropeptidergic regulation of behavior with single cell resolution.

NEUROPEPTIDE GPCRs IN *C. ELEGANS*

Since the publication of the *C. elegans* genome, many predictions have been made about the number of neuropeptide GPCRs it contains. These predictions are usually based on sequence similarities to vertebrate and insect neuropeptide GPCRs (Bargmann, 1998; Fredriksson and Schiöth, 2005). Compared to other *C. elegans* GPCRs, neuropeptide GPCRs appear to be less closely related to their vertebrate counterparts. This agrees with the apparently low conservation of the *C. elegans* neuropeptides (Bargmann, 1998). A crucial step in the characterization of a predicted neuropeptide GPCR is the identification of its natural ligand(s). For this purpose, a reverse pharmacology approach (see Finding Neuropeptide Ligands for Orphan GPCRs) can be applied (Mertens et al., 2004; Beets et al., 2011). Another way to predict neuropeptide GPCRs is to use all deorphanized neuropeptide GPCRs as a seeding set in a Multiple Expectation Maximization for Motif Elicitation/Motif Alignment and Search Tool (MEME/MAST) analysis. Doing so, a list of 125 potential neuropeptide receptors could be obtained (Janssen et al., 2010). Since this prediction, the number of deorphanized neuropeptide GPCRs has increased from 6 to 23. We enhanced this MEME/MAST analysis by use of an updated seeding set containing all newly deorphanized neuropeptide GPCRs and merged our predictions with the list of neuropeptide GPCRs from WormAtlas et al. (2002–2012). Manual verification of every receptor ensured a reliable, revised list of potential neuropeptide GPCRs in *C. elegans* (**Table 1**).

All predicted neuropeptide GPCRs can be grouped in the rhodopsin and secretin families according to the GRAFS classification system. Rhodopsin GPCRs are subdivided based on their resemblance to insect and mammalian neuropeptide GPCRs. The neuropeptide Y (NPY)/RFamide-like receptor family, containing 41 receptors, represents the best characterized group. Twelve of its representatives have been deorphanized and all are activated by FMRFamide like peptides (NPR-1, NPR-3, NPR-4, NPR-5a/b, NPR-6, NPR-10a/b, NPR-11, FRPR-3, and FRPR-18a/b). Their corresponding signaling pathways are involved in a multitude of functions such as locomotion, feeding, energy metabolism, and reproduction. So far, none of the 24 receptors belonging to the somatostatin and galanin-like receptor group have been deorphanized. Only RNAi phenotypes with respect to locomotion and fat metabolism have been observed for this poorly studied group. The tachykinin (neurokinin)-like receptor group contains 12 receptors. Mertens et al. (2006) deorphanized one of these receptors, namely NPR-22a. Remarkably, this GPCR was not activated by the predicted *C. elegans* tachykinin-like peptide but by a handful of FMRFamide-related peptides (FaRPs). The cholecystokinin (CCK)/gastrin-like receptor and gonadotropin releasing hormone (GnRH), oxytocin (OT), vasopressin (VP)-like receptor groups contain 3 and 14 receptors, respectively. Deorphanization of CKR-2a/b and GNRR-1a supports the theory of receptor-ligand coevolution (Janssen et al., 2010). Although no clear CCK or

Table 1 | List of orphan and deorphanized neuropeptide GPCRs in *C. elegans* (adapted from WormAtlas et al., 2002–2012).

Receptor group	Gene sequence name	Protein	WormBase ID	Ligand-encoding precursor gene (Ligand[a])	Putative role in	Reference
RHODOPSIN FAMILY OF GPCRs						
Neuropeptide Y/RFamide-like receptors	C39E6.6	NPR-1	WP:CE06941	*flp-18* (FLP-18-1, FLP-18-2, FLP-18-3, FLP-18-4, FLP-18-5, FLP-18-6); *flp-21* (FLP-21)	Feeding behavior; aerotaxis; thermal avoidance; ethanol tolerance; innate immunity	de Bono and Bargmann (1998), Kubiak et al. (2003), Rogers et al. (2003), Davies et al. (2004), Cheung et al. (2005), Rogers et al. (2006), Gloria-Soria and Azevedo (2008), Styer et al. (2008), Glauser et al. (2011), Milward et al. (2011)[c]
	T05A1.1a	NPR-2a	WP:CE32924	/	Fat storage;	Keating et al. (2003),
	T05A1.1b	NPR-2b	WP.CE32925	/	locomotion[b]	Cohen et al. (2009)[c]
	C10C6.2	NPR-3	WP:CE08056	*flp-15* (FLP-15-1, FLP-15-2)	Locomotion[b]	Keating et al. (2003), Kubiak et al. (2003)[c]
	C16D6.2	NPR-4	WP:CE37317	*flp-1* (FLP-1-6); *flp-4* (FLP-4-2); *flp-18* (FLP-18-1, FLP-18-2, FLP-18-3, FLP-18-4, FLP-18-5, FLP-18-6)	Fat storage; olfaction; foraging; reproduction[b]	Keating et al. (2003), Lowery et al. (2003), Cohen et al. (2009)[c]
	Y58G8A.4a	NPR-5a	WP:CE33345	*flp-1* (FLP-1-2); *flp-3* (FLP-3-1, FLP-3-3, FLP-3-6, FLP-3-8); *flp-18* (FLP-18-1, FLP-18-2, FLP-18-3, FLP-18-4, FLP-18-5, FLP-18-6); *flp-21* (FLP-21)	Fat storage; dauer formation	Kubiak et al. (2008), Cohen et al. (2009)[c]
	Y58G8A.4b	NPR-5b	WP:CE36962	*flp-1* (FLP-1-2); *flp-3* (FLP-3-1, FLP-3-3, FLP-3-6, FLP-3-8); *flp-4* (FLP-4-2); *flp-18* (FLP-18-1, FLP-18-2, FLP-18-3, FLP-18-4, FLP-18-5, FLP-18-6); *flp-21* (FLP-21)		Lowery et al. (2003), Kubiak et al. (2008)[c]
	F41E7.3	NPR-6	WP:CE31509 WP:CE31509	*flp-18* (FLP-18-3, FLP-18-6); *flp-21* (FLP-21)	Reproduction[b]	Keating et al. (2003); Lowery et al. (2003); [c]
	F35G8.1	NPR-7	WP:CE30408	/	Fat storage; locomotion[b]	Keating et al. (2003), Cohen et al. (2009)[c]
	C56G3.1a	NPR-8a	WP:CE04283	/	/	[c]
	C56G3.1b	NPR-8b	WP:CE30923	/	/	[c]
	C53C7.1a	NPR-10a	WP:CE19767	*flp-3* (FLP-3-1, FLP-3-3, FLP-3-5, FLP-3-6, FLP-3-7, FLP-3-8); *flp-18* (FLP-18-1, FLP-18-3, FLP-18-4, FLP-18-5, FLP-18-6)	/	Lowery et al. (2003)[c]
	C53C7.1b	NPR-10b	WP:CE36989		/	
	C25G6.5	NPR-11	WP:CE47199	*flp-1* (FLP-1-6); *flp-5* (FLP-5-2); *flp-14* (FLP-14); *flp-18* (FLP-18-3); *flp-21* (FLP-21); *nlp-1* (MDANAFRMSFamide)	Local search behavior; olfactory adaptation, reproduction[b]	Keating et al. (2003), Lowery et al. (2003), Chalasani et al. (2010)[c]
	T22D1.12	NPR-12	WP:CE17256	/	Reproduction[b]	Rual et al. (2004)[c]
	ZC412.1	NPR-13	WP:CE35920	/	/	[c]
	W05B5.2	NPR-14	WP:CE42751	/	/	[c]
	T07D4.1	NPR-20	WP:CE46449	/	/	[c]
	T23C6.5	NPR-21	WP:CE35783	/	/	[c]
	C02B8.5	FRPR-1	WP:CE47103	/	/	
	C05E7.4	FRPR-2	WP:CE46227	/	/	
	C26F1.6	FRPR-3	WP:CE06880	*flp-7* (FLP-7-1, FLP-7-2, FLP-7-3); *flp-11* (FLP-11-1)	Reproduction[b]	Keating et al. (2003), Mertens et al. (2004)[c]
	C54A12.2	FRPR-4	WP:CE36809	/	/	[c]
	C56A3.3a	FRPR-5a	WP:CE45431	/	/	[c]

(Continued)

Table 1 | Continued

Receptor group	Gene sequence name	Protein	WormBase ID	Ligand-encoding precursor gene (Ligand[a])	Putative role in	Reference
	C56A3.3b	FRPR-5b	WP:CE45452	/	/	c
	F21C10.12	FRPR-6	WP:CE32868	/	/	c
	F53A9.5	FRPR-8	WP:CE43844	/	/	c
	F53B7.2a	FRPR-9a	WP:CE44099	/	/	c
	F53B7.2b	FRPR-9b	WP:CE44063	/	/	c
	K06C4.8	FRPR-11	WP:CE11816	/	/	c
	K06C4.9	FRPR-12	WP:CE29506	/	/	c
	K07E8.5	FRPR-14	WP:CE35992	/	/	c
	K10C8.2	FRPR-15	WP:CE42140	/	/	c
	R12C12.3	FRPR-16	WP:CE02848	/	/	c
	T14C1.1	FRPR-17	WP:CE34212	/	/	
	T19F4.1a	FRPR-18a	WP:CE29348	*flp-2* (FLP-2-1, FLP-2-2)	/	Mertens et al. (2005)[c]
	T19F4.1b	FRPR-18b	WP:CE29349		/	
	Y41D4A.8	FRPR-19	WP:CE21846	/	/	c
	C30B5.5	FRPR-20	WP:CE02524	/	/	c
	C09F12.3	C09F12.3	WP:CE33973	/	/	d
	D1014.2	D1014.2	WP:CE44520	/	/	
Somatostatin and galanin-like receptors	ZK455.3	NPR-9	WP:CE03814	/	Fat storage; roaming behavior	Bendena et al. (2008)[c]
	F56B6.5a	NPR-16a	WP:CE31186	/	Lipid metabolism[b]	Ashrafi et al. (2003)[c]
	F56B6.5b	NPR-16b	WP:CE39375	/		
	C06G4.5	NPR-17	WP:CE38997	/	/	c
	C43C3.2a	NPR-18a	WP:CE01524	/	/	c
	C43C3.2b	NPR-18b	WP:CE47537	/	/	c
	C43C3.2c	NPR-18c	WP:CE47497	/	/	c
	C43C3.2d	NPR-18d	WP:CE47523	/	/	c
	C43C3.2e	NPR-18e	WP:CE47594	/	/	c
	C43C3.2f	NPR-18f	WP:CE47636	/	/	c
	C43C3.2g	NPR-18g	WP:CE47570	/	/	c
	R106.2	NPR-24	WP:CE39612	/	/	c
	T02E9.1	NPR-25	WP:CE13062	/	Locomotion[b]	Keating et al. (2003)[c]
	T02D1.6	NPR-26	WP:CE30684	/	/	c
	F42C5.2	NPR-27	WP:CE47648	/	/	c
	F55E10.7	NPR-28	WP:CE40072	/	/	
	ZC84.4	NPR-29	WP:CE24711	/	/	
	H10E21.2	NPR-30	WP:CE43737	/	/	
	Y116A8B.5	NPR-32	WP:CE46735	/	/	
	Y54E2A.1	Y54E2A.1	WP:CE31259	/	/	c
	C17H11.1	C17H11.1	WP:CE29584	/	/	d
	C24B5.1	C24B5.1	WP:CE36981	/	/	d
	F57A8.4	F57A8.4	WP:CE05985	/	/	c
	W10C4.1	W10C4.1	WP:CE39426	/	/	d
Tachykinin (neurokinin)-like receptors	C38C10.1	TKR-1	WP:CE44282	/	Lipid metabolism[b]	Ashrafi et al. (2003)[c]
	AC7.1a	TKR-3a	WP:CE38261	/	Reproduction[b]	Kamath et al. (2003), Simmer et al. (2003), Green et al. (2011)[c]
	AC7.1b	TKR-3b	WP:CE38262	/		
	T27D1.3	NPR-15	WP:CE43181	/	/	c
	Y59H11AL.1a	NPR-22a	WP:CE31260	*flp-1* (FLP-1-6); *flp-7* (FLP-7-1, FLP-7-2, FLP-7-3, FLP-7-4); *flp-9* (FLP-9); *flp-11* (FLP-11-1, FLP-11-2, FLP-11-3); *flp-13* (FLP-13-4); *flp-22* (FLP-22)	/	Mertens et al. (2006)[c]

(Continued)

Table 1 | Continued

Receptor group	Gene sequence name	Protein	WormBase ID	Ligand-encoding precursor gene (Ligand[a])	Putative role in	Reference
	Y59H11AL.1b	NPR-22b	WP:CE38456	/	/	[c]
	C49A9.7	C49A9.7	WP:CE16937	/	/	[c]
	C50F7.1a	C50F7.1a	WP:CE33574	/	/	[c]
	C50F7.1b	C50F7.1b	WP:CE04239	/	/	[c]
	F31B9.1	NPR-33	WP:CE17727	/	/	[c]
	T11F9.1a	T11F9.1a	WP:CE47396	/	/	[c]
	T11F9.1b	T11F9.1b	WP:CE47310	/	/	[c]
Cholecysto-kinin/gastrin-like receptors	T23B3.4	CKR-1	WP:CE45656	/	Reproduction[b]	Rual et al. (2004)[c]
	Y39A3B.5c/b	CKR-2a	(GenBank database accession number EU346943)	*flp-1* (FLP-1-1); *nlp-12* (DYRPLQ Famide, DGYRPLQFamide); *nlp-13* (SSSMYDRDIMSFamide); *nlp-14* (ALDGLDGSGFGFD)	Locomotion; fat storage; amylase activity/secretion	Janssen et al. (2008a), Hu et al. (2011)[c]
	Y39A3B.5c/d	CKR-2b	(GenBank database EU346944 accession number)			
Gonadotropin releasing hormone, oxytocin, vasopressin-like receptors	F54D7.3a	GNRR-1a	WP:CE17102	*nlp-47* (NLP-47)	Reproduction[b]	Lindemans et al. (2009a)[c]
	F45D7.3b	GNRR-1b	WP:CE46861	/	/	[c]
	C15H11.2a	GNRR-2a	WP:CE08179	/	/	
	C15H11.2b	GNRR-2b	WP:CE45186	/	/	
	ZC374.1	GNRR-3	WP:CE40886	/	/	
	C41G11.4a	GNRR-4a	WP:CE29716	/	/	
	C41G11.4b	GNRR-4b	WP:CE30896	/	/	
	C41G11.4c	GNRR-4c	WP:CE35428	/	/	
	H22D07.1	GNRR-5	WP:CE33129	/	/	
	F13D2.2	GNRR-6	WP:CE03194	/	Locomotion[b]	Kamath et al. (2003)
	F13D2.3	GNRR-7	WP:CE33996	/	/	
	Y105C5A.23	GNRR-8	WP:CE24056	/	Reproduction[b]	Ceron et al. (2007)
	T07D10.2	NTR-1	WP:CE13377	*ntc-1* (CFLNSCPYRRYamide)	Gustatory associative learning, reproduction	Beets et al. (2012), Garrison et al. (2012)[c]
	F14F4.1	NTR-2	WP:CE17670	/	/	[c]
Neurotensin, neuromedin U, growth hormone secretagogue, thyrotropin releasing hormone-like receptors	C48C5.1	NMUR-1	WP:CE45664	/	/	[c]
	K10B4.4	NMUR-2	WP:CE38395	*nlp-44* (AFFYTPRIamide)	/	Lindemans et al. (2009b)[c]
	F02E8.2a	NMUR-3a	WP:CE33990	/	/	[c]
	F02E8.2b	NMUR-3b	WP:CE07017	/	/	[c]
	C30F12.6	NMUR-4	WP:CE16886	/	Reproduction[b]	Ceron et al. (2007)
	F57H12.4	FRPR-10	WP:CE43724	/	/	[c]
	F57B7.1a	DMSR-1a	WP:CE05989	/	/	[e]
	F57B7.1b	DMSR-1b	WP:CE31009	/	/	[e]
	C46F4.1a	EGL-6a	WP:CE04219	*flp-10* (FLP-10); *flp-17* (FLP-17-1, FLP-17-2)	Reproduction	Trent et al. (1983), Ringstad and Horvitz (2008)
	C46F4.1b	EGL-6b	WP:CE43400			
	B0563.6a	B0563.6a	WP:CE29551	/	/	[e]
	B0563.6b	B0563.6b	WP:CE33513	/	/	[e]
	B0563.6c	B0563.6c	WP:CE41751	/	/	[e]

(Continued)

Table 1 | Continued

Receptor group	Gene sequence name	Protein	WormBase ID	Ligand-encoding precursor gene (Ligand[a])	Putative role in	Reference
	R03A10.6	SPRR-1	WP:CE43810	/	/	d
	F42D1.3	SPRR-2	WP:CE31511	/	/	d
	F39B3.2	FRPR-7	WP:CE30978	/	/	d
	K03H6.5	K03H6.5	WP:CE39585	/	/	d
/	C48C5.3	AEXR-3	WP:CE04226	/	/	c
/	T10E10.3	T10E10.3	WP:CE35766	/	/	d
/	T21H3.5	T21H3.5	WP:CE13906	/	/	d
/	Y70D2A.1	Y70D2A.1	WP:CE34231	/	/	d
/	ZK1307.7a	ZK1307.7a	WP:CE37863	/	/	d
/	ZK1307.7b	ZK1307.7b	WP:CE46539	/	/	d
/	B0034.5	B0034.5	WP:CE45030	/	/	d
/	B0334.6	B0334.6	WP:CE30473	/	/	d
SECRETIN FAMILY OF GPCRs						
/	C18B12.2	SEB-3	WP:CE23557CE23557		Locomotion; stress response; ethanol tolerance	Jee et al. (2012)
	B0457.1a	LAT-1a	WP:CE02945	/	/	f
	B0457.1b	LAT-1b	WP:CE32789	/	/	f
	B0286.2a	LAT-2a	WP:CE36968	/	/	f
	C18B12.2	C18B12.2	WP:CE23557	/	/	f,g
	ZK643.3a	SECR-1a	WP:CE33750	/	/	f,g
	ZK643.3b	SECR-1b	WP:CE01112	/	/	f,g
	C13B9.4a	PDFR-1a	WP:CE30860	*pdf-1* (PDF-1a, PDF-1b); *pdf-2* (PDF-2)	Locomotion; reproduction	Janssen et al. (2008b), Meelkop et al. (2012)
	C13B9.4b	PDFR-1b	WP:CE370787			
	C13B9.4c	PDFR-1c	WP:CE37088			

*GPCRs are ranked according to the GRAFS classification system. Deorphanized neuropeptide GPCRs are marked in gray. Underlined neuropeptides are most potent to be the endogenous ligands ([a]see **Table A1** in Appendix for neuropeptide ligand sequences). [b]Putative roles supported by RNAi. Neuropeptide GPCRs are predicted in [c]Janssen et al. (2010), [e]Hewes and Taghert (2001), [f]Harmar (2001), and [g]Cardoso et al. (2006). [d]To complete the list of neuropeptide GPCR we performed a MEME/MAST analysis as described in Janssen et al. (2010).*

sulfakinin orthologs could be identified through *in silico* searches, library-based screening led to the identification of NLP-12a and NLP-12b as the endogenous ligands of CKR-2a/b. Alignment of these peptides to vertebrate CCK/gastrin hormones and arthropod sulfakinins revealed their similarity. The endogenous ligand of GNRR-1a was found using an *in silico* approach. GNRR-1a and its ligand, NLP-47, are both involved in reproduction as shown by RNAi experiments (Lindemans et al., 2009a). The VP/OT-like receptor NTR-1 has only recently been identified and deorphanized. The VP/OT-related signaling system is involved in gustatory associative learning and male reproduction (Beets et al., 2012; Garrison et al., 2012). The group of neurotensin, neuromedin U (NMU), growth hormone secretagogue, and thyrotropin releasing hormone (TRH)-like receptors contains 17 receptors, of which three have been deorphanized: NMUR-2 and EGL-6a/b. Only the EGL-6a/b receptors are functionally characterized and they proved to be involved in the regulation of egg-laying (Ringstad and Horvitz, 2008). The secretin family of GPCRs contains nine receptors. Of these, the three pigment dispersing factor (PDF) GPCRs are deorphanized and play a role in locomotion and egg-laying (Janssen et al., 2008a; Meelkop et al., 2012).

G PROTEIN SIGNALING IN *C. ELEGANS*

G protein-coupled signaling pathways are highly conserved among *C. elegans* and mammals. In the classical G protein signaling pathway (**Figure 1**), the inactive receptor is bound to the heterotrimeric $G\alpha\beta\gamma$ protein. Upon binding of an activating ligand, the receptor changes its confirmation and acts as a guanine nucleotide exchange factor (GEF) by catalyzing the release of GDP and binding of GTP by the $G\alpha$ subunit. The now activated heterotrimeric $G\alpha\beta\gamma$ protein dissociates from the receptor and splits into a $G\alpha$-GTP and a $G\beta\gamma$ subunit. $G\alpha$-GTP regulates different effectors depending on the $G\alpha$ subtype ($G\alpha_s$, $G\alpha_{i/o}$, $G\alpha_q$, and $G\alpha_{12/13}$). $G\alpha_q$ is known for its activation of phospholipase $C\beta$ ($PLC\beta$), which splits phosphatidylinositol 4,5-bisphosphate (PIP2) into diacylglycerol (DAG) and inositol-1,4,5-trisphosphate (IP3). Binding of IP3 to IP3 dependent calcium channels leads to an increase in calcium, and DAG will bind and activate protein kinase C (PKC). $G\alpha_s$ and $G\alpha_{i/o}$ act through adenylyl cyclase by stimulating ($G\alpha_s$) or inhibiting ($G\alpha_{i/o}$) its activity and thereby regulating the concentration of cyclic AMP, which activates protein kinase A (PKA). $G\alpha_{12/13}$ activates Rho dependent pathways. The $G\beta\gamma$ subunit also regulates certain downstream effectors such as ion channels and

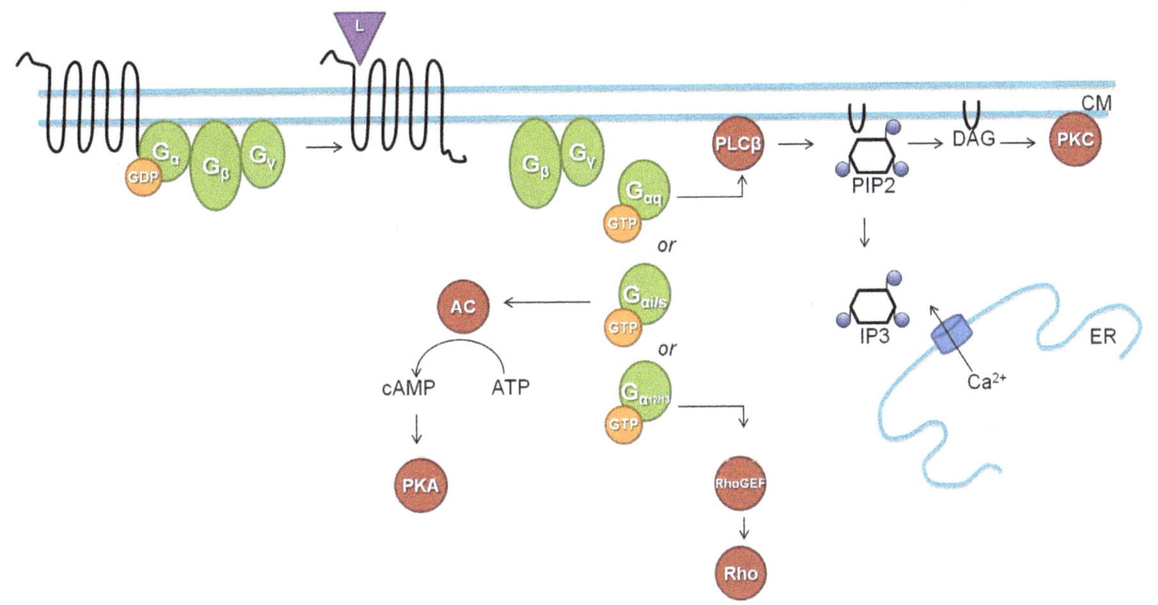

FIGURE 1 | The classical G protein signaling pathway (L, ligand; CM, cell membrane; GDP, guanosine diphosphate; GTP, guanosine triphosphate; AC, adenylate cyclase; cAMP, cyclic adenosine monophosphate; ATP, adenosine triphosphate; PKA, protein kinase A; PLCβ, phospholipase Cβ; PIP2, phosphatidylinositol 4,5-bisphosphate; DAG, diacylglycerol; IP3, inositol-1,4,5-trisphosphate; ER, endoplasmic reticulum; PKC, protein kinase C; GEF, guanine nucleotide exchange factor).

PLCβ. G protein signaling is terminated by internalization of the GPCR, which is initiated by phosphorylation through GPCR kinases (GRKs; Ritter and Hall, 2009).

C. elegans has homologs for most of the above described G proteins and downstream second messengers. The worm has 21 Gα, 2 Gβ (GPB-1 and GPB-2), and 2 Gγ (GPC-1 and GPC-2) proteins. GPB-1 and GPC-2 seem to be mediators in the classical G protein signaling as the homologs of Gβ and Gγ respectively. For each of the four mammalian Gα subtypes there is a homologous Gα protein in *C. elegans* [GSA-1 ($G\alpha_s$), GOA-1 ($G\alpha_{i/o}$), EGL-30 ($G\alpha_q$), and GPA-12 ($G\alpha_{12/13}$)]. The remaining *C. elegans* Gα subtypes are believed to be specific for chemosensory GPCRs (Jansen et al., 1999; Bastiani and Mendel, 2006). EGL-30 and GSA-1 are the only Gα proteins for which the conservation of their downstream targets has been demonstrated. The classical role of the EGL-30 $G\alpha_q$ protein is intensively studied in neuromuscular junctions where it stimulates the release of the neurotransmitter ACh. EGL-30 binds and activates EGL-8, the PLCβ homolog, which splits PIP2 into IP3 and DAG. In neuromuscular junctions, DAG binds to UNC-13 which regulates synaptic vesicle release of ACh through syntaxin (Lackner et al., 1999). IP3 on the other hand can bind to the IP3 dependent calcium channel ITR-1 which leads to a calcium response (Bastiani et al., 2003; Baylis and Vázquez-Manrique, 2012). The $G\alpha_s$ protein homolog GSA-1 seems to function through the adenylate cyclase ACY-1. GSA-1 is an essential protein but constitutive activation of GSA-1 in the presence of ACY-1 causes neurodegeneration (Korswagen et al., 1997; Berger et al., 1998). Constitutive expression of rat $G\alpha_s$ correspondingly causes the same neurodegenerative phenotype.

FINDING NEUROPEPTIDE LIGANDS FOR ORPHAN GPCRs

To find the activating ligand(s) of a GPCR, a reverse pharmacology approach can be applied. In this approach, the orphan GPCR is expressed in a heterologous expression system. Often Chinese hamster ovary (CHO) or human embryonic kidney (HEK) cells are the recombinant systems of choice because of their ease of use and proven history of functional GPCR expression (Szekeres, 2002). Subsequently, receptor expressing cells are challenged with a library of compounds and activation of the GPCR of interest is measured. The compound library is usually compiled based on bioinformatic predictions and peptidomic analyses of RP-HPLC fractions of a tissue extract (Beets et al., 2011). In the past few years, several successful strategies have been developed for receptor deorphanization (Mertens et al., 2004; Beets et al., 2011). One of the most frequently used methods is probably the calcium mobilization assay based on the detection of intracellular calcium that is released from storage sites upon receptor activation. This method is often combined with the co-expression of a promiscuous G protein, such as the $G\alpha_{16}$ subunit, which can direct the intracellular signaling cascade of the activated receptor through a calcium flux (Offermanns and Simon, 1995). Alternatively, chimeric G proteins can be used to lead the signal cascade to a pathway of choice (Milligan and Rees, 1999). The resulting calcium flux can then be detected by bioluminescent proteins such as aequorin, or by fluorescent calcium indicators (e.g., Fluo-4). In the bioluminescent assay, cells expressing the apoaequorin protein are charged prior to the assay with the cofactor coelenterazine to form a calcium-sensitive aquorin complex. When calcium binds to aequorin, the complex is oxidized and blue light is omitted. Similar to the luminescence assay, receptor expressing cells can be loaded with a fluorophore, of which the fluorescence increases upon binding of calcium (Mertens et al., 2004). Thanks to the development of automated systems for simultaneous compound addition and signal detection in various well-plate formats, such as the FLEXstation® (Molecular Devices, CA, USA) fluorescent plate reader, calcium mobilization methods can be used in high-throughput screening assays. Once the activating ligand(s) of a receptor are found, the endogenous Gα signaling protein is identified by omitting the promiscuous $G\alpha_{16}$ protein. Coupling of a receptor with $G\alpha_q$, $G\alpha_s$, or $G\alpha_i$ can be visualized by respectively measuring the calcium increase or cAMP in-/decrease.

CHARACTERIZED NEUROPEPTIDERGIC SIGNALING PATHWAYS

NPR-1 SIGNALING: INHIBITION OF AGGREGATION AND AEROTAXIS

The neuropeptide receptor 1 (NPR-1) was the first neuropeptide GPCR to be deorphanized in *C. elegans* (Kubiak et al., 2003; Rogers et al., 2003). This receptor shows homology to the vertebrate NPY receptor family that is implicated in a variety of physiological processes such as food intake and stress (Heilig, 2004; Arora and Anubhuti, 2006). In the nematode *C. elegans*, NPR-1 is involved in a multitude of functions such as food-dependent behaviors, thermal avoidance, ethanol tolerance, and innate immunity (de Bono and Bargmann, 1998; Davies et al., 2004; Gray et al., 2004; Cheung et al., 2005; Rogers et al., 2006; Gloria-Soria and Azevedo, 2008; Styer et al., 2008; Glauser et al., 2011; Milward et al., 2011; Jang et al., 2012).

The most explicit function of NPR-1 was elucidated with the observation of aggregating and solitary feeders in wild type isolates of *C. elegans* (de Bono and Bargmann, 1998). This behavioral difference could be attributed to a single amino acid difference. Aggregating isolates carry an *npr-1* Phe-215 allele whereas solitary feeders possess an *npr-1* Val-215 allele. Since a functional null mutation of *npr-1* converts the solitary wild type N2 lab strain into an aggregating one, NPR-1 activity is suggested to suppress aggregating behavior. The RMG inter/motor neuron seems to be the cellular hub of this NPR-1 mediated feeding behavior, as demonstrated by the full rescue of the solitary behavior through RMG-specific expression of NPR-1 in an *npr-1* knockout mutant (Macosko et al., 2009). The RMG neuron is the hub of a gap junction network that connects five sensory neurons which are known to trigger aggregation, while NPR-1 inhibits this gap junction driven activation of RMG (**Figure 2**).

Reduced NPR-1 activity in the RMG-hub-and-spoke circuit also contributes to thermal avoidance and sex-specific pheromone responses in *C. elegans*. Deletion of the NPR-1 receptor increases the threshold for heat avoidance, and cell-specific rescue of *npr-1* demonstrates the role of the RMG interneuron in the regulation of heat avoidance behavior (Glauser et al., 2011). Similarly, RMG-specific rescue of *npr-1* restores pheromone avoidance defects in the *npr-1* mutant background (Jang et al., 2012). Therefore, the RMG neural network can be considered a multifunctional sensory circuit that uses neuropeptide GPCR signaling amongst others to coordinate behavioral output.

In insects and mollusks FaRPs are reported as ligands for NPR-1-like receptors (Tensen et al., 1998; Feng et al., 2003). In 2003, two independent groups were able to deorphanize the NPR-1 receptor by using *C. elegans* and other invertebrate FaRPs. Both FLP-21 and FLP-18 peptides activated the solitary Val-215 receptor. The social Phe-215 receptor variant could only be activated by FLP-21. NPR-1 signaling occurs through a $G\alpha_{i/o}$ type of G protein (Kubiak et al., 2003; Rogers et al., 2003). Deorphanization of the NPR-1 receptor supports its role in repressing aggregation, since the solitary Val-215 receptor variant displayed higher binding and functional activity than the Phe-215 receptor variant.

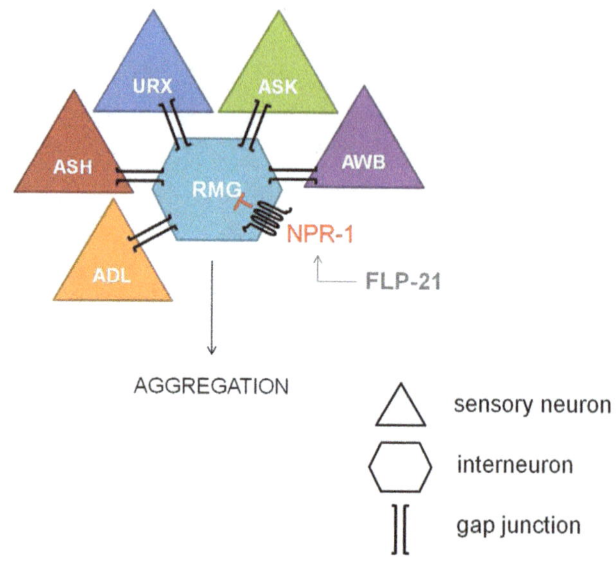

FIGURE 2 | Inhibiton of the RMG inter/motor neuron by NPR-1. The RMG neuron is the hub of a gap junction network connecting the ADL, ASH, URX, ASK, and AWB sensory neurons, which are known to trigger aggregation. NPR-1 inhibits this gap junction driven activation of RMG (figure adapted from Macosko et al., 2009).

Besides its role in feeding behavior, NPR-1 also regulates aerotaxis (**Figure 3**). *C. elegans* exhibits a strong behavioral preference for 5–12% oxygen, avoiding higher and lower oxygen levels. Oxygen levels are sensed by the URX, PQR, AQR, and SDQ neurons (Gray et al., 2004). Oxygen sensing in these neurons is mediated by soluble guanylate cyclase homologs (GCY-35 and GCY-36). When ambient oxygen levels decrease, cGMP levels rise and the cGMP gated TAX-2/TAX-4 ion channel opens, leading to the depolarization of the neurons. Activation of NPR-1 in the presence of food inhibits the activation of these neurons (Cheung et al., 2005; Chang et al., 2006; Rogers et al., 2006). Oxygen binding globins such as GLB-5 further tune the behavioral responses to varying oxygen concentrations, and this effect is again modified by the NPR-1 receptor (Persson et al., 2009). In addition, it has also been shown that the NPR-1 expressing neurons AQR, PQR, and URX contribute to the enhancement of the worm's sensory perception under hypoxic conditions (Pocock and Hobert, 2010). PQR, AQR, and URX were recently reported to act as tonic receptors that cause long-lasting changes in neural circuit activity that sets *C. elegans* behavior according to ambient oxygen concentrations (Busch et al., 2012), which is also reflected in optimal foraging strategies (Milward et al., 2011). A Ca^{2+} relay involving the L-type voltage-gated Ca^{2+} channel subunit EGL-19, the ryanodine receptor UNC-68, and the inositol-1-4,5-trisphosphate receptor

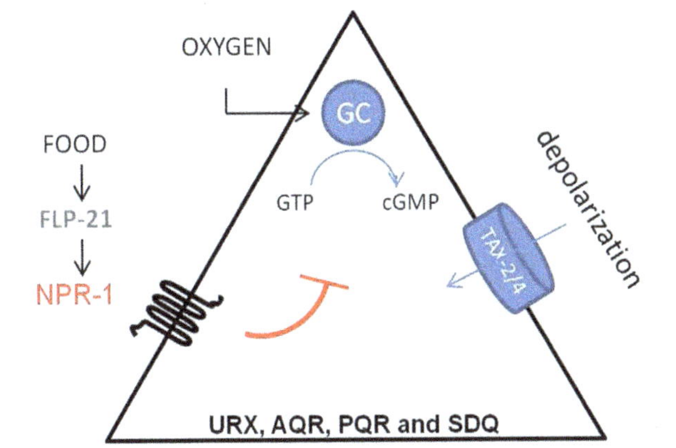

FIGURE 3 | Regulation of aerotaxis by NPR-1. *C. elegans* detects oxygen through the URX, PQR, AQR, SDQ neurons. Oxygen sensing in these neurons is mediated by soluble guanylate cyclase homologs (sGC-35 and sGC-36). When ambient oxygen levels decrease, cGMP levels rise and the cGMP gated TAX-2/TAX-4 ion channel opens, which leads to the depolarization of the neurons. Activation of NPR-1 in the presence of food inhibits this activation (Cheung et al., 2005; Chang et al., 2006).

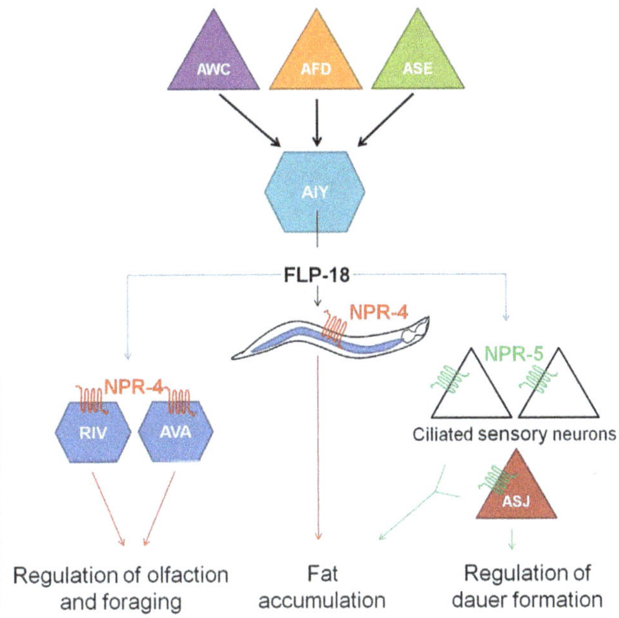

FIGURE 4 | Hypothetical model in which the detection of nutrition by sensory neurons (AWC, AFD, and ASE) is coupled to the release of FLP-18 neuropeptides from AIY interneurons and subsequent signaling through the RFamide-like receptors NPR-4 and NPR-5. By acting on NPR-4 in the intestine and NPR-5 in ciliated neurons, FLP-18 neuropeptides control fat storage. Signaling through NPR-4 in RIV and AVA neurons also modulates responses to odor and foraging behavior. Another food-dependent decision, dauer formation, is regulated by FLP-18 action on NPR-5 in the ASJ neurons (figure adapted from Cohen et al., 2009).

ITR-1 mediate tonic signaling from AQR, PQR, and URX, evoking continuous neuropeptide release.

The role of NPR-1 in the worm's innate immunity was elucidated by Styer et al. (2008), who uncovered an immune inhibitory function for this receptor. Mutations in the *npr-1* gene directly affect the expression of innate immunity markers, suggesting that neuropeptide GPCRs participate in the neuronal regulation of immune responses. In addition, polymorphisms in the *npr-1* gene have been correlated with the worm's pathogen avoidance and susceptibility (Aballay, 2009; Reddy et al., 2009, 2011).

RFAMIDE-LIKE RECEPTOR SIGNALING: FLP-18 SIGNALING THROUGH NPR-4 AND NPR-5

Both a reverse pharmacology study expressing orphan receptors in CHO cells and an independent *Xenopus laevis* oocyte assay demonstrated that the *flp-18*-encoded peptides are the most potent ligands of NPR-5a and NPR-5b, the splice variants of *npr-5* (Kubiak et al., 2008; Cohen et al., 2009). The latter study also showed that another member of the GPCR rhodopsin family, NPR-4, is also activated by FLP-18 peptides (Cohen et al., 2009), which in addition to their activation of NPR-1 (Kubiak et al., 2003) indicates these are widely deployed ligands of GPCRs. NPR-5a and NPR-5b seem to transduce the FLP-18 signal mainly through a $G\alpha_q$ type G protein, while NPR-4 might use a different cellular signaling machinery.

flp-18(db99) loss-of-function mutants display chemosensory, dauer formation, and foraging defects, accumulate excess intestinal fat and exhibit reduced aerobic metabolism. Distinct subsets of these phenotypes are phenocopied by *npr-4(tm1782)* and *npr-5(ok1583)* deletion mutants. Each one of the FLP-18 receptors regulates fat metabolism in response to the release of FLP-18 peptides from AIY and RIG interneurons in the head, some of the multiple expression sites of *flp-18*. NPR-4 mediated regulation of intestinal fat occurs at the level of the gut, while NPR-5 modulates the activity of a number of amphid sensory neurons. FLP-18 neurohormones released from AIY interneurons act on NPR-4 in AVA and RIV interneurons and appear to be implicated in odor responses and foraging behavior. The chemosensory ASJ neurons regulate dauer formation through activation of NPR-5. All of these observations led to the proposition of a model (**Figure 4**) in which sensory detection of nutritional availability is coupled to adequate responses such as foraging behavior and metabolic alterations via RFamide-like receptor signaling (Cohen et al., 2009).

OFF-FOOD SEARCH BEHAVIOR: FEEDBACK SIGNALING THROUGH NPR-11

Characterization of the neuropeptide GPCR NPR-11 is a good example of how the knowledge of the entire neuronal wiring diagram makes *C. elegans* a favorable model organism. When worms are removed from a food source, they display a local search behavior characterized by increased turning rates during the first 15 min. This behavior is known to depend on the activity of the AWC olfactory neurons, which release both glutamate and the neuropeptide NLP-1. Glutamate is necessary for increased turning rates during the off-food search behavior of the worm, a behavioral change that is also observed in knockout mutants of *nlp-1*. In glutamate-depleted mutants no increase is noticed, suggesting that NLP-1 acts as a co-transmitter for glutamate by decreasing its effect (Chalasani et al., 2010).

To identify the receptor through which NLP-1 is signaling, Chalasani et al. (2010) looked for orphan GPCRs expressed in neurons that are connected to the AWC sensory neurons. A knockout mutation of NPR-11, resulted in a similar phenotype as displayed by the *nlp-1* mutant. A calcium based assay confirmed the NLP-1/NPR-1 interaction.

Comparison of the calcium response of AWC neurons during the local search behavior upon food removal suggested that NPR-11 activation by NLP-1 evokes a negative feedback loop which dampens AWC activity (**Figure 5**). NPR-1 is expressed in the AIA interneurons which also express the insulin-like peptide INS-1. Indeed, an *ins-1* mutant shows the same increase in turning rates upon food removal as the *nlp-1* and *npr-11* mutants. Calcium imaging of the AWC neurons could confirm the role of INS-1 as a suppressor of AWC activity (Chalasani et al., 2010).

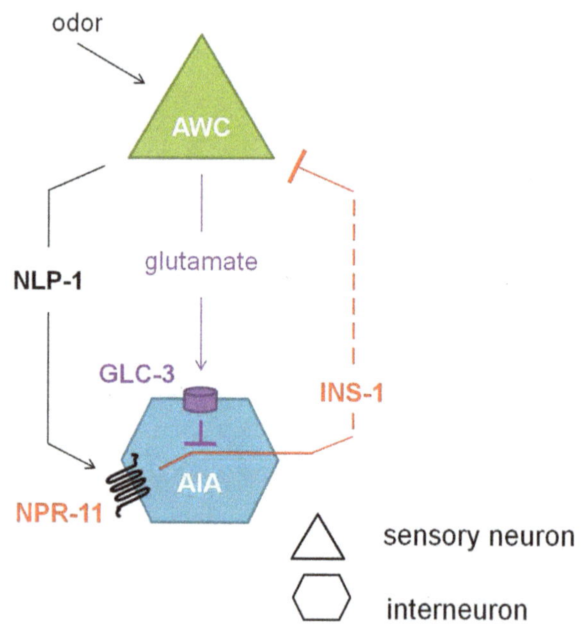

FIGURE 5 | Neuropeptide feedback regulation of the AWC sensory neurons. The AIA interneurons are inhibited via the glutamate-gated chloride channel GLC-3 upon release of the neurotransmitter glutamate from the AWC neurons. Alternatively, when odor is sensed, the AWC neurons release NLP-1, which in turn activates NPR-11 on the AIA interneurons. Upon activation of NPR-11, INS-1 is released, inhibiting AWC activity and thereby reducing its inhibition on AIA (adapted from Chalasani et al., 2010).

CONSERVATION OF GnRH SIGNALING

Gonadotropin releasing hormone is mainly known for its role in reproduction in vertebrates (Kah et al., 2007). The GnRH receptor and its ligand are highly conserved in vertebrates and homologs of the receptor are predicted in a variety of invertebrates (Roch et al., 2011). Remarkably, insect GnRH receptor orthologs are activated by adipokinetic hormone (AKH), corazonin, and AKH/corazonin-related peptide (ACP), which are known to be involved in energy metabolism, pigmentation, and cardiac regulation (Park et al., 2002; Staubli et al., 2002; Hansen et al., 2010; Lindemans et al., 2011; Roch et al., 2011). The genome of *C. elegans* is predicted to encode for a family of eight GnRH-related receptor genes (*gnrr-1* to *gnrr-8*). Only one of these receptors (GNRR-1, isoform a) has been deorphanized (Lindemans et al., 2009a). Since *Drosophila melanogaster* AKH (*Dm*-AKH) was capable of activating this receptor, the authors performed an *in silico* search for an AKH-GnRH-like peptide in *C. elegans*. This way, they were able to identify the decapeptide NLP-47 (pQMTFTDQWT) as the endogenous ligand for GNRR-1a ($EC_{50} = 150$ nM; Lindemans et al., 2009a). AKH is known to regulate lipid mobilization during flight in insects (Gäde and Auerwald, 2003). Fat contents were examined by performing an RNAi knockdown of *gnrr-1* and/or *nlp-47*. Unfortunately, no significant differences between knockdowns and wild type were observed (Lindemans et al., 2009a). Nevertheless, injection of synthetic *Ce*-AKH-GnRH into the cockroach *Periplaneta americana* resulted in a significant increase in the levels of hemolymph carbohydrates. A delay in egg-laying could be observed after both *gnrr-1* and *nlp-47* knockdown (Lindemans et al., 2009a). The identification of an AKH-GNRH-like signaling system involved in reproduction is an interesting finding and could be a key to the interplay between reproduction and energy metabolism.

Since no clear ortholog for GnRH was found in insects and nematodes, it was proposed that GnRH has been preserved in lophotrochozoans, but lost in the ecdysozoans (Tsai and Zhang, 2008). Nevertheless, phylogenetic analysis of the ligands of the ecdysozoan GnRH receptors suggests that AKH and corazonin share a common ancestor with GnRH (Lindemans et al., 2011; Roch et al., 2011).

THE NMU-LIKE SIGNALING PATHWAY

In vertebrates, NMU is a highly conserved neuropeptide that plays a fundamental role in key physiological processes such as smooth muscle contraction, regulation of blood pressure, feeding and energy homeostasis, stress responses, and immune regulation (Brighton et al., 2004). All NMU peptides isolated in vertebrates have an identical C-terminal pentapeptide (FRPRNamide; Brighton et al., 2004). The presence of an NMU-like receptor in invertebrates was first reported for the fruitfly *D. melanogaster*. The fruitfly genome encodes four NMU receptor homologs. These receptors are activated by pyrokinin neuropeptides (PRXamide) and are involved in many functions such as feeding behavior and visceral muscle contraction (Schoofs et al., 1993; Park et al., 2002; Melcher and Pankratz, 2005).

The *C. elegans* genome encodes four NMU receptor homologs. To date, only NMUR-1 has an assigned phenotype. Wild type *C. elegans* display an altered lifespan depending on the type of food source they live on. In 2010, NMUR-1 was demonstrated to be involved in this food source dependent regulation of lifespan (Maier et al., 2010). So far, the activating ligand of NMUR-1 has not yet been identified. In contrast, though still a receptor of unknown function, NMUR-2 has recently been deorphanized based on an *in silico* search for *C. elegans* homologs of the *Drosophila* pyrokinin peptides. This revealed three putative PRXamide peptides, all encoded by the same peptide precursor gene *nlp-44*. Only one of these peptides, AFFYTPRI-NH2, could activate NMUR-2 (Lindemans et al., 2009b).

PDF-LIKE SIGNALING: LOCOMOTION AND REPRODUCTION

In *C. elegans*, the G protein-coupled PDF receptors of the secretin receptor family PDFR-1a, b, c, d, and e represent five splice isoforms of *pdfr-1* (Janssen et al., 2008a; Barrios et al., 2012). Their endogenous neuropeptide ligands PDF-1a, PDF-1b, and PDF-2, encoded by *pdf-1* and *pdf-2*, are all of the NLP-type. All three PDF peptides are able to bind PDFR-1a, b and c; though with significant differences in affinity (Janssen et al., 2008a). PDFR-1a and PDFR-1b signaling occurs via a $G\alpha_s$ type of G protein, while PDFR-1c signaling occurs through a $G\alpha_{i/o}$ type of G protein (Janssen et al., 2009). PDFR-1d and e were only recently recovered from cDNA (Barrios et al., 2012), and have not yet been characterized in detail. The PDF-like neuropeptide pathway is highly conserved in nematodes, and PDF neuropeptides are also found in insects and crustaceans. In the latter, they were initially discovered and named pigment dispersing hormones (PDHs; Rao and Riehm, 1993; Janssen et al., 2009; Meelkop et al., 2011; Temmerman et al., 2011). Furthermore, all three *C. elegans* PDF receptors are closely related to insect orthologs, such as the *D. melanogaster* PDF receptor, and are distantly related to the vertebrate calcitonin GPCRs and vasoactive intestinal peptide (VIP) receptors (Janssen et al., 2008a). In *C. elegans*, the *pdfr-1* gene is expressed in every body wall muscle cell and, like *pdf-1* and *pdf-2*, in neuronal cells that are involved in the sensing and integration of environmental stimuli and the control of locomotion (Janssen et al., 2008a, 2009).

So far, functional characterization reveals that the PDF signaling system of *C. elegans* is involved in both locomotion and egg-laying, which stresses the pleiotropic nature of its biological functions. The *pdf-1(tm1996)* loss-of-function mutant shows locomotion defects by moving slower and executing more reversals than wild type worms. This locomotion phenotype is recapitulated by the overexpression of PDF-2 (Janssen et al., 2008a). *pdf-2 (tm4393)* deletion mutants conduct fewer backward/forward transitions than wild type animals, suggesting that PDF-1 and PDF-2 neuropeptides exert antagonistic effects on locomotion via PDFR-1. Furthermore, the PDF receptor loss-of-function mutant *pdfr-1(lst34)* turned out to have similar locomotion defects as the *pdf-1(tm1996)* mutant. Three splice variants of *pdfr-1* (a, b, c) were proven to be involved in the regulation of locomotion (Meelkop et al., 2012). The PDF system is also implicated in reproduction, as the timing of egg-laying appears to be delayed in *C. elegans pdf-1(tm1996)*, *pdf-2(tm4393)*, and *pdf-2(tm4780)* deletion mutants (Meelkop et al., 2012). The b and d isoforms could rescue a male-specific defect in mate-searching behavior. This defect is mediated through PDF-1 peptides, but not PDF-2; and seems to be needed in gender-shared neurons for the regulation of this sex-specific behavior (Barrios et al., 2012). Functions for PDF signaling in locomotion and reproduction have been demonstrated in other invertebrate species as well (Renn et al., 1999; Helfrich-Forster et al., 2000; Hamanaka et al., 2005). Recently, proteomic analysis proposed the involvement of PDF signaling in lipid metabolism and stress resistance (Temmerman et al., 2012).

THE CCK/GASTRIN-LIKE SIGNALING SYSTEM: FOOD METABOLISM

Cholecystokinin and gastrin are well-characterized peptide hormones in vertebrates. By acting on two conserved GPCRs, CCK1R, and CCK2R; they are implicated in a variety of digestive functions including the stimulation of digestive enzyme production, intestinal motility, and the promotion of satiety in order to regulate food intake (Konturek et al., 2003; Dufresne et al., 2006; Clerc et al., 2007). In arthropods, the sulfakinin (SK) family of neuropeptides is both structurally and functionally related to the well-conserved vertebrate CCK and gastrin peptides (Schoofs and Nachman, 2006). A Basic Local Alignment Search Tool (BLAST) analysis of the *C. elegans* genome revealed *ckr-1* and *ckr-2* as the homologous genes of the vertebrate CCK/gastrin receptors and their SK counterparts in insects (Kubiak et al., 2002; Meeusen et al., 2003; McKay et al., 2007). The *ckr-2* gene encodes two splice isoform receptors, CKR-2a and CKR-2b, which belong to the rhodopsin GPCR family. By use of a reverse pharmacology approach, the endogenous *C. elegans* NLP-12a and NLP-12b neuropeptides – encoded by the *nlp-12* gene – were appointed the CCK/gastrin-like ligands of CKR-2a and CKR-2b (Janssen et al., 2008b). Signaling of the CCK receptors occurs through a $G\alpha_q$ type of G protein. The *nlp-12* gene is expressed in a single tail neuron, identified as DVA, while *ckr-2* is expressed in cholinergic and GABAergic motor neurons (Janssen et al., 2008b; Hu et al., 2011).

The *C. elegans ckr-2(tm3082)* receptor mutant displays decreased intestinal amylase activity/secretion relative to wild type worms, suggesting the involvement of CKR-2 signaling in the stimulation of digestive enzyme secretion. The CCK/gastrin signaling system also appears to be involved in the control of fat storage since *ckr-2(tm3082)* as well as *nlp-12(ok335)* deletion mutants show an increased fat content compared to wild type animals (Janssen et al., 2008b). Both observations are in accordance with the functions attributed to the CCK/gastrin signaling system in vertebrates and the SK signaling system in arthropods. Recently, Hu et al. (2011) suggested a mechanosensory feedback loop (**Figure 6**) for proprioceptive control of normal locomotion, whereby muscle contraction aids the secretion of NLP-12 by the stretch-activated DVA neuron. Subsequent signaling of NLP-12 through CKR-2 enhances presynaptic ACh release to potentiate transmission at neuromuscular junctions and as such adjust the pattern of locomotion. Correspondingly, a significantly reduced locomotion rate was observed for both the *ckr-2(tm3082)* and *nlp-12(ok335)* mutants compared to wild type worm.

AN FaRP SIGNALING PATHWAY INVOLVED IN EGG-LAYING BEHAVIOR

The *egl-6* gene encodes two GPCR isoforms that are both involved in the inhibition of egg-laying. In comparison with wild type, *egl-6(n592)* and *egl-6* overexpression mutants display slower egg-laying rates and longer retention of embryos. Allele *n592* appeared to be a gain-of-function mutation in *egl-6*, increasing its inhibiting activity (Ringstad and Horvitz, 2008). Similar to NPR-11, ligands for EGL-6 were first suggested by looking at neuropeptides displaying the defective egg-laying phenotype of *egl-6* overexpression when they are overexpressed in wild type worms but not in *egl-6* deletion mutants. This way, *flp-10* and *flp-17* turned out to encode for the ligands of EGL-6. In addition, a *Xenopus laevis* oocyte assay demonstrated that FLP-10, FLP-17-1, and FLP-17-2 were able to unambiguously activate the EGL-6 GPCR at nanomolar concentrations (Ringstad and Horvitz, 2008). These FaRPs signal from multiple cell types via EGL-6 in a $G\alpha_{i/o}$-dependent manner to inhibit egg-laying (**Figure 7**). In response to environmental cues, FLP-17 neurohormones are principally expressed in BAG sensory neurons and thought to modulate egg-laying behavior by acting

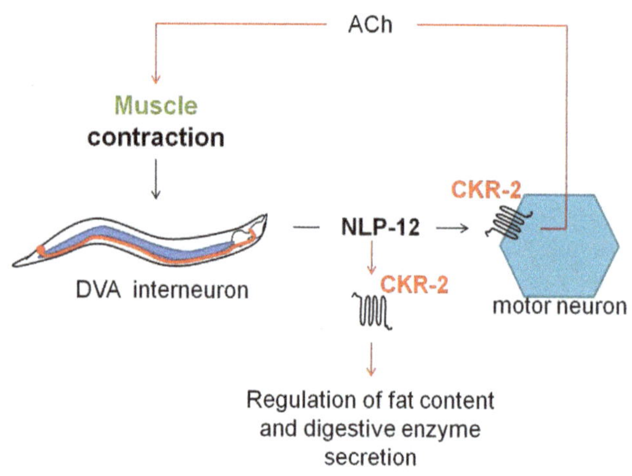

FIGURE 6 | Upon muscle contraction, NLP-12 neuropeptides are released by a single tail neuron, DVA. Subsequent activation of the NLP-12 receptor, CKR-2, potentiates transmission at cholinergic neuromuscular junctions, thereby providing a mechanism for proprioceptive control of locomotion (Hu et al., 2011). NLP-12 signaling through CKR-2 also appears to be involved in the regulation of fat storage and digestive enzyme production (Janssen et al., 2008b).

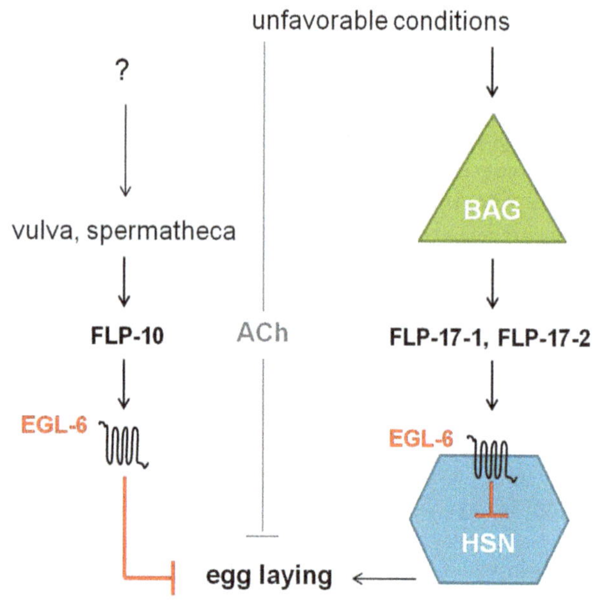

FIGURE 7 | Unfavorable conditions cause the release of FLP-17 neuropeptides from BAG neurons. These neurohormones activate EGL-6 in HSN neurons in order to inhibit egg-laying. Release of FLP-10 by the vulva and spermatheca along with subsequent signaling via EGL-6 also inhibits egg-laying. How parts of the hermaphrodite's reproductive system might inhibit egg-laying is not yet fully understood. In parallel to peptidergic inhibition, cholinergic signals inhibit egg-laying upon unfavorable conditions (Ringstad and Horvitz, 2008).

on EGL-6 in HSN motor neurons. The latter neurons are known to stimulate the action of vulval muscles and are involved in egg-laying (Trent et al., 1983; White et al., 1986). The non-neuronal expression of FLP-10 peptides in parts of the hermaphrodite's reproductive system also inhibits egg-laying (Kim and Li, 2004; Ringstad and Horvitz, 2008). Upon unfavorable conditions, signaling through ACh also inhibits egg-laying in parallel to the aforementioned peptidergic inhibition (Ringstad and Horvitz, 2008).

VP/OT SIGNALING: GUSTATORY ASSOCIATIVE LEARNING AND REPRODUCTION

Recently, a VP/OT-related signaling system has been identified in *C. elegans*. In mammals, this system is involved in a plethora of peripheral hormonal functions including water homeostasis, reproduction, and stress responses (van Kesteren et al., 1995; Aikins et al., 2008). These neuropeptides also function as neuromodulators in the central nervous system influencing social cognition and behavior, memory and learning (de Wied et al., 1993; Young and Wang, 2004; Meyer-Lindenberg et al., 2011). In the roundworm, a single VP/OT-like peptide, named nematocin (NTC-1), and two nematocin receptors (NTR-1 and NTR-2) are identified. The NTR-1 receptor is activated by the nematocin peptide in a dose-dependent way. On the other hand, the NTR-2 receptor is not directly activated by NTC-1 but co-expression of NTR-1 and NTR-2 is suggested to affect the intracellular levels of cAMP upon nematocin binding (Beets et al., 2012; Garrison et al., 2012).

In hermaphrodites, the *ntc-1* gene is mainly expressed in the DVA and AVK neurons. Since *ntr-1* is expressed in the left ASE (ASEL) gustatory neurons, the ASH and ADF chemosensory neurons, which function in chemotaxis toward water-soluble cues, Beets et al. (2012) studied the salt chemotaxis behavior of *ntc-1* and *ntr-1* mutants. Similar to wild type worms, *ntc-1* and *ntr-1* mutants are attracted to low NaCl concentrations. When pre-exposed to these low NaCl concentrations in the absence of food, wild type worms show reduced attraction to or avoidance of NaCl, a behavioral switch termed gustatory plasticity (Hukema et al., 2008). However, the aversive response of pre-exposed worms is reduced in *ntc-1* and *ntr-1* mutants. These results indicate that nematocin signaling is implicated in gustatory associative learning, similar to the effects of VP and OT on mammalian cognition. Moreover, AVK-specific expression of *ntc-1* and ASEL-specific expression of *ntr-1* in the *ntc-1* and *ntr-1* mutant background, respectively, partially restored gustatory plasticity. Genetic analysis and supplementation studies indicated that the TRPV channel protein OSM-9, the Gγ-subunit GPC-1 and serotonin and dopamine signaling interact with the nematocin pathway in regulating gustatory plasticity (Beets et al., 2012).

ntc-1, *ntr-1*, and *ntr-2* are expressed in sexually dimorphic patterns and have been shown to function in male mating behavior. *ntc-1*, *ntr-1*, and *ntr-2* mutant males perform poorly in several types of mating behaviors compared with wild type worms. Mutations in the NTR-1 and NTR-2 receptor cause partly overlapping defects in the mating response. Remarkably, cell-specific knockout of nematocin in the mechanosensory DVA neuron, which is not male-specific, seems to be responsible for most of the male mating defects. These findings indicate that nematocin signaling is necessary to coordinate male mating behaviors (Garrison et al., 2012).

CONCLUSION

Despite the simplicity of its nervous system, *C. elegans* displays complex behaviors with a high level of plasticity and striking similarities to the functioning of "higher" nervous systems. The completely defined anatomy and wiring of the worm's nervous system, combined with a rapid life cycle and powerful molecular and genetic tools, have allowed the dissection of neuropeptidergic signaling networks with single cell resolution. As in other animals, neuropeptides in *C elegans* signal through GPCRs. Many predictions have been made about neuropeptide GPCR encoding genes in the *C. elegans* genome. This review brings the number of predicted neuropeptide GPCRs up to 128. High-throughput RNAi and mutagenesis studies of orphan neuropeptide GPCRs in *C. elegans* revealed their involvement in a broad repertoire of behaviors. However, cognate ligands for only 22 of the predicted neuropeptide GPCRs have been identified and only eight of these receptors are functionally characterized. These well-defined neuropeptidergic signaling systems play crucial roles in key physiological processes such as reproduction, locomotion, and lipid metabolism, as well as in social and foraging behaviors. The broad functioning of these neuropeptide GPCRs in nematode physiology emphasizes the pivotal role of neuropeptidergic signaling in *C. elegans*. The development of high-throughput deorphanization systems in combination with an advanced genetic toolbox will allow further functional characterization of neuropeptide GPCRs in *C elegans*, likely increasing our understanding of peptidergic signaling systems in other organisms as well.

ACKNOWLEDGMENTS

The authors acknowledge the Research Foundation Flanders (FWO-Vlaanderen, Belgium, G.0767.09 and G.0601.11) and the KU Leuven Research Foundation GOA/11/002. Isabel Beets, Liesbet Temmerman, Tom Janssen, and Steven J. Husson are research fellows of the FWO-Vlaanderen.

REFERENCES

Aballay, A. (2009). Neural regulation of immunity: role of NPR-1 in pathogen avoidance and regulation of innate immunity. *Cell Cycle* 8, 966–969.

Aikins, M. J., Schooley, D. A., Begum, K., Detheux, M., Beeman, R. W., and Park, Y. (2008). Vasopressin-like peptide and its receptor function in an indirect diuretic signaling pathway in the red flour beetle. *Insect Biochem. Mol. Biol.* 38, 740–748.

Arora, S., and Anubhuti. (2006). Role of neuropeptides in appetite regulation and obesity – a review. *Neuropeptides* 40, 375–401.

Ashrafi, K., Chang, F. Y., Watts, J. L., Fraser, A. G., Kamath, R. S., Ahringer, J., et al. (2003). Genome-wide RNAi analysis of *Caenorhabditis elegans* fat regulatory genes. *Nature* 421, 268–272.

Avery, L. (2010). *Caenorhabditis elegans* behavioral genetics: where are the knobs? *BMC Biol.* 8:69. doi:10.1186/1741-7007-8-69

Bargmann, C. I. (1998). Neurobiology of the *Caenorhabditis elegans* genome. *Science* 282, 2028–2033.

Barrios, A., Ghosh, R., Fang, C., Emmons, S. W., and Barr, M. M. (2012). PDF-1 neuropeptide signaling modulates a neural circuit for mate-searching behavior in *C. elegans*. *Nat. Neurosci.* 15, 1675–7682.

Bastiani, C. A., Gharib, S., Simon, M. I., and Sternberg, P. W. (2003). *Caenorhabditis elegans* Gαq regulates egg-laying behavior via a PLC β-independent and serotonin-dependent signaling pathway and likely functions both in the nervous system and in muscle. *Genetics* 165, 1805–1822.

Bastiani, C. A., and Mendel, J. (2006). "Heterotrimeric G proteins in *C. elegans*," in *WormBook*, ed. The *C. elegans* Research Community, WormBook. doi:10.1895/wormbook.1.75.1. Available at: http://www.wormbook.org

Baylis, H. A., and Vázquez-Manrique, R. P. (2012). Genetic analysis of IP(3) and calcium signalling pathways in *C. elegans*. *Biochim. Biophys. Acta* 1820, 1253–1268.

Beets, I., Janssen, T., Meelkop, E., Temmerman, L., Suetens, N., Rademakers, S., et al. (2012). Vasopressin/oxytocin-related signaling regulates gustatory associative learning in *C. elegans*. *Science* 338, 543–545.

Beets, I., Lindemans, M., Janssen, T., and Verleyen, P. (2011). Deorphanizing G protein-coupled receptors by a calcium mobilization assay. *Methods Mol. Biol.* 789, 377–391.

Bendena, W. G., Boudreau, J. R., Papanicolaou, T., Maltby, M, Tobe, S. S., and Chin-Sang, I. (2008). A *Caenorhabditis elegans* allatostatin/galanin-like receptor NPR-9 inhibits local search behavior in response to feeding cues. *Proc. Natl. Acad. Sci. U.S.A.* 105, 1339–1342.

Berger, J., Hart, C., and Kaplan, J. M. (1998). G alphas-induced neurodegeneration in *Caenorhabditis elegans*. *J. Neurosci.* 18, 2871–2880.

Brenner, S. (1974). The genetics of *Caenorhabditis elegans*. *Genetics* 77, 71–94.

Brighton, P. J., Szekeres, P. G., and Willars, G. B. (2004). Neuromedin U and its receptors: structure, function, and physiological roles. *Pharmacol. Rev.* 56, 231–248.

Brownlee, D. J. A., and Fairweather, I. (1999). Exploring the neurotransmitter labyrinth in nematodes. *Trends Neurosci.* 22, 16–24.

Busch, K. E., Laurent, P., Soltesz, Z., Murphy, R. J., Faivre, O., Hedwig, B., et al. (2012). Tonic signaling from O(2) sensors sets neural circuit activity and behavioral state. *Nat. Neurosci.* 15, 581–591.

Cardoso, J. C., Pinto, V. C., Vieira, F. A., Clark, M. S., and Power, D. M. (2006). Evolution of secretin family GPCR members in the metazoa. *BMC Evol. Biol.* 6:108. doi:10.1186/1471-2148-6-108

Ceron, J., Rual, J. F., Chandra, A., Dupuy, D., Vidal, M., and van den Heuvel, S. (2007). Large-scale RNAi screens identify novel genes that interact with the *C. elegans* retinoblastoma pathway as well as splicing-related components with synMuv B activity. *BMC Dev. Biol.* 7:30. doi:10.1186/1471-213X-7-30

Chalasani, S. H., Kato, S., Albrecht, D. R., Nakagawa, T., Abbott, L. F., and Bargmann, C. I. (2010). Neuropeptide feedback modifies odor-evoked dynamics in *Caenorhabditis elegans* olfactory neurons. *Nat. Neurosci.* 13, 615–621.

Chang, A. J., Chronis, N., Karow, D. S., Marletta, M. A., and Bargmann, C. I. (2006). A distributed chemosensory circuit for oxygen preference in *C. elegans*. *PLoS Biol.* 4:e274. doi:10.1371/journal.pbio.0040274

Cheung, B. H. H., Cohen, M., Rogers, C., Albayram, O., and de Bono, M. (2005). Experience-dependent modulation of *C. elegans* behavior by ambient oxygen. *Curr. Biol.* 15, 905–917.

Clerc, P., Coll Constans, M. G., Lulka, H., Broussaud, S., Guigne, C., Leung-Theung-Long, S., et al. (2007). Involvement of cholecystokinin 2 receptor in food intake regulation: hyperphagia and increased fat deposition in cholecystokinin 2 receptor-deficient mice. *Endocrinology* 148, 1039–1049.

Cohen, M., Reale, V., Olofsson, B., Knights, A., Evans, P., and de Bono, M. (2009). Coordinated regulation of foraging and metabolism in *C. elegans* by RFamide neuropeptide signaling. *Cell Metabolism* 9, 375–385.

Davies, A. G., Bettinger, J. C., Thiele, T. R., Judy, M. E., and McIntire, S. L. (2004). Natural variation in the npr-1 gene modifies ethanol responses of wild strains of *C. elegans*. *Neuron* 42, 731–743.

de Bono, M., and Bargmann, C. I. (1998). Natural variation in a neuropeptide Y receptor homolog modifies social behavior and food response in *C. elegans*. *Cell* 94, 679–689.

de Wied, D., Diamant, M., and Fodor, M. (1993). Central nervous system effects of the neurohypophyseal hormones and related peptides. *Front. Neuroendocrinol.* 14, 251–302.

Dufresne, M., Seva, C., and Fourmy, D. (2006). Cholecystokinin and gastrin receptors. *Physiol. Rev.* 86, 805–847.

Feng, G., Reale, V., Chatwin, H., Kennedy, K., Venard, R., Ericsson, C., et al. (2003). Functional characterization of a neuropeptide F-like receptor from *Drosophila melanogaster*. *Eur. J. Neurosci.* 18, 227–238.

Fredriksson, R., and Schiöth, H. B. (2005). The repertoire of G-protein-coupled receptors in fully sequenced genomes. *Mol. Pharmacol.* 67, 1414–1425.

Gäde, G., and Auerwald, L. (2003). Mode of action of neuropeptides from the adipokinetic hormone family. *Gen. Comp. Endocrinol.* 132, 10–20.

Garrison, J. L., Macosko, E. Z., Bernstein, S., Pokala, N., Albrecht, D. R., and Bargmann, C. I. (2012). Oxytocin/vasopressin-related peptides have an ancient role in reproductive behavior. *Science* 338, 540–543.

Gasnier, B. (2000). The loading of neurotransmitters into synaptic vesicles. *Biochimie* 82, 327–337.

Glauser, D. A., Chen, W. C., Agin, R., Macinnis, B. L., Hellman, A. B., Garrity, P. A., et al. (2011). Heat avoidance is regulated by transient receptor potential (TRP) channels and a neuropeptide signaling pathway in Caenorhabditis elegans. *Genetics* 188, 91–103.

Gloria-Soria, A., and Azevedo, R. B. (2008). npr-1 regulates foraging and dispersal strategies in *Caenorhabditis elegans. Curr. Biol.* 18, 1694–1699.

Gray, J. M., Karow, D. S., Lu, H., Chang, A. J., Chang, J. S., Ellis, R. E., et al. (2004). Oxygen sensation and social feeding mediated by a *C. elegans* guanylate cyclase homologue. *Nature* 430, 317–322.

Green, R. A., Kao, H. L., Audhya, A., Arur, S., Mayers, J. R., Fridolfsson, H. N., et al. (2011). A high-resolution *C. elegans* essential gene network based on phenotypic profiling of a complex tissue. *Cell* 145, 470–482.

Hamanaka, Y., Yasuyama, K., Numata, H., and Shiga, S. (2005). Synaptic connections between pigment-dispersing factor-immunoreactive neurons and neurons in the pars lateralis of the blow fly *Protophormia terraenovae. J. Comp. Neurol.* 491, 390–399.

Hansen, K. K., Stafflinger, E., Schneider, M., Hauser, F., Cazzamali, G., Williamson, M., et al. (2010). Discovery of a novel insect neuropeptide signaling system closely related to the insect adipokinetic hormone and corazonin hormonal systems. *J. Biol. Chem.* 285, 10736–10747.

Harmar, A. J. (2001). Family-B G-protein-coupled receptors. *Genome Biol.* 2, reviews3013.1–reviews3013.10.

Hartenstein, V. (2006). The neuroendocrine system of invertebrates: a developmental and evolutionary perspective. *J. Endocrinol.* 190, 555–570.

Heilig, M. (2004). The NPY system in stress, anxiety and depression. *Neuropeptides* 38, 213–224.

Helfrich-Forster, C., Tauber, M., Park, J. H., Muhlig-Versen, M., Schneuwly, S., and Hofbauer, A. (2000). Ectopic expression of the neuropeptide pigment-dispersing factor alters behavioral rhythms in *Drosophila melanogaster. J. Neurosci.* 20, 3339–3353.

Hewes, R. S., and Taghert, P. H. (2001). Neuropeptides and neuropeptide receptors in the *Drosophila melanogaster* genome. *Genome Res.* 11, 126–142.

Holden-Dye, L., and Walker, R. J. (2012). The roles of neuropeptides in *Caenorhabditis elegans* including their importance in the regulation of feeding and metabolism. *Protein Pept. Lett.* [Epub ahead of print].

Hu, Z., Pym, E. C. G., Babu, K., Murray, A. B. V., and Kaplan, J. M. (2011). A neuropeptide-mediated stretch response links muscle contraction to changes in neurotransmitter release. *Neuron* 71, 92–102.

Hukema, R. K., Rademakers, S., and Jansen, G. (2008). Gustatory plasticity in *C. elegans* involves integration of negative cues and NaCl taste mediated by serotonin, dopamine, and glutamate. *Learn. Mem.* 15, 829–836.

Husson, S. J., Clynen, E., Baggerman, G., De Loof, A., and Schoofs, L. (2005). Discovering neuropeptides in *Caenorhabditis elegans* by two dimensional liquid chromatography and mass spectrometry. *Biochem. Biophys. Res. Commun.* 335, 76–86.

Husson, S. J., Clynen, E., Baggerman, G., Janssen, T., and Schoofs, L. (2006). Defective processing of neuropeptide precursors in *Caenorhabditis elegans* lacking proprotein convertase 2 (KPC-2/EGL-3): mutant analysis by mass spectrometry. *J. Neurochem.* 98, 1999–2012.

Husson, S. J., Mertens, I., Janssen, T., Lindemans, M., and Schoofs, L. (2007a). Neuropeptidergic signaling in the nematode *Caenorhabditis elegans. Prog. Neurobiol.* 82, 33–55.

Husson, S. J., Janssen, T., Baggerman, G., Bogert, B., Kahn-Kirby, A., Ashrafi, K., et al. (2007b). Impaired processing of FLP and NLP peptides in carboxypeptidase E (EGL-21)-deficient *Caenorhabditis elegans* as analyzed by mass spectrometry. *J. Neurochem.* 102, 246–260.

Husson, S. J., and Schoofs, L. (2007). Altered neuropeptide profile of *Caenorhabditis elegans* lacking the chaperone protein 7B2 as analyzed by mass spectrometry. *FEBS Lett.* 581, 4288–4292.

Jang, H., Kim, K., Neal, S. J., Macosko, E., Kim, D., Butcher, R. A., et al. (2012). Neuromodulatory state and sex specify alternative behaviors through antagonistic synaptic pathways in *C. elegans. Neuron* 75, 585–592.

Jansen, G., Thijssen, K. L., Werner, P., Horst, M. V. D., Hazendonk, E., and Plasterk, R. H. A. (1999). The complete family of genes encoding G proteins of *Caenorhabditis elegans. Nat. Genet.* 21, 414–419.

Janssen, T., Husson, S. J., Lindemans, M., Mertens, I., Rademakers, S., Ver Donck, K., et al. (2008a). Functional characterization of three G protein-coupled receptors for pigment dispersing factors in *Caenorhabditis elegans. J. Biol. Chem.* 283, 15241–15249.

Janssen, T., Meelkop, E., Lindemans, M., Verstraelen, K., Husson, S. J., Temmerman, L., et al. (2008b). Discovery of a cholecystokinin-gastrin-like signaling system in nematodes. *Endocrinology* 149, 2826–2839.

Janssen, T., Husson, S. J., Meelkop, E., Temmerman, L., Lindemans, M., Verstraelen, K., et al. (2009). Discovery and characterization of a conserved pigment dispersing factor-like neuropeptide pathway in *Caenorhabditis elegans. J. Neurochem.* 111, 228–241.

Janssen, T., Lindemans, M., Meelkop, E., Temmerman, L., and Schoofs, L. (2010). Coevolution of neuropeptidergic signaling systems: from worm to man. *Ann. N. Y. Acad. Sci.* 1200, 1–14.

Jarrell, T. A., Wang, Y., Bloniarz, A. E., Brittin, C. A., Xu, M., Thomson, J. N., et al. (2012). The connectome of a decision-making neural network. *Science* 337, 437–444.

Jee, C., Lee, J., Lim, J. P., Parry, D., Messing, R. O., and McIntire, S. L. (2012). SEB-3, a CRF receptor-like GPCR, regulates locomotor activity states, stress responses and ethanol tolerance in *Caenorhabditis elegans. Genes Brain Behav.* [Epub ahead of print].

Kah, O., Lethimonier, C., Somoza, G., Guilgur, L. G., Vaillant, C., and Lareyre, J. J. (2007). GnRH and GnRH receptors in metazoa: a historical, comparative, and evolutive perspective. *Gen. Comp. Endocrinol.* 153, 346–364.

Kamath, R. S., Fraser, A. G., Dong, Y., Poulin, G., Durbin, R., Gotta, M., et al. (2003). Systematic functional analysis of the *Caenorhabditis elegans* genome using RNAi. *Nature* 421, 231–237.

Keating, C. D., Kriek, N., Daniels, M., Ashcroft, N. R., Hopper, N. A., Siney, E. J., et al. (2003). Whole-genome analysis of 60 G protein-coupled receptors in *Caenorhabditis elegans* by gene knockout with RNAi. *Curr. Biol.* 13, 1715–1720.

Kim, K., and Li, C. (2004). Expression and regulation of an FMRFamide-related neuropeptide gene family in *Caenorhabditis elegans. J. Comp. Neurol.* 475, 540–550.

Konturek, S. J., Pepera, J., Zabielski, K., Konturek, P. C., Pawlik, T., Szlachcic, A., et al. (2003). Brain-gut axis in pancreatic secretion and appetite control. *J. Physiol. Pharmacol.* 54, 293–317.

Korswagen, H. C., Park, J. H., Ohshima, Y., and Plasterk, R. H. (1997). An activating mutation in a *Caenorhabditis elegans* Gs protein induces neural degeneration. *Genes Dev.* 11, 1493–1503.

Krishnan, A., Almén, M. S., Fredriksson, R., and Schiöth, H. B. (2012). The origin of GPCRs: identification of mammalian like Rhodopsin, Adhesion, Glutamate and Frizzled GPCRs in fungi. *PLoS ONE* 7:e29817. doi:10.1371/journal.pone.0029817

Kubiak, T. M., Larsen, M. J., Bowman, J. W., Geary, T. G., and Lowery, D. E. (2008). FMRFamide-like peptides encoded on the flp-18 precursor gene activate two isoforms of the orphan *Caenorhabditis elegans* G-protein-coupled receptor Y58G8A.4 heterologously expressed in mammalian cells. *Biopolymers* 90, 339–348.

Kubiak, T. M., Larsen, M. J., Burton, K. J., Bannow, C. A., Martin, R. A., Zantello, M. R., et al. (2002). Cloning and functional expression of the first *Drosophila melanogaster* sulfakinin receptor DSK-R1. *Biochem. Biophys. Res. Commun.* 291, 313–320.

Kubiak, T. M., Larsen, M. J., Nulf, S. C., Zantello, M. R., Burton, K. J., Bowman, J. W., et al. (2003). Differential activation of "social" and "solitary" variants of the *Caenorhabditis elegans* G protein-coupled receptor NPR-1 by its cognate ligand AF9. *J. Biol. Chem.* 278, 33724–33729.

Lackner, M. R., Nurrish, S. J., and Kaplan, J. M. (1999). Facilitation of synaptic transmission by EGL-30 Gαq and EGL-8 PLCβ: DAG binding to UNC-13 is required to stimulate acetylcholine release. *Neuron* 24, 335–346.

Li, C., and Kim, K. (2008). "Neuropeptides," in *WormBook*, ed. The *C. elegans* Research Community, WormBook. doi:10.1895/wormbook.1.142.1. Available at: http://www.wormbook.org

Li, C., and Kim, K. (2010). Neuropeptide gene families in *Caenorhabditis elegans. Adv. Exp. Med. Biol.* 692, 98–137.

Li, C., Kim, K., and Nelson, L. S. (1999). FMRFamide-related neuropeptide gene family in *Caenorhabditis elegans. Brain Res.* 848, 26–34.

Lindemans, M., Janssen, T., Beets, I., Temmerman, L., Meelkop, E., and Schoofs, L. (2011). Gonadotropin-releasing hormone and adipokinetic hormone signaling systems share a common evolutionary origin. *Front. Endocrinol.* 2:16. doi:10.3389/fendo.2011.00016

Lindemans, M., Liu, F., Janssen, T., Husson, S. J., Mertens, I., Gäde, G., et al. (2009a). Adipokinetic hormone signaling through the gonadotropin-releasing hormone receptor modulates egg-laying in *Caenorhabditis elegans. Proc. Natl. Acad. Sci. U.S.A.* 106, 1642–1647.

Lindemans, M., Janssen, T., Husson, S. J., Meelkop, E., Temmerman, L., Clynen, E., et al. (2009b). Discovery and characterization of a nematode pyrokinin receptor in *Caenorhabditis elegans. Biochem. Biophys. Res. Commun.* 379, 760–764.

Lowery, D. E., Geary, T. G., Kubiak, T. M., and Larsen, M. J. (2003). *Pharmacia and Upjohn Company, G Protein-Coupled Receptor-like Receptors and Modulators Thereof.* United States Patent 6632621.

Macosko, E. Z., Pokala, N., Feinberg, E. H., Chalasani, S. H., Butcher, R., Clardy, J., et al. (2009). A hub-and-spoke circuit drives pheromone attraction and social behaviour in *C. elegans. Nature* 458, 1171–1175.

Maier, W., Adilov, B., Regenass, M., and Alcedo, J. (2010). A neuromedin U receptor acts with the sensory system to modulate food type-dependent effects on *C. elegans* lifespan. *PLoS Biol.* 8:e1000376. doi:10.1371/journal.pbio.1000376

McKay, R. M., McKay, J. P., Suh, J. M., Avery, L., and Graff, J. M. (2007). Tripeptidyl peptidase II promotes fat formation in a conserved fashion. *EMBO Rep.* 8, 1183–1189.

Meelkop, E., Temmerman, L., Janssen, T., Suetens, N., Beets, I., Van Rompay, L., et al. (2012). PDF receptor signaling in *Caenorhabditis elegans* modulates locomotion and egg-laying. *Mol. Cell. Endocrinol.* 361, 232–240.

Meelkop, E., Temmerman, L., Schoofs, L., and Janssen, T. (2011). Signalling through pigment dispersing hormone-like peptides in invertebrates. *Prog. Neurobiol.* 93, 125–147.

Meeusen, T., Mertens, I., De Loof, A., and Schoofs, L. (2003). G protein-coupled receptors in invertebrates: a state of the art. *Int. Rev. Cytol.* 230, 189–261.

Melcher, C., and Pankratz, M. J. (2005). Candidate gustatory interneurons modulating feeding behavior in the *Drosophila* brain. *PLoS Biol.* 3:e305. doi:10.1371/journal.pbio.0030305

Mertens, I., Clinckspoor, I., Janssen, T., Nachman, R., and Schoofs, L. (2006). FMRFamide related peptide ligands activate the *Caenorhabditis elegans* orphan GPCR Y59H11AL.1. *Peptides* 27, 1291–1296.

Mertens, I., Meeusen, T., Janssen, T., Nachman, R., and Schoofs, L. (2005). Molecular characterization of two G protein-coupled receptor splice variants as FLP2 receptors in *Caenorhabditis elegans. Biochem. Biophys. Res. Commun.* 330, 967–974.

Mertens, I., Vandingenen, A., Meeusen, T., De Loof, A., Schoofs, L., and Meeusen, T. (2004). Postgenomic characterization of G-protein-coupled receptors. *Pharmacogenomics* 5, 657–672.

Meyer-Lindenberg, A., Domes, G., Kirsch, P., and Heinrichs, M. (2011). Oxytocin and vasopressin in the human brain: social neuropeptides for translational medicine. *Nat. Rev. Neurosci.* 12, 524–538.

Milligan, G., and Rees, S. (1999). Chimaeric G alpha proteins: their potential use in drug discovery. *Trends Pharmacol. Sci.* 20, 118–124.

Milward, K., Busch, K. E., Murphy, R. J., de Bono, M., and Olofsson, B. (2011). Neuronal and molecular substrates for optimal foraging in *Caenorhabditis elegans. Proc. Natl. Acad. Sci. U.S.A.* 108, 20672–20677.

Mitchell, P., Mould, R., Dillon, J., Glautier, S., Andrianakis, I., James, C., et al. (2010). A differential role for neuropeptides in acute and chronic adaptive responses to alcohol: behavioural and genetic analysis in *Caenorhabditis elegans. PLoS ONE* 5:e10422. doi:10.1371/journal.pone.0010422

Nathoo, N., Moeller, R., Westlund, B., and Hart, C. (2001). Identification of neuropeptide-like protein gene families in *Caenorhabditis elegans* and other species. *Proc. Natl. Acad. Sci. U.S.A.* 98, 14000–14005.

Offermanns, S., and Simon, M. I. (1995). G alpha 15 and G alpha 16 couple a wide variety of receptors to phospholipase C. *J. Biol. Chem.* 270, 15175–15180.

Park, Y., Kim, Y. J., and Adams, M. E. (2002). Identification of G protein-coupled receptors for *Drosophila* PRXamide peptides, CCAP, corazonin, and AKH supports a theory of ligand-receptor coevolution. *Proc. Natl. Acad. Sci. U.S.A.* 99, 11423–11428.

Persson, A., Gross, E., Laurent, P., Busch, K. E., Bretes, H., and de Bono, M. (2009). Natural variation in a neural globin tunes oxygen sensing in wild *Caenorhabditis elegans. Nature* 458, 1030–1033.

Pierce, S. B., Costa, M., Wisotzkey, R., Devadhar, S., Homburger, S. A., Buchman, A. R., et al. (2001). Regulation of DAF-2 receptor signaling by human insulin and ins-1, a member of the unusually large and diverse *C. elegans* insulin gene family. *Genes Dev.* 15, 672–686.

Pin, J. P. (2000). Molecular tinkering of G protein-coupled receptors: an evolutionary success. *EMBO J.* 18, 1723–1729.

Pocock, R., and Hobert, O. (2010). Hypoxia activates a latent circuit for processing gustatory information in *C. elegans. Nat. Neurosci.* 13, 610–661.

Rao, K. R., and Riehm, J. P. (1993). Pigment-dispersing hormones. *Ann. N. Y. Acad. Sci.* 680, 78–88.

Reddy, K. C., Andersen, E. C., Kruglyak, L., and Kim, D. H. (2009). A polymorphism in npr-1 is a behavioral determinant of pathogen susceptibility in *C. elegans. Science* 323, 382–384.

Reddy, K. C., Hunter, R. C., Bhatla, N., Newman, D. K., and Kim, D. H. (2011). *Caenorhabditis elegans* NPR-1-mediated behaviors are suppressed in the presence of mucoid bacteria. *Proc. Natl. Acad. Sci. U.S.A.* 108, 12887–12892.

Renn, S. C., Park, J. H., Rosbash, M., Hall, J. C., and Taghert, P. H. (1999). A pdf neuropeptide gene mutation and ablation of PDF neurons each cause severe abnormalities of behavioral circadian rhythms in *Drosophila. Cell* 99, 791–802.

Ringstad, N., and Horvitz, H. R. (2008). FMRFamide neuropeptides and acetylcholine synergistically inhibit egg-laying by *C. elegans. Nat. Neurosci.* 11, 1168–1176.

Ritter, S. L., and Hall, R. A. (2009). Fine-tuning of GPCR activity by receptor-interacting proteins. *Nat. Rev. Mol. Cell Biol.* 10, 819–830.

Roch, G. J., Busby, E. R., and Sherwood, N. M. (2011). Evolution of GnRH: diving deeper. *Gen. Comp. Endocrinol.* 171, 1–16.

Rogers, C., Persson, A., Cheung, B., and de Bono, M. (2006). Behavioral motifs and neural pathways coordinating O2 responses and aggregation in *C. elegans. Curr. Biol.* 16, 649–659.

Rogers, C., Reale, V., Kim, K., Chatwin, H., Li, C., Evans, P., et al. (2003). Inhibition of *Caenorhabditis elegans* social feeding by FMRFamide-related peptide activation of NPR-1. *Nat. Neurosci.* 6, 1178–1185.

Rual, J. F., Ceron, J., Koreth, J., Hao, T., Nicot, A. S., Hirozane-Kishikawa, T., et al. (2004). Toward improving *Caenorhabditis elegans* phenome mapping with an ORFeome-based RNAi library. *Genome Res.* 14, 2162–2168.

Scalettar, B. A. (2006). How neurosecretory vesicles release their cargo. *Neuroscientist* 12, 164–176.

Schiöth, H. B., and Fredriksson, R. (2005). The GRAFS classification system of G-protein coupled receptors in comparative perspective. *Gen. Comp. Endocrinol.* 142, 94–101.

Schoofs, L., and Nachman, R. J. (2006). "Sulfakinins," in *Handbook of Biologically Active Peptides*, ed. A. Kastin (New York: Elsevier), 183–189.

Schoofs, L., Vanden Broeck, J., and De Loof, A. (1993). The myotropic peptides of *Locusta migratoria*: structures, distribution, functions and receptors. *Insect Biochem. Mol. Biol.* 23, 859–881.

Simmer, F., Moorman, C., Van Der Linden, A. M., Kuijk, E., Van Den Berghe, P. V., Kamath, R., et al. (2003). Genome-wide RNAi of *C. elegans* using the hypersensitive *rrf-3* strain reveals novel gene functions. *PLoS Biol.* 1:e12. doi:10.1371/journal.pbio.0000012

Staubli, F., Jorgensen, T. J., Cazzamali, G., Williamson, M., Lenz, C., Sondergaard, L., et al. (2002). Molecular identification of the insect adipokinetic hormone receptors. *Proc. Natl. Acad. Sci. U.S.A.* 99, 3446–3451.

Styer, K. L., Singh, V., Macosko, E., Steele, S. E., Bargmann, C. I., and Aballay, A. (2008). Innate immunity in *Caenorhabditis elegans* is regulated by neurons expressing NPR-1/GPCR. *Science* 322, 460–464.

Sulston, J. E., Schierenberg, E., White, J. G., and Thomson, J. N. (1983). The embryonic cell lineage of the nematode *Caenorhabditis elegans. Dev. Biol.* 100, 64–119.

Szekeres, P. G. (2002). Functional assays for identifying ligands at orphan G protein-coupled receptors. *Recept. Channels* 8, 297–308.

Temmerman, L., Bogaerts, A., Meelkop, E., Cardoen, D., Boerjan, B., Janssen, T., et al. (2012). A proteomic approach to neuropeptide function elucidation. *Peptides* 34, 3–9.

Temmerman, L., Meelkop, E., Janssen, T., Bogaerts, A., Lindemans, M., Husson, S. J., et al. (2011). *C. elegans* homologs of insect clock proteins: a tale of many stories. *Ann. N. Y. Acad. Sci.* 1220, 137–148.

Tensen, C. P., Cox, K. J., Burke, J. F., Leurs, R., van der Schors, R. C., Geraerts, W. P., et al. (1998). Molecular cloning and characterization of an invertebrate homologue of a neuropeptide Y receptor. *Eur. J. Neurosci.* 10, 3409–3416.

The *C. elegans* Sequencing Consortium. (1998). Genome sequence of the nematode *C. elegans*: a platform for investigating biology. *Science* 282, 2012–2018.

Thomas, J. H., and Robertson, H. M. (2008). The *Caenorhabditis* chemoreceptor gene families. *BMC Biol.* 6:42. doi:10.1186/1741-7007-6-42

Trent, C., Tsung, N., and Horvitz, H. R. (1983). Egg-laying defective mutants of the nematode *Caenorhabditis elegans*. *Genetics* 104, 619–647.

Tsai, P. S., and Zhang, L. (2008). The emergence and loss of gonadotropin-releasing hormone in protostomes: orthology, phylogeny, structure, and function. *Biol. Reprod.* 79, 798–805.

van Kesteren, R. E., Tensen, C. P., Smit, A. B., van Minnen, J., van Soest, P. F., Kits, K. S., et al. (1995). A novel G protein-coupled receptor mediating both vasopressin- and oxytocin-like functions of Lys-conopressin in *Lymnaea stagnalis*. *Neuron* 15, 897–908.

Weimer, R. M., and Jorgensen, E. M. (2003). Controversies in synaptic vesicle exocytosis. *J. Cell Sci.* 116, 3661–3666.

White, J. G., Southgate, E., Thomson, J. N., and Brenner, S. (1986). The structure of the nervous system of the nematode *C. elegans*. *Philos. Trans. R. Soc. Lond. B Biol. Sci.* 314, 1–340.

WormAtlas, Altun, Z. F., Herndon, L. A., Crocker, C., Lints, R., and Hall, D. H. (eds). (2002–2012). Available at: http://www.wormatlas.org

Young, L. J., and Wang, Z. (2004). The neurobiology of pair bonding. *Nat. Neurosci.* 7, 1048–1045.

APPENDIX

Table A1 | List of sequences of neuropeptide ligands produced by neuropeptide precursors and sorted according to the neuropeptide *C. elegans* GPCRs they activate.

Neuropeptide GPCR	Neuropeptide gene	Neuropeptide precursor gene	Neuropeptide sequence
NPR-1	*flp-18*	FLP-18-1	(DFD)GAMPGVLRFG
		FLP-18-2	EMPGVLRFG
		FLP-18-3	(SYFDEKK)SVPGVLRFG
		FLP-18-4	EIPGVLRFG
		FLP-18-5	SEVPGVLRFG
		FLP-18-6	DVPGVLRFG
	flp-21	FLP-21	GLGPRPLRFG
NPR-3	*flp-15*	FLP-15-1	GGPQGPLRFG
		FLP-15-2	RGPSGPLRFG
NPR-4	*flp-1*	FLP-1-6	(K)PNFLRFG
	flp-4	FLP-4-2	ASPSFIRFG
	flp-18	FLP-18-1	(DFD)GAMPGVLRFG
		FLP-18-2	EMPGVLRFG
		FLP-18-3	(SYFDEKK)SVPGVLRFG
		FLP-18-4	EIPGVLRFG
		FLP-18-5	SEVPGVLRFG
		FLP-18-6	DVPGVLRFG
NPR-5a	*flp-1*	FLP-1-2	SQPNFLRFG
	flp-3	FLP-3-1	SPLGTMRFG
		FLP-3-3	SAEPFGTMRFG
		FLP-3-6	EDGNAPFGTMRFG
		FLP-3-8	SADDSAPFGTMRFG
	flp-18	FLP-18-1	(DFD)GAMPGVLRFG
		FLP-18-2	EMPGVLRFG
		FLP-18-3	(SYFDEKK)SVPGVLRFG
		FLP-18-4	EIPGVLRFG
		FLP-18-5	SEVPGVLRFG
		FLP-18-6	DVPGVLRFG
	flp-21	FLP-21	GLGPRPLRFG
NPR-5b	*flp-1*	FLP-1-2	SQPNFLRFG
	flp-3	FLP-3-1	SPLGTMRFG
		FLP-3-3	SAEPFGTMRFG
		FLP-3-6	EDGNAPFGTMRFG
		FLP-3-8	SADDSAPFGTMRFG
	flp-4	FLP-4-2	ASPSFIRFG
	flp-18	FLP-18-1	(DFD)GAMPGVLRFG
		FLP-18-2	EMPGVLRFG
		FLP-18-3	(SYFDEKK)SVPGVLRFG
		FLP-18-4	EIPGVLRFG
		FLP-18-5	SEVPGVLRFG
		FLP-18-6	DVPGVLRFG
	flp-21	FLP-21	GLGPRPLRFG
NPR-6	*flp-18*	FLP-18-3	(SYFDEKK)SVPGVLRFG
		FLP-18-6	DVPGVLRFG
	flp-21	FLP-21	GLGPRPLRFG
NPR-10a	*flp-3*	FLP-3-1	SPLGTMRFG
		FLP-3-3	SAEPFGTMRFG
		FLP-3-5	ASEDALFGTMRFG

(Continued)

Table A1 | Continued

Neuropeptide GPCR	Neuropeptide gene	Neuropeptide precursor gene	Neuropeptide sequence
		FLP-3-6	EDGNAPFGTMRFG
		FLP-3-7	EAEEPLGTMRFG
		FLP-3-8	SADDSAPFGTMRFG
NPR-10b	*flp-18*	FLP-18-1	(DFD)GAMPGVLRFG
		FLP-18-3	(SYFDEKK)SVPGVLRFG
		FLP-18-4	EIPGVLRFG
		FLP-18-5	SEVPGVLRFG
		FLP-18-6	DVPGVLRFG
NPR-11	*flp-1*	FLP-1-6	(K)PNFLRFG
	flp-5	FLP-5-2	AGAKFIRFG
	flp-14	FLP-14	KHEYLRFG
	flp-18	FLP-18-3	(SYFDEKK)SVPGVLRFG
	flp-21	FLP-21	GLGPRPLRFG
	nlp-1		MDANAFRMSFG
FRPR-3	*flp-7*	FLP-7-1	TPMQRSSMVRFG
		FLP-7-2	SPMQRSSMVRFG
		FLP-7-3	SPMERSAMVRFG
	flp-11	FLP-11-1	AMRNALVRFG
FRPR-18a	*flp-2*	FLP-2-1	LRGEPIRFG
FRPR-18b		FLP-2-2	SPREPIRFG
NPR-22a	*flp-1*	FLP-1-6	(K)PNFLRFG
	flp-7	FLP-7-1	TPMQRSSMVRFG
		FLP-7-2	SPMQRSSMVRFG
		FLP-7-3	SPMERSAMVRFG
		FLP-7-4	SPMDRSKMVRFG
	flp-9	FLP-9	KPSFVRFG
	flp-11	FLP-11-1	AMRNALVRFG
		FLP-11-2	ASGGMRNALVRFG
		FLP-11-3	NGAPQPFVRFG
	flp-13	FLP-13-4	AADGAPLIRFG
	flp-22	FLP-22	SPSAKWMRFG
CKR-2a	*flp-1*	FLP-1-1	SADPNFLRFG
	nlp-12		DYRPLQFG
			DGYRPLQFG
CKR-2b	*nlp-13*		SSSMYDRDIMSFG
	nlp-14		ALDGLDGSGFGFD
GNRR-1a	*nlp-47*	NLP-47	pQMTFTDQWT
NTR-1	*ntc-1*	NTC-1	CFLNSCPYRRYG
NMUR-2	*nlp-44*		AFFYTPRIG
EGL-6a	*flp-10*	FLP-10	QPKARSGYIRFG
EGL-6b	*flp-17*	FLP-17-1	KSAFVRFG
		FLP-17-2	KSQYIRFG
PDFR-1a	*pdf-1*	PDF-1a	SNAELINGLIGMDLGKLSAVG
PDFR-1b		PDF-1b	SNAELINGLLSMNLNKLSGAG
PDFR-1c	*pdf-2*	PDF-2	NNAEVVNHILKNFGALDRLGDVG

Permissions

All chapters in this book were first published in NGPCRSN, by Frontiers; hereby published with permission under the Creative Commons Attribution License or equivalent. Every chapter published in this book has been scrutinized by our experts. Their significance has been extensively debated. The topics covered herein carry significant findings which will fuel the growth of the discipline. They may even be implemented as practical applications or may be referred to as a beginning point for another development.

The contributors of this book come from diverse backgrounds, making this book a truly international effort. This book will bring forth new frontiers with its revolutionizing research information and detailed analysis of the nascent developments around the world.

We would like to thank all the contributing authors for lending their expertise to make the book truly unique. They have played a crucial role in the development of this book. Without their invaluable contributions this book wouldn't have been possible. They have made vital efforts to compile up to date information on the varied aspects of this subject to make this book a valuable addition to the collection of many professionals and students.

This book was conceptualized with the vision of imparting up-to-date information and advanced data in this field. To ensure the same, a matchless editorial board was set up. Every individual on the board went through rigorous rounds of assessment to prove their worth. After which they invested a large part of their time researching and compiling the most relevant data for our readers.

The editorial board has been involved in producing this book since its inception. They have spent rigorous hours researching and exploring the diverse topics which have resulted in the successful publishing of this book. They have passed on their knowledge of decades through this book. To expedite this challenging task, the publisher supported the team at every step. A small team of assistant editors was also appointed to further simplify the editing procedure and attain best results for the readers.

Apart from the editorial board, the designing team has also invested a significant amount of their time in understanding the subject and creating the most relevant covers. They scrutinized every image to scout for the most suitable representation of the subject and create an appropriate cover for the book.

The publishing team has been an ardent support to the editorial, designing and production team. Their endless efforts to recruit the best for this project, has resulted in the accomplishment of this book. They are a veteran in the field of academics and their pool of knowledge is as vast as their experience in printing. Their expertise and guidance has proved useful at every step. Their uncompromising quality standards have made this book an exceptional effort. Their encouragement from time to time has been an inspiration for everyone.

The publisher and the editorial board hope that this book will prove to be a valuable piece of knowledge for researchers, students, practitioners and scholars across the globe.

List of Contributors

Akie Hamamoto, Tomoko Saho and Yumiko Saito
Graduate School of Integrated Arts and Sciences, Hiroshima University, Hiroshima, Japan

Manabu Horikawa
Bioorganic Research Institute, Suntory Foundation for Life Sciences, Osaka, Japan

Shwetha Ramachandrappa, Rebecca J. Gorrigan, Adrian J. L. Clark and Li F. Chan
Centre for Endocrinology, William Harvey Research Institute,Queen Mary University of London, Bartsand The London School of Medicine and Dentistry, London, UK

Zherui Wu, and Patricia Forgez
INSERM-UPMC UMR_S938, Hôpital Saint-Antoine, Paris, France

Daniel Martinez-Fong
Departamento de Fisiología, Biofísicay Neurociencias, Centro de Investigación y de Estudios Avanzados del Instituto Politécnico Nacional, Mexico City, Mexico

Jean Trédaniel
INSERM-UPMC UMR_S938, Hôpital Saint-Antoine, Paris, France
Unité de Cancérologie Thoracique, Groupe Hospitalier Paris Saint Joseph/Université Paris Descartes, Paris, France

Xavier Pedragosa-Badia, Jan Stichel and Annette G.Beck-Sickinger
Institute of Biochemistry, Faculty of Biosciences, Pharmacy and Psychology, Universität Leipzig, Leipzig, Germany

David Chatenet, Thi-Tuyet M. Nguyen, Myriam Létourneau and Alain Fournier
Laboratoire d'études moléculaires et pharmacologiques des peptides, INRS - Institut Armand-Frappier, Université du Québec, Ville de Laval, QC, Canada
Laboratoire International Associé Samuel de Champlain (INSERM/INRS-Université de Rouen), France

Nanthakumar Thirunarayanan and Bruce M. Raakaand Marvin C. Gershengorn
Laboratory of Endocrinology and Receptor Biology, National Institute of Diabetes and Digestive and Kidney Diseases, National Institutes of Health, Bethesda, MD, USA

Anne-Laure Schang, Bruno Quérat, Violaine Simon, Ghislaine Garrel, Christian Bleux, Raymond Counis, Joëlle Cohen-Tannoudji and Jean-Noël Laverrière
Physiologie de l'Axe Gonadotrope, Biologie Fonctionnelle et Adaptative, EAC CNRS 4413, Sorbonne Paris Cité, Université Paris Diderot-Paris 7, Paris, France

Aditya J. Desai and Laurence J. Miller
Department of Molecular Pharmacology and Experimental Therapeutics, MayoClinic, Scottsdale, AZ, USA

Patricia M. Hinkle
Department of Pharmacology and Physiology, University of Rochester Medical Center, Rochester, NY, USA

Austin U. Gehret
Department of Science and Mathematics, National Technical Institute for the Deaf, Rochester Institute of Technology, Rochester, NY, USA

Brian W. Jones
Department of Pharmacology, University of Washington, Seattle, WA, USA

Despina E. Ganella
The Florey Institute of Neuroscience and Mental Health, The University of Melbourne, Melbourne, VIC, Australia
Department of Biochemistry and Molecular Biology, The University of Melbourne, Melbourne, VIC, Australia

Sherie Ma
The Florey Institute of Neuroscience and Mental Health, The University of Melbourne, Melbourne, VIC, Australia

AndrewL . Gundlach
The Florey Institute of Neuroscience and Mental Health, The University of Melbourne, Melbourne, VIC, Australia
Florey Department of Neuroscience and Mental Health, The University of Melbourne, Melbourne, VIC, Australia
Department of Anatomy and Neuroscience, The University of Melbourne, Melbourne, VIC, Australia

Kjell Fuxe, Dasiel O. Borroto-Escuela, Wilber Romero-Fernandez and Feliciano Calvo
Department of Neuroscience, Karolinska Institutet, Stockholm, Sweden

Alexander O. Tarakanov
St. Petersburg Institute for Informatics and Automation, Russian Academy of Sciences, Saint Petersburg, Russia

Pere Garriga and Mercé Tena
Centre de Biotecnologia Molecular, Departament d´ Enginyeria Química, Universitat Politécnica de Catalunya, Barcelona, Spain

Manuel Narvaez, Carmelo Millón, José A. Narvaez and Zaida Díaz-Cabiale
Department of Physiology, School of Medicine, University of Málaga, Málaga, Spain

Concepción Parrado
Department of Histology, School of Medicine, University of Málaga, Málaga, Spain

Francisco Ciruela
Unitat de Farmacologia, Departament Patologiai Terapéutica Experimental, Universitatde Barcelona, Barcelona, Spain

Luigi F. Agnati
Department of Biomedical Sciences, University of Modena and Reggio Emilia, Modena, Italy
Istituto di Ricovero e Curaa Carattere Scientifico, Lido Venice, Italy

Michihiro Mieda, Natsuko Tsujino and Takeshi Sakurai
Department of Molecular Neuroscience and Integrative Physiology, Graduate School of Medical Science, Kanazawa University, Kanazawa, Ishikawa, Japan

Grégory Conductier
UMR7275, Institutde Pharmacologie Moléculaire et Cellulaire, Centre National de la Recherche Scientifique, Valbonne, France
University of Nice Sophia Antipolis, Nice, France

Sonia Jego, Raphaël Lavoie and Antoine Adamantidis
Douglas Mental Health University Institute, Montreal, QC, Canada

Agnès O. Martin, Chrystel Lafont and Patrice Mollard
UMR5203, Institut de Génomique Fonctionnelle, Centre National de la Recherche Scientifique, Montpellier, France

U661, INSERM, Montpellier and France
UMR-5203, Universités de Montpellier 1 & 2, Montpellier, France

Jean-Louis Nahon
UMR7275, Institutde Pharmacologie Moléculaire et Cellulaire, Centre National de la Recherche Scientifique, Valbonne, France
University of Nice Sophia Antipolis, Nice, France
Station de Primatologie, UPS 846, Centre National de la Recherche Scientifique, Roussetsur Arc, France

Pierre-Yves Risold
Laboratoire d' Histologie, IFR 133, Faculté de Médecine et de Pharmacie, Besançon, France

Dan Larhammar and Christina A. Bergqvist
Unit of Pharmacology, Department of Neuroscience, Science for Life Laboratory-Uppsala University, Uppsala, Sweden

Takanori Ida and Hatsumi Tominaga
Interdisciplinary Research Organization, University of Miyazaki, Miyazaki, Japan

Tomoko Takahashi
Department of Biology, School of Medicine, Kurume University, Fukuoka, Japan

Takahiro Sato, Hiroko Sano and Masayasu Kojima
Molecular Genetics, Institute of Life Sciences, Kurume University, Fukuoka, Japan

Kazuhiko Kume
Department of Stem Cell Biology, Institute of Molecular Embryology and Genetics, Kumamoto University, Kumamoto, Japan

Mamiko Ozaki, Tetsutaro Hiraguchi, Hajime Shiotani, Saki Terajima and Yuki Nakamura,
Department of Biology, Graduate School of Science, Kobe University, Hyogo, Japan

Kenji Mori, Morikatsu Yoshida, Mikiya Miyazato and Kenji Kangawa
Department of Biochemistry, National Cerebral and Cardiovascular Center Research Institute, Osaka, Japan

Johji Kato
Frontier Science Research Center, University of Miyazaki, Miyazaki, Japan

Noboru Murakami
Department of Veterinary Physiology, Faculty of Agriculture, University of Miyazaki, Miyazaki, Japan

Jelle Caers, Heleen Verlinden, Sven Zels, Hans Peter Vandersmissen, Kristel Vuerinckx and Liliane Schoofs
Animal Physiology and Neurobiology, Department of Biology, Zoological Institute, KU Leuven, Leuven, Belgium

Lotte Frooninckx, Liesbeth Van Rompay, Liesbet Temmerman, Elien Van Sinay, Isabel Beets, Tom Janssen, Steven J. Husson and Liliane Schoofs
Laboratory of Functional Genomics and Proteomics, Department of Biology, Katholieke Universiteit Leuven, Leuven, Belgium

Index

www.ingramcontent.com/pod-product-compliance
Lightning Source LLC
LaVergne TN
LVHW061513220926
848485LV00018B/881